Principles of Medicinal Chemistry

Principles of Medicinal Chemistry

Edited by
Thomas Haldane

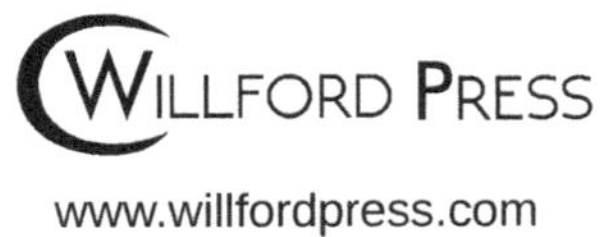

www.willfordpress.com

Published by Willford Press,
118-35 Queens Blvd., Suite 400,
Forest Hills, NY 11375, USA

ISBN: 978-1-68285-407-5

Cataloging-in-Publication Data

Principles of medicinal chemistry / edited by Thomas Haldane.
p. cm.
Includes bibliographical references and index.
ISBN 978-1-68285-407-5
1. Pharmaceutical chemistry. 2. Chemistry. I. Haldane, Thomas.
RS403 .P75 2018
615.19--dc23

For information on all Willford Press publications
visit our website at www.willfordpress.com

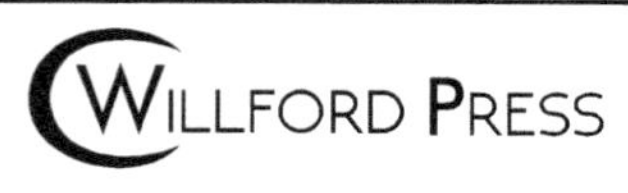

Contents

Preface

Medicinal chemistry studies the chemical syntheses that leads to the development of new therapeutic agents. Medicinal chemistry is an important branch of chemistry. It identifies and alters new chemical entities to transform them into suitable components for drug manufacture. New and efficient drug designing is one of the fundamental processes of this field. For all those who are interested in medicinal chemistry, this book can prove to be an essential guide. Students and researchers in the fields of pharmaceutics, medicinal chemistry and toxicology will find this book helpful.

This book is a result of research of several months to collate the most relevant data in the field.

When I was approached with the idea of this book and the proposal to edit it, I was overwhelmed. It gave me an opportunity to reach out to all those who share a common interest with me in this field. I had 3 main parameters for editing this text:

1. Accuracy - The data and information provided in this book should be up-to-date and valuable to the readers.
2. Structure - The data must be presented in a structured format for easy understanding and better grasping of the readers.
3. Universal Approach - This book not only targets students but also experts and innovators in the field, thus my aim was to present topics which are of use to all.

Thus, it took me a couple of months to finish the editing of this book.

I would like to make a special mention of my publisher who considered me worthy of this opportunity and also supported me throughout the editing process. I would also like to thank the editing team at the back-end who extended their help whenever required.

Editor

1

Novel sialic acid derivatives lock open the 150-loop of an influenza A virus group-1 sialidase

Santosh Rudrawar[1], Jeffrey C. Dyason[1], Marie-Anne Rameix-Welti[2,3,4], Faith J. Rose[1], Philip S. Kerry[5], Rupert J.M. Russell[5], Sylvie van der Werf[2,3,4], Robin J. Thomson[1], Nadia Naffakh[2,3,4] & Mark von Itzstein[1]

Influenza virus sialidase has an essential role in the virus' life cycle. Two distinct groups of influenza A virus sialidases have been established, that differ in the flexibility of the '150-loop', providing a more open active site in the *apo* form of the group-1 compared to group-2 enzymes. In this study we show, through a multidisciplinary approach, that novel sialic acid-based derivatives can exploit this structural difference and selectively inhibit the activity of group-1 sialidases. We also demonstrate that group-1 sialidases from drug-resistant mutant influenza viruses are sensitive to these designed compounds. Moreover, we have determined, by protein X-ray crystallography, that these inhibitors lock open the group-1 sialidase flexible 150-loop, in agreement with our molecular modelling prediction. This is the first direct proof that compounds may be developed to selectively target the pandemic A/H1N1, avian A/H5N1 and other group-1 sialidase-containing viruses, based on an open 150-loop conformation of the enzyme.

[1] Institute for Glycomics, Gold Coast Campus, Griffith University, Queensland 4222, Australia. [2] Institut Pasteur, Unité de Génétique Moléculaire des Virus à ARN, Département de Virologie, Paris F-75015, France. [3] CNRS URA3015, Paris F-75015, France. [4] Université Paris Diderot, Paris F-75013, France. [5] Interdisciplinary Centre for Human and Avian Influenza Research, University of St Andrews, North Haugh, St Andrews, Fife KY16 9ST, UK. Correspondence and requests for materials should be addressed to M.v.I. (email: m.vonitzstein@griffith.edu.au).

Influenza remains a serious health concern to humanity, with high morbidity and mortality rates[1 2] and the recent influenza A/H1N1 pandemic underscores the potential threat of this highly adaptive virus[3]. The sialidase (neuraminidase) of influenza virus has a major role in the virus' life cycle by facilitating release of virus progeny from the infected cell[4]. Two phylogenetically distinct groups[5] of influenza A virus sialidases, group-1 (N1, 4, 5 and 8) and group-2 (N2, 3, 6, 7 and 9), have been established. The anti-influenza drugs[6] (Fig. 1) Relenza (zanamivir, **1**) and Tamiflu (oseltamivir, **2**), through its active form oseltamivir carboxylate (OC, **3**), efficiently block the activity of both influenza A virus group-1 and group-2 sialidases, resulting in the virus progeny remaining clumped at the infected cell's surface. Noteworthy is that the discovery of these inhibitors was based exclusively on group-2 sialidase structures[6].

The recently solved[5] structures of group-1 sialidases showed an unexpected structural difference between group-1 and group-2 sialidases, with the group-1 sialidases having a loop, the so-called '150-loop', that is flexible compared with the identical loop of the group-2 sialidases. This protein loop can provide either a more open (group-1) or closed (group-2) active site architecture in the *apo* form of the enzyme. Furthermore, the 150-loop, in initially complexed structures of **3**–group-1 sialidase[5], has been observed in the more open orientation and eventually closes and tightly coordinates **3**. In contrast, a very recent structural investigation on the 2009 pandemic H1N1 sialidase concluded that this group-1 enzyme seems to lack a 150-cavity[7]. It has been proposed that the more open enzyme architecture and consequently larger active site cavity in the *apo* structures of the group-1 sialidases could provide new opportunities for inhibitor design[5,6,8,9]. In the context of the recent pandemic swine origin A/H1N1 and the pandemic 1918 A/H1N1 influenza viruses, as well as the continuing threat of avian A/H5N1, such inhibitors could lead to new anti-influenza drugs that would add to the very limited number of treatment options available.

The potent influenza virus sialidase inhibitors **1** and **3** show essentially comparable inhibition of influenza A virus group-1 and 2 sialidases[8]. This is not surprising as these inhibitors do not have the capacity to maintain the 150-loop of group-1 sialidases in an open orientation. An important question remains to be answered—could the 150-loop of influenza A virus group-1 sialidases be locked open to provide new opportunities in influenza virus sialidase inhibitor design? Moreover, could such 'designer' compounds that lock open this loop also selectively inhibit group-1 sialidases, including the pandemic swine origin H1N1 sialidase. Interestingly, C-4-modified zanamivir (**1**) derivatives have been recently reported that are believed to take advantage of this open 150-loop feature, although neither selectivity nor structural data have been presented in support of this conclusion[10]. More recently OC (**3**) analogues have been reported[11] that efficiently inhibit and are selective for a group-1 influenza virus sialidase. These compounds are thought to access the 150-cavity, and preliminary nuclear magnetic resonance (NMR) spectroscopic evidence for this conclusion is reported.

To probe and attempt to lock open the 150-loop of influenza virus group-1 sialidases, we have undertaken a multidisciplinary study that used molecular modelling, chemical synthesis, enzyme and cell-based assays and protein X-ray crystallography. We have successfully designed and synthesized novel C-3-substituted sialic acid-based derivatives that efficiently and selectively inhibit group-1 sialidase activity by locking open the flexible 150-loop. These derivatives contain the zanamivir (**1**) core structure, although they lack the C-4 guanidino moiety, and incorporate a hydrophobic entity at the C-3 position. Moreover, we have demonstrated that these inhibitors are also effective against influenza virus clinical isolates containing mutations in the sialidase glycoprotein that convey resistance to oseltamivir (**2**) and reduced sensitivity to zanamivir (**1**).

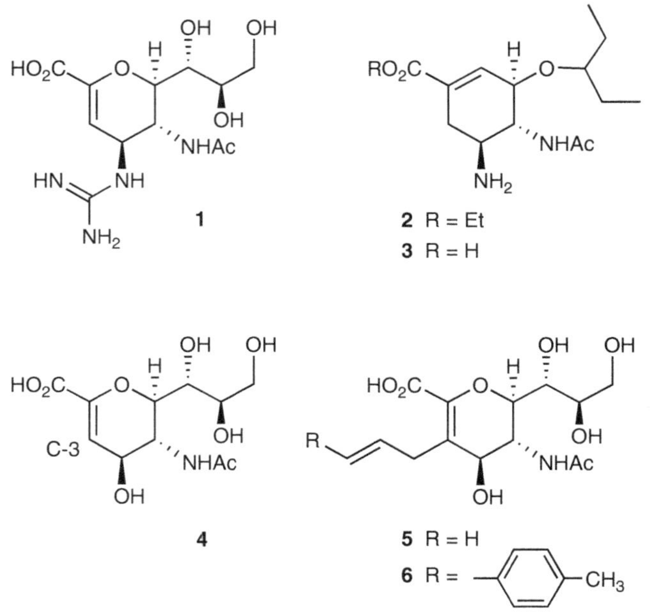

Figure 1 | Chemical structures of anti-influenza viral drugs and influenza virus sialidase inhibitors. Zanamivir (**1**), oseltamivir (**2**), oseltamivir carboxylate (**3**), Neu5Ac2en (**4**), 3-allyl-Neu5Ac2en (**5**) and 3-(*p*-tolyl)allyl-Neu5Ac2en (**6**).

Results

Molecular modelling study of a group-1 sialidase. Our modelling study commenced with the superimposition of two group-1 sialidase N8 structures, *apo* N8 (2ht5) and the N8–**4** complex (2htr), which contain an open and closed 150-loop, respectively. This provided an opportunity to view the well-known sialidase inhibitor 5-acetamido-2,6-anhydro-3,5-dideoxy-D-*glycero*-D-*galacto*-non-2-enonic acid (Neu5Ac2en, **4**, Fig. 1) modelled in the context of a sialidase active site with an open 150-loop conformation. We concluded from this inspection that carbon-3 (C-3) of Neu5Ac2en (**4**) is oriented towards the 150-cavity in the more open form of the enzyme. As a consequence, we then used **4** as a template (Methods) to design probes of this cavity. This design study suggested that **4** modified at C-3 should be able to bind to the active site of *apo*-N8 with minimal distortion of the normal binding mode. Moreover, our modelling indicated that hydrophobic functionalities, such as an allyl or arylallyl group, introduced at C-3 on template **4**, should be accommodated in the 150-cavity. Finally, our modelling study also suggested that such functionalities would lock open the 150-loop and, as a direct outcome, should be selective for the influenza A virus group-1 sialidases. Interestingly, the C-3 position on **4**, to the best of our knowledge, has never been functionalized.

Synthesis of novel sialic acid derivatives. To explore novel functionalization of the C-3 position of **4**, we chose chemistries that would introduce a functional group that could be readily elaborated. We believed that introduction of an allyl group would provide significant opportunity to elaborate the new functionality through olefin cross-metathesis reactions[12]. Our strategy to access this novel class of chemical probe utilized the per-*O*-acetylated, methyl ester derivative of **4** (Fig. 2, Supplementary Methods). From this derivative, we were able to readily prepare the target compounds (Fig. 1), 3-allyl-Neu5Ac2en (**5**) and 3-(*p*-tolyl)allyl-Neu5Ac2en (**6**).

Biological evaluation of sialic acid derivatives. To assess the ability of these compounds to selectively block the enzyme activity of group-1 influenza A virus sialidases, **5** and **6** have been evaluated in an *in vitro* fluorometric assay[13] against both wild-type and mutant group-1 (N1) and a wild-type group-2 (N2) viral sialidase (Methods). As anticipated, both probes **5** and **6** indeed showed selectivity for the group-1 (N1) sialidases compared with the group-2 (N2) sialidase (Table 1), with a micromolar level of inhibition determined for **6** against the N1 sialidases. This is in distinct contrast to the parent inhibitor Neu5Ac2en (**4**), also a micromolar inhibitor, that shows comparable inhibition of both group-1 and group-2 sialidases. These data support the notion that **5** and **6** access a novel subsite within the influenza virus group-1 sialidase active site, such as that observed in the open 150-loop conformation[5]. Moreover, both of the sialic acid-based probes displayed activity against N1 sialidases associated with clinically relevant viruses[8] with mutations that affect sensitivity to both **1** and **2** (Table 1). Finally, the selectivity for inhibition of N1 over N2 sialidase activity, shown by **5** and **6**, was confirmed by plaque reduction assay studies (Supplementary Fig. S1) and 50% effective concentration (EC_{50}) determinations (Supplementary Table S1).

Structures of group-1 sialidase N8–5 and 6 complexes. Influenza virus sialidase N8 [A/duck/Ukraine/1/63 (H3N8)] was used as a convenient and representative group-1 sialidase for structural studies. Both probes **5** and **6** were successfully complexed with N8 and structures readily determined. Both inhibitors **5** and **6** in

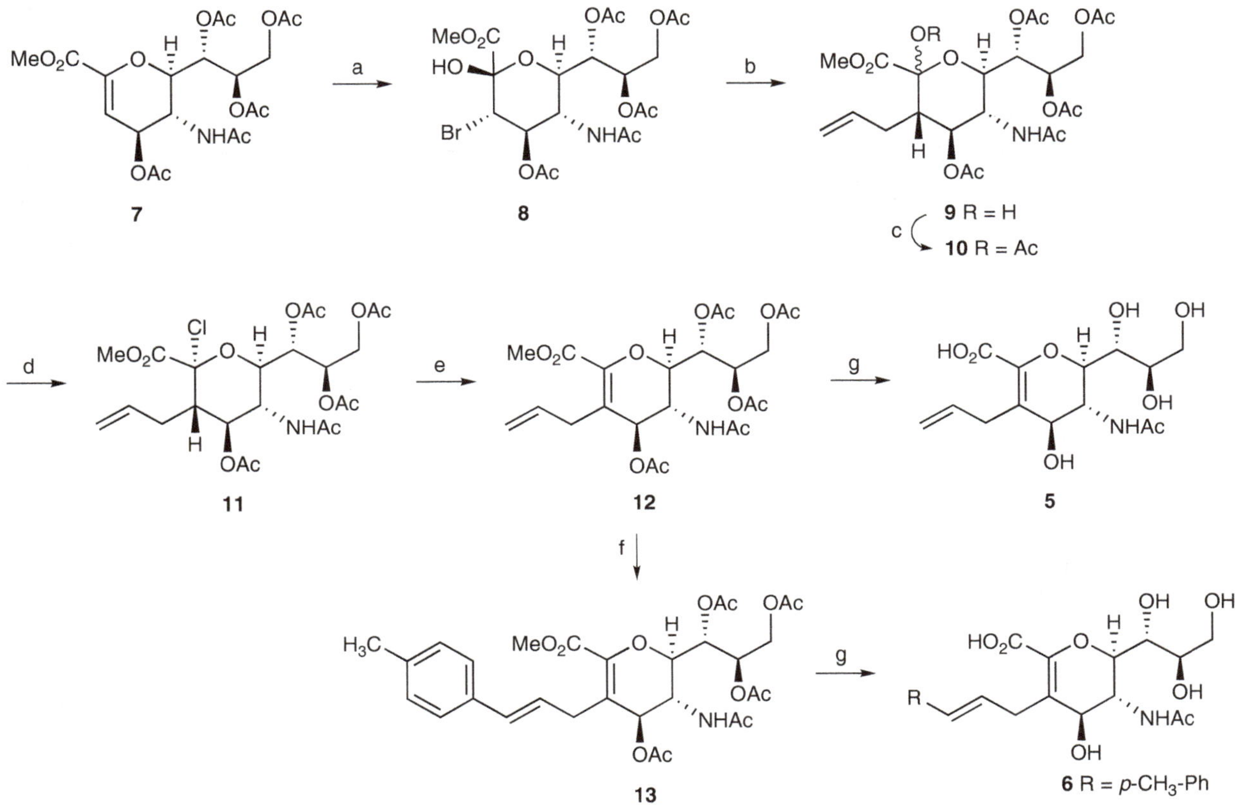

Figure 2 | Preparation of 3-allyl-Neu5Ac2en (5) and 3-(*p*-tolyl)allyl-Neu5Ac2en (6). Reagents and conditions: (**a**) NBS, DMSO/H_2O (2.5:1), −30 °C, 2 h (38% di-equatorial bromohydrin **8**, 28% di-axial bromohydrin); (**b**) Bu_3SnAll, AIBN, dry toluene, N_2, 100 °C, 8 h (57%); (**c**) Ac_2O, dry pyridine, DMAP, N_2, room temperature, 16 h (95%); (**d**) AcCl, dry MeOH, dry DCM, 5 °C to room temperature, 48 h; (**e**) DBU, dry DCM, N_2, room temperature, 8 h (91% over steps d and e, based on recovered starting material); (**f**) Grubbs' catalyst second generation, 4-methylstyrene, dry DCM, N_2, 40 °C, 24 h (69%; 77% based on recovered starting material). (**g**) 1 M aq. NaOH, MeOH, 5 °C to room temperature, 12–16 h (**5** and **6**, 60%, based on recovered starting material, and 94%, respectively).

Table 1 | Selective inhibition of influenza A group-1 sialidase by locking open the 150-loop.

Sialidase type	K_i (μM)*			
	5	**6**	**4**	**1**
N1 (A/HongKong/156/97 (H5N1))	222 ± 17	7.3±0.8	0.97±0.15	$0.17\pm0.08\times10^{-3}$
N1 (A/Paris/2590/2009 (H1N1 pandemic))	153 ± 18	1.7±0.2	0.67±0.08	$0.13\pm0.01\times10^{-3}$
N2 (A/Paris/908/97 (H3N2))	3629 ± 2130	219±30	1.24±0.23	$0.56\pm0.16\times10^{-3}$
N1 (A/HongKong/156/97 (H5N1) H274Y)	459 ± 92	11±0.9	1.43±0.17	$0.38\pm0.14\times10^{-3}$
N1 (A/Paris/2590/2009 (H1N1 pandemic) H274Y)	232 ± 15	2.9±0.1	0.91±0.05	$0.23\pm0.04\times10^{-3}$
N1 (A/HongKong/156/97 (H5N1) N294S)	980 ± 50	25±3.1	3.90±0.5	$0.71\pm0.04\times10^{-3}$
N1 (A/HongKong/156/97 (H5N1) Q136K)	16.8 ± 2.5	2.6±0.4	1.37±0.15	$13.6\pm1.3\times10^{-3}$

Inhibition of wild-type N1, H274Y, N294S and Q136K mutant N1 sialidases, and an N2 sialidase by **5** and **6** compared with parent template **4** and zanamivir (**1**).
*Results are given as means ± s.d. (see Methods—Inhibition Assays for details).

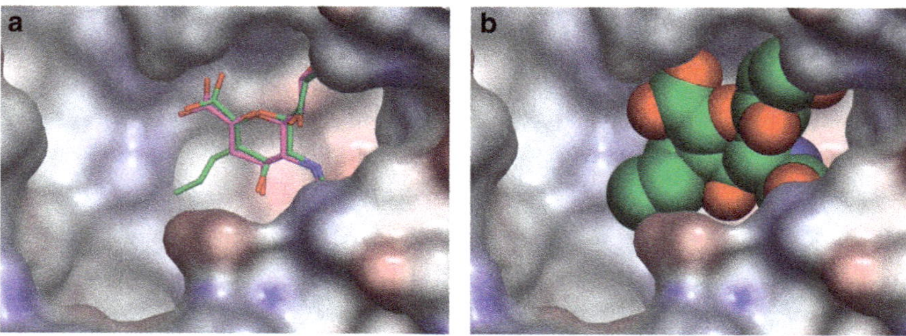

Figure 3 | N8–5 complex. (**a**) Superimposition of N8-inhibitor complexes of 3-allyl-Neu5Ac2en (**5**, green) and Neu5Ac2en (**4**, magenta; 2htr). (**b**) N8-**5** complex with open 150-loop (**5** in CPK format). The N8-**5** complex maintains the open conformation of the 150-loop seen in the *apo* structure[5] (**a**, **b**).

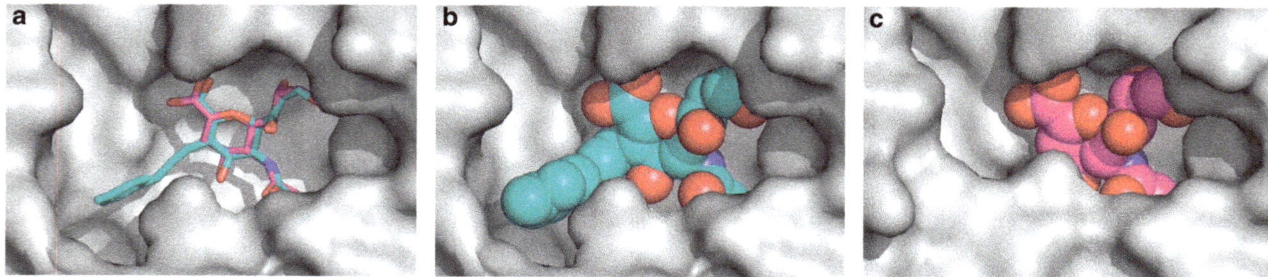

Figure 4 | N8–6 complex. (**a**) Superimposition of N8-inhibitor complexes of 3-(*p*-tolyl)allyl-Neu5Ac2en (**6**, cyan) and Neu5Ac2en (**4**, magenta; 2htr). (**b**) N8-**6** complex with an open 150-loop (**6** in CPK format). (**c**) N8-**4** complex with a closed 150-loop[5] (**4** in CPK format). The N8-**6** complex maintains an open conformation of the 150-loop seen in the *apo* structure[5] (**a**, **b**), in contrast to the complex with **4** where the 150-loop is closed (**c**).

complex with N8 (N8–**5**, Fig. 3, Supplementary Fig. S2, Supplementary Movie 1; N8–**6**, Fig. 4, Supplementary Fig. S3, Supplementary Movie 2) clearly demonstrated that the C-3 functionalities occupied the cavity formed by the open 150-loop.

Discussion

On the basis of our structure-assisted studies, we identified 3-allyl-Neu5Ac2en (**5**) as an important versatile chemical intermediate for influenza virus sialidase inhibitor development. Our synthetic strategy to access **5** required the corresponding 3-substituted *N*-acetylneuraminic acid derivative, fully protected 3-allyl-Neu5Ac (**10**) (Fig. 2). This derivative was synthesized from fully protected Neu-5Ac2en (**7**) through bromohydroxylation[14], and subsequent reaction of the di-equatorial bromohydrin **8** with allyltributyltin[15]. Reacting **8** with allyltributyltin in toluene at elevated temperature in the presence of the free radical initiator AIBN resulted in an improved yield of **9** (57%) compared with that reported[15] for the ultraviolet light-catalysed reaction (34%). Acetylation of **9** provided intermediate **10** in good yield (95%). Chlorination of **10** at C-2 provided **11**, with subsequent β-elimination of HCl in the presence of 1,8-diazabicyclo-[5.4.0]undec-7-ene (DBU), resulting in the formation of the novel C-3-substituted 2,3-unsaturated derivative **12**. The side chain at C-3 could be efficiently extended using an olefin cross-metathesis reaction[12]. Accordingly, reaction of allyl derivative **12** with 4-methylstyrene in the presence of Grubbs' catalyst (second generation)[16] produced the 3-(*p*-tolyl)allyl derivative **13** in 69% isolated yield (corrected to 77% based on recovered **12**). We observed that the cross-metathesis reaction was stereoselective and provided the thermodynamically more stable (*E*)-isomer. This was confirmed by a ^{1}H NMR coupling constant ($J_{1,2}$) for the *trans*-olefinic hydrogens of 15.9 Hz. Exposure of **12** and **13** to standard base-catalysed deprotection conditions gave the target 3-allyl-Neu5Ac2en (**5**) in a 51% yield (60% yield based on recovered **12**), and 3-(*p*-tolyl)allyl-Neu5Ac2en (**6**) in a 94% yield, following isolation and purification.

Our initial biological evaluation of **5** and **6** against wild-type influenza virus sialidases confirmed that both compounds were selective inhibitors of group-1 sialidases (Table 1). Plaque reduction assay and EC_{50} determinations confirmed that **6** selectively inhibited the growth of wild-type N1-containing viruses compared with a wild-type N2-containing virus (Supplementary Fig. S1 and Supplementary Table S1). Importantly, our data revealed that the 2009 pandemic H1N1 virus and N1 sialidase are as sensitive to these C-3 functionalized sialic acid derivatives as the other evaluated group-1 viruses and sialidases. This observation contrasts a very recent report[7], in which the conclusion reached was that this particular group-1 sialidase lacks a 150-cavity. Therefore, we propose that the 2009 pandemic H1N1 sialidase does have an accessible 150-cavity that is exposed to some extent upon the binding of an appropriate inhibitor such as **5** or **6**.

Oseltamivir (**2**) resistance among influenza A/H1N1 viruses has rapidly emerged over the previous two influenza seasons[17]. The observation[8,17] of significant resistance development to oseltamivir (**2**) and apparent reduced[18] sensitivity to zanamivir (**1**) led us to investigate the affinity of these novel sialic acid derivatives for three influenza virus sialidases that contain well-characterized key mutations. Each of these sialidases contained one of the following mutations (N2 numbering), H274Y (H275Y in N1 numbering), N294S, or Q136K, which influence the efficacy of the sialidase-targeting drugs. Our data (Table 1) suggest that N1 with an H274Y mutation, which significantly reduces OC (**3**) sensitivity[8,17], remains sensitive to **5** and **6**. The level of inhibition for these compounds follows the same apparent trend (approximately a factor of 2 poorer affinity compared with wild-type enzyme) that is observed for both zanamivir (**1**) and Neu5Ac2en (**4**). The N294S mutation reduces sensitivity to **5** and **6** by approximately the same factor (~3.5) determined for **1** and **4**. Strikingly, the Q136K mutation, that reduces sensitivity to zanamivir (**1**) and to a lesser extent **4**, significantly increases sensitivity to the novel sialic acid derivatives **5** and **6**. This improvement in sensitivity may be the result of an increase in hydrophobicity, contributed by the lysine side chain, of the active site region that consequently better accommodates the lipophilic moiety at C-3 of **5** and **6**.

These data taken together suggest that a C-3-modified sialic acid derivative, such as **6**, may provide a valuable lead compound for next generation anti-influenza drug discovery. Moreover, the introduction of the additional hydrophobic character may provide opportunity for these compounds, unlike zanamivir (**1**), to be developed as orally bioavailable drugs.

To provide direct proof of the binding mode of **5** and **6** with a group-1 sialidase, the compounds were soaked into preformed crystals of N8 sialidase [A/duck/Ukraine/1/63 (H3N8)], in which the 150-loop is in the open conformation[5]. The N8–**5** (Fig. 3a and b, Supplementary Fig. S2 and Supplementary Movie 1) and N8–**6** (Fig. 4a and b, Supplementary Fig. S3, and Supplementary Movie 2) complexes obtained after a 60-min soak show that both **5** and **6** are positioned in the active site as anticipated. In both complexes, the dihydropyran ring, the C-6 glycerol side chain (showing a bidentate interaction between the C-8 and C-9 hydroxyl groups and Glu-276), and the C-4 hydroxyl and C-5 acetamido groups are oriented essentially as seen with Neu5Ac2en (**4**) (PDB:2htr)[5]. The C-3 allyl and (*p*-tolyl)allyl group of **5** and **6**, respectively, extend into the 150-cavity, as predicted, locking the 150-loop open. Under similar soaking conditions, the N8–**4** complex (Fig. 4c) has the 150-loop in a closed conformation[5]. An interesting difference observed in the N8–**5** complex (Fig. 3), compared with the *apo* structure or the open 150-loop complex with **3** (ref. 5), is the position of Arg-118, one of the three arginine residues that normally complexes the Neu5Ac2en carboxylate group. In the N8–**5** complex, Arg-118 is oriented away from the position seen in the other two open 150-loop structures and as a consequence no longer forms a hydrogen bond with the carboxylate group of **5** (Fig. 5). This observation suggests that there is more flexibility in this region of the active site than previously thought and may provide additional direction in future influenza virus sialidase inhibitor development. In a previous molecular modelling study[19], the notion of flexibility in this region of the active site was predicted. In another study[20], the triarginyl cluster interaction with the sialic acid carboxylate group has been calculated to contribute ~50% of the overall binding energy and so represents one of the strongest influences on substrate binding to the sialidase active site. The loss of interaction with Arg-118 could be expected to contribute to the *in vitro* sialidase inhibition observed for **5** in comparison with inhibitors that have interaction with all three residues of the triarginyl cluster.

Although movement of Arg-118 was observed in the N8–**5** complex (Figs 3 and 5), compared with the *apo* structure or the open 150-loop complex with **3** (ref. 5), the N8–**6** complex (Figs 4 and 5) clearly shows that **6** binds in a manner that does not induce any significant reorientation of active site amino-acid residues. The 150-loop structure, the triarginyl cluster that forms a hydrogen bond with the carboxylate group of **6** and other key amino acids are all in a similar orientation[5] to that seen in the *apo* open 150-loop structure (2ht5) (Fig. 5). Interestingly, the amino-acid residue Glu-119 in the *apo* form and in both the N8–**5** and N8–**6** complexes has a very similar orientation, and is quite distinct from the closed loop form, as observed in the N8–**4** complex (Fig. 5). Clearly, a reorientation of this residue occurs as the active site closes around inhibitor **4**. The fact that both the parent inhibitor **4** and **6** are micromolar inhibitors suggests that the loss of interactions between the C-4 hydroxyl group of **4** and active site residue Glu-119 of the closed 150-loop form[5] is almost completely compensated for by new hydrophobic interactions between the aromatic moiety at C-3 in **6** and the 150-cavity (Fig. 6). Compound **6** provides a lead scaffold that, guided by structural analysis, can be further modified at the C-3 functionality itself or the C-4 position, as was the case for zanamivir. As can be seen in Figure 6, the open cavity has significant positive charge character and provides scope for introduction of negatively charged substituents. Such modifications offer considerable opportunity for the development of potent influenza virus sialidase inhibitors.

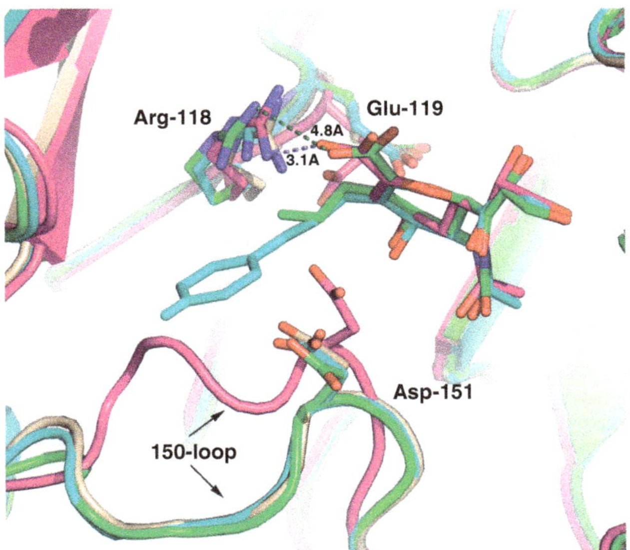

Figure 5 | Superimposition of N8 structures. Superimposition of the open 150-loop of N8-**6** (cyan) and N8-**5** (green), *apo*-N8 (pale orange; 2ht5) complexes, and the closed 150-loop of N8-**4** (magenta; 2htr).

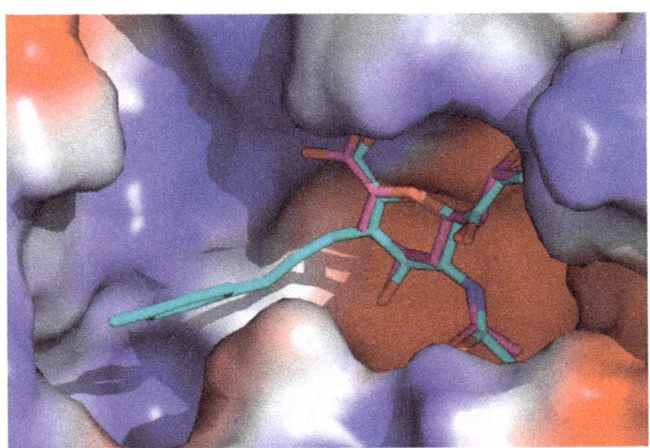

Figure 6 | Electrostatic potential map of the N8-6 complex. N8-**6** complex showing electrostatic potential on the protein surface (red, negative; blue, positive; and white, neutral/hydrophobic). Neu5Ac2en (**4**), in magenta, is superimposed on **6**.

In conclusion, we have demonstrated that it is possible, using appropriately substituted Neu5Ac2en derivatives, to lock open the flexible 150-loop of influenza A virus group-1 sialidases. Moreover, these derivatives demonstrate selectivity for an influenza A virus group-1 sialidase compared with a group-2 sialidase and the capacity to inhibit oseltamivir-resistant influenza virus sialidases. Further studies using the C-3-substituted Neu5Ac2en template may help to determine whether group-2 sialidases also possess, as suggested by molecular dynamics simulations[19,21], some plasticity or flexibility in this area of the protein. Finally, the most recent and the most devastating pandemic influenza A viruses, swine origin H1N1 and the 1918 H1N1 respectively, both contain a group-1 sialidase. This study may provide and inform new direction in the discovery of novel influenza virus sialidase inhibitors as next generation, first-line-of-defence, anti-influenza drugs to specifically tackle such viruses.

Methods

Molecular modelling. Superimposition of the influenza A virus sialidase *apo*-N8 structure (2ht5) and the N8–**4** structure (2htr) using DeepView (Swiss-PDB-Viewer)[22] was visually inspected in Astex Viewer[23]. Several Neu5Ac2en (**4**) derivatives substituted at the C-3 position, including **5** and **6**, were then built in InsightII[24] and docked using AutoDock 3.0.5 (ref. 25) into the active site of the *apo*-N8 structure (2ht5). Specifically, the protein was prepared in the standard manner using AutoDock Tools (version 1.4.5) (ref. 26) and a grid of 70 Å × 60 Å × 60 Å was constructed with a spacing of 0.375 points per Å, centred around the active site. The following parameters were used in the AutoDocking calculations: ga_pop_size = 250, ga_num_evals = 20,000,000, and 250 docking conformations were generated. The results were processed using the utilities provided with AutoDock[25] and visualized using AstexViewer[23]. AutoDock has been successfully used to predict the binding pose and energy of interaction of known inhibitors in the influenza virus sialidase active site and confirms that AutoDock is able to reproduce experimentally determined binding modes with a high degree of accuracy[27].

Synthesis of sialic acid derivatives. The sialic acid derivatives **5** and **6** were prepared according to Figure 2, using protocols described in the Supplementary Information. ^{1}H NMR spectra for the key compounds are provided (Supplementary Figs S4–S7).

Viruses. Influenza virus A/Hong Kong/156/97 (H5N1) and influenza virus A/California/07/2009 (H1N1 pdm) were kindly provided by Alan Hay (NIMR) and by Nancy Cox (Centers for Disease Control), respectively. The influenza viruses A/Paris/0497/2007 (H1N1), A/Paris/2590/2009 (H1N1 pdm) and A/Paris/908/97 (H3N2) were isolated by the National Influenza Center (Northern France) at the Institut Pasteur in Paris (France).

Sialidase inhibition assay. The sequence encoding the sialidase was amplified from viral RNA by reverse transcription–PCR, and cloned into the pCI vector (Invitrogen), using standard procedures. Two independent clones were selected for the neuraminidase of each of the three wild-type viruses included in the study. The H274Y, N294S and Q136K mutations were each introduced into a plasmidic clone encoding the N1 of A/Hong Kong/156/97 or A/Paris/2590/2009, using a QuickChange site-directed mutagenesis kit (Stratagene). All constructs were verified by sequencing using a Big Dye terminator sequencing kit and an automated sequencer (Perkin Elmer). Sialidase inhibition assays were carried out on MES-β-dodecyl-D-maltoside cell extracts prepared from 293T cells transiently expressing the viral enzyme, as previously described[13]. Sialidase enzymatic activity was measured using the fluorogenic substrate 2-α-(4-methylumbelliferyl)-D-*N*-acetylneuraminic acid (Sigma), according to the method of Potier *et al.*[28] Final concentration of the substrate ranged from 5 to 100 µM. Fluorescence was monitored every 45 s for 20 to 30 min at 37 °C, using a Xenius spectrofluorometer (SAFAS) with excitation and emission wavelengths of 330 and 450 nm, respectively. To measure the inhibitory effect of compounds, cells were preincubated for 30 min at 37 °C in the presence of variable concentrations of the compounds (0.01–10 nM for zanamivir (**1**), or 25 nM to 2 µM when tested on the Q136K mutant N1; 0.1–100 µM for Neu5Ac2en (**4**); 6.125–800 µM for **5**; 1–400 µM for **6**), and the substrate was added at a final concentration of 20 µM. Measurements are the mean of 2–8 experimentally determined values. The kinetic parameters V_{max}, K_m and K_i were calculated by fitting the data to the appropriate Michaelis Menten equations, using the Levenberg–Marquardt algorithm as provided in the commercially available KaleidaGraph software package (Synergy Software).

Cell-based virus inhibition assay. The plaque phenotype of the indicated viruses was assayed on MDCK-SIAT cells[29] in the presence of serial dilutions of zanamivir (**1**, 0.1 nM to 10 µM), Neu5Ac2en (**4**, 10 nM to 1 mM), **5** (500 nM to 5 mM) or **6** (10 nM to 1 mM), using a plaque assay protocol adapted from a published procedure[30]. Cells were stained with crystal violet after 72 h of incubation at 35 °C. For each inhibitor, the average plaque diameters were plotted against the inhibitor concentrations. The EC_{50} was determined graphically as the concentration of inhibitor that induced a 50% reduction in the average plaque diameter. The A/California/07/2009 H1N1 pandemic strain was used in the plaque reduction assay due to its capacity to form larger plaques compared with the corresponding A/Paris/2590/2009 H1N1 pandemic strain.

Protein X-ray crystallography. N8 sialidase from A/Duck/Ukraine/1/63 (H3N8) was prepared from virus grown in hens' eggs. Sialidase was released from the viruses by bromelain digestion, and further purified, as previously described[5]. N8 sialidase crystals were grown by vapour diffusion in hanging drops consisting of 2 µl of reservoir solution (0.1 M imidazole, pH 8.0 and 35% (±)-2-methyl-2,4-pentanediol (MPD)) and 2 µl of concentrated protein solution (10 mg ml^{-1} in 10 mM Tris–HCl, pH 8.0). A crystal of N8 sialidase was soaked in 1 mM **5** or **6** for 60 min. Data were collected on an in-house rotating anode (RA Micro7 HFM) and a Saturn944 CCD at 100 K and processed with d*Trek[31]. Standard refinement was carried out with a combination of Refmac[32] and PHENIX[33], together with manual model building with O[34] or Coot[35]. Statistical support for the N8–**5** and N8–**6** structures is presented in Supplementary Table S2. Structural data have been deposited with the Protein Data Bank with accession codes 3O9J (N8–**5**) and 3O9K (N8–**6**).

References

1. Zambon, M. C. The pathogenesis of influenza in humans. *Rev. Med. Virol.* **11,** 227–241 (2001).
2. World Health Organisation — Fact sheet No 211 (2009) Influenza. http://www.who.int/mediacentre/factsheets/fs211/en/.
3. Sullivan, S. J., Jacobson, R. M., Dowdle, W. R. & Poland, G. A. 2009 H1N1 influenza. *Mayo Clin. Proc.* **85,** 64–76 (2010).
4. Wagner, R., Matrosovich, M. & Klenk, H.- D. Functional balance between haemagglutinin and neuraminidase in influenza virus infections. *Rev. Med. Virol.* **12,** 159–166 (2002).
5. Russell, R. J. *et al.* The structure of H5N1 avian influenza neuraminidase suggests new opportunities for drug design. *Nature* **443,** 45–49 (2006).
6. von Itzstein, M. The war against influenza: discovery and development of sialidase inhibitors. *Nat. Rev. Drug Discov.* **6,** 967–974 (2007).
7. Li, Q. *et al.* The 2009 pandemic H1N1 neuraminidase N1 lacks the 150-cavity in its active site. *Nat. Struct. Mol. Biol.* **17,** 1266–1268 (2010).
8. von Itzstein, M. & Thomson, R. J. Anti-influenza drugs: the development of sialidase inhibitors. *Handb. Exp. Pharmacol.* **189,** 111–154 (2009).
9. De Clercq, E. Antiviral agents active against influenza A viruses. *Nat. Rev. Drug Discov.* **5,** 1015–1025 (2006).
10. Wen, W. H. *et al.* Analogs of zanamivir with modified C4-substituents as the inhibitors against the group-1 neuraminidases of influenza viruses. *Bioorg. Med. Chem.* **18,** 4074–4084 (2010).
11. Mohan, S., McAtamney, S., Haselhorst, T., von Itzstein, M. & Pinto, B. M. Carbocycles related to oseltamivir as influenza virus group-1-specific neuraminidase inhibitors. binding to N1 enzymes in the context of virus-like particles. *J. Med. Chem.* **53,** 7377–7391 (2010).
12. Nolan, S. P. & Clavier, H. Chemoselective olefin metathesis transformations mediated by ruthenium complexes. *Chem. Soc. Rev.* **39,** 3305–3316 (2010).
13. Rameix-Welti, M. A. *et al.* Natural variation can significantly alter the sensitivity of influenza A (H5N1) viruses to oseltamivir. *Antimicrob. Agents Chemotherap.* **50,** 3809–3815 (2006).
14. Okamoto, K., Kondo, T. & Goto, T. Functionalization of 2-deoxy-2,3-dehydro-*N*-acetylneuraminic acid methyl ester. *Bull. Chem. Soc. Jpn.* **60,** 631–636 (1987).
15. Paulsen, H. & Matschulat, P. Synthese von *C*-glycosiden der *N*-acetyl-neuraminsäure und weiteren derivaten. *Liebigs Ann. Chem.* **5,** 487–495 (1991).
16. Scholl, M., Ding, S., Lee, C. W. & Grubbs, R. H. Synthesis and activity of a new generation of ruthenium-based olefin metathesis catalysts coordinated with 1,3-dimesityl-4,5-dihydroimidazol-2-ylidene ligands. *Org. Lett.* **1,** 953–956 (1999).
17. Okomo-Adhiambo, M. *et al.* Host cell selection of influenza neuraminidase variants: implications for drug resistance monitoring in A(H1N1) viruses. *Antiviral Res.* **85,** 381–388 (2010).
18. Hurt, A. C., Holien, J. K., Parker, M., Kelso, A. & Barr, I. G. Zanamivir-resistant influenza viruses with a novel neuraminidase mutation. *J. Virol.* **83,** 10366–10373 (2009).
19. Amaro, R. E. *et al.* Remarkable loop flexibility in avian influenza N1 and its implications for antiviral drug design. *J. Am. Chem. Soc.* **129,** 7764–7765 (2007).
20. Taylor, N. R. & von Itzstein, M. Molecular modeling studies on ligand binding to sialidase from influenza virus and the mechanism of catalysis. *J. Med. Chem.* **37,** 616–624 (1994).
21. Amaro, R. E., Cheng, X., Ivanov, I., Xu, D. & McCammon, J. A. Characterizing loop dynamics and ligand recognition in human- and avian-type influenza neuraminidases via generalized born molecular dynamics and end-point free energy calculations. *J. Am. Chem. Soc.* **131,** 4702–4709 (2009).
22. Guex, N. & Peitsch, M. C. SWISS-MODEL and the Swiss-PdbViewer: an environment for comparative protein modeling. *Electrophoresis* **18,** 2714–2723 (1997).
23. Hartshorn, M. J. AstexViewer: a visualisation aid for structure-based drug design. *J. Comput. Aided Mol. Des.* **16,** 871–881 (2002).
24. Accelrys. *InsightII* (Accelrys, 2001).
25. Goodsell, D. S., Morris, G. M. & Olson, A. J. Automated docking of flexible ligands: applications of AutoDock. *J. Mol. Recognit.* **9,** 1–5 (1996).
26. Sanner, M. F. Python: a programming language for software integration and development. *J. Mol. Graph. Model* **17,** 57–61 (1999).
27. Cheng, L. S. *et al.* Ensemble-based virtual screening reveals potential novel antiviral compounds for avian influenza neuraminidase. *J. Med. Chem.* **51,** 3878–3894 (2008).
28. Potier, M. *et al.* Fluorometric assay of neuraminidase with a sodium (4-methylumbelliferyl-α-D-*N*-acetylneuraminate) substrate. *Anal. Biochem.* **94,** 287–296 (1979).
29. Matrosovich, M. *et al.* Overexpression of the α-2,6-sialyltransferase in MDCK cells increases influenza virus sensitivity to neuraminidase inhibitors. *J. Virol.* **77,** 8418–8425 (2003).
30. Matrosovich, M., Matrosovich, T., Garten, W. & Klenk, H. D. New low-viscosity overlay medium for viral plaque assays. *Virol. J.* **3,** 63 (2006).
31. Pflugrath, J. W. The finer things in X-ray diffraction data collection. *Acta Crystallogr. D Biol. Crystallogr.* **55,** 1718–1725 (1999).

32. Collaborative Computational Project, Number 4. The CCP4 suite: programs for protein crystallography. *Acta Crystallogr. D Biol. Crystallogr.* **50,** 760–763 (1994).
33. Adams, P. D. *et al.* PHENIX: building new software for automated crystallographic structure determination. *Acta Crystallogr. D Biol. Crystallogr.* **58,** 1948–1954 (2002).
34. Jones, T. A., Zou, J. Y., Cowan, S. W. & Kjeldgaard, M. Improved methods for building protein models in electron density maps and the location of errors in these models. *Acta Crystallogr. A.* **47,** 110–119 (1991).
35. Emsley, P. & Cowtan, K. Coot: model-building tools for molecular graphics. *Acta Crystallogr. D Biol. Crystallogr.* **60,** 2126–2132 (2004).

Acknowledgments

M.v.I. gratefully acknowledges the financial support of the Honda Foundation (Australia) in a grant to the Institute for Glycomics, and the Australian Research Council (ARC) through the award of an Australian Federation Fellowship. R.J.M.R. thanks the Medical Research Council and the Scottish Funding Council for financial support. N.N., M.-A.R.-W. and S.v.d.W. thank F. Agou (Institut Pasteur) for providing access to a Xenius spectrofluorometer and for helpful advice, Xingyi Ge for generating the Q136K mutant constructs and Georges Abou Jaoude for providing the expression plasmids for the N1 of A/Paris/2590/2009. Finally, we thank John Skehel, David Stevens and Patrick Collins of the MRC-National Institute for Medical Research, UK, for the kind provision of N8 NA protein.

Author contributions

S.R. contributed to the design and analysis of the chemical aspects of the study, carried out all of the described chemistry and contributed to the preparation of the manuscript. J.C.D. contributed to the design of the molecular modelling studies, carried out all of the computational chemistry and contributed to the preparation of the manuscript. F.J.R. carried out the purification of the designed and synthesized compounds. M.-A.R.-W., S.v.d.W. and N.N. contributed to the design and/or carried out the described biological assays and contributed to the preparation of the manuscript. P.S.K. and R.J.M.R. carried out the design, execution and analysis of the described structural studies and contributed to the preparation of the manuscript. R.J.T. contributed to the design and analysis of the chemical aspects of the study and preparation of the manuscript. M.v.I conceived the project, contributed to the design and analysis of the described studies and the preparation of the manuscript.

Additional information

Competing financial interests: The authors declare no competing financial interests.

2

Glycopeptide analogues of PSGL-1 inhibit P-selectin *in vitro* and *in vivo*

Venkata R. Krishnamurthy[1,2], Mohammed Y. R. Sardar[1,2], Yu Ying[3], Xuezheng Song[3], Carolyn Haller[1,2], Erbin Dai[1,2], Xiaocong Wang[4], Donny Hanjaya-Putra[1,2], Lijun Sun[1], Vasilios Morikis[5], Scott I. Simon[5], Robert J. Woods[4,6], Richard D. Cummings[3] & Elliot L. Chaikof[1,2]

Blockade of P-selectin (P-sel)/PSGL-1 interactions holds significant potential for treatment of disorders of innate immunity, thrombosis and cancer. Current inhibitors remain limited due to low binding affinity or by the recognized disadvantages inherent to chronic administration of antibody therapeutics. Here we report an efficient approach for generating glycosulfopeptide mimics of N-terminal PSGL-1 through development of a stereoselective route for multi-gram scale synthesis of the C2 O-glycan building block and replacement of hydrolytically labile tyrosine sulfates with isosteric sulfonate analogues. Library screening afforded a compound of exceptional stability, GSnP-6, that binds to human P-sel with nanomolar affinity ($K_d \sim 22$ nM). Molecular dynamics simulation defines the origin of this affinity in terms of a number of critical structural contributions. GSnP-6 potently blocks P-sel/PSGL-1 interactions *in vitro* and *in vivo* and represents a promising candidate for the treatment of diseases driven by acute and chronic inflammation.

[1] Department of Surgery, Center for Drug Discovery and Translational Research, Beth Israel Deaconess Medical Center, Harvard Medical School, 110 Francis Street, Suite 9F, Boston, Massachusetts 02215, USA. [2] Wyss Institute of Biologically Inspired Engineering, Harvard University, 110 Francis Street, Suite 9F, Boston, Massachusetts 02115, USA. [3] Department of Biochemistry, Emory University, Atlanta, Georgia 30322, USA. [4] Complex Carbohydrate Research Center, University of Georgia, Athens, Georgia 30602, USA. [5] Department of Biomedical Engineering, University of California Davis, Davis, California 95616, USA. [6] School of Chemistry, National University of Ireland, Galway, University Road, Galway, Ireland. Correspondence and requests for materials should be addressed to E.L.C. (email: echaikof@bidmc.harvard.edu).

The vascular endothelium forms a dynamic interface between blood elements and peripheral tissues. Characteristically, leukocyte–endothelial interactions are mediated by transient tethering, followed by rapid integrin activation and subsequent transendothelial migration[1,2]. The recruitment of leukocytes to sites of inflammation is mediated by selectin adhesion molecules and their ligands[3]. P-selectin (P-sel)[4,5], found on activated platelets and vascular endothelium, is rapidly translocated to the cell surface within minutes of an inflammatory stimulus, E-sel[6] is expressed on endothelial cells after *de novo* synthesis within a few hours of activation, while L-sel is expressed on most leukocytes and functions as a homing receptor to mediate binding of lymphocytes to high endothelial venules of peripheral lymph nodes[7]. Excessive trafficking of leukocytes to extravascular locations can lead to tissue injury contributing to the development of inflammatory bowel disease, chronic obstructive pulmonary disease, atherosclerosis and post-thrombotic syndrome, among a variety of other disorders. Thus, selectins, as a mediator of early adhesion and intracellular signalling events in the inflammatory cascade, represent a promising target for the design of agents that limit adverse inflammatory responses.

While structurally diverse glycoprotein counter-receptors bind selectins with high affinity, the most well characterized ligand is P-sel-glycoprotein-ligand-1 (PSGL-1)[8]. PSGL-1 binds all three selectins, but with highest affinity to P-sel[9]. Ligation of P-sel expressed on endothelial cells by PSGL-1 constitutes the initial 'capture and rolling' step in the leukocyte–endothelial cell adhesion cascade[10]. Likewise, the interaction of PSGL-1 with P-sel on activated platelets promotes formation of leukocyte–platelet aggregates that contributes to adhesion and infiltration of inflammatory cells and both activated platelets and soluble P-sel promote leukocyte infiltration[11–13]. Significantly, the engagement of PSGL-1 to P-sel activates intracellular signalling pathways that induces the β2-integrin LFA-1 to adopt an extended conformation associated with the intermediate affinity state, which supports leukocyte deceleration and cell arrest onto the endothelium[14]. PSGL-1 also activates the expression of intracellular protein kinases, such as Rho/Rock kinase, which mediates cell migration, and MAPK kinase that controls expression of pro-inflammatory cytokines[15,16]. Blockade of P-sel/PSGL-1 interactions holds significant potential for the treatment of disorders due to maladaptive acute or chronic inflammatory responses[17–19].

The role of P-sel/PSGL-1 in a number of disease states has led to the design of a variety of biologics, small molecules and glycopeptide mimics to target these interactions. Although P-sel and PSGL-1 blocking antibodies are undergoing clinical evaluation for the treatment of sickle cell disease and Crohn's disease, they are expensive to manufacture, limited in shelf-life and the development of antibodies against monoclonal therapeutics, including chimeric and humanized monoclonal antibodies, continues to limit the effectiveness of antibody therapy especially when there is need for daily or long-term administration[20]. Small molecule inhibitors designed through modifications of sialyl Lewis x (sLe^x) continue to be limited by their low potency and off-target toxicity. For example, GMI-1070 has demonstrated efficacy in treating sickle cell disease, but its low activity to P-sel ($IC_{50} \sim 423\,\mu M$) requires infusion of ~2 g of drug per day[21]. Likewise, PSI-697 only weakly inhibits human platelet–monocyte aggregation, which is almost certainly attributable to its low $K_d \sim 200\,\mu M$ (ref. 22). Similarly, the glycomimetic, bimosiamose (TBC1269), is a pan-sel inhibitor with an IC_{50} of 70 μM against P-sel and an IC_{50} of >500 μM against E- and L-sel[23]. Most existing P-sel inhibitors have been designed to mimic the core-2 *O*-glycan (C2 *O*-glycan) bearing sLe^x moiety, but often fail to account for the crucial contributions of multiple clustered tyrosine sulfates[21,24,25]. Indeed, Leppänen *et al.*[26–28] have shown that high affinity binding of P-sel to PSGL-1 requires stereospecific interactions with both clustered tyrosine sulfates (Tyr-SO_3H) and a nearby C2 *O*-glycan bearing a sLe^x-containing hexasaccharide epitope (C_2-*O*-sLe^x). To date, attempts to synthesize mimics of the N terminus of PSGL-1 have been limited by the acid sensitivity of tyrosine sulfates[29,30], poor selectivity in key glycosylation steps[31] and incompatible protecting groups for oligosaccharide synthesis[32].

We report an efficient approach for the generation of a diverse set of glycopeptide mimics of PSGL-1. Key features of this synthesis include an efficient stereoselective route that has lead to multi-gram scale synthesis of the C2 *O*-glycan and replacement of hydrolytically labile tyrosine sulfates with stable, isosteric sulfonate analogues affording compounds with high affinity to P-sel (K_d 14–22 nM). In the process, we identified a high affinity, chemically stable compound, termed GSnP-6 that blocks PSGL-1/P-sel interactions *in vitro* and *in vivo*.

Results

Compound design and strategy. In our approach, we envisaged a building block containing protecting groups fully compatible with peptide synthesis, after which sLe^x would be incorporated. Appendages were selected so that the resulting compounds could be selectively extended by glycosyltransferases to provide a diverse array of glycopeptide mimetics of PSGL-1. In this regard, we previously identified a threonine-derived C2 *O*-glycan as an appropriate building block for such studies[33]. However, attempts to synthesize the glycoamino acid building block suffered from suboptimal regioselectivity (α/β: 1:2:6) in the key glycosylation step. Furthermore, use of a glycosyl imidate donor required a triflic azide-mediated diazotransfer step, which is potentially explosive, thus prohibiting deployment of this scheme for preparative scale synthesis (>50 g). As a result, the C2 *O*-glycan was only obtained on milligram scale. To circumvent these problems, a more efficient scheme was developed that lead to multi-gram scale synthesis of this key compound. Synthesis began from 3,4,6 tri-*O*-acetyl-D-galactal, which can be readily converted to a halide via a one-pot azidochlorination step (Fig. 1). Although previously reported[34], direct coupling of the chloride intermediate with a Fmoc-threonine acceptor was unsuccessful due to its rapid decomposition. Therefore, this intermediate was converted *in situ* to the thioglycoside donor **1**. Significantly, this two-step, one-pot procedure could be safely carried out on a preparative scale (>50 g) to provide donor **1** in 67% yield. Azidochlorination does not completely eliminate explosive risk, but it is substantially reduced and greatly facilitates safe, large-scale production. Coupling with the Fmoc-threonine acceptor afforded **2** in 78% yield with high α selectivity (α/β: 95:5). Glycoamino acid **2** was then converted to diol **5** by following previously reported steps[33]. Significantly, this new scheme provided acceptor **5** in less than seven steps with 21% overall yield, which established this route for this key building block as the most efficient and convenient to date[31–33].

In the key glycosylation step with acceptor **5**, we anticipated that the axial 4-OH group would be of low reactivity, especially when carrying a substituent at O-3. However, an undesired tetrasaccharide was identified in ~20% yield[33]. Both desired and undesired compounds had similar retention factor values. Thus, chromatographic separation was challenging and laborious, particularly at a preparative scale. To address this problem, we performed low temperature activation (−10 °C) with glucosamine donor **6** at 0.8 equiv. (as opposed to 1.2 equiv.), which produced only the β-glycoside **7** in 79% yield

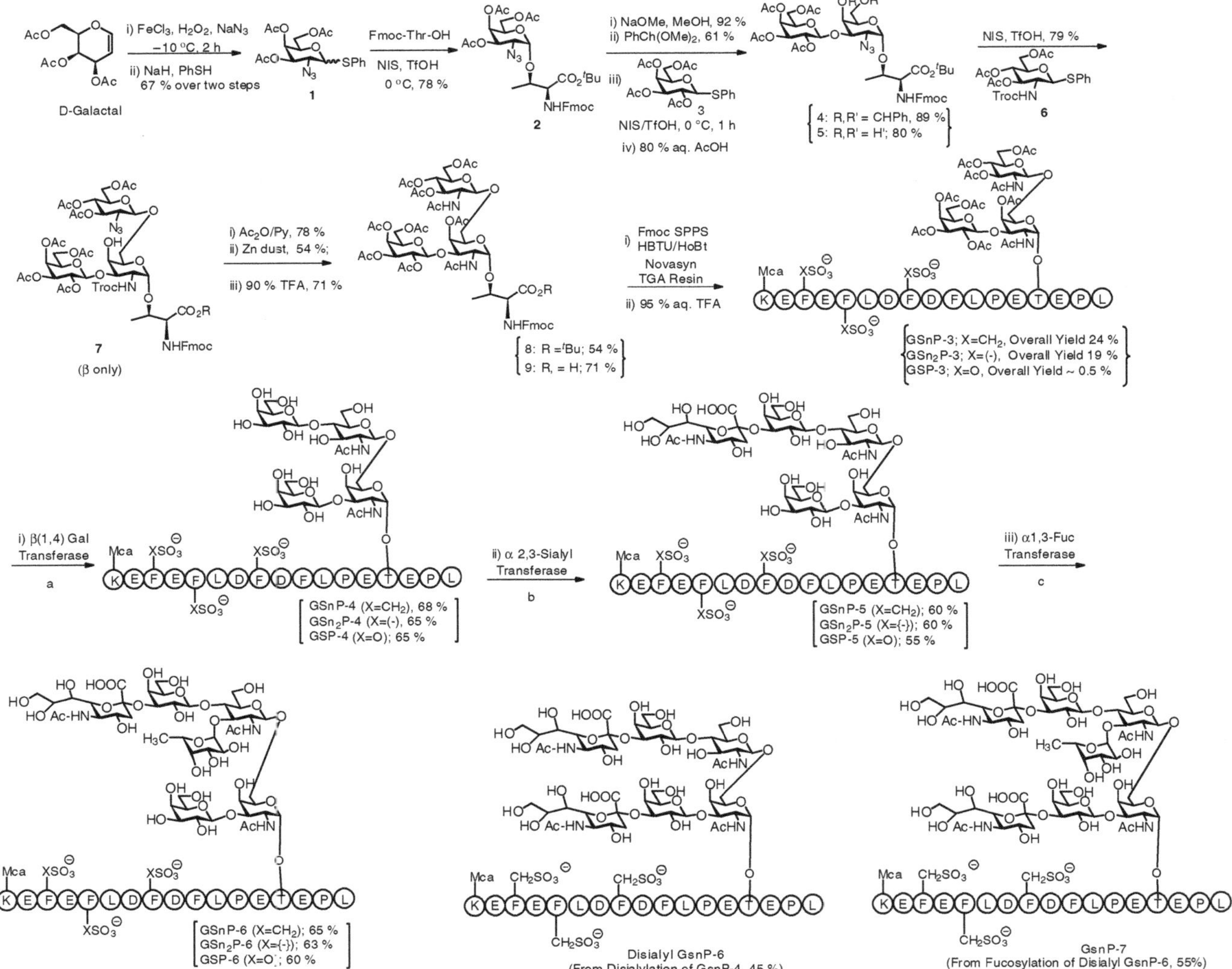

Figure 1 | Synthesis of the Core-2 glycan and subsequent enzymatic steps to afford a family of 17 glycopeptide mimetics of PSGL-1. Enzymatic steps (**a**) UDP-Gal, β-1,4-GalT (bovine), alkaline phosphatase, 130 mM HEPES, pH 7.4, 40 mM sodium cacodylate, pH 7.0, 20 mM $MnCl_2$ and 0.02% NaN_3; (**b**) α 2,3-(*N*)-sialylT CMP-NeuAc 50 mM MOPS, pH 7.4, 0.1% bovine serum albumin and 0.02% NaN_3, 14 h; (**c**) GDP-Fuc, α1,3-FucT-VI, 50 mM MOPS, pH 7.4, 20 mM $MnCl_2$ and 0.02% NaN_3, 16 h. The desialylated GSnP-6 was obtained from GSnP-4 in 45% yield. GSnP-7 was obtained in 55% yield by fucosylation of disialylated GSnP-6. 4-(Sulfomethyl)phenylalanine series (*n*): GSnP-6 (X: CH_2; R = H); GSnP-7 (X: CH_2; R = Sialyl); 4-(Sulfo)phenylalanine series (n_2): GSn_2P-6 (X: bond; R = H); Tyrosine O-sulfate series: GSP-6 (X: O; R = H). The last numeral refers to the size of the glycan (for example, 6 for hexasaccharide).

(Supplementary Figs 1 and 2). The (1→6)-linkage in **7** was confirmed by nuclear Överhauser enhancement spectroscopy (NOESY) spectrum, which displayed a cross-peak between H-1 of the glucosamine residue and H-6 of the galactosamine residue. gHMBC nuclear magnetic resonance (NMR) of **7** confirmed that O-6 was glycosylated in revealing cross-peaks from 101.3 p.p.m. (C-1 of the glucosamine residue, A-C1) and 4.02 p.p.m. (H-6 of the galactosamine residue, BH6), as well as from 4.70 p.p.m. (H-1 of the glucosamine residue, A-H1) and 69.5 p.p.m. (C-6 of the galactosamine residue, B-C6) (Supplementary Figs 3–7). Acetylation of **7** with Py/Ac_2O, zinc reduction and TFA-mediated *t*-butyl ester deprotection provided the C2 *O*-glycan **9** (Supplementary Figs 8 and 9). This new route improved not only selectivity and yield, but also enabled the production of gram quantities of intermediate **9** and facilitated the synthesis of a broad range of structural mimics of PSGL-1.

With the availability of this glycoamino acid building block, glycopeptide mimics of the N-terminal domain of PSGL-1 were synthesized using a Fmoc-assisted SPPS strategy (Fig. 1). Coupling reactions were performed using 2-(1H-benzotriazole-1-yl)-1,1,3,3-tetramethyluronium hexafluorophosphate (HBTU) and 1-hydroxy-benzotriazol (HOBt) and the deprotection step was carried out with 20% piperidine. Addition of the sterically hindered C2 glycoamino acid **9** proceeded smoothly without formation of any side products. However, the incorporation of Fmoc-Tyr (O-SO_3^-) amino acid in peptide synthesis is extremely challenging owing to its acid lability[35]. As an alternative approach, enzymatic sulfation has been proven less than ideal since tyrosine sulfotransferase is not commercially available, and while the enzymatic reaction is optimal at 30 °C tyrosine sulfotransferase is unstable >20 °C (ref. 36). Chemical sulfation of tyrosine residues after peptide synthesis also suffers from low specificity[30], incomplete reaction with sulfating reagents[37], and low yield[38]. Together, these factors place significant limitations on the use of Tyr (O-SO_3^-), which has limited their broad application in drug design. Therefore, we elected to replace the acid labile Tyr (O-SO_3^-) moiety with bioiosteric, hydrolytically stabile analogues, namely, Fmoc-Phe (*p*-CH_2SO_3H)[39,40] and Fmoc-Phe (*p*-SO_3H)[41]. Such sulfonate mimics can be readily incorporated in solid phase peptide synthesis without the need for any side-chain protecting groups using standard HBTU coupling conditions. The chromogenic amino acid Fmoc-Lys(Mca)-OH was also incorporated at the N terminus of the PSGL-1 sequence for facile detection and quantification. After peptide synthesis, the deprotection of sulfonate mimics could be readily carried out with 95% aqueous TFA at room temperature. Saponification of O-acetate groups in $GS_{(n)}P$-3 was achieved with catalytic NaOMe to afford the glycopeptide mimics, which were further purified by reversed-phase high-performance liquid chromatography (RP-HPLC). In synthesizing the native tyrosine O-sulfate sequence, glycosulfopeptide-3 (GSP-3), deprotection was performed at 0 °C to suppress the degradation of tyrosine O-sulfates[42]. When tyrosine O-sulfates were employed in peptide synthesis, overall yield of GSP-3 was <0.5%, indicating the labile nature of tyrosine sulfates[36,43]. In contrast, use of hydrolytically stable tyrosine sulfonate analogues resulted in a dramatic improvement in overall yield to afford GSnP-3 and GSn_2P-3 in 24% and 19% yields, respectively.

The sLe^x moiety was incorporated into $GS_{(n)}P$-3 by using glycosyltransferases in stepwise order to sequentially add galactose, sialic acid and fucose. The highly efficient β1,4-galactosyltransferase (β1,4-GalT) is commercially available and was used to initially install β1,4-galactose. Since sialyltransferases have low efficiency towards a fucosylated Le^x structure, fucose was installed after sialylation. Thus, galactose was first appended in a β1,4 linkage to GlcNAc by treatment with β1,4-GalT in the presence of UDP-Galactose to produce GS(n)P-4. Similarly, addition of sialic acid was achieved by incubation of GSnP-4 with α2,3-sialyltransferase (α,2,3-(N)-sialylT) in the presence of CMP-NeuAc to obtain GSnP-5. The sLe^x structure was completed by incubation of $GS_{(n)}P$-5 with human α1,3-fucosyltransferase V and GDP-Fucose to produce $GS_{(n)}P$-6. All enzymatic steps proceeded with 60 to 70% yield without observed interference of the sulfonate residues[44]. In addition, desialylated glycopeptide mimics were generated through additional sialylation of GSnP-4 to provide disialyl GSnP-6 (45% yield) followed by fucosylation to provide GSnP-7 in 55% yield. Using this approach, a diverse array of 17 glycopeptide mimics of PSGL-1 was synthesized including GSnP[3–6], disialyl GSnP-6, GSnP-7, GSn_2P[3–6], GSP[3–6] and three GSnP C1 peptides (Fig. 1, Supplementary Figs 10–17).

GSnP-6 demonstrates nanomolar affinity to P-sel. The binding affinity of this set of glycopeptide mimics towards P-, L- and E-sel was initially screened using microarray technology. The 17 glycopeptide mimics along with five glycan standards (sLe^x, NA2, NA2,3, NA2,6 and LNnT) were printed on a NHS-activated glass slide. The slide was then incubated with recombinant immunoglobulin (Ig) chimeras of P-, L- or E-sel (5–20 $\mu g\,ml^{-1}$) followed by Alexa-488-labelled anti-human IgG antibody (5 $\mu g\,ml^{-1}$). Similar to the native, N-terminal PSGL-1 sequence containing tyrosine sulfate (GSP-6), GSnP-6 bound to P-sel more strongly than to E- or L-sel (Fig. 2a–c, Supplementary Fig. 18). Likewise, GSnP-7, a sialylated extension of GSnP-6, showed higher affinity to P-sel. However, disialyl GSnP-6, lacking the fucosyl residue displayed lower affinity to P-sel, consistent with the key contribution of α1,3-fucose. Binding of glycopeptide mimics was Ca^{2+} dependent and inhibited by EDTA.

Dissociation constants (K_d) were determined using a Biacore binding assay after initial capture of biotinylated $GS_{(n)}P$-6 onto streptavidin-coated sensor chips followed by flow through of P-, L- or E-sel-Ig (2.5–60 $\mu g\,ml^{-1}$). Dissociation constants for GSnP-6 and GSn_2P-6 to human P-sel were 22 and 14 nM (Fig. 2d), respectively, compared with the reported K_d of 73 nM for native PSGL-1 (ref. 9). The K_d of GSnP-6 to murine P-sel was approximately ninefold lower than to human P-sel (Fig. 2e). GSnP-6 bound to E- and L-sel with lower affinity (Supplementary Fig. 19), consistent with reports of PSGL-1 binding to E- and L-sel at a K_d of 2 to 5 μM (ref. 28).

Sulfotyrosine exhibits poor stability under acid and near neutral conditions, thereby limiting its use in drug development. For example, rapid decomposition occurs at 37 °C on exposure to TFA and other scavengers used in peptide synthesis and the hydrolysis rate of sulfotyrosine increases with increasing temperature[42,43]. Consistent with these observations, the native N-terminal PSGL-1 sequence, GSP-6, rapidly degraded under low pH conditions (pH ~ 5; T = 37 °C). In contrast, the GS_nP-6 mimic demonstrated superior stability when subjected to both low pH (pH ~ 5; T = 37 °C) and high temperature (pH7 ~ 7.5; T = 60 °C), without observed degradation products as detected by RP-HPLC (Fig. 2f).

Molecular dynamics simulations. Computational simulations were used to predict key structural residues responsible for P-sel/GSnP-6 interactions. Molecular dynamics (MD) simulations were first validated by reproducing all structural attributes of the PSGL-1/P-sel interaction, as defined by crystallographic data and experimental investigations. The positions of the glycan and the peptide components of PSGL-1 were monitored over the course of simulating its interaction with P-sel (Supplementary Fig. 20). Simulations confirmed that the ligand remained stable in the binding site, with the glycan displaying less positional variation than the peptide. In addition, all experimentally observed hydrogen bonds and salt bridges between the ligand and the protein were observed during the MD simulations. Of note, the dynamic motions of the system weakened some of these interactions relative to others (Supplementary Table 2). In particular, while the hydrogen bonds associated with the glycan appeared markedly stable, the interactions between the tyrosine sulfate residues and the P-sel surface residues were relatively unstable and depended heavily on the protonation state of H114. This is consistent with a recent report by Cao *et al.*[45], who demonstrated that the protonation state of H114 impacts the binding affinity of PSGL-1 to P-sel. As expected, full protonation of this histidine enhanced the stability of these interactions, particularly those associated with tyrosine sulfate (Y607) and H114. Similarly, the structure (Fig. 3) and stability (Supplementary Fig. 20) of GSnP-6 in the fully protonated H114 complex was comparable to that observed for the native PSGL-1 sequence, and retained all of the key non-covalent interactions (Supplementary Table 1). In the case of neutral H114, the interactions between the tyrosine sulfonates and the protein were unstable, leading to orientation disruption of the peptide component in GSnP-6. The frequency of the rebinding interaction was too low to observe statistical convergence in the MD simulation (Supplementary Fig. 20). Thus, only simulations with fully protonated H114 were employed in the subsequent analysis of interaction energies.

Combinations of five GB parameterizations and protein dielectric constant values (ε) ranging from 1 to 5 were initially evaluated to determine which, if any, set of conditions reproduced the relative contributions of PSGL-1 constituent features to P-sel-binding affinity. Optimal conditions were then employed to assess the interaction energies of GSnP-6 with P-sel, as well as the contributions of distinct structural features of the analogue. The molecular mechanics-generalized born solvent-accessible surface area (MM/GBSA) calculations using either the GB_2^{OBC} or GB_1^{OBC} model produced comparable results with $\varepsilon = 4.0$, in agreement

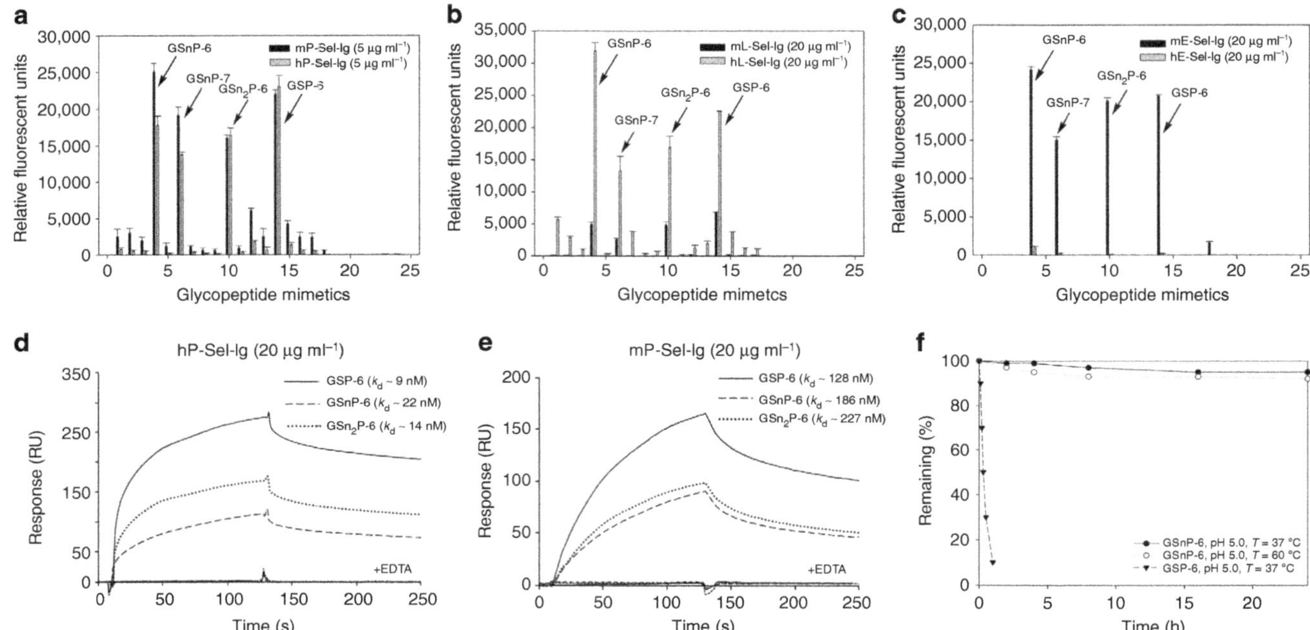

Figure 2 | Binding of P-, E- or L-selectin to PSGL-1 glycopeptide mimics and GSnP-6 stability analysis. Microarray binding studies of glycopeptide mimics towards (**a**) human and mouse P-selectin (5 $\mu g\,ml^{-1}$), (**b**) human and mouse L-selectin (20 $\mu g\,ml^{-1}$) and (**c**) human and mouse E-selectin (20 $\mu g\,ml^{-1}$). The compounds printed on the microarray in the order depicted here in **a–c** are detailed in Supplementary Fig. 18. Reference compounds included sialyl Lewis x (sLe^x), the biantennary glycans NA2, NA2,3, NA2,6, as well as lacto-*N*-neo-tetraose (LNnT) and biotin. Bound selectin-Igs were detected using Alexa-488-labelled anti-human IgG antibody (5 $\mu g\,ml^{-1}$). Three lectins RCA-1, AAL and PNA were used to confirm the sequence of enzymatic steps. Monoclonal antibodies CHO131, PSG2 antibody and PL-1 were used to confirm the presence of sLe^x, tyrosine sulfates and the peptide sequence, respectively. Biacore binding analysis to human P-selectin with observed rate constants for (**d**) GSnP-6, k_{on} $3.1 \times 10^5\,M^{-1}s^{-1}$, k_{off} $6.9 \times 10^3\,s^{-1}$; GSn$_2$P-6, k_{on} $6.4 \times 10^5\,M^{-1}s^{-1}$, k_{off} $6.8 \times 10^3\,s^{-1}$. Biacore binding analysis to *mouse* P-selectin with observed rate constants for (**e**) GsnP-6, k_{on} $4.9 \times 10^4\,M^{-1}s^{-1}$, k_{off} $8.0 \times 10^3\,s^{-1}$; GSn$_2$P-6 k_{on} $5.3 \times 10^4\,M^{-1}s^{-1}$, k_{off} $9.0 \times 10^3\,s^{-1}$. (**f**) Temperature- and pH-dependent stability studies of GSnP-6.

with relative experimental values (Supplementary Table 2). Since the GB$_1^{OBC}$ parameterization has been successfully employed to compute interaction energies in other carbohydrate–protein systems involving charged moieties, it was selected over the GB$_2^{OBC}$ parameterization (Supplementary Fig. 21)[46]. This combination was able to correctly rank the relative contributions to binding, with Fuc $\approx$ total sulfate > Neu5Ac, and identified that the second sulfate made a larger contribution (by -1.3 to $-1.6\,kcal\,mol^{-1}$) than the other two.

The experimental interaction energies of P-sel with PSGL-1 ligand and the analogue GSnP-6 were similar at $-9.8\,kcal\,mol^{-1}$ ($K_d = 73\,nM$) and $-10.5\,kcal\,mol^{-1}$ (22 nM), respectively. Using the combination of GB$_1^{OBC}$ with $\varepsilon = 4.0$, the absolute interaction energies of P-sel with PSGL-1 and GSnP-6 were predicted to be $-45.1 \pm 3.4\,kcal\,mol^{-1}$ and $-44.6 \pm 3.1\,kcal\,mol^{-1}$, respectively (Table 1). As anticipated, due to the omission of entropic penalties, predicted interaction energies were almost fourfold larger than experimental values[47–49]. Nonetheless, interaction energies were statistically equivalent, which is in agreement with experimental data. To facilitate detection on binding microarrays, GSnP-6 was chemically derivatized with a 7-amino-4-methylcoumarin (MCA) tag, which alters net charge, as well as local properties of the terminal lysine. The MCA tag was not included in the modelling, which employed only a lysine residue. The remaining residues in the peptide sequence of PSGL-1 and GSnP-6 render essentially identical contributions to the interaction energies. Due to the similarities of the two ligands, the relative contributions of the glycans to binding affinity were also indistinguishable within standard deviations. Likewise, the individual contributions from each sulfate group were comparable for each ligand, despite chemical differences (Table 1). An unexpected and potentially significant observation concerns the second tyrosine sulfate residue (607), whose strong affinity (-8.4 to $-9.5\,kcal\,mol^{-1}$) appears to arise predominantly from van der Waals interactions (-6.6 to $-7.0\,kcal\,mol^{-1}$). In summary, computational analysis reproduced salient structural and energetic features of PSGL-1/P-sel interactions and predicted that GSnP-6 would behave comparably, consistent with observed affinity data (Fig. 3).

GSnP-6 inhibits P- and L-sel binding to PSGL-1. Flow cytometry was initially used to characterize the ability of GSnP-6 to block binding of sel Fc chimeras to murine and human leukocytes. Recombinant mouse P-, L- or E-sel-Fc chimera (2 $\mu g\,ml^{-1}$) were incubated with murine leukocytes and GSnP-6 (0–30 μM). Likewise, recombinant human P-, L- or E-sel-Fc chimera (2 $\mu g\,ml^{-1}$) were incubated with human peripheral blood leukocytes, as well as the human U937 cell line in the presence of GSnP-6 (0–30 μM). Binding of selectin chimeras was detected with phycoerythrin (PE)-conjugated anti-Fc antibody, quantified as mean fluorescent intensity and plotted as per cent inhibition. Specificity was confirmed with PSGL-1 blocking antibodies. GSnP-6 inhibited P-sel-dependent interactions in a dose-dependent manner in both human and mouse leukocytes, including human neutrophils ($IC_{50} \sim 14\,\mu M$), human monocytes ($IC_{50} \sim 20\,\mu M$), mouse neutrophils ($IC_{50} \sim 19\,\mu M$) and mouse monocytes ($IC_{50} \sim 28\,\mu M$) (Fig. 4a,b). GSnP-6 also inhibited PSGL-1/L-sel interactions at a somewhat lower potency ($IC_{50} \sim 30\,\mu M$) for human and mouse leukocytes (Fig. 4c).

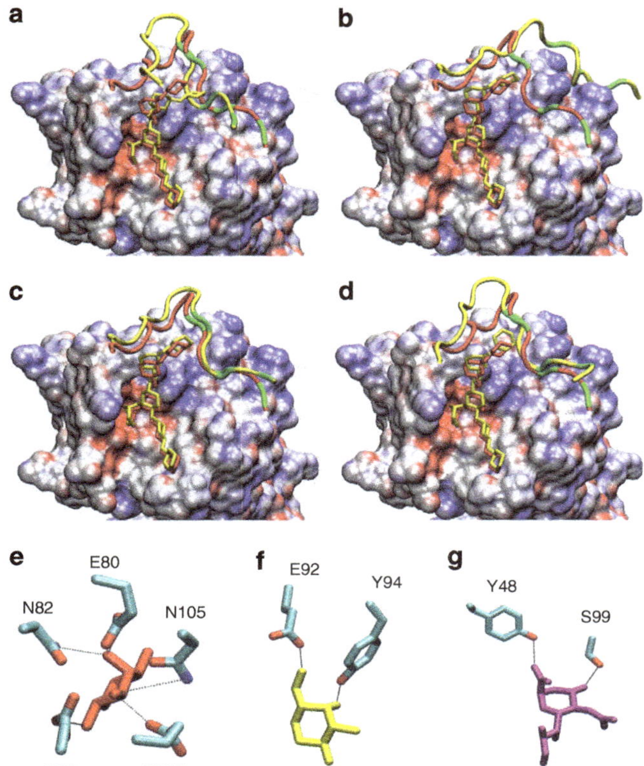

Figure 3 | Interactions of the N terminus of PSGL-1 and GSnP-6 bound to P-selectin, as a function of the protonation state of H114. Conformation of PSGL-1 (**a**) and GSnP-6 (**b**) ligands most similar to the average shape acquired from MD simulations performed with neutral H114. The crystal structure of the PSGL-1 ligand is shown in red with a splined representation of the peptide backbone, sulfated amino acid positions in green and a stick representation for monosaccharide rings. Assuming that H114 is fully protonated leads to optimal reproduction of the crystallographic data for PSGL-1 (**c**) and leads to similar binding for GSnP-6 (**d**). The solvent-accessible surface of P-selectin is coloured according to the electrostatic potential (acidic region: red; basic region: blue). (**e**-**g**) Hydrogen bonds between Fuc (red), Core-2Gal (yellow), and Neu5Ac (purple) and P-selectin residues.

Inhibition of E-sel interactions was not observed over this concentration range (Supplementary Fig. 22), which is consistent with the lower binding affinity of PSGL-1 for E-sel and the notion that leukocytes interact with E-sel through alternate ligands including CD44 and ESL-1 on mouse, and L-sel on human leukocytes[50,51].

GSnP-6 inhibits leukocyte rolling and arrest. PSGL-1 interactions with P-sel have been shown to signal activation of CD18 (β2-integrin) to adopt a high affinity extended conformation resulting in integrin-dependent deceleration and cell arrest. Inhibition of this interaction leads to an increase in rolling velocity and a reduction in cell arrest[51]. Human neutrophils and monocytes were incubated with GSnP-6 (0–30 μM) or PBS vehicle for 10 min and perfused through a microfluidic flow chamber at 2 dyn cm^{-2} over glass substrates coated with ICAM-1 and P-sel-Fc chimeras[52]. Total cell capture, defined as the number of cells that rolled or arrested (velocity $\leq 1\,\mu m\,s^{-1}$), was determined, along with leukocyte rolling velocity. Videomicroscopic analysis demonstrated that GSnP-6 lead to a dose-dependent inhibition of monocyte and neutrophil capture in shear flow, with an IC50 of 3 μM and 5 μM, respectively (Fig. 4d). At a concentration as low as 2 μM, GSnP-6 increased the rolling velocity of human neutrophils and monocytes and resulted in 80% inhibition at 6 μM, a dose that abrogated the fraction achieving arrest (Fig. 4d–f). In contrast, incubation with the sulfated polysaccharide, fucoidan, at a concentration of up to 50 μg ml^{-1} (~50 μM) did not affect the efficiency of capture, rolling or arrest when compared with PBS control (data not shown). GSnP-6 at concentrations as high as 30 μM did not perturb leukocyte rolling and arrest on substrates coated with ICAM-1 and E-sel (Supplementary Fig. 23). This implies that GSnP-6 specifically inhibits the interaction between PSGL-1 and P-sel in neutrophils and monocytes over this concentration range.

Intravital microscopy was performed within 30 min of surgical stimulation of the murine cremaster muscle to determine the ability of GsnP-6 to inhibit leukocyte binding to microvascular endothelium *in vivo*[53]. Seven venules per mouse ($n = 4$, saline control; $n = 3$, GSnP-6, 4 μmol kg^{-1} i.v.) with a diameter of 30–40 μm were analyzed and the velocities of 5–10 rolling leukocytes were determined in each venule by individually tracking leukocyte distance/time (μm s^{-1}). A significant increase in mean rolling velocity was observed after intravenous administration of GSnP-6 when compared with saline vehicle control (Fig. 4g,h, saline: $40.8 \pm 1.7\,\mu m\,s^{-1}$ versus GSnP-6: $74.9 \pm 3.4\,\mu m\,s^{-1}$; $P \leq 0.01$; Student's *t*-test). Cumulative frequency histogram analysis demonstrated a twofold increase in median rolling velocities (Fig. 4i, saline: 35.5 μm s^{-1} versus GSnP-6: 64.0 μm s^{-1}; Supplementary Fig. 24).

GSnP-6 inhibits thromboinflammatory events *in vivo*. PSGL-1/P-sel interactions are responsible for the formation of leukocyte–platelet aggregates, which promotes the infiltration of leukocytes, as well as the release of neutrophil extracellular traps and other procoagulant factors[54]. Human and murine platelet–leukocyte aggregates were quantified in whole blood using dual-label flow cytometry[55]. Human or mouse blood was stimulated with a thrombin receptor-activating peptide to induce platelet P-sel expression and dosed with 40 μM GSnP-6. GSnP-6 inhibited 65% of platelet–neutrophil and 72% of platelet–monocyte aggregate formation in human blood (Fig. 5a,b; $P < 0.05$; Student's *t*-test) and 42% of platelet–neutrophil and 47% of platelet–monocyte aggregate formation in murine blood (Fig. 5c,d; $P < 0.05$; Student's *t*-test).

The capacity of GSnP-6 to inhibit early thromboinflammatory events *in vivo* was characterized by platelet adhesion to leukocytes and platelet aggregation in a cremaster model of tumour-necrosis factor-α (TNF-α)-induced venular inflammation[56]. TNF-α was administered intrascrotally (0.5 μg) to male mice (6–8 weeks old, C57BL/6) 3 h prior to imaging. P-sel blocking antibody (RB40.34), GSnP-6, or saline was subsequently administered at the time of imaging and platelet microaggregate formation and platelet–neutrophil binding was monitored in venules (*d* 30–45 μm, 8–10 venules per mouse, $n = 5$ mice per test group) over 2 min intervals through visualization of platelets and neutrophils labelled with Dylight 649-anti-CD42b and Alexa Fluor 488-anti-Gr-1 antibodies, respectively. Three hours after intrascrotal administration of TNF-α, venule endothelial cells display ~700 mm^2 adherent neutrophils and limited rolling flux (~1 white blood cells per min) (Supplementary Fig. 25). Although administration of anti-CD62P or GSnP-6 at this stage would not be expected to alter established populations of adherent leukocytes, leukocyte–platelet interactions and platelet aggregate formation can be examined. Platelet accumulation was quantified by calculating median integrated fluorescence intensity, normalized to vessel surface area. GSnP-6 significantly reduced platelet–neutrophil interactions and platelet thrombi

Table 1 | Per-residue MM/GBSA interaction energies* for interactions of P-selectin with residues in PSGL-1 and GSnP-6.

	PSGL-1	GSnP-6		PSGL-1	GSnP-6
Y/YC 605†	−1.4 ± 0.6	−1.3 ± 0.6	Neu5Ac	−2.7 ± 0.8	−2.6 ± 0.8
Y/YC 607†	−5.5 ± 0.7	−6.0 ± 0.6	Core-2 Gal	−4.2 ± 0.7	−4.2 ± 0.7
Y/YC 610†	−0.8 ± 0.4	−0.6 ± 0.3	GlcNAc	−3.3 ± 0.6	−3.2 ± 0.5
SO_3^- 605‡	−1.9 ± 0.8	−2.3 ± 0.9	Fuc	−4.8 ± 1.3	−4.7 ± 1.3
SO_3^- 607‡	−2.9 ± 0.9	−3.5 ± 0.8	GalNAc	−0.6 ± 0.3	−0.4 ± 0.2
SO_3^- 610‡	−0.8 ± 0.6	−0.8 ± 0.4	Gal	0.1 ± 0.1	0.1 ± 0.1
Subtotal	−13.3 ± 1.7	−14.1 ± 1.5	Subtotal	−15.5 ± 1.8	−15.0 ± 1.8
	Amino acids				
K603§	NA	1.3 ± 0.1	L613	−4.1 ± 1.1	−3.4 ± 1.2
E604	0.1 ± 0.2	−0.6 ± 0.1	P614	−1.9 ± 1.2	−1.3 ± 1.0
E606	−1.2 ± 0.4	−1.2 ± 0.3	E615	−0.9 ± 0.2	−0.9 ± 0.2
L608	−2.2 ± 1.2	−3.3 ± 0.8	T616‖	−1.4 ± 0.3	−1.3 ± 0.4
D609	−1.8 ± 0.7	−1.9 ± 0.7	E617	−0.6 ± 0.3	−0.5 ± 0.3
D611	−0.7 ± 0.1	−0.7 ± 0.1	P618	−0.4 ± 0.1	−0.4 ± 0.2
F612	−1.2 ± 0.6	−0.9 ± 0.5			
Total interaction energy	−45.1 ± 3.4	−44.6 ± 3.1	Subtotal	−16.3 ± 2.3	−15.1 ± 2.1

NA, not applicable.
*All results are in kcal mol^{-1}. The entropy contributions are not included in these results.
†Contribution from tyrosine sulfate (YS) or tyrosine sulfonate (YCS) not including the SO_3^- group.
‡SO_3^- is counted as a residue in the energy decomposition, instead of $-O\text{-}SO_3^-$ or $-CH_2\text{-}SO_3^-$.
§Numbering based on the crystal structure.
‖Glycosylation site.

formation, similar to that observed after administration of a P-sel blocking antibody ($*P<0.05$, Student's *t*-test; Fig. 5c; Supplementary Fig. 25).

Discussion

The PSGL-1/P-sel pathway plays a critical role in disorders of innate immunity[12,17,57,58], thrombosis[19,59] and cancer[60,61] and, as a consequence, the pharmacological blockade of this pathway represents an important therapeutic target. While the PSGL-1 glycan is a critical component of a diverse set of cell–cell recognition processes, as a complex glycoconjugate its recognition occurs in the context of other aglycone components that support leukocyte recruitment under shear stress of blood flow. Specifically, PSGL-1 is representative of a novel class of GSP that includes GPIbα[62] and endoglycan[63], among many other important biomacromolecules. Detailed structural and mechanistic studies of PSGL-1 have revealed that high affinity recognition requires stereospecific interactions with both clustered tyrosine sulfates and a C2 *O*-glycan that bears a sLe^x-containing hexasaccharide epitope[26–28]. Thus, while first generation small molecule inhibitors of P-sel/PSGL-1 interactions designed to mimic the sLe^x moiety have proven valuable in validating targets, they have yet to achieve clinical benefit, which is likely related to their low binding affinity to selectins.

Despite the potential of sLe^x-GSPs, such as PSGL-1, to serve as tools for biological studies and the promise of PSGL-1 glycopeptide mimetics as therapeutic agents, their utility has been limited by low yield and limited stability. For example, synthesis of the C2 *O*-glycan typically suffers from suboptimal regioselectivity and may involve a triflic azide-mediated diazotransfer step, which is potentially explosive; thus, prohibiting preparative scale synthesis (> 50 g). Likewise, the desire to generate clustered tyrosine sulfates by direct incorporation of Fmoc-Tyr (O-SO3-) amino acids during peptide synthesis is extremely challenging, owing to its acid lability. Alternatively, the sulfation of tyrosine residues by enzymatic sulfation is hindered by the instability of tyrosine sulfotransferase >20 °C and chemical sulfation is limited by low specificity, incomplete reaction and low yield.

This report highlights three important milestones that effectively circumvent these problems. First, we have developed an efficient stereoselective route that has lead to multi-gram scale synthesis of the C2 *O*-glycan. This scheme is the shortest and most convenient reported to date, which has facilitated the synthesis of a broad range of GSP mimics. Second, we have determined that the acid labile Tyr (O-SO3-) moiety can be readily replaced with bioisosteric, hydrolytically stable Phe (p-CH2SO3H) and Phe (p-SO3H), increasing overall yield from <0.5 to 24%. The significance of these new synthetic strategies was demonstrated by the identification and production of a PSGL-1 glycopeptide mimic, GSnP-6, from a GSP library, which is very stable and has the highest affinity (K_d 22 nM) to P-sel reported to date. Our studies have confirmed that GSnP-6 potently blocks in a dose-dependent manner, the adhesion of platelet and leukocyte subsets implicated in the pathogenesis of variety of diseases. Finally, we have used GSnP-6 to establish a MD model as an important tool for providing new structural insights for the design and evaluation of additional novel PSGL-1 glycomimetics.

In conclusion, a combination of chemical and enzymatic synthesis provided a diverse array of glycopeptide mimetics of PSGL-1. In the process, GSnP-6 was identified as a chemically stable compound that potently inhibits P-sel/PSGL-1 interactions both in the microvasculature and in model systems that reveal its antagonist specificity in blocking platelet, monocyte and neutrophil thromboinflammatory adhesion. A key discovery was the incorporation of stable sulfonated isosters, which permits facile peptide synthesis and provides a greater therapeutic window than the parent physiological ligand with considerable potential for application in disease states characterized by both acute and chronic inflammation.

Methods

General. All reagents were purchased from commercial sources and used as received, unless otherwise indicated. All solvents were dried and distilled by standard protocols. All reactions were performed under an inert atmosphere of argon or nitrogen, unless otherwise indicated. For peptide synthesis, Fmoc-Leu Novasyn TGA resin (resin loading: 0.3 mmol g^{-1}), DMF (Biotech grade) and

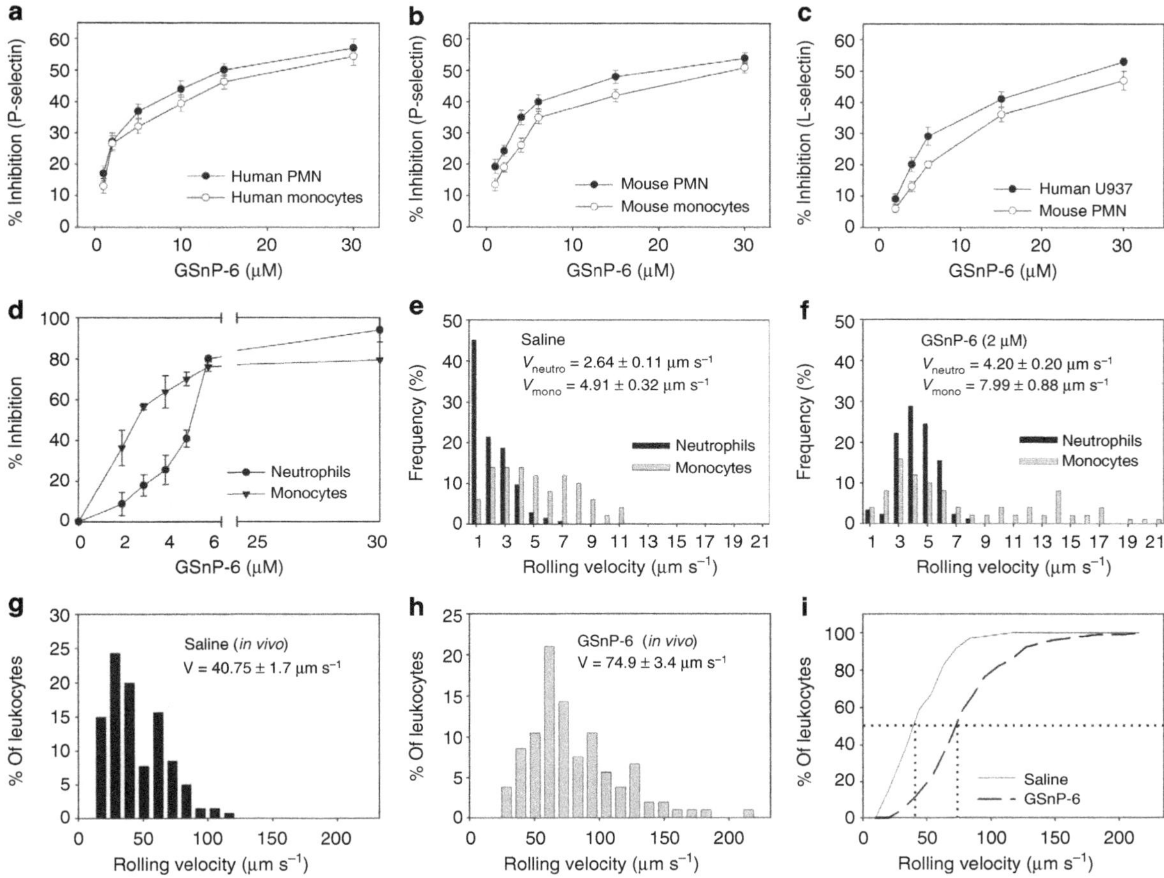

Figure 4 | GSnP-6 inhibits selectin adhesive interactions *in vitro* and *in vivo*. (**a**,**b**) GSnP-6 (0–30 μM) was incubated with (**a**) human circulating PMN and monocytes or (**b**) mouse circulating PMN and monocytes and species appropriate P-selectin chimera, analyzed by flow cytometry and plotted as per cent inhibition versus PBS control. GSnP-6 inhibited P-selectin-dependent interactions in a dose-dependent manner in human and mouse leukocytes, including human neutrophils ($IC_{50}\sim$14 μM), human monocytes ($IC_{50}\sim$20 μM), mouse neutrophils ($IC_{50}\sim$19 μM) and mouse monocytes ($IC_{50}\sim$28 μM). (**c**) GSnP-6 inhibited PSGL-1/L-selectin interactions to human U937 and mouse neutrophils with a lower potency ($IC_{50}\sim$30 μM). Data are represented as mean ± s.e.m., $n=3$. (**d-f**) GSnP-6 inhibits P-selectin/PSGL-1 adhesion under shear *in vitro*. (**d**) GSnP-6 (0–6 μM) exhibits dose-dependent inhibition of human neutrophil and human monocyte rolling and arrest on a recombinant ICAM-1/P-selectin substrate in the presence of shear; $n=3$ PBS, $n=3$ per GSnP-6 dose, velocities (μm s^{-1}) of 120 cells per condition were measured, data are plotted as mean ± s.e.m. (**e**,**f**) GSnP-6 increases rolling velocity of neutrophils and monocytes, cumulative frequency histograms are shown for PBS vehicle control (**e**) and 2 μM GSnP-6 (**f**); *V*neutrophil: saline versus GSnP-6, $P<0.0001$ (Student's *t*-test); *V*monocyte: saline versus GSnP-6, $P<0.0001$ (Student's *t*-test). (**g-i**) GSnP-6 (4 μmol kg^{-1}, $n=4$ mice, 5 leukocytes per vessel analyzed in 28 vessels) or saline control ($n=3$ mice, 5 leukocytes per vessel analyzed in 21 vessels) were delivered i.v. and leukocyte rolling velocity was recorded 15–25 min post surgical stimulation of the mouse cremaster to characterize P-selectin-dependent responses *in vivo*; *V*mean: saline versus GSnP-6, $P<0.01$ (Student's *t*-test). (**i**) Cumulative frequency histogram of leukocyte rolling velocities, median values indicated by vertical lines (median velocity saline = 35.5 μm s^{-1}, median velocity GSnP-6 = 64.0 μm s^{-1}).

piperidine were purchased from Novabiochem. Fmoc-Phe(CH_2SO_3H)-OH and Fmoc-Phe(SO_3H)-OH amino acids were purchased from RSP Amino Acids LLC. Coupling agents HBTU, HOBt and all other Fmoc-protected amino acids were purchased from EMD chemicals. Free reducing glycans, used as standards, were obtained from V-LABS Inc. (Covington, LA, USA). EZ-link NHS-biotin was purchased from Thermo Scientific (Rockford, IL, USA). Biotinylated lectins were from Vector Labs (Burlingame, CA, USA). Cyanine 5- and Alexa-488-labelled Streptavidin, Alexa488- and Alexa633-labelled secondary antibodies were purchased from Life Technologies (Woburn, MA, USA). Recombinant human ST3Gal IV and ST3Gal 1 were kind gifts from Dr Kelley Moremen at the University of Georgia. Studies with the anti-sulfotyrosine monoclonal antibody PSG2 were kindly performed with help from Dr Kevin Moore, Oklahoma Medical Research Foundation. Recombinant selectin Fc chimeras were purchased from R&D systems (Minneapolis, MN, USA). Protein A/G was purchased from Fischer Scientific (PI-21186). Fucoidan control was obtained from Sigma-Aldrich. The NHS-activated NEXTERION Slide H slides were purchased from Schott North America (Louisville, KY, USA). ^1H and ^{13}C were recorded with Inova 600 MHz spectrometer. High Resolution MALDI spectra were recorded by Harvard University Mass Spectrometry Center Waters Micro MX MALDI-TOF instrument. Optical rotation values were recorded using Perkin Elmer Polarimeter. All organic extracts were dried over sodium sulfate and concentrated under aspirator vacuum.

All experimental protocols for compound synthesis, characterization data sets for all compounds, including NMR, HPLC and MALDI profiles, as well as details of computational and biological studies are provided in Supplementary Information.

Microarray printing, binding assay and scanning. For a multi-panel experiment on a single slide, the array layout was designed using Piezoarray software according to the dimension of a standard 14-chamber adaptor. The adaptor was applied on the slide to separate a single slide to 14 chambers sealed from each other during the experiment. All glycopeptides and control samples were printed on a NHS-activated glass slide in phosphate buffer (300 mM sodium phosphates, pH 8.5). The average spot volume was within 10% variation (intra-tip) of 0.33 nl. The average spot size was 100 μm. The following glycans were derivatized with 2-amino-N-(2-aminoethyl)-benzamide (AEAB)[64]: asialobiantennary N-glycan NA2 (Galβ1–4GlcNAcβ1–2Manα1–6(Galβ1–4GlcNAcβ1–2Manα1–3)Manβ1–4GlcNAcβ1–4GlcNAc), the 2,3-disiaylated biantennary N-glycan NA2,3 (Neu5Acα2–3Galβ1–4GlcNAcβ1–2Manα1–6(Neu5Acα2–3Galβ1–4GlcNAcβ1–2Manα1–3)Manβ1–4GlcNAcβ1–4GlcNAc), the 2,6-disialylated biantennary N-glycan NA2,6 (Neu5Acα2–6Galβ1–4GlcNAcβ1–2Manα1–6(Neu5Acα2–6Galβ1–4GlcNAcβ1–2Manα1–3)Manβ1–4GlcNAcβ1–4GlcNAc) and lacto-N-neo-tetraose (LNnT) (Galβ1–4GlcNAcβ1–3Galβ1–4Glc). These AEAB derivatives and biotin–$NHNH_2$,

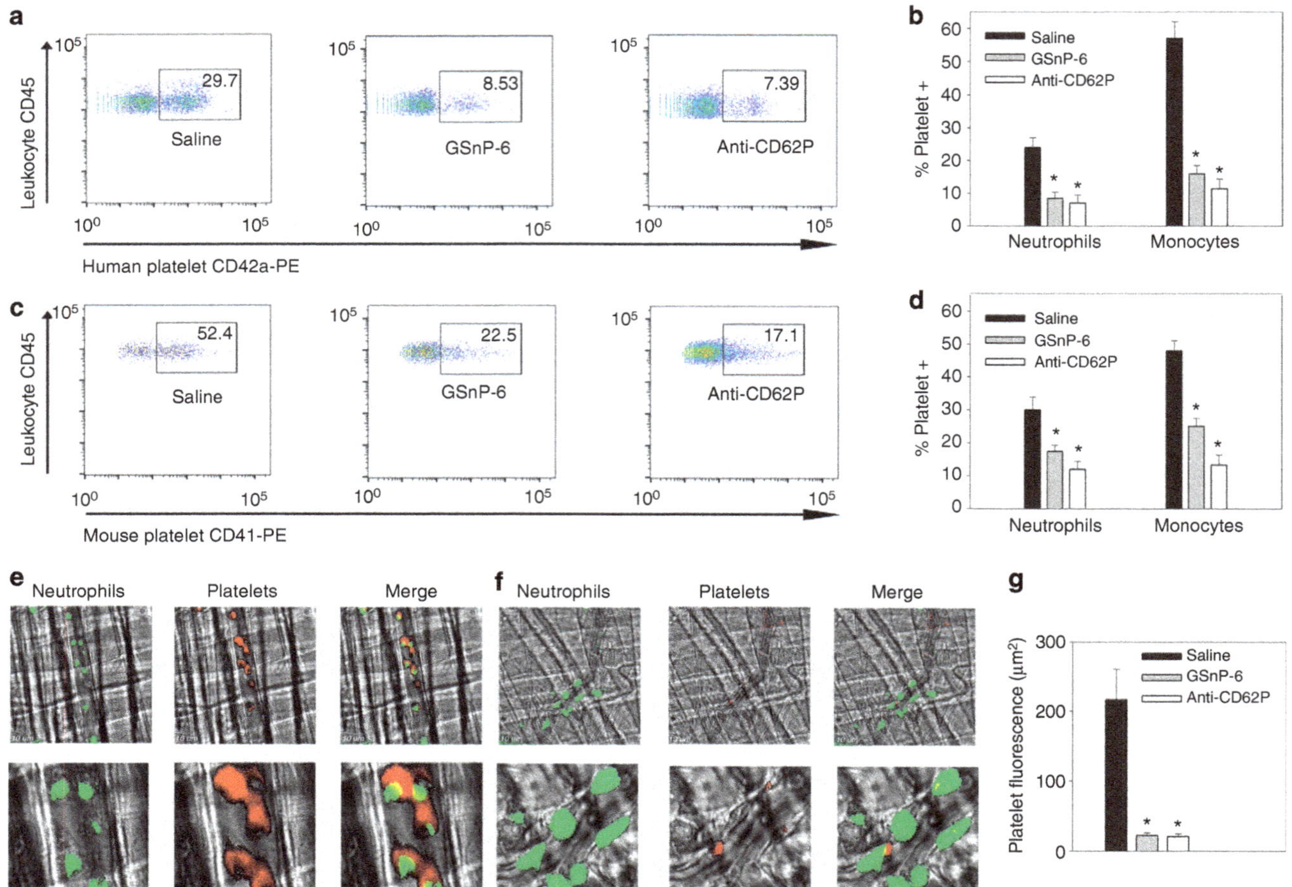

Figure 5 | GSnP-6 limits platelet-leukocyte aggregation *in vitro* and *in vivo*. (**a**-**d**) Anti-coagulated human or mouse blood was dosed with 40 μM GSnP-6 at room temperature and stimulated for platelet P-selectin expression with thrombin receptor-activating peptide (40 μM human PAR_1-activating peptide, 200 μM mouse PAR_4-activating peptide). Platelet-leukocyte aggregates were quantified by two-colour flow cytometry; $CD45^+$ monocyte and neutrophil populations were discerned through characteristic side scatter and quantified as % Platelet positive in saline control, 40 μM GSnP-6, and anti-CD62P (5 μg ml^{-1} human KPL-1, 5 μg ml^{-1} mouse RB40.34) treated samples. (**a**) Representative scatter plot of human samples incubated with anti-CD42a-PE and anti-CD45-APC, (**b**) % Platelet-positive neutrophils and monocytes in human samples, GSnP-6 inhibited 65% of platelet-neutrophil and 72% of platelet-monocyte aggregate formation in human blood. (**c**) Representative scatter plot of mouse samples incubated with anti-CD41-PE and anti-CD45-APC, (**d**) % Platelet-positive neutrophils and monocytes in mouse samples, GSnP-6 inhibited 42% of platelet-neutrophil and 47% of platelet-monocyte aggregate formation in mouse blood. Data representative of triplicate sample mean ± s.e.m., $^*P < 0.05$ versus saline control (Student's *t*-test). (**e**-**g**) *In vivo* platelet-leukocyte aggregation in a TNF-α model of venular inflammation. (**e**) Intravital microscopy of venular inflammation 3 h after administration of TNF-α demonstrates platelet aggregation and platelet-PMN binding after administration of saline control (PMN green; platelet red). (**f**) Platelet aggregation and platelet-PMN binding are not observed after administration of GSnP-6 (4 μmol kg^{-1} iv). (**g**) The platelet inhibitory effect of GSnP-6 was equivalent to that observed for anti-CD62P, a P-selectin blocking antibody (75 μg per mouse i.v.) and was significantly less than saline control ($^*P < 0.05$ versus saline (Student's *t*-test), $n = 5$ mice per treatment, 8-10 venules per mouse analyzed; error bars are represented as s.e.m.).

all at 50 μM concentration were printed on the microarray as controls and reference standards. After printing, the slide was placed in a high moisture chamber at 50 °C and incubated for 1 h. The slide was subsequently washed and blocked with 50 mM ethanolamine in 0.1 M Tris buffer (pH 8.0) for 1 h, dried by centrifugation and stored desiccated at −20 °C prior to use. The binding assay was performed by incubating the slide with human or mouse P-, E- or L- selectin (5 μg ml^{-1} in calcium buffer (pH 8.0). Binding is Ca^{2+} dependent and was quantitatively inhibited by addition of EDTA. Detection was accomplished using Alexa 488 goat anti-Human IgG (5 μg ml^{-1}). The slide was subsequently washed (TSM Buffer, five times), centrifuged and analyzed with a Perkin Elmer ProScanArray microarray scanner equipped with four lasers covering an excitation range from 488 to 637 nm. The scanned images were analyzed using ScanArray Express software (Supplementary Fig. 18).

Biacore binding assay of PSGL-1 mimics. Biotinylated $GS_{(n)}P$-6 was first captured quantitatively on a streptavidin-coated sensor chip (GE Healthcare). Different amounts of P-, L- or E-sel-Ig were incubated in the wells (2.5–60 μg ml^{-1}) and bound selectins were detected using fluorescently labelled anti-human IgG. PL1 and CHO131 (Santa Cruz, CA, USA) are mAbs that recognize the peptide sequence and C2 sLe^x, respectively, which were used to confirm the immobilization step and to compare the relative amount of glycopeptides on the chip (Supplementary Fig. 19). The bound mAbs and selectins were removed from the sensor chip by injecting 10 mM glycine-HCl, pH 2.0, and 50 mM EDTA, respectively, at 20 μl/min for 30 s. The kinetic parameters were obtained by plotting the curves using a 1:1 binding model provided by the Biacore evaluation software.

At low GSnP-6 density (<5 response units (RU)), no plateau was observed even at highest concentrations of L- or E- Sel-Ig (60 μg ml^{-1}). By contrast P-Sel (P-Sel-Ig), generated a saturated binding curve irrespective of the GsnP-6-coated densities used (<5–60 RU), indicating that affinity of P-Sel-Ig for GSnP-6 is less dependent on the density of the immobilized ligand. The comparison of GSnP's densities (<5 RU versus 60 RU) indicate that binding of L- or E-Sel-Ig has ~25-fold lower affinity for the immobilized GSnP-6 than P-Sel-Ig.

MD simulation studies. Force field parameters for the oligosaccharide and SO_3^- moiety in the tyrosine sulfate (YS) and tyrosine sulfonate (YCS) residues were taken from the GLYCAM06 (version h)[65] parameter set, while those for the protein came from AMBER12 (ff99sb)[66]. Parameters for the linkage between the SO_3^- group and the amino acid side chains were approximated from existing terms in two parameter sets (Supplementary Table 3). Ensemble-averaged partial atomic charges for the YS and YCS residues were developed according to the standard GLYCAM protocol[65], from a collection of 300 snapshots extracted at 0.1-ns intervals from MD simulations (30 ns) performed in explicit solvent (TIP3P) for the zwitterionic forms of each amino acid. The initial coordinates for the charge calculations were based on the crystal structure of a monomer of the P-sel/PSGL-1 complex obtained from the Protein Data Bank (PDB entry code: 1G1S). The coordinates for the YCS residues were generated by replacing the phenolic oxygen atom in the YS residue with a methylene group. Molecular electrostatic potentials were computed at the HF/6-31G*//HF/6-31G* level with the Gaussian03 software package[67], and restrained electrostatic potential charge fitting was performed using the RESP procedure with a restraint weight of 0.01. During charge fitting, the amino acid backbone charges were constrained to the standard values employed in ff99sb. The MD simulations were initiated with RESP charge sets computed for single conformations of each residue. The MD simulations were performed under nPT conditions (12 Å TIP3P water buffer in a cubic box, covalent bonds involving hydrogen atoms constrained using the SHAKE algorithm, a time step of 2 fs with heating from 5 to 300 K over a period of 50 ps controlled by the Berendsen thermostat). Prior to MD simulation, the systems were subjected to energy minimization under nVT conditions (500 steps steepest descent (sd), followed by 24,500 steps of conjugate-gradient minimization).

Prior to simulation, water molecules and sodium ions in the crystal structure were removed, and the strontium ion substituted by magnesium, because parameters for strontium ion are not available in AMBER. Missing residue E604 was added to Y605 at the N terminus of the ligand using the LEaP module in AMBER12 with the backbone conformation copied from the E154-Y155 sequence. Sodium counter ions were added to each protein–glycopeptide complex to achieve neutrality using LEaP, prior to solvation with TIP3P water (8 Å buffer in an octahedral box). Energy minimization of the solvated complexes was performed in two steps under nVT conditions. Initially, the positions of water molecules and counter ions were minimized (500 steps sd followed by 24,500 steps conjugate gradient), during which all other solute atoms were restrained (100 kcal mol^{-1} Å^2). In the second step, all restraints were removed with the exception of those on the protein backbone, and the minimization cycle was repeated. Subsequently, heating to 300 K was performed over 50 ps (nVT) with a weak restraint (10 kcal mol^{-1} Å^2) on the backbone atoms of P-Selectin only. Systems were then equilibrated at 300 K for 0.5 ns (nPT ensemble, with the Berendsen thermostat) prior to production MD, under the same conditions (covalent bonds involving hydrogen atoms constrained using SHAKE, 2-fs time step). Production MD simulations were for 250 ns performed with the GPU implementation of PMEMD from AMBER12. In all MD simulations, a non-bonded cut-off of 8 Å was applied to van der Waals interactions, with long-range electrostatics treated with the particle mesh Ewald approximation, and mixed 1–4 non-bonded scale factors applied, as recommended for systems containing both carbohydrates and proteins (SCEE = SCNB = 1.0 for the oligosaccharide and SCEE = 1.2 and SCNB = 2.0 for the protein)[65].

MM/GBSA calculations were carried out on 10,000 snapshots extracted evenly from the entire simulation trajectory using the single-trajectory method[68] with the MMPBSA.py.MPI module. The ability to correctly predict the relative per residue contributions to affinity is essential if the MM-GBSA calculations are to be employed in the rational design of inhibitors based on the PSGL-1 structure. There are several parameterizations of the GBSA model, none of which has been established as optimal for use in analyzing glycopeptide–protein binding. Further, estimating the affinity of PSGL-1/P-sel interactions faces the additional challenge of quantifying the potentially highly polarizing influence of multiple charge–charge interactions. In a non-polarizable classical force field, one approach for addressing this limitation is to employ an internal dielectric constant (ε) greater than unity in the MM-GBSA analysis. Again, as in the case of the GB approximation, no optimal value for ε has been reported for this type of interaction, although typical values < 4.0 D. Last, entropic effects arising from changes in conformational flexibility may be estimated separately, but may require very long MD simulations to achieve convergence, and are frequently omitted when computing estimates of relative affinity[69]. Because of the novel nature of interactions involving YS and YCS, the suitability of five different GB implementations was examined, specifically: (1) the Hawkins, Cramer, Truhlar pairwise generalized Born model with parameters described by Tsui and Case (GB^{HCT} model, igb = 1); the modified GB model developed by Onufriev, Bashford and Case, with the following values for α, β and γ: GB_1^{OBC} ($\alpha = 0.8$, $\beta = 0.0$, $\gamma = 2.909125$, igb = 2) and GB_2^{OBC} ($\alpha = 1.0$, $\beta = 0.8$, $\gamma = 4.8$, igb = 5); the GBn models described by Mongan, Simmerling, McCammon, Case and Onufriev: GBn_1, igb = 7; GBn_2, igb = 8. In addition, six different internal dielectric (ε) values (ε = 1.0, 1.5, 2.0, 3.0, 4.0 and 5.0) were considered in the MM/GBSA calculations.

Flow cytometry. Flow cytometry was used to quantify binding inhibition of (P-, L-, E-) selectin chimeras to human and mouse leukocytes[58]. Heparinized whole mouse blood was collected via cardiac puncture under the approval of the Animal Care and Use Committee of Beth Israel Deaconess Medical Center (BIDMC). Normal human blood draws were collected in citrate under approval of the BIDMC Institutional Review Board. The human monocyte cell line U937 was obtained from ATCC and cultured according to supplied protocols. Cells were incubated with increasing concentrations of GSnP-6 (0–30 μM) and Fc chimeras of human or mouse P-, L-, and E-sel (R&D Systems, 2 μg ml^{-1}) followed by PE-conjugated anti-Fc (1:100). The interaction of the selectins with mouse leukocytes, human leukocytes, or human U937 was analyzed by flow cytometry (BD LSR II) and quantified (FlowJo) as mean fluorescent intensity and plotted as per cent inhibition. PSGL-1 specificity was examined in the presence of blocking antibodies KPL-1 (anti-human PSGL-1) and 4RA10 (anti-mouse PSGL-1). Inhibition experiments were performed in triplicate. GSnP-6 inhibited binding of P- and L-sel-IgG chimeras in a dose-dependent manner. The P-sel inhibitor KF38789 was included as a reference compound. Inhibition of E-sel-IgG binding was not observed over the examined concentration range (Supplementary Fig. 22).

***In vitro* flow assay.** Recombinant human ICAM-1-Fc, P-sel-Fc, and E-sel-Fc were purchased from R&D Systems (Lot #: DLA0914011, FDA0913111, and BGU0413091 respectively). Neutrophils and monocytes were isolated from freshly collected human blood from healthy donors consented through an approved UC Davis institutional review board protocol. Whole blood was layered over neutrophil or mononuclear cell separation media, Polymophoprep, an Axis Shield formulation purchased from Cosmo Bio USA. After centrifugation myeloid cells were extracted and washed with 4-(2-hydroxyethyl)-1-piperazineethanesulfonic acid buffered salt solution. Coverslips were prepared as follows: 25 mm diameter, #1.5 glass coverslips were Piranha etched to remove organic molecules and to deposit hydroxyl group molecules on the surface. The etched coverslips were submerged in acetone with 1% 3-aminopropyltriethoxysilane (APTES) to add aminosilane groups. Recombinant human ICAM-1-Fc along with either P-sel-Fc or E-sel-Fc were absorbed at 5 μg ml^{-1} for 1 h prior to the experiment. Human neutrophils were suspended at a concentration of 10^6 cells per ml in 4-(2-hydroxyethyl)-1-piperazineethanesulfonic acid buffered salt solution and allowed to incubate for 10 min with PBS (vehicle control), 2, 3, 4, 5, 6 and 30 μM concentrations of GSnP-6. Treated cells were perfused through a microfluidic flow chamber at a calculated shear stress of 2 dyn cm^{-2} and cell motion recorded at three to five fields of view at 7.5 frames per s for 2 min along the centerline of the channel using a Matrox Meteor II and ImagePro Plus software to analyze cell kinetics. To further observe neutrophil behaviour, buffer was infused and images were collected at two additional locations along the channel. Rolling and arrested neutrophils were determined by tracking the cell centroid over 10 s increments utilizing MTrack2 software plugin for ImageJ. Neutrophils moving at a velocity of < 1 μm s^{-1} were considered to be arrested.

Intravital microscopy. Surgical preparation of the mouse cremaster was performed as previously described. All experiments were performed in the BIDMC Center for Hemostasis and Thrombosis Research Core and were approved by the Animal Care and Use Committee of the BIDMC. Mice were anesthetized with an i.p. injection of ketamine HCl (125 mg kg^{-1}), xylazine (12.5 mg kg^{-1}) and atropine (0.25 mg ml^{-1}), and placed on a 37 °C surgical blanket. The jugular vein was cannulated with PE 10 tubing to allow introduction of reagents, including GSnP-6 (4 μmol kg^{-1} in saline), saline vehicle control or 0.5 μm Dragon Green microspheres (Bangs Laboratories, Inc) for the measurement of centerline velocity. The trachea was intubated with PE90 to facilitate breathing. The cremaster muscle was exteriorized, pinned to the stage and superfused with thermocontrolled bicarbonate-buffered saline equilibrated with 5% CO_2 in N_2. The surgical procedure was accomplished within 10 min. Microvessel data were obtained using an Olympus AX microscope with × 60 or × 40 water immersion objectives recorded with a Hamamatsu C9300-201/Gen III videoscope image intensifier interface. Coordinated image acquisition and offline data analyses were carried out using SlideBook software (Intelligent Imaging Innovations). At the termination of the experiment, blood was drawn via cardiac puncture and analyzed for complete blood count. Venules (30–40 μm in diameter) were observed 15 to 25 min after surgical stimulation of tissue to study P-sel-dependent rolling. Vessel diameter was measured using SlideBook ruler. Centerline blood flow velocity (V_{cl}) was determined by measuring frame-to-frame displacement of single fluorescent microspheres in the centre of the vessel wall. Volumetric blood flow rate (Q) was calculated using the equation $Q = (V_{cl} \times 0.625 \times A_{cs})$, where A_{cs} is the cross-sectional area of the vessel (πr^2) and 0.625 is an empirical correction factor. Wall shear rate (γ_w) was calculated as $\gamma_w = 2.12 \times [(8 \times 0.625 \times V_{cl})/D_v)]$, where D_v is the vessel diameter. Haemodynamic parameters are reported in Supplementary Table 4. Recordings of each vessel were analyzed in brightfield for 30 to 60 s and leukocyte rolling flux was characterized as the number of leukocytes passing a plane perpendicular to the vessel axis (Supplementary Fig. 24). Total leukocyte flux was determined as a product of systemic leukocyte concentration (cells per μl) and volumetric blood flow rate (μl s^{-1}). Leukocyte rolling was characterized as the rolling flux fraction, which is the number of rolling leukocytes reported as a percentage of total leukocyte flux. Rolling velocity (μm s^{-1}) was measured by tracking individual leukocyte translation over 2 s.

Assessment of platelet–leukocyte aggregation *in vitro*. Platelet–leukocyte aggregates were quantified in whole blood using dual-label flow cytometry[55]. Anti-coagulated human or mouse blood was incubated with 40 μM GSnP-6 at room temperature and stimulated with thrombin receptor-activating peptide (human PAR_1-activating peptide 40 µM; mouse PAR_4-activating peptide 200 µM) to induce platelet P-sel expression. Platelet–leukocyte aggregates were quantified by two-colour flow cytometry by incubating human samples with anti-CD42a-PE and anti-CD45-APC and mouse samples with anti-CD41-PE and anti-CD45-APC. CD45+ monocyte and neutrophil populations were discerned through characteristic side scatter and quantified as % Platelet positive in saline control, GSnP-6 (40 µM) or anti-CD62P (human KPL-1 (5 µg ml^{-1}), mouse RB40.34 (5 µg ml^{-1}) treated samples.

Assessment of platelet-leukocyte interactions *in vivo*. TNF-α was administered intrascrotally (0.5 µg) to male mice (6–8 weeks old, C57BL/6) 3 h prior to surgical preparation and imaging. Surgical preparation of the cremaster was performed, as described above. Agents were administered through the jugular cannula just prior to cremaster exposure and imaging, including saline vehicle control, GSnP-4 (4 µmol kg^{-1}), anti-CD62P blocking antibody (clone RB40.34, 3 mg kg^{-1}), anti-platelet Dylight 649-anti-CD42b (Emfret, 1 µl g^{-1}) and Alexa Fluor 488 anti-Gr-1 (0.5 µg g^{-1}). Microvessel data were obtained using an Olympus AX microscope with a ×60 water immersion objective recorded with a Hamamatsu C9300-201/Gen III videoscope image intensifier interface. Coordinated image acquisition and offline data analyses were carried out using SlideBook software. For each treatment condition, platelet accumulation was characterized as median integrated fluorescence plotted during a 2-min time interval from 5 mice (8–10 venules per mouse). The platelet signal was quantified as area under the curve for each individual capture, plotted against time and normalized to vessel surface area. Platelet aggregation and platelet–PMN binding is observed in saline control vessels while limited platelet signal is captured in GSnP-6- and anti-CD62P-treated animals (Supplementary Fig. 25A–D). Characterization of leukocyte–endothelial interactions at 3 h post-TNFα activation revealed minimal rolling flux and similar levels of adherent leukocytes between all groups (Supplementary Fig. 25E,F).

References

1. Kolaczkowska, E. & Kubes, P. Neutrophil recruitment and function in health and inflammation. *Nat. Rev. Immunol.* **13,** 159–175 (2013).
2. Ley, K., Laudanna, C., Cybulsky, M. I. & Nourshargh, S. Getting to the site of inflammation: the leukocyte adhesion cascade updated. *Nat. Rev. Immunol.* **7,** 678–689 (2007).
3. Zarbock, A., Ley, K., McEver, R. P. & Hidalgo, A. Leukocyte ligands for endothelial selectins: specialized glycoconjugates that mediate rolling and signaling under flow. *Blood* **118,** 6743–6751 (2011).
4. Palabrica, T. *et al.* Leukocyte accumulation promoting fibrin deposition is mediated *in vivo* by P-selectin on adherent platelets. *Nature* **359,** 848–851 (1992).
5. Mayadas, T. N., Johnson, R. C., Rayburn, H., Hynes, R. O. & Wagner, D. D. Leukocyte rolling and extravasation are severely compromised in P selectin-deficient mice. *Cell* **74,** 541–554 (1993).
6. Weller, A., Isenmann, S. & Vestweber, D. Cloning of the mouse endothelial selectins. Expression of both E- and P-selectin is inducible by tumor necrosis factor alpha. *J. Biol. Chem.* **267,** 15176–15183 (1992).
7. Girard, J. P., Moussion, C. & Forster, R. HEVs, lymphatics and homeostatic immune cell trafficking in lymph nodes. *Nat. Rev. Immunol.* **12,** 762–773 (2012).
8. Carlow, D. A. *et al.* PSGL-1 function in immunity and steady state homeostasis. *Immunol. Rev.* **230,** 75–96 (2009).
9. Mehta, P., Cummings, R. D. & McEver, R. P. Affinity and kinetic analysis of P-selectin binding to P-selectin glycoprotein ligand-1. *J. Biol. Chem.* **273,** 32506–32513 (1998).
10. McEver, R. P. & Cummings, R. D. Role of PSGL-1 binding to selectins in leukocyte recruitment. *J. Clin. Invest.* **100,** 485–491 (1997).
11. Wang, H. B. *et al.* P-selectin primes leukocyte integrin activation during inflammation. *Nat. Immunol.* **8,** 882–892 (2007).
12. Sreeramkumar, V. *et al.* Neutrophils scan for activated platelets to initiate inflammation. *Science* **346,** 1234–1238 (2014).
13. da Costa Martins, P. *et al.* Platelet-monocyte complexes support monocyte adhesion to endothelium by enhancing secondary tethering and cluster formation. *Arterioscler. Thromb. Vasc. Biol.* **24,** 193–199 (2004).
14. Ma, Y. Q., Plow, E. F. & Geng, J. G. P-selectin binding to P-selectin glycoprotein ligand-1 induces an intermediate state of alphaMbeta2 activation and acts cooperatively with extracellular stimuli to support maximal adhesion of human neutrophils. *Blood* **104,** 2549–2556 (2004).
15. Fox, R. *et al.* PSGL-1 and mTOR regulate translation of ROCK-1 and physiological functions of macrophages. *EMBO J.* **26,** 505–515 (2007).
16. Hidari, K. I., Weyrich, A. S., Zimmerman, G. A. & McEver, R. P. Engagement of P-selectin glycoprotein ligand-1 enhances tyrosine phosphorylation and activates mitogen-activated protein kinases in human neutrophils. *J. Biol. Chem.* **272,** 28750–28756 (1997).
17. Dong, Z. M., Brown, A. A. & Wagner, D. D. Prominent role of P-selectin in the development of advanced atherosclerosis in ApoE-deficient mice. *Circulation* **101,** 2290–2295 (2000).
18. Sato, C. *et al.* P-selectin glycoprotein ligand-1 deficiency is protective against obesity-related insulin resistance. *Diabetes* **60,** 189–199 (2011).
19. von Bruhl, M. L. *et al.* Monocytes, neutrophils, and platelets cooperate to initiate and propagate venous thrombosis in mice *in vivo*. *J. Exp. Med.* **209,** 819–835 (2012).
20. Baert, F. *et al.* Influence of immunogenicity on the long-term efficacy of infliximab in Crohn's disease. *N. Engl. J. Med.* **348,** 601–608 (2003).
21. Chang, J. *et al.* GMI-1070, a novel pan-selectin antagonist, reverses acute vascular occlusions in sickle cell mice. *Blood* **116,** 1779–1786 (2010).
22. Japp, A. G. *et al.* Effect of PSI-697, a novel P-selectin inhibitor, on platelet-monocyte aggregate formation in humans. *J. Am. Heart Assoc.* **2,** 1–6 (2013).
23. Beeh, K. M. *et al.* Bimosiamose, an inhaled small-molecule pan-selectin antagonist, attenuates late asthmatic reactions following allergen challenge in mild asthmatics: a randomized, double-blind, placebo-controlled clinical cross-over-trial. *Pulm. Pharmacol. Ther.* **19,** 233–241 (2006).
24. Kranich, R. *et al.* Rational design of novel, potent small molecule pan-selectin antagonists. *J. Med. Chem.* **50,** 1101–1115 (2007).
25. Huang, A. *et al.* Discovery of 2-[1-(4-Chlorophenyl)cyclopropyl]-3-hydroxy-8-(trifluoromethyl)quinoline-4-carboxylic acid (PSI-421), a P-selectin Inhibitor with improved pharmacokinetic properties and oral efficacy in models of vascular injury. *J. Med. Chem.* **53,** 6003–6017 (2010).
26. Leppänen, A. *et al.* A novel glycosulfopeptide binds to P-selectin and inhibits leukocyte adhesion to P-selectin. *J. Biol. Chem.* **274,** 24838–24848 (1999).
27. Leppänen, A., White, S. P., Helin, J., McEver, R. P. & Cummings, R. D. Binding of glycosulfopeptides to P-selectin requires stereospecific contributions of individual tyrosine sulfate and sugar residues. *J. Biol. Chem.* **275,** 39569–39578 (2000).
28. Leppänen, A., Yago, T., Otto, V. I., McEver, R. P. & Cummings, R. D. Model glycosulfopeptides from P-selectin glycoprotein ligand-1 require tyrosine sulfation and a core 2-branched O-glycan to bind to L-selectin. *J. Biol. Chem.* **278,** 26391–26400 (2003).
29. Koeller, K. M., Smith, M. E. B., Huang, R.-F. & Wong, C.-H. Chemoenzymatic synthesis of a PSGL-1N-terminal glycopeptide containing tyrosine sulfate and α-O-linked sialyl Lewis X. *J. Am. Chem. Soc.* **122,** 4241–4242 (2000).
30. Huang, K.-T. *et al.* Multi-enzyme one-pot strategy for the synthesis of sialyl Lewis X-containing PSGL-1 glycopeptide. *Carbohydr. Res.* **341,** 2151–2155 (2006).
31. Baumann, K., Kowalczyk, D. & Kunz, H. Total synthesis of the glycopeptide recognition domain of the P-selectin glycoprotein ligand 1. *Angew. Chem. Int. Ed.* **47,** 3445–3449 (2008).
32. Vohra, Y., Buskas, T. & Boons, G.-J. Rapid assembly of oligosaccharides: a highly convergent strategy for the assembly of a glycosylated amino acid derived from PSGL-1. *J. Org. Chem.* **74,** 6064–6071 (2009).
33. Krishnamurthy, V. R. *et al.* Synthesis of an Fmoc-threonine bearing core-2 glycan: a building block for PSGL-1 via Fmoc-assisted solid-phase peptide synthesis. *Carbohydr. Res.* **345,** 1541–1547 (2010).
34. Plattner, C., Höfener, M. & Sewald, N. One-pot azidochlorination of glycals. *Org. Lett.* **13,** 545–547 (2011).
35. Yagami, T., Kitagawa, K., Aida, C., Fujiwara, H. & Futaki, S. Stabilization of a tyrosine O-sulfate residue by a cationic functional group: formation of a conjugate acid-base pair. *J. Pept. Res.* **56,** 239–249 (2000).
36. Baumann, K. *et al.* Sulfated and non-sulfated glycopeptide recognition domains of P-selectin glycoprotein ligand 1 and their binding to P- and E-selectin. *Angew. Chem. Int. Ed.* **48,** 3174–3178 (2009).
37. Bunschoten, A. *et al.* A general sequence independent solid phase method for the site specific synthesis of multiple sulfated-tyrosine containing peptides. *Chem. Commun.* 2999–3001 (2009).
38. Simpson, L. S. & Widlanski, T. S. A comprehensive approach to the synthesis of sulfate esters. *J. Am. Chem. Soc.* **128,** 1605–1610 (2006).
39. Roosenburg, S. *et al.* Stabilized (111)in-labeled sCCK8 analogues for targeting CCK2-receptor positive tumors: Synthesis and evaluation. *Bioconjug. Chem.* **21,** 663–670 (2010).
40. Lam, S. N., Acharya, P., Wyatt, R., Kwong, P. D. & Bewley, C. A. Tyrosine-sulfate isosteres of CCR5 N-terminus as tools for studying HIV-1 entry. *Bioorg. Med. Chem.* **16,** 10113–10120 (2008).
41. Acharya, P. *et al.* Structure-based identification and neutralization mechanism of tyrosine-sulfate mimetics that inhibit HIV-1 entry. *ACS Chem. Biol.* **6,** 1069–1077 (2011).
42. Yagami, T., Shiwa, S., Futaki, S. & Kitagawa, K. Evaluation of the final deprotection system for the solid-phase synthesis of Tyr(SO3H)-containing peptides with 9-fluorenylmethyloxycarbonyl (Fmoc)-strategy and its application to the synthesis of cholecystokinin (CCK)-12. *Chem. Pharm. Bull.* **41,** 376–380 (1993).
43. Balsved, D., Bundgaard, J. R. & Sen, J. W. Stability of tyrosine sulfate in acidic solutions. *Anal. Biochem.* **363,** 70–76 (2007).

44. Koeller, K. M., Smith, M. E. B. & Wong, C.-H. Tyrosine sulfation on a PSGL-1 glycopeptide influences the reactivity of glycosyltransferases responsible for synthesis of the attached O-glycan. *J. Am. Chem. Soc.* **122,** 742–743 (2000).
45. Cao, T. M., Takatani, T. & King, M. R. Effect of extracellular pH on selectin adhesion: theory and experiment. *Biophys. J.* **104,** 292–299 (2013).
46. Hou, T., Wang, J., Li, Y. & Wang, W. Assessing the performance of the MM/PBSA and MM/GBSA methods. 1. The accuracy of binding free energy calculations based on molecular dynamics simulations. *J. Chem. Inf. Model.* **51,** 69–82 (2011).
47. Massova, I. & Kollman, P. A. Computational alanine scanning to probe protein – protein interactions: A novel approach to evaluate binding free energies. *J. Am. Chem. Soc.* **121,** 8133–8143 (1999).
48. Wang, J. M., Morin, P., Wang, W. & Kollman, P. A. Use of MM-PBSA in reproducing the binding free energies to HIV-1 RT of TIBO derivatives and predicting the binding mode to HIV-1 RT of efavirenz by docking and MM-PBSA. *J. Am. Chem. Soc.* **123,** 5221–5230 (2001).
49. Wong, S., Amaro, R. E. & McCammon, J. A. MM-PBSA captures key role of intercalating water molecules at a protein-protein interface. *J. Chem. Theory Comput.* **5,** 422–429 (2009).
50. Simon, S. I., Hu, Y., Vestweber, D. & Smith, C. W. Neutrophil tethering on E-selectin activates beta 2 integrin binding to ICAM-1 through a mitogen-activated protein kinase signal transduction pathway. *J. Immunol.* **164,** 4348–4358 (2000).
51. Yago, T. *et al.* E-selectin engages PSGL-1 and CD44 through a common signaling pathway to induce integrin alphaLbeta2-mediated slow leukocyte rolling. *Blood* **116,** 485–494 (2010).
52. Altman, S. M., Dixit, N. & Simon, S. I. Detection of bidirectional signaling during integrin activation and neutrophil adhesion. *Methods Mol. Biol.* **1124,** 235–248 (2014).
53. Ridger, V. C., Hellewell, P. G. & Norman, K. E. L- and P-selectins collaborate to support leukocyte rolling *in vivo* when high-affinity P-selectin-P-selectin glycoprotein ligand-1 interaction is inhibited. *Am. J. Pathol.* **166,** 945–952 (2005).
54. Clark, S. R. *et al.* Platelet TLR4 activates neutrophil extracellular traps to ensnare bacteria in septic blood. *Nat. Med.* **13,** 463–469 (2007).
55. Kling, D. *et al.* Pharmacological control of platelet-leukocyte interactions by the human anti-P-selectin antibody inclacumab—Preclinical and clinical studies. *Thromb. Res.* **131,** 401–410 (2013).
56. Li, J. *et al.* Neutrophil AKT2 regulates heterotypic cell-cell interactions during vascular inflammation. *J. Clin. Invest.* **124,** 1483–1496 (2014).
57. Mulligan, M. S. *et al.* Neutrophil-dependent acute lung injury. Requirement for P-selectin (GMP-140). *J. Clin. Invest.* **90,** 1600–1607 (1992).
58. An, G. *et al.* P-selectin glycoprotein ligand-1 is highly expressed on Ly-6Chi monocytes and a major determinant for Ly-6Chi monocyte recruitment to sites of atherosclerosis in mice. *Circulation* **117,** 3227–3237 (2008).
59. Falati, S. *et al.* Accumulation of tissue factor into developing thrombi *in vivo* is dependent upon microparticle P-selectin glycoprotein ligand 1 and platelet P-selectin. *J. Exp. Med.* **197,** 1585–1598 (2003).
60. Laubli, H. & Borsig, L. Selectins promote tumor metastasis. *Semin. Cancer Biol.* **20,** 169–177 (2010).
61. Labelle, M., Beguma, S. & Hynes, R. O. Platelets guide the formation of early metastatic niches. *Proc. Natl Acad. Sci. USA* **111,** E3053–E3061 (2014).
62. Lopez, J. A. *et al.* The alpha and beta chains of human platelet glycoprotein Ib are both transmembrane proteins containing a leucine-rich amino acid sequence. *Proc. Natl Acad. Sci. USA* **85,** 2135–2139 (1988).
63. Fieger, C. B., Sassetti, C. M. & Rosen, S. D. Endoglycan, a member of the CD34 family, functions as an L-selectin ligand through modification with tyrosine sulfation and sialyl Lewis x. *J. Biol. Chem.* **278,** 27390–27398 (2003).
64. Song, X. *et al.* Novel fluorescent glycan microarray strategy reveals ligands for galectins. *Chem. Biol.* **30,** 36–47 (2009).
65. Kirschner, K. N. *et al.* GLYCAM06: a generalizable biomolecular force field. Carbohydrates. *J. Comput. Chem.* **29,** 622–655 (2008).
66. Case, D. A. *et al.* The Amber biomolecular simulation programs. *J. Comput. Chem.* **26,** 1668–1688 (2005).
67. Frisch, M. J. *et al. Gaussian 03* (Gaussian, Inc., 2004).
68. Kollman, P. A. *et al.* Calculating structures and free energies of complex molecules: combining molecular mechanics and continuum models. *Acc. Chem. Res.* **33,** 889–897 (2000).
69. Hou, T., Wang, J., Li, Y. & Wang, W. Assessing the performance of the molecular mechanics/Poisson Boltzmann surface area and molecular mechanics/generalized Born surface area methods. II. The accuracy of ranking poses generated from docking. *J. Comput. Chem.* **32,** 866–877 (2011).

Acknowledgements

We acknowledge support from the National Institutes of Health (DK069275, HL106018, GM103694, HL60963, AI047294, HL085607, GM094919 and GM103390), the Science Foundation of Ireland (08/IN.1/B2070) and the European Research Development Fund. V.R.K. thanks Dr Sunia Trauger (Harvard University, *FAS*-Center for Systems Biology) and Dr Jim Lee (DFCI, Molecular Biology Core Facility) for help with mass spectrometry. C.H. thanks Glenn Merrill-Skoloff (BIDMC Center for Hemostasis and Thrombosis Research Core) for assistance with intravital microscopy.

Author contributions

V.R.K., R.D.C. and E.L.C. jointly conceived the project, and directed the chemistry and biology, respectively. M.Y.R.S. was responsible for execution of the chemistry. Y.Y. and X.S. are responsible for the execution of enzymatic steps and binding affinity studies. Molecular modelling was directed by R.W. and carried out by X.W. C.H., E.D. and D.H.-P. carried out cellular and *in vivo* studies. V.M. and S.I.S. carried out *in vitro* shear studies. All authors contributed to the preparation of the manuscript.

Additional information

Competing financial interests: A patent based on these investigations has been filed by V.R.K., M.Y.R.S., R.D.C. and E.L.C. The remaining authors declare no conflict of interest.

Octapod iron oxide nanoparticles as high-performance T_2 contrast agents for magnetic resonance imaging

Zhenghuan Zhao[1], Zijian Zhou[1], Jianfeng Bao[2], Zhenyu Wang[2], Juan Hu[1], Xiaoqin Chi[3], Kaiyuan Ni[1], Ruifang Wang[2], Xiaoyuan Chen[4], Zhong Chen[2] & Jinhao Gao[1,5]

Spherical superparamagnetic iron oxide nanoparticles have been developed as T_2-negative contrast agents for magnetic resonance imaging in clinical use because of their biocompatibility and ease of synthesis; however, they exhibit relatively low transverse relaxivity. Here we report a new strategy to achieve high transverse relaxivity by controlling the morphology of iron oxide nanoparticles. We successfully fabricate size-controllable octapod iron oxide nanoparticles by introducing chloride anions. The octapod iron oxide nanoparticles (edge length of 30 nm) exhibit an ultrahigh transverse relaxivity value ($679.3 \pm 30\ mM^{-1}s^{-1}$), indicating that these octapod iron oxide nanoparticles are much more effective T_2 contrast agents for *in vivo* imaging and small tumour detection in comparison with conventional iron oxide nanoparticles, which holds great promise for highly sensitive, early stage and accurate detection of cancer in the clinic.

[1] State Key Laboratory of Physical Chemistry of Solid Surfaces, The Key Laboratory for Chemical Biology of Fujian Province, and Department of Chemical Biology, College of Chemistry and Chemical Engineering, Xiamen University, Xiamen 361005, China. [2] Department of Physics and Electronic Science, Fujian Key Laboratory of Plasma and Magnetic Resonance, Xiamen University, Xiamen 361005, China. [3] Fujian Provincial Key Laboratory of Chronic Liver Disease and Hepatocellular Carcinoma, Zhongshan Hospital, Xiamen University, Xiamen 361004, China. [4] Laboratory of Molecular Imaging and Nanomedicine, National Institute of Biomedical Imaging and Bioengineering, National Institutes of Health, Bethesda, Maryland 20892, USA. [5] Center for Molecular Imaging and Translational Medicine, School of Public Health, Xiamen University, Xiamen 361005, China. Correspondence and requests for materials should be addressed to J.G. (email: jhgao@xmu.edu.cn).

Magnetic resonance imaging (MRI) has a critically important role in molecular imaging and clinical diagnosis, because it is non-invasive and is capable of producing images with high spatial and temporal resolution[1–3]. Approximately 35% of clinical MR scans need contrast agents to improve their sensitivity and diagnostic accuracy[4]. For example, superparamagnetic iron oxide nanoparticles are the prevailing T_2 contrast agents, especially for the imaging and detection of lesions in normal tissues[5–8]. However, there are several challenges for using T_2 contrast agents (for example, Feridex and Resovist) in the clinic. As they are intrinsically negative contrast agents, false-positive diagnosis may be found in the hypointense areas, such as blood pooling, calcification and metal deposition[9–11]. In particular, these commercially available T_2 contrast agents were synthesized in aqueous media and, consequently, exhibit poor crystallinity and relatively low relaxivity[12]. Thus, the primary limitation of MRI is the relatively low sensitivity of the contrast agents[13,14]. The development of new T_2 contrast agents with high relaxivity for high-performance MRI diagnosis is required. Considering that the ability of iron oxide nanoparticles for MRI applications is strongly dependent on their sizes and magnetic characteristics, strategies for making iron oxide nanoparticles based on size control and metal doping have been developed[15–18]. Usually, the larger spherical iron oxide nanoparticles have stronger saturated magnetization (M_s) and higher T_2 relaxivity (r_2). However, the spherical iron oxide nanoparticles with large size would show ferri/ferromagnetic properties at room temperature, resulting in interparticle agglomeration even in the absence of external magnetic field[12]. On the basis of the quantum mechanical outer sphere theory, the T_2 relaxivity is highly dependent on both the M_s value and the effective radius of typically superparamagnetic core[19–21]. In the motional average regime[22,23], the relaxivity r_2 is given by (where all of the nanoparticle contrast agents were simulated as spheres)[24]

$$r_2 = \left(256\pi^2\gamma^2/405\right)\kappa M_s^2 r^2/D(1+L/r) \quad (1)$$

where M_s and r are saturation magnetization and effective radius of magnetic nanostructure, respectively, D is the diffusivity of water molecules, L is the thickness of an impermeable surface coating, and κ is the conversion factor ($\kappa = V^*/C_{Fe}$, V^* is the volume fraction, C_{Fe} is the concentration of Fe element; for more details, see Supplementary Note 1). According to equation (1), we can predict that an increased M_s value or larger effective magnetic core radius will result in a higher r_2 value. Although maintaining the M_s value (the maximum M_s of bulk magnetite is about 92 emu g^{-1} at room temperature), one can still further achieve a much higher T_2 relaxivity by increasing the effective radius of the magnetic core, which is largely morphology dependent.

In the past two decades, controlled synthesis (for example, ion-assisted methods) of unusual and sophisticated metallic nanostructures (for example, octahedral, tetrahexahedral and concave)[25–29] is prevailing compared with that of metal oxide nanostructures[30–32]. However, the investigation of iron oxide nanoparticles with different morphologies is rare, probably because it is difficult to prepare iron oxide nanoparticles with diverse shapes. The nanostructure-activity relationship of iron oxide nanoparticles as MRI contrast agents has not been extensively exploited[33,34]. Herein, we report a novel strategy to strongly increase T_2 relaxivity by tuning the effective magnetic core radius through morphology control. We successfully synthesize octapod-shaped iron oxide nanoparticles by introducing chloride ions in the reaction system under thermal decomposition conditions. The octapod iron oxide nanoparticles (edge length of 30 nm) exhibit relatively moderate M_s (~71 emu g^{-1}) but ultrahigh r_2 relaxivity (679.3 ± 30 mM^{-1} s^{-1}) because of the unique structure and highly effective boundary radius. The animal study shows that the octapod iron oxide nanoparticles are suitable as high-performance T_2 contrast agents for *in vivo* MRI and early tumour detection, particularly for liver lesions.

Results

Synthesis and characterization. The octapod iron oxide nanoparticles were prepared via decomposition of iron oleate in the presence of sodium chloride (NaCl). Briefly, the iron oleate was decomposed at 320 °C for 2 h in 1-octadecene solvent containing oleic acid as the surfactant and NaCl as the capping agent. Transmission electron microscopy (TEM) images (Fig. 1a,b) showed that the as-prepared product consists of uniform four-

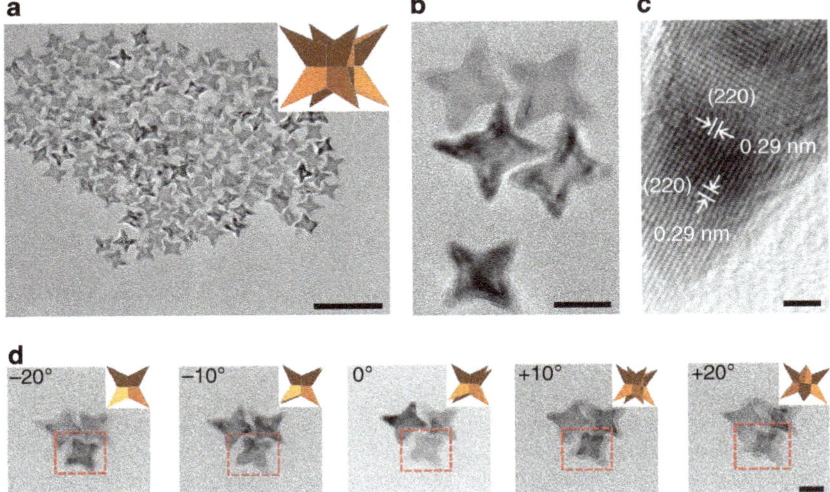

Figure 1 | TEM analyses of octapod iron oxide nanoparticles. (**a**) TEM image of Octapod-30 consisted of uniform four-armed star-like particles (inset: geometric model). Scale bar, 100 nm. (**b**) The higher magnification TEM image of Octapod-30. Scale bar, 20 nm. (**c**) high-resolution TEM image of Octapod-30, showing the single crystallinity with the lattice fringes across the entire nanoparticles correspond to Fe_3O_4 (220). Scale bar, 2 nm. (**d**) Tilted TEM images of three Octapod-30. Along with the tilting, the nanoparticles (red dotted squares) change from four-armed star-like to elongated six-armed stars, indicating that the geometric shape of Octapod-30 is a concave octapod owning eight trigonal pyramidal arms (insets: corresponding geometric models). Scale bar, 20 nm.

armed star-like iron oxide particles with high yield (>95%). The average edge length between two nearby armed points is about 30 nm. We observed uniform lattice fringes across the entire nanoparticles with spacing corresponding to Fe_3O_4 (220) in high-resolution TEM images (Fig. 1c). After carefully surveying these unique nanoparticles, we found some shadows likely belong to the four arms of star-like particles, indicating the possible presence of concave feature in the particles. To better visualize the three-dimensional structure of the nanoparticles, we tilted the sample away from the direction perpendicular to the electron beam. Along with the tilting, the nanoparticles changes from four-armed star-like to elongated six-armed stars (Fig. 1d), which fits to the feature of octapod nanoparticles owning eight trigonal pyramidal arms[27]. On the basis of these observations, we proposed a concave polyhedral model of this unique iron oxide nanostructure (Fig. 1a, inset). To confirm this proposed structure, we characterized an individual octapod nanoparticle by high-resolution TEM and relevant selected-area electron diffraction measurements. Both the outlines and angles between the edges of individual nanoparticle are consistent with the geometric models of concave bounded by [311] high-index facets (Supplementary Fig. S1). The X-ray powder diffraction pattern of octapod nanoparticles matched well with magnetite Fe_3O_4 reference values (JCPDS number 82-1533) without any iron phase, suggesting the octapod iron oxide nanoparticles are pure magnetite with inversed spinel crystal structure (Supplementary Fig. S2).

Controlled synthesis of octapod iron oxide nanoparticles. As expected, NaCl may be essential in the synthesis of octapod iron oxide nanoparticles. We obtained the uniform octapod iron oxide nanoparticles by supplying a certain amount of NaCl (0.17 mmol of NaCl to 0.86 mmol of iron oleate) to a 10 ml of reaction solution. When the amount of NaCl was reduced to 0.085 mmol, the yield of octapod iron oxide nanoparticles was significantly reduced. There were very few octapod iron oxide nanoparticles when the amount of NaCl was further decreased to 0.034 mmol (Supplementary Fig. S3). These results suggest that NaCl may have an important role in the formation of octapod iron oxide nanoparticles. To understand the effects of chloride anions and sodium cations in the formation of octapod iron oxide nanoparticles, we conducted a number of control experiments. When using NaOH and Na oleate instead of NaCl, the products were mainly the mixture of spherical and cubic iron oxide nanoparticles. Similarly, we did not obtain the octapod structure after adding either NaF or KBr in reactions (Supplementary Fig. S4), indicating that the chloride ions are more critical in the formation of octapod iron oxide nanoparticles than of sodium ions. Furthermore, we used hexadecyl trimethyl ammonium chloride, KCl, hexadecyl trimethyl ammonium bromide and KBr instead of NaCl to investigate the structures of final products (Supplementary Fig. S5). The similar octapod products were obtained by adding hexadecyl trimethyl ammonium chloride or KCl, whereas no desired octapod structures were obtained in the presence of hexadecyl trimethyl ammonium bromide or KBr. These results further confirm that the chloride ions are the key inducer of the formation of octapod iron oxide nanoparticles. We were also able to control the sizes of octapod nanoparticles by varying the reaction time in the presence of NaCl. The octapod nanoparticles with average edge lengths of 14, 20, 30 and 36 nm were formed by reaction for 0.5, 1, 2 and 2.5 h, respectively (Fig. 2a–d), suggesting that the chloride ions may affect the formation of octapod nanoparticles throughout the particle growth process. One possible mechanism of forming octapod iron oxide nanoparticles was that the chloride ions were selectively bound to iron ions exposed on the high-index facets (probably [311]) of iron oxide during the particle growth (Fig. 2e,f). Such a chloride ion-assisted formation mechanism was supported by finding the presence of a trace amount of chlorine on the octapod iron oxide nanoparticles using energy-dispersive X-ray spectroscopy and X-ray photoelectron spectroscopy (Fig. 2e and Supplementary Fig. S6). To the best of our knowledge, this is the first report on the controlled synthesis of unique octapod iron oxide nanostructures with high surface-to-volume ratio (Supplementary Note 2).

Structure and properties of octapod iron oxide nanoparticles. Sophisticated morphology of nanostructures may alter the effective radii of particle cores. According to the quantum mechanical outer sphere theory, we simulated a spherical ball covering the full octapod iron oxide nanoparticle as a model to represent the objective existence of octapod nanoparticles under an external magnetic field B_0 (Fig. 3a). Thus, the diameter of the model shows the effective diameters of octapod iron oxide nanoparticles. We found the effective radii of octapod iron oxide nanoparticles to be ~2.4 times as large as that of spherical nanoparticles having the same geometric core volumes (Supplementary Fig. S7 and Supplementary Note 2), demonstrating that the octapod morphology can significantly increase the effective radii of nanoparticles and indicating that octapod iron oxide nanoparticles may possess much higher T_2 relaxivity than the spherical nanoparticles with similar geometric volumes. To investigate the MRI contrast ability of octapod and spherical iron oxide nanoparticles with the same geometric volumes, we chose the octapod iron oxide nanoparticles with average edge lengths of 30 nm (denoted as Octapod-30) and 20 nm (denoted as Octapod-20) as two representative examples. Accordingly, spherical nanoparticles with mean diameters of 16 nm (denoted as Spherical-16) and 10 nm (denoted as Spherical-10) were used for comparison because of the similarity in volume (that is, Octapod-30 with Spherical-16 and Octapod-20 with Spherical-10). We then tested the magnetic properties of octapod and spherical iron oxide nanoparticles by a superconducting quantum interference device. Octapod-30, Octapod-20, Spherical-16 and Spherical-10 all showed a smooth M–H curve with no hysteresis at ambient temperature (Fig. 3b). The blocking temperature of Octapod-30 and Octapod-20 were 290 K and 240 K, respectively (Supplementary Fig. S8), which further confirmed that Octapod-30 and Octapod-20 exhibited superparamagnetic behaviours at room temperature, enabling these nanoparticles for many biomedical applications (for example, biological separation and MRI contrast enhancement). The M_s values of Octapod-30, Octapod-20, Spherical-16 and Spherical-10 were about 71, 51, 67 and 55 emu g^{-1}, respectively. The slightly higher M_s value of Octapod-30 than that of Spherical-16 may be due to the reduced spin canting effect in octapod morphology comparing with spherical particle[35]. Despite of similar M_s values, the shape anisotropy in these octapod magnetite nanostructures and significantly increased effective radii of the magnetic cores may be responsible for the distinctly high T_2 relaxivities.

As the as-prepared nanoparticles were hydrophobic and unsuitable for biomedical applications, we transferred the nanoparticles to aqueous media using the conjugates of dendritic molecules and 1-hexadecylamine (denoted as HDA-G_2) by a hydrophobic–hydrophobic interaction[36]. The encapsulated nanoparticles showed excellent colloidal stability in aqueous solution. We did not observe any aggregations or morphology alteration after storage for more than 1 month (Supplementary Fig. S9). Furthermore, we measured the hydrodynamic diameters (HDs) of all the samples by dynamic light scattering. The HDs of

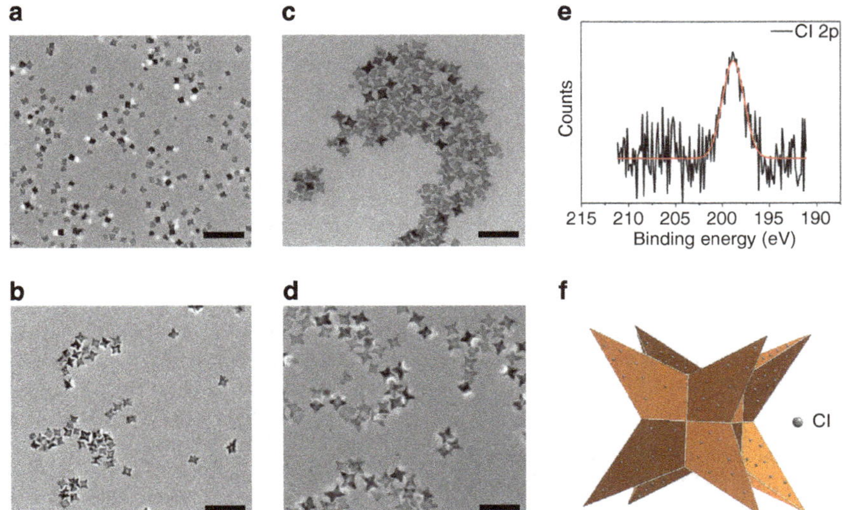

Figure 2 | Controlled synthesis of octapod iron oxide nanoparticles with different edge lengths. The octapod iron oxide nanoparticles with edge lengths of (**a**) 14, (**b**) 20, (**c**) 30 and (**d**) 36 nm formed after 1, 1.5, 2 and 2.5 h reaction times in the presence of NaCl, respectively. (**e**) X-ray photoelectron spectroscopy analysis of octapod iron oxide nanoparticles showed the Cl 2p3/2 peak at 198.9 eV, corresponding to the binding energy of Cl-Fe(III). The red line is a fitted result of the spectrum. (**f**) The model illustrated that the Cl ions may selectively bind to Fe ions on the surface of octapod iron oxide nanoparticles during size growth. Scale bar, 100 nm.

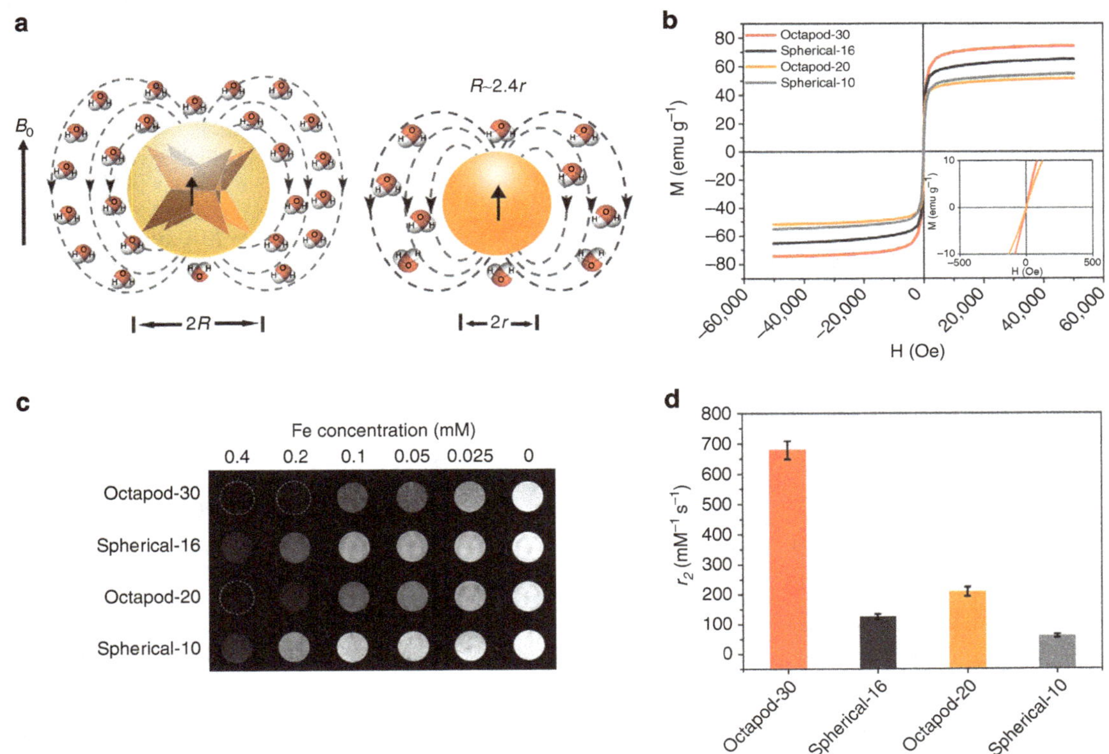

Figure 3 | MR contrast effect of octapod iron oxide nanoparticles. (**a**) Schematic cartoon shows the ball models of octapod and spherical iron oxide nanoparticles with the same geometric volume (the black dotted lines represents the magnetic field of the octapod and spherical iron oxide nanoparticles. The same length of black arrow means the same M_s of octapod and spherical iron oxide nanoparticles). With the same geometric core volume, the octapod nanoparticles have much larger effective volume (radius, R) than the spherical nanoparticles (radius, r) with $R \sim 2.4r$ under an external magnetic field B_0. (**b**) The smooth M-H curves of Octapod-30, Octapod-20, Spherical-16 and Spherical-10 measured at 300 K using a superconducting quantum interference device magnetometer (inset: M-H curves of Octapod-30 and Octapod-20 in low-magnetic field areas). The M_s values of Octapod-30, Octapod-20, Spherical-16 and Spherical-10 are about 71, 51, 67 and 55 emu g^{-1}, respectively. (**c**) T_2-weigthed MR images of Octapod-30, Octapod-20, Spherical-16 and Spherical-10 in aqueous solution with 1% agarose at various concentrations of iron using a Varian 7T microMRI scanner. (**d**) Comparison of r_2 values of Octapod-30, Octapod-20, Spherical-16 and Spherical-10. The error bars represent ± s.d. of five independent experiments.

Spherical-10, Spherical-16, Octapod-20 and Octapod-30 were 22 ± 2, 30 ± 3, 49 ± 5 and 58 ± 2 nm, respectively (Supplementary Fig. S9), suggesting that the iron oxide nanoparticles were monodisperse in water without any clustering and aggregation. Moreover, there are a large number of free amine groups available on the surface of the water-dispersible octapod nanoparticles, allowing for further modification and functionalization. It is of note that the HD of Octapod-30 is about twice as much as that of Spherical-16, which is consistent with the proposed model (Fig. 3a). In addition, the physical surface-to-volume ratio of Octapod-30 in aqueous medium is larger than that of the simulated spherical model because of the unique octapod structure. Hence, it is expected that the effective surface area of Octapod-30 for diffusion of water molecules may be more than four times greater than that of Spherical-16.

Transverse relaxivity of octapod iron oxide nanoparticles. We then tested the transverse relaxivity (r_2) values of the above four samples by a 7T MR scanner. With the increase of Fe concentrations, the signal intensity of T_2-weighted phantom images obviously decreased (Fig. 3c), indicating that all the samples have the potential to generate MRI contrast enhancement on T_2-weighted sequences. Notably, the octapod iron oxide nanoparticles exhibited stronger T_2 contrast effects than spherical iron oxide nanoparticles, suggesting that the octapod iron oxide nanoparticles may serve as highly sensitive T_2 contrast agents. The r_2 values of Octapod-30, Octapod-20, Spherical-16 and Spherical-10 were about 679.25 ± 30, 209.03 ± 15, 125.86 ± 9 and $59.91 \pm 6\,mM^{-1}\,s^{-1}$, respectively (Fig. 3d and Supplementary Figs S10 and S11). Because of the increased effective radii of octapod iron oxide cores, the r_2 value of Octapod-30 was ~ 5.4 times larger than that of Spherical-16. Meanwhile, Octapod-20 has a higher r_2 value than Spherical-10 (about 3.5 times) as well. It should be mentioned that the M_s values and geometric volumes of both octapod iron oxide nanoparticles were very close to the corresponding spherical iron oxide nanoparticles (that is, Octapod-30 to Spherical-16 and Octapod-20 to Spherical-10). Our results demonstrate that structurally increasing the effective radii of iron oxide through morphology control is an attractive alternative to existing strategies, such as metal doping and particle clustering[18,37–39] to increase the T_2 relaxivity of iron oxide nanoparticles.

Liver MRI using octapod iron oxide nanoparticles. Iron oxide nanoparticles as T_2 contrast agents have been extensively used in liver MRI. Before the animal study, we first tested the cytotoxicity of water-dispersible octapod iron oxide nanoparticles using HepG2 cell line as a model. The MTT (3-(4,5-dimethylthiazol-2-yl)-2,5-diphenyltetrazolium bromide) assay indicated that octapod iron oxide nanoparticles have no appreciable cytotoxicity for 24 h even at concentration up to 100 μg Fe per ml, suggesting the high biocompatibility of the octapod iron oxide nanoparticles (Supplementary Fig. S12). To verify that octapod iron oxide nanoparticles display better contrast effects than traditional spherical iron oxide nanoparticles *in vivo*, we chose Octapod-30 and Spherical-16 as representative samples and conducted T_2-weigthed MRI of liver using BALB/c mouse as a model. After intravenous injection of Octapod-30 and Spherical-16 samples at a dose of 1 mg Fe per kg of mouse body weight, we indeed observed significant signal attenuation in the liver region for both nanoparticles (Fig. 4a) at 0.5 h post injection (p.i.). To quantify the contrast, we identified the liver as the region of interest and calculated the signal-to-noise ratio (SNR) and SNR_{post}/SNR_{pre} value for each animal (Fig. 4b and Supplementary Table S1). It appears that the Octapod-30 exhibited much higher contrast (63.9 ± 3.2 and $67.3 \pm 1.3\%$ at 0.5 and 1 h p.i., respectively) than Spherical-16 (39.8 ± 1.5 and $53.5 \pm 1.6\%$ at 0.5 and 1 h p.i., respectively), suggesting that Octapod-30 with higher r_2 value is more sensitive than Spherical-16 in T_2 imaging of liver *in vivo*. Prussian blue staining detected blue spots throughout the liver sections after administration of Octapod-30 and Spherical-16 (Supplementary Fig. S13), confirming that the signal attenuation in the liver was caused by iron oxide nanoparticle accumulation. The inductively coupled plasma mass spectrometry analysis (Supplementary Fig. S14) indicates that the liver uptake of Octapod-30 and Spherical-16 is in a comparable manner, demonstrating that the much better contrast is due to the higher r_2 value of Octapod-30. In MRI, lower dose of contrast agents may imply lower cost and less side effect, which pledges greater prospects in clinical diagnosis. The high contrast of Octapod-30 prompted us to conduct liver MRI at a lower dose. By reducing the injection dose of Octapod-30 to 0.5 mg Fe per kg, the contrast ($39.9 \pm 2.5\%$ at 0.5 h and $56.2 \pm 1.9\%$ at 1 h) was still slightly higher than that when Spherical-16 at $1\,mg\,kg^{-1}$ does (Supplementary Fig. S15 and Supplementary Table S1).

Detection of liver cancer by MRI. To further evaluate the ability of Octapod-30 for liver cancer imaging, we conducted a T_2-weigthted MRI on an orthotopic HepG2 tumour model. We established the orthotopic liver tumour model by inoculation of small subcutaneous HepG2 tumour fragments into the liver of nude mice. When the hepatic carcinoma reached 3–5 mm in diameter, we intravenously injected Octapod-30 and Spherical-16 into the nude mice (2 mg Fe per kg) and scanned the animals at a 7T microMRI scanner. As hepatic tumours contain much less active Kupffer cells and macrophages[36], they do not accumulate iron oxide nanoparticles as efficiently as normal liver tissues do[40,41]. Thus, the hepatic tumours would show pseudo-positive contrast as compared with normal liver tissues. Both particles caused obvious contrast enhancement in the tumour sites after intravenous administration (Fig. 4c). Moreover, the injection of Octapod-30 resulted in higher MR contrast in the tumour site than Spherical-16, leading to easy differentiation between the liver lesions and normal liver tissues in the MR images. The tumour-to-liver contrast increased over time and was as high as 136.9 ± 8.5 and $64.5 \pm 2.7\%$ at 4 h p.i. for Octapod-30 and Spherical-16, respectively (Fig. 4d and Supplementary Table S2), indicating that Octapod-30 exhibited much higher signal changes for liver tumour imaging and detection limit than Spherical-16. The use of Octapod-30 with ultrahigh T_2 relaxivity as contrast agent may significantly improve the sensitivity of T_2 imaging, which should be extremely important for accurate detection and early diagnosis of cancer.

Discussion

We further compared the r_2 values of spherical nanoparticles with mean diameter of 25 nm (donated as Spherical-25) and Octapod-20, which have the similar effective diameters (HDs). The results demonstrated that the r_2 value of Octapod-20 is somewhat higher than that of Spherical-25, although the M_s value of Spherical-25 is larger than that of Octapod-20 (Supplementary Fig. S11). This phenomenon may be attributed to the strong inhomogeneity of the local magnetic fields induced by the unique octapod-shaped iron oxide nanoparticles, suggesting that the outer sphere theory may have limitations when applied to nanoparticles with significant anisotropy[21]. Because of the unique morphology of octapod iron oxide nanoparticles, the local magnetic field induced by an octapod iron oxide nanoparticle under an external magnetic field (B_0) may be more inhomogeneous than that of a spherical one, which may further induce proton dephasing and

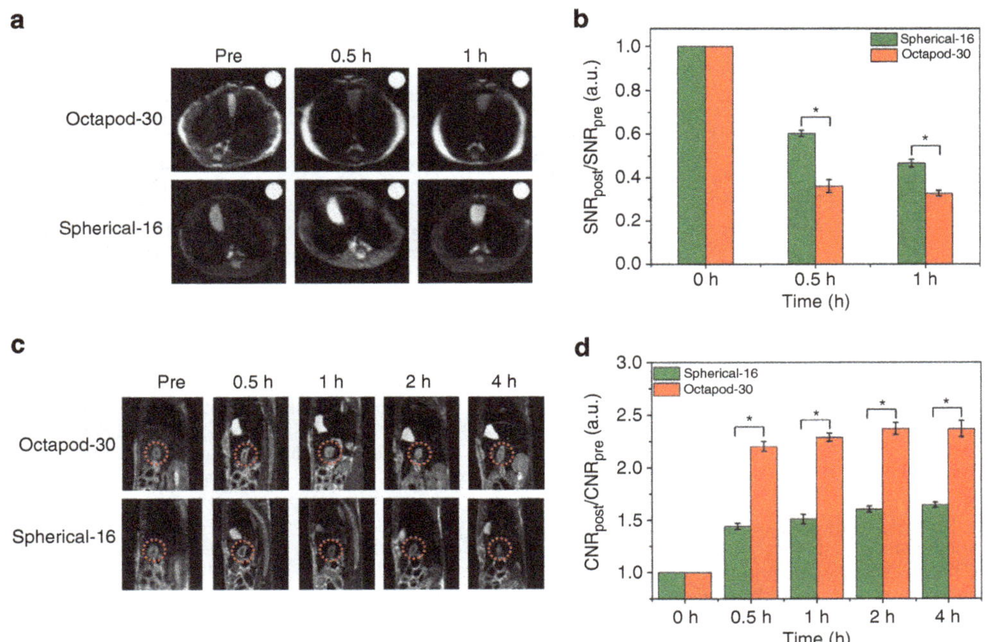

Figure 4 | *In vivo* MRI. (**a**) *In vivo* MR images of BALB/c mice at 0, 0.5 and 1 h after intravenous injection of Octapod-30 (upper) and Spherical-16 (lower) in transverse plane, respectively (the white dot is the signal reference using water in an NMR tube). (**b**) Quantification of liver contrast collected at 0, 0.5 and 1 h after accumulation of Octapod-30 and Spherical-16 in BALB/c mice at dose of 1.0 mg Fe per kg, respectively ($^*P<0.01$). (**c**) *In vivo* MR images of orthotopic xenograft liver tumour model at 0, 0.5, 1, 2 and 4 h after intravenous injection of Octapod-30 and Spherical-16 in sagittal plane. (**d**) Quantification of contrast-to-noise ratio (CNR) of tumour-to-liver contrast at 0, 0.5, 1, 2 and 4 h after administration of Octapod-30 and Spherical-16, with a dose of 2.0 mg Fe per kg, respectively ($^*P<0.01$).

enhance the T_2 shortening[42]. On the basis of the calculations using the Landau–Lifshitz–Gilbert equation, we found that the octapod morphology did result in a significantly more inhomogeneous induced magnetic field than the spherical one as expected, whereas the induced magnetic field in the far field (micrometer away) is negligible ($\sim 10^{-3}$ Oe) and almost the same regardless of the nanoparticle shape (Supplementary Fig. S16 and Supplementary Table S3). These results indicate that octapod iron oxide nanoparticles could further increase the r_2 value by inducing a more inhomogeneous magnetic field. The fact that the r_2 value of Spherical-25 is close to that of Octapod-20 manifests that the increased effective radius is the main reason to improve the transverse relaxivity of octapod iron oxide nanoparticles.

In summary, we have demonstrated a novel strategy for designing concave octapod iron oxide nanoparticles with ultrahigh r_2 values as T_2 contrast agents. The key to successful fabrication of size-controllable octapod iron oxide nanoparticles is the presence of chloride anions. It turns out that by increasing the effective radius and local field inhomogeneity of the magnetic core, the octapod iron oxide nanoparticles exhibit an incredibly high T_2 contrast enhancement effect. The controlled synthesis of octapod iron oxide nanoparticles is facile, highly reproducible and amenable to scale up, thereby rendering these novel iron oxide nanoparticles promising T_2 contrast agents for MRI. This new strategy of achieving extremely high T_2 relaxivity of iron oxide nanoparticles by increasing the effective radii of iron oxide cores rather than the magnetization values is believed to be critically important in developing highly sensitive second-generation contrast agents for MRI (Supplementary Table S4), especially for the early and accurate diagnosis of liver cancer in patients. Moreover, the controllable synthesis of novel octapod iron oxide nanoparticles, together with other morphologies (for example, sphere, cube and rod), certainly facilitates the applications of magnetic nanoparticles in high-density data storage, hyperthermia treatment and magnetically guided drug delivery.

Methods

Synthesis of octapod iron oxide nanoparticles. In a typical synthesis of octapod iron oxide nanoparticles, iron oleate (0.8 g, 0.86 mmol), NaCl (10 mg, 0.17 mmol), oleic acid (110 μl, 0.35 mmol) and distilled water (60 μl) were mixed together with 10 ml of 1-octadecene. The resulting solution was degassed in vacuum for 30 min and backfilled with argon to remove any low volatile impurities and oxygen at room temperature. And then, we heated the reaction solution to 320 °C with a constant heating rate of 3.3 °C min^{-1}, and were kept at the temperature for 2 h. The colour of the solution changed from reddish-brown to transparent orange and finally brownish-black. Then, the solution was cooled to room temperature and mixed with 30 ml of isopropanol to precipitate the nanoparticles. The nanoparticles were separated by centrifugation and washed three times with ethanol. The final product was dissolved in hexane for long-term storage at 4 °C. See Supplementary Methods for further details of synthesis procedures.

Measurement of T_2 relaxivities. To measure the T_2 relaxivity, Octapod-30, Octapod-20, Spherical-16 and Spherical-10 with different iron concentrations were dispersed in 1% agarose solution. The samples were scanned (at 300 K) using a T_2-weighted fast spin-echo multi-slice sequence (fSEMS) (TR/TE = 2,000/20, 40, 60, 80, 100 ms, slice thickness = 2 mm) by a 7T MRI scanner (Varian 7T microMRI System).

***In vivo* liver MRI.** Animal experiments were executed according to the protocol approved by Institutional Animal Care and Use Committee of Xiamen University. We performed the *in vivo* MRI of liver by using BALB/c mouse as a model. After intravenous injection of iron oxide nanoparticles at a dose of 1 mg Fe per kg of mouse body weight, the coronal and transverse plane MR images were scanned using an fSEMS (TR/TE = 3,000/40 ms, 256 × 256 matrices, averages = 1) on a Varian 7T microMRI scanner. The MR images were obtained at pre-injection, 0.5 and 1 h p.i. ($n = 3$ per group). To qualify the signal enhancement, we calculated the SNR by the equation: $SNR_{liver} = SI_{liver}/SD_{noise}$, where SI represents signal intensity and SD represents s.d.

***In vivo* liver tumour imaging.** We established the orthotopic liver tumour model by inoculation of small subcutaneous HepG2 tumour fragments into the liver of nude mice. When the tumour reached 3–5 mm in diameter, mice were intravenously injected with Octapod-30 and Spherical-16 at a dose of 2 mg Fe per kg. The coronal and transverse plane MR images were acquired using an fSEMS (TR/TE = 3,000/40 ms, 256 × 256 matrices, averages = 1) on a 7T MRI scanner. The MR images were sequentially obtained at 0, 0.5, 1, 2 and 4 h p.i. ($n = 3$ per group). To qualify the efficacy of contrast enhancement, we introduced the CNR (contrast-to-noise ratio), which was given by $CNR = (SNR_{tumour}-SNR_{liver})/SNR_{tumour}$.

References

1. Laurent, S. *et al.* Magnetic iron oxide nanoparticles: Synthesis, stabilization, vectorization, physicochemical characterizations, and biological applications. *Chem. Rev.* **108,** 2064–2110 (2008).
2. Tassa, C., Shaw, S. Y. & Weissleder, R. Dextran-coated iron oxide nanoparticles: a versatile platform for targeted molecular imaging, molecular diagnostics, and therapy. *Acc. Chem. Res.* **44,** 842–852 (2011).
3. Corot, C., Robert, P., Idee, J. M. & Port, M. Recent advances in iron oxide nanocrystal technology for medical imaging. *Adv. Drug Deliv. Rev.* **58,** 1471–1504 (2006).
4. Major, J. L. & Meade, T. J. Bioresponsive, cell-penetrating, and multimeric MR contrast agents. *Acc. Chem. Res.* **42,** 893–903 (2009).
5. Weissleder, R. *et al.* Ultrasmall superparamagnetic iron oxide - characterization of a new class of contrast agnets for MR imaging. *Radiology* **175,** 489–493 (1990).
6. Bulte, J. W. M. & Kraitchman, D. L. Iron oxide MR contrast agents for molecular and cellular imaging. *NMR Biomed.* **17,** 484–499 (2004).
7. Harisinghani, M. G. *et al.* Noninvasive detection of clinically occult lymph-node metastases in prostate cancer. *N. Engl. J. Med.* **348,** 2491–2495 (2003).
8. Gao, J. H., Gu, H. W. & Xu, B. Multifunctional magnetic nanoparticles: design, synthesis, and biomedical applications. *Acc. Chem. Res.* **42,** 1097–1107 (2009).
9. Terreno, E., Castelli, D. D., Viale, A. & Aime, S. Challenges for molecular magnetic resonanceimaging. *Chem. Rev.* **110,** 3019–3042 (2010).
10. Kim, B. H. *et al.* Large-scale synthesis of uniform and extremely small-sized iron oxide nanoparticles for high-resolution T_1 magnetic resonance imaging contrast agents. *J. Am. Chem. Soc.* **133,** 12624–12631 (2011).
11. Lee, N. & Hyeon, T. Designed synthesis of uniformly sized iron oxide nanoparticles for efficient magnetic resonance imaging contrast agents. *Chem. Soc. Rev.* **41,** 2575–2589 (2012).
12. Lee, N. *et al.* Magnetosome-like ferrimagnetic iron oxide nanocubes for highly sensitive MRI of single cells and transplanted pancreatic islets. *Proc. Natl Acad. Sci. USA* **108,** 2662–2667 (2011).
13. Ananta, J. S. *et al.* Geometrical confinement of gadolinium-based contrast agents in nanoporous particles enhances T1 contrast. *Nat. Nanotech.* **5,** 815–821 (2010).
14. Ghosh, D. *et al.* M13-templated magnetic nanoparticles for targeted in vivo imaging of prostate cancer. *Nat. Nanotech.* **7,** 677–682 (2012).
15. Sun, S. H. & Zeng, H. Size-controlled synthesis of magnetite nanoparticles. *J. Am. Chem. Soc.* **124,** 8204–8205 (2002).
16. Park, J. *et al.* Ultra-large-scale syntheses of monodisperse nanocrystals. *Nat. Mater.* **3,** 891–895 (2004).
17. Lee, J.-H. *et al.* Artificially engineered magnetic nanoparticles for ultra-sensitive molecular imaging. *Nat. Med.* **13,** 95–99 (2007).
18. Jang, J.-t. *et al.* Critical enhancements of MRI contrast and hyperthermic effects by dopant-controlled magnetic nanoparticles. *Angew. Chem. Int. Ed.* **48,** 1234–1238 (2009).
19. Yoo, D., Lee, J.-H., Shin, T.-H. & Cheon, J. Theranostic magnetic nanoparticles. *Acc. Chem. Res.* **44,** 863–874 (2011).
20. Koenig, S. H. & Kellar, K. E. Theory of $1/T_1$ and $1/T_2$ NMRD profiles of solutions of magnetic nanoparticles. *Magn. Reson. Med.* **34,** 227–233 (1995).
21. Roch, A., Muller, R. N. & Gillis, P. Theory of proton relaxation induced by superparamagnetic particles. *J. Chem. Phys.* **110,** 5403–5411 (1999).
22. Vuong, Q. L., Berret, J.-F., Fresnais, J., Gossuin, Y. & Sandre, O. A universal scaling law to predict the efficiency of magnetic nanoparticles as MRI T_2-contrast agents. *Adv. Healthcare Mater.* **1,** 502–512 (2012).
23. Gillis, P., Moiny, F. & Brooks, R. A. On T_2-shortening by strongly magnetized spheres: a partial refocusing model. *Magn. Reson. Med.* **47,** 257–263 (2002).
24. Tong, S., Hou, S., Zheng, Z., Zhou, J. & Bao, G. Coating optimization of superparamagnetic iron oxide nanoparticles for high T_2 relaxivity. *Nano Lett.* **10,** 4607–4613 (2010).
25. Tian, N., Zhou, Z. Y., Sun, S. G., Ding, Y. & Wang, Z. L. Synthesis of tetrahexahedral platinum nanocrystals with high-index facets and high electro-oxidation activity. *Science* **316,** 732–735 (2007).
26. Lim, B., Xiong, Y. & Xia, Y. A water-based synthesis of octahedral, decahedral, and icosahedral Pd nanocrystals. *Angew. Chem. Int. Ed.* **46,** 9279–9282 (2007).
27. Huang, X., Zhao, Z., Fan, J., Tan, Y. & Zheng, N. Amine-assisted synthesis of concave polyhedral platinum nanocrystals having [411] high-index facets. *J. Am. Chem. Soc.* **133,** 4718–4721 (2011).
28. Zhang, J. *et al.* Concave cubic gold nanocrystals with high-index facets. *J. Am. Chem. Soc.* **132,** 14012–14014 (2010).
29. Huang, X. *et al.* Freestanding palladium nanosheets with plasmonic and catalytic properties. *Nat. Nanotech.* **6,** 28–32 (2011).
30. Yin, J. *et al.* Low-symmetry iron oxide nanocrystals bound by high-index facets. *Angew. Chem. Int. Ed.* **49,** 6328–6332 (2010).
31. Hofmann, C. *et al.* Shape control of new Fe_xO-Fe_3O_4 and $Fe_{1-y}Mn_yO$-$Fe_{3-z}Mn_zO_4$ nanostructures. *Adv. Funct. Mater.* **18,** 1661–1667 (2008).
32. Hou, Y. L., Xu, Z. C. & Sun, S. H. Controlled synthesis and chemical conversions of FeO nanoparticles. *Angew. Chem. Int. Ed.* **46,** 6329–6332 (2007).
33. Zabow, G., Dodd, S., Moreland, J. & Koretsky, A. Micro-engineered local field control for high-sensitivity multispectral MRI. *Nature* **453,** 1058–1063 (2008).
34. Zabow, G., Dodd, S. J., Moreland, J. & Koretsky, A. P. The fabrication of uniform cylindrical nanoshells and their use as spectrally tunable MRI contrast agents. *Nanotechnology* **20,** 385301 (2009).
35. Noh, S.-H. *et al.* Nanoscale magnetism control via surface and exchange anisotropy for optimized ferrimagnetic hysteresis. *Nano Lett.* **12,** 3716–3721 (2012).
36. Zhou, Z. J. *et al.* A synergistically enhanced T_1–T_2 dual-modal contrast agent. *Adv. Mater.* **24,** 6223–6228 (2012).
37. Ai, H. *et al.* Magnetite-loaded polymeric micelles as ultrasensitive magnetic-resonance probes. *Adv. Mater.* **17,** 1949–1952 (2005).
38. Bruns, O. T. *et al.* Real-time magnetic resonance imaging and quantification of lipoprotein metabolism in vivo using nanocrystals. *Nat. Nanotech.* **4,** 193–201 (2009).
39. Yoon, T.-J., Lee, H., Shao, H. & Weissleder, R. Highly magnetic core–shell nanoparticles with a unique magnetization mechanism. *Angew. Chem. Int. Ed.* **50,** 4663–4666 (2011).
40. Huang, J. *et al.* Effects of nanoparticle size on cellular uptake and liver MRI with polyvinylpyrrolidone-coated iron oxide nanoparticles. *ACS Nano* **4,** 7151–7160 (2010).
41. Ba-Ssalamah, A. *et al.* Clinical value of MRI liver-specific contrast agents: a tailored examination for a confident non-invasive diagnosis of focal liver lesions. *Eur. Radiol.* **19,** 342–357 (2009).
42. Bjørnerud, A. & Johansson, L. The utility of superparamagnetic contrast agents in MRI: theoretical consideration and applications in the cardiovascular system. *NMR Biomed.* **17,** 465–477 (2004).

Acknowledgements

This work was supported by the National Key Basic Research Program of China (2013CB933901 and 2013CB733802), National Natural Science Foundation of China (21222106, 21021061, 81000662, 81201805 and J1210014), Natural Science Foundation of Fujian (2013J06005) and the Program for New Century Excellent Talents in University (NCET-10-0709). We thank B. Xu, L.S. Zheng, E. Meggers and C.B. Cai for the fruitful discussions.

Author contributions

J.G. and Z. Zhao conceived and designed the experiments; Z. Zhao, Z. Zhou, J.B., J.H., X. Chi. and K.N. performed the experiments; J.G., Z. Zhao and Z.C. analysed the data; Z.W. and R.W. did the theoretical calculations; and J.G., X. Chen and Z. Zhao co-wrote the paper. All authors discussed the results and commented on the manuscript.

Additional information

Competing financial interests: The authors declare no competing financial interests.

4

Structure-guided discovery of potent and dual-acting human parainfluenza virus haemagglutinin-neuraminidase inhibitors

Patrice Guillon[1,*,**], Larissa Dirr[1,*], Ibrahim M. El-Deeb[1,*,**], Moritz Winger[1,*,**], Benjamin Bailly[1], Thomas Haselhorst[1], Jeffrey C. Dyason[1] & Mark von Itzstein[1,*,**]

Human parainfluenza viruses (hPIVs) cause upper and lower respiratory tract disease in children that results in a significant number of hospitalizations and impacts health systems worldwide. To date, neither antiviral drugs nor vaccines are approved for clinical use against parainfluenza virus, which reinforces the urgent need for new therapeutic discovery strategies. Here we use a multidisciplinary approach to develop potent inhibitors that target a structural feature within the hPIV type 3 haemagglutinin-neuraminidase (hPIV-3 HN). These dual-acting designer inhibitors represent the most potent designer compounds and efficiently block both hPIV cell entry and virion progeny release. We also define the binding mode of these inhibitors in the presence of whole-inactivated hPIV and recombinantly expressed hPIV-3 HN by Saturation Transfer Difference NMR spectroscopy. Collectively, our study provides an antiviral preclinical candidate and a new direction towards the discovery of potential anti-parainfluenza drugs.

[1] Institute for Glycomics, Gold Coast Campus, Griffith University, Gold Coast, Queensland 4222, Australia. * These authors contributed equally to this work. ** Joint senior authors. Correspondence and requests for materials should be addressed to M.v.I. (email: m.vonitzstein@griffith.edu.au).

The *Paramyxoviridae* family contains viruses that are clinically significant in both medical and veterinary settings[1]. Human parainfluenza viruses types 1 to 3 (hPIV-1, 2 and 3), members of this family, are the leading cause of upper and lower respiratory tract disease in infants and young children and also impact the elderly and immunocompromised[2–5]. Significantly, it is estimated that in the United States alone, up to five million lower respiratory tract infections occur each year in children who are below 5 years, and hPIV has been isolated in approximately one-third of these cases[6,7]. There are currently neither vaccines[8] nor specific antiviral therapy[9] to prevent or treat hPIV infections, respectively, despite continuing efforts[10]. Some of the more recent approaches have focused on an entry blockade[11] and the triggering of premature virus fusion by a small molecule[12]. An initial interaction of parainfluenza virus with the host cell is through its surface glycoprotein, haemagglutinin–neuraminidase (HN)[13] and involves the recognition of *N*-acetylneuraminic acid (**1**)-containing glycoconjugates[14–16] (Fig. 1a). The parainfluenza virus HN is a multifunctional protein that encompasses the functions of receptor binding (for cell adhesion) and receptor destruction (facilitating virus release), not only within the one protein, but apparently in a single binding site[13]. In addition, the HN is involved in the activation of the viral surface fusion (F) protein necessary to initiate infection of the target host cell[13,17]. The essential triple role of HN in viral pathogenesis makes it an ideal target for the development of hPIV-specific therapeutics. A limited number of unsaturated neuraminic acid-based HN inhibitors (**2–6**, Fig. 1a) have been reported[18–23], although none of these inhibitors have advanced as clinical candidates presumably due to the lack of sufficient antiviral effect. One of the most potent and widely investigated hPIV type 3 haemagglutinin–neuraminidase (hPIV-3 HN) inhibitors[18,20,21] to date, **6**, has a neuraminidase IC_{50} value of $\sim 20\,\mu M$. This inhibitor incorporates an isobutyramido group at C5, demonstrating that hPIV-3 HN can accommodate larger acylamino groups in the C5-binding domain, and an azide functionality at C4 on the unsaturated neuraminic acid-based template.

We have recently described[24] significant flexibility associated with the hPIV-3 HN 216 loop that borders the active site region. This flexible loop can establish a more open cavity, the 216 cavity, and provides new opportunities for inhibitor discovery. Here we successfully explore this exciting opportunity using a multidisciplinary approach that employs, structure-based computational chemistry, synthetic chemistry, NMR-based structural and biological techniques to discover potent inhibitors of hPIV-3 HN activity and cell infection.

Results

Computational chemistry and inhibitor design. The characterization of the hPIV-3 HN 216 loop flexibility[24] motivated us to explore the potential of designing Neu5Ac2en derivatives with bulky C4 substituents that could be accommodated in and lock open the 216 cavity within the active site. Accordingly, molecular dynamics (MD) simulations have been employed to design and assess Neu5Ac2en derivatives that incorporate C4-functionalized triazoles. From our initial study of 216 loop flexibility and the resultant 216 cavity dimensions, it was clear that relatively bulky C4 substituents on the unsaturated neuraminic acid-based

a

1: *N*-Acetylneuraminic acid

2: R = OH Neu5Ac2en
3: R = N_3
4: R = $NHC(NH)NH_2$ zanamivir

5: R = OH
6: R = N_3 BCX 2798

7: R = CH_2OCH_3
8: R = Ph

9: R = CH_2OCH_3
10: R = Ph

b

11: R = Methyl
12: R = Isopropyl

i: R_2—≡
ii

13: R_1 = Methyl, $R_2 = CH_2OCH_3$
14: R_1 = Methyl, R_2 = Ph
15: R_1 = Isopropyl, $R_2 = CH_2OCH_3$
16: R_1 = Isopropyl, R_2 = Ph

7: R_1 = Methyl, $R_2 = CH_2OCH_3$
8: R_1 = Methyl, R_2 = Ph
9: R_1 = Isopropyl, $R_2 = CH_2OCH_3$
10: R_1 = Isopropyl, R_2 = Ph

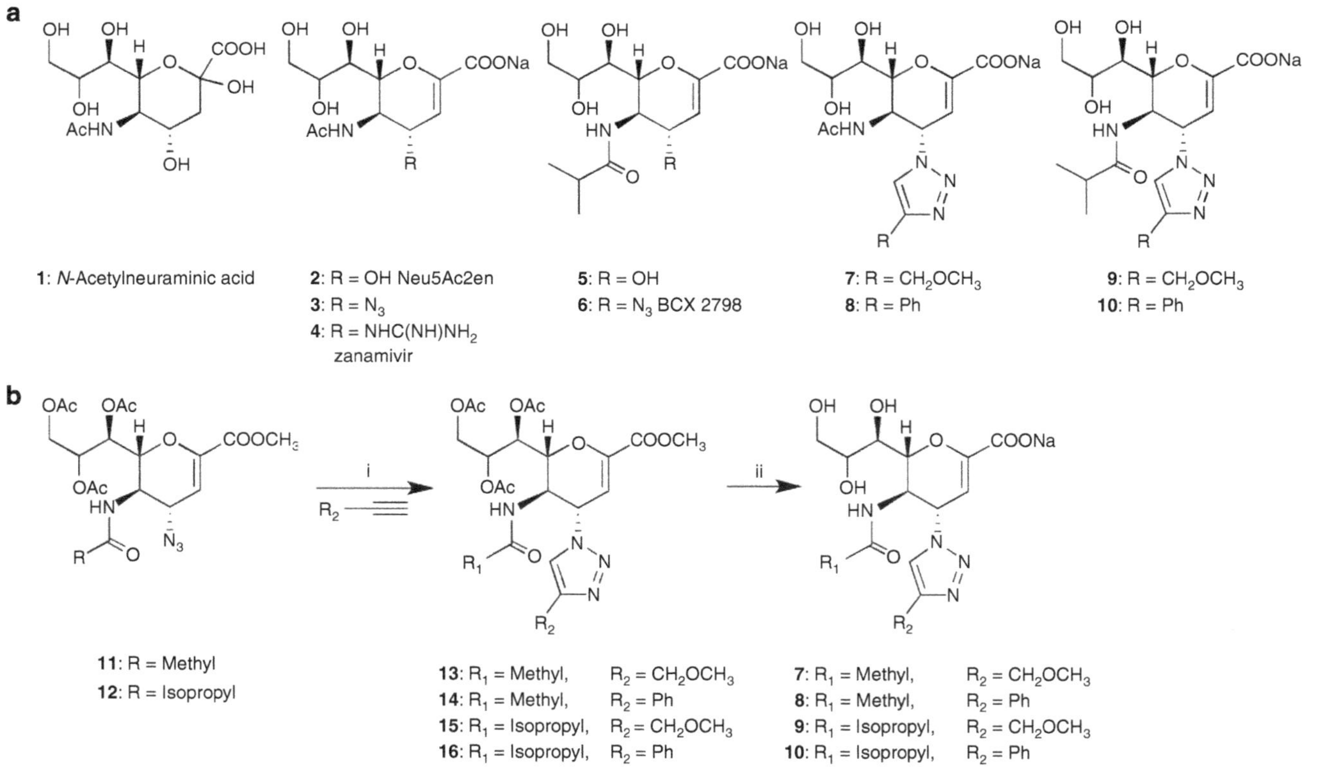

Figure 1 | Structures of reference sialidase inhibitors, the novel hPIV inhibitors and the synthetic strategy. (**a**) Structures of *N*-acetylneuraminic acid (**1**), the naturally occurring sialidase inhibitor Neu5Ac2en (**2**), 4-azido-4-deoxy-Neu5Ac2en (**3**), the potent influenza virus sialidase inhibitor zanamivir (**4**), the C5 isobutyramido analogue of Neu5Ac2en (**5**), the reference hPIV inhibitor BCX 2798 (**6**) and the novel inhibitors **7-10**. (**b**) Synthesis of the novel hPIV inhibitors **7-10**. (i) $CuSO_4$, sodium ascorbate, *tert*-butanol/H_2O (1:1), 45 °C, 6 h (**13**, 78%; **14**, 82%; **15**, 71%; **16**, 84%); (ii) NaOH, MeOH/H_2O (1:1), RT, o/n (**7**, 85%; **8**, 96%; **9**, 92%; **10**, 89%).

template (**7–10**, Fig. 1a) could be well tolerated within the open 216 cavity. Furthermore, modelling of these C4 triazole-substituted inhibitors in complex with hPIV-3 HN led us to conclude that both an acetamido (**7**, **8**) and an isobutyramido (**9**, **10**) moiety at C5 on the template could also be well accommodated simultaneously within the C5-binding domain. We specifically assessed, using MD simulations, the capacity of the bulkier triazole compounds (**8** and **10**) to efficiently lock open the 216 loop in hPIV-3 HN. Finally, we determined relative interaction energies of **8** and **10** in complex with hPIV-3 HN to predict if the bulkier C5 acylamino moiety, in combination with the bulky C4 substituent, would be expected to improve inhibitor affinity.

Compound 8 as an hPIV-3 HN inhibitor model. The simulation of the available hPIV-3 HN crystal structure (PDB accession code 1V3E) (ref. 25) in complex with **8**, using a defined parameter set (Supplementary Table 1a–e), allowed an analysis of the dynamic behaviour of the protein relative to the zanamivir (**4**)-bound structure. Atom-positional root mean square deviations (r.m.s.d.) of the hPIV-3 HN backbone atoms (C_α, N, C) for the 216 loop from the simulations of the hPIV-3 HN–**4** and –**8** complexes are presented in Fig. 2a. From this study, it is apparent that the 216 loop undergoes more significant deviations from the crystal structure in the case of the hPIV-3 HN–**8** complex (black curve). r.m.s.d. values greater than 0.5 nm are observed for the simulation of the hPIV-3 HN–**8** complex, whereas the structure deviates less (0.4 nm) for the hPIV-3 HN–**4** complex.

This notion is further supported by the root mean square fluctuations (r.m.s.f.) observed for the C_α atoms of the backbone for residues associated with the 216 loop (residues 205–225, Fig. 2b). Increased r.m.s.f. are observed for the residues of the second half of the 216 loop (215–220), where values of ~0.3 nm are reached, indicating a substantial conformational rearrangement within that domain compared with the starting hPIV-3 HN reference X-ray crystal structure (PDB accession code IV3E) (ref. 25). Table 1 shows a selection of r.m.s.f. values of residues comprised in the 216 loop.

Our data suggest that loop flexibility, present under physiological simulation conditions, has been significantly underestimated in crystal structures and provides an exciting opportunity for anti-parainfluenza virus drug discovery. Comparison of the hPIV-3 HN–**4** complex and the hPIV-3 HN–**8** complex simulations demonstrates that the C4 substituent on **8** induces significant movement in the hPIV-3 HN 216 loop. The induced loop opening can be seen from the solvent-accessible surface plots of the final structures obtained from 10-ns simulations of hPIV-3 HN–**4** complex (Fig. 2c, left panel) and hPIV-3 HN–**8** complex (Fig. 2c, right panel).

One of the most populated conformational clusters from the MD simulations of hPIV-3 HN in complex with **4** and **8**, are shown in Fig. 3a, while the superposition of the final conformations from the simulations of hPIV-3 HN in complex with **4** and **8** are shown in Fig. 3b. The difference in 216 loop conformation can clearly be seen (coloured loops: 1V3E–**4** (magenta) and 1V3E–**8** (green)). The 216 cavity adopts a more open conformation when in complex with the more sterically encumbered inhibitor **8**. Generally, a wider cavity is observed for the simulation of hPIV-3 HN–**8** complex. The most populated cluster from the simulation of the hPIV-3 HN–**4** complex has a slightly smaller cavity volume (654 Å^3) compared with the simulated hPIV-3 HN–**8** complex (717 Å^3).

To evaluate if a bulkier C5 acylamino moiety would be accommodated in the presence of the C4-functionalized triazole, we undertook an identical analysis of **10** in complex with hPIV-3 HN (Supplementary Movie 1). Our preliminary analysis led us to conclude that a C5 isobutyramido moiety is well accommodated within the C5-binding domain in the presence of the C4-functionalized triazole (Fig. 3c).

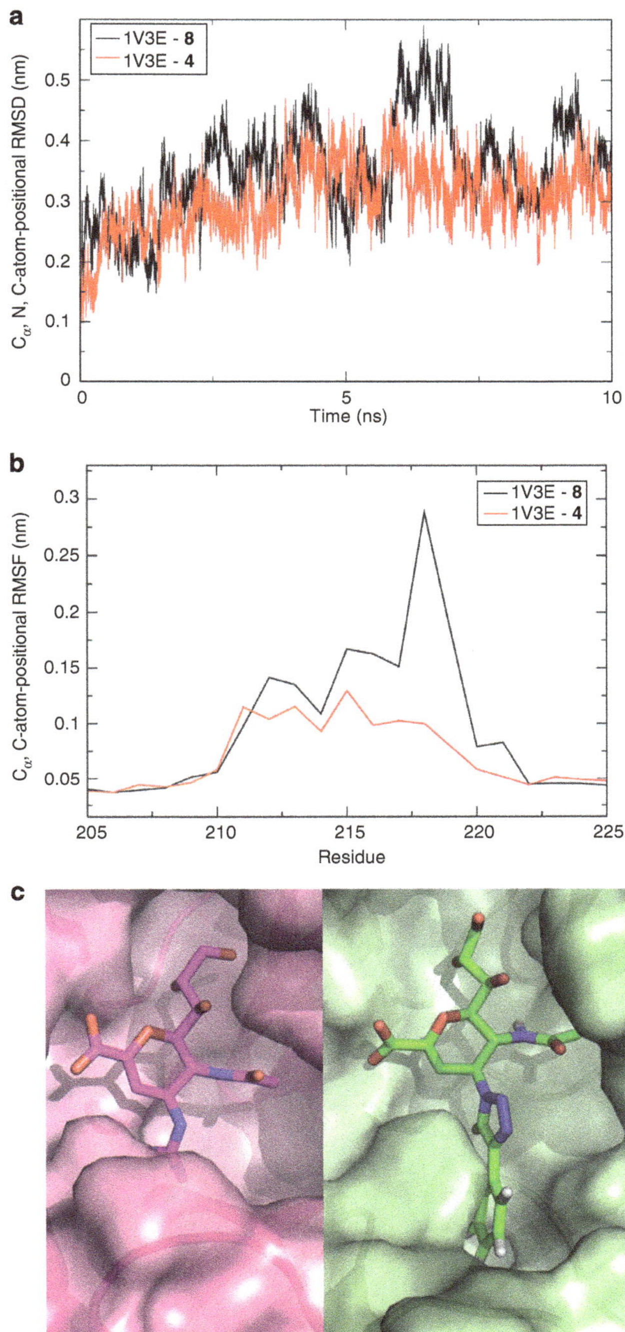

Figure 2 | The predicted influence of 4 and 8 complexation on HN 216 loop conformation. (**a**) Atom-positional r.m.s.d. of the 216 loop's backbone atoms (C_α, N, C) with respect to the crystal structure of hPIV-3 HN (1V3E) bound to zanamivir. (**b**) Atom-positional r.m.s.f. of the C_α atoms of the residues in the 216 loop, hPIV-3 HN (1V3E) bound to **4** (red) and hPIV-3 HN (1V3E) bound to **8** (black). The least-squares superposition involved all C_α atoms of the protein backbone. (**c**) Solvent-accessible surface plots of the final coordinates of hPIV-3 HN (1V3E) bound to **4** (left) and bound to **8** (right). **8** can be accommodated in an open-loop structure of hPIV-3 HN.

Inhibitor-relative interaction energies. To quantify the extent of inhibitor engagement with hPIV-3 HN, we have used our MD simulations approach to determine theoretical averaged interaction energies for the known inhibitor **2**, based on a previous study[24], as well as the novel C5 acetamido and C5 isobutyramido inhibitors, **8** and **10,** respectively. Average interaction energy (E_{avI}) values of -609.38 ± 10.92, -733.96 ± 15.49 and $-821.88 \pm 10.93\ \mathrm{kJ\ mol^{-1}}$ for **2, 8** and **10,** respectively, in complex with hPIV-3 HN (PDB accession code 1V3E) (ref. 25) were determined. Most importantly, these calculations support the notion that the replacement of the acetamido moiety in **8** with an isobutyramido moiety in **10** significantly improves the absolute E_{avI} value of the inhibitor in complex with the protein. Consequently, **10** is predicted to be a more potent hPIV-3 HN inhibitor than **8**. Further analysis of the MD simulation and extraction of the lowest ($-1{,}078.13\ \mathrm{kJ\ mol^{-1}}$) interaction energy structure of **10** in complex with hPIV-3 HN (1V3E) revealed that **10** makes several key interactions, in this orientation, within the binding pocket (Fig. 3d). Noteworthy is the electrostatic interaction between the ligand's carboxylate and the triarginyl cluster (Arg192, Arg424,

Table 1 | Root mean square fluctuations of selected residues comprised in the 216 loop for the 1V3E-4 and 1V3E-8 simulated systems, in nanometres, compared with the reference X-ray structure (PDB accession code 1V3E).

Residue	Reference X-ray structure (1V3E)	1V3E-4	1V3E-8
210	0.036	0.059	0.056
212	0.046	0.104	0.141
214	0.048	0.093	0.109
216	0.057	0.111	0.162
218	0.060	0.134	0.289
220	0.041	0.070	0.079

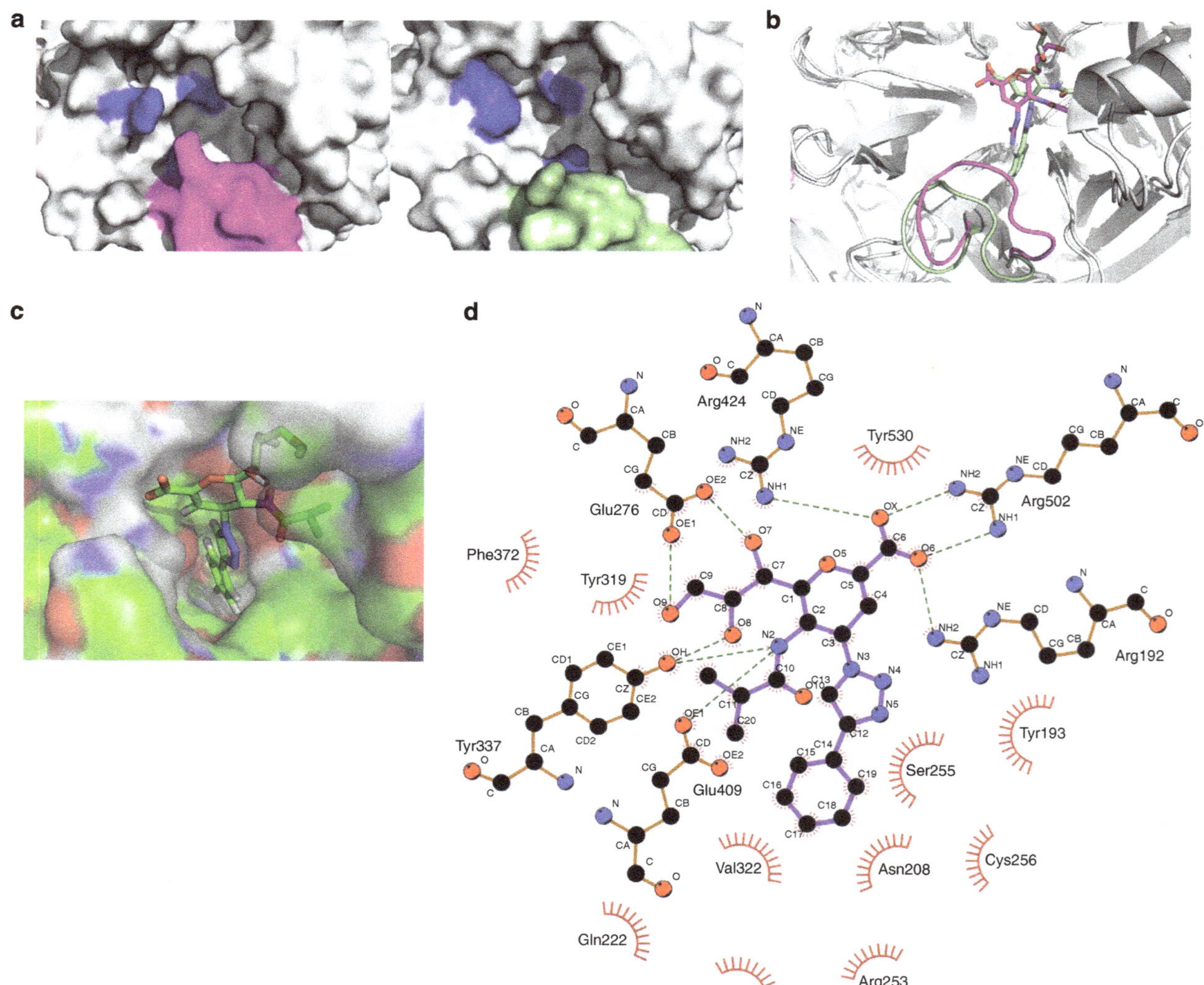

Figure 3 | The predicted structure of the HN active site in complex with 4 and 8. (**a**) Solvent-accessible surface plots of the most populated conformational clusters of hPIV-3 HN (1V3E) bound to **4** (left) and bound to **8** (right). The residues comprised in the 216 loop (205–225) are coloured in magenta (1V3E-**4**) and green (1V3E-**8**), respectively. Arginines associated with inhibitor binding are coloured in blue. (**b**) Superposition of snapshots of the final trajectories of hPIV-3 HN bound to **4** and **8** after 10 ns of MD simulation. The 216 loop is highlighted in colour (green: 1V3E-**8**, magenta: 1V3E-**4**). **4** (magenta) and **8** (atomic colours) are shown in stick representation. (**c**) Solvent-accessible surface plot of the final coordinates of hPIV-3 HN (1V3E) bound to **10**. Both the C4-functionalized triazole and the C5 isobutyramido moiety are well accommodated in an open 216-loop structure of hPIV-3 HN. (**d**) Key interactions between **10** and hPIV-3 HN. The triarginyl cluster (Arg192, Arg424, Arg502) engages the inhibitor's negatively charged carboxylate, the C7 hydroxyl group engages Glu276 in a hydrogen bond interaction as does the C5 isobutyramido NH with Tyr337 and Glu409. Hydrophobic interactions are observed for both the C4 aromatic and C5 isobutyl functionalities.

Arg502), hydrogen bond interactions between the C7 hydroxyl group and Glu276 and the C5 isobutyramido NH and Tyr337 and Glu409. Furthermore, additional hydrophobic interactions are observed for both the C4 aromatic and C5 isobutyl functionalities, particularly with the peptide backbone, within the C4- and C5-binding domains, respectively.

Synthesis of the target triazoles 7–10. Guided by our computational analysis, we synthesized the identified C4-functionalized triazole unsaturated *N*-acetylneuraminic acid derivatives **7–10** to further explore their capacity to inhibit hPIV-3 HN function by accessing an open 216 loop within the hPIV-3 HN-binding site. The synthesis of the triazoles **7–10** was achieved using the known[26–29] 4-azido-4-deoxy-Neu5Ac2en-based intermediates **11** and **12**. Thus, each of the two intermediates was exposed to either methylpropargyl ether or ethynylbenzene under typical click azide–alkyne coupling conditions[27,28] (heating a mixture of the 4-azido-4-deoxy-Neu5Ac2en derivative, alkyne, $CuSO_4$ and sodium ascorbate in a (1:1) mixture of water and *tert*-butanol for 6 h) to afford the triazole derivative (Fig. 1b).

Triazoles **13** and **14** (starting from **11**) and the triazole derivatives **15** and **16** (starting from **12**) were isolated in yields of 78, 82, 71 and 84%, respectively. The resulting per-*O*-acetylated triazole derivatives **13–16** were then deprotected by treatment with aqueous methanol (50%) adjusted to pH 13–14 at room temperature (RT) for 24 h to yield the final products **7–10** as sodium salts in 85, 96, 92 and 89% yields, respectively. The novel compounds were appropriately characterized (Supplementary Methods) and all compounds were determined, by ^1H and ^{13}C NMR spectroscopy, to be of high purity (Supplementary Fig. 3a–t).

Inhibitor screening with hPIV-3 HN. The reference inhibitors **2**, **3**, **5** and **6**, as well as the novel inhibitors **7–10**, were evaluated for their capacity to inhibit both the neuraminidase and haemagglutinin functions of the hPIV-3 HN protein using neuraminidase inhibition (NI) and haemagglutination inhibition (HI) assays. Thus, NI was assessed by an end point fluorescence-based assay employing the substrate 2′-(4-methylumbelliferyl) α-D-*N*-acetylneuraminide (MUN)[18,30–32]. The HI evaluation methodology[18,33] utilized both guinea pig red blood cells (gp RBC) and human red blood cells (h RBC) to determine virus-mediated agglutination of erythrocytes.

A comparison of the potency of the synthesized C4-modified Neu5Ac2en derivatives against hPIV-3 HN was undertaken and, for convenience sake, the IC_{50} values were divided into two groups based on the acylamino group present at C5. Group 1 inhibitors have a C5 acetamido functionality and Group 2 inhibitors have a C5 isobutyramido functionality (Fig. 4, Supplementary Fig. 4 and Supplementary Table 2). The benchmark and well-characterized broad spectrum neuraminidase inhibitor Neu5Ac2en (**2**) showed the weakest inhibition with IC_{50} values of 1,565 μM and 1,438 μM for hPIV-3 HN NI and HI, respectively. The inhibition observed for **3**, the C5 acetamido analogue of BCX 2798 (**6**), was improved when compared with **2**, although it was still in the high micromolar range with IC_{50} values of 138 μM and 210 μM for hPIV-3 HN NI and HI, respectively. These IC_{50} values were similar to those observed for our novel inhibitor **7**, a C4 methoxymethyl-functionalized triazole Neu5Ac2en derivative, with experimentally determined hPIV-3 HN NI and HI IC_{50} values of 154 and 313 μM, respectively. A significant improvement in potency was observed on replacement of the C4 triazole's methoxymethyl moiety (**7**) with a bulkier phenyl group (**8**). IC_{50} values of 6.5 and 4.6 μM were determined for hPIV-3 HN NI and HI for **8**, respectively.

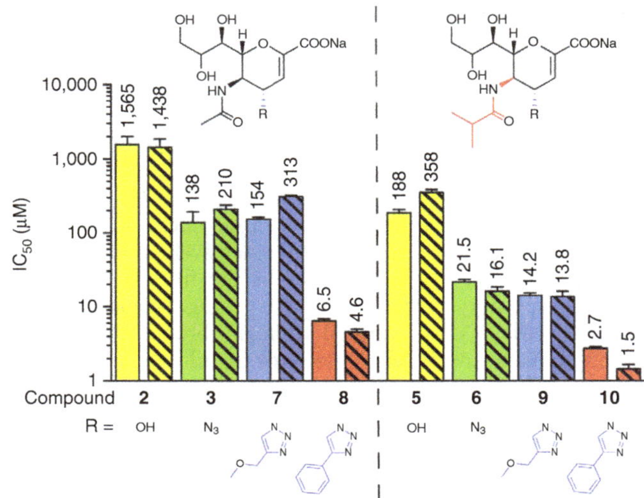

Figure 4 | NI (solid) and HI (dashed) IC_{50} values for the Neu5Ac2en derivatives 2, 3, 5–10. Inhibitors **2**, **3**, **7**, **8** with a C5 acetamido group (left panel, group 1) and inhibitors **5**, **6**, **9**, **10** with a C5 isobutyramido group (right panel, group 2). These values are the means of determinations from three independent experiments and error bars correspond to calculated s.d.

In the second group of inhibitors, which contain a C5 isobutyramido functionality, it was obvious that the affinity of each inhibitor was improved relative to its C5 acetamido analogue. The order of potency, not unexpectedly, was identical within the same group. Thus, the weakest inhibition was found for **5**, the C5 isobutyramido analogue of Neu5Ac2en, with IC_{50} values of 188 and 358 μM for NI and HI, respectively, and IC_{50} values of 21.5 and 16.1 μM for NI and HI, respectively, were determined for the reference hPIV inhibitor BCX 2798 (**6**). Inhibitor **9**, with the relatively small methoxymethyl substituent on the triazole ring, had IC_{50} values close to those determined for the C4 azido analogue **6** (IC_{50} = 14.2 and 13.8 μM for NI and HI, respectively). Similarly, as observed in the C5 acetamido-containing Group 1 inhibitors, increasing the substituent size from the methoxymethyl group in inhibitor **9** to a bulkier phenyl moiety as in inhibitor **10** resulted in a remarkable improvement in potency with IC_{50} values of 2.7 and 1.5 μM for NI and HI, respectively. Interestingly, an improvement in HI IC_{50} values was observed when h RBCs were used instead of gp RBCs (Supplementary Fig. 5). This improvement most likely reflects sialic acid content and/or linkage presentation differences between human and guinea pig red blood cells. For example, it is well known that human tissues and cells, including red blood cells, only express *N*-acetylneuraminic acid-containing glycoconjugate receptors, whereas other animals also express *N*-glycolylneuraminic acid-based receptors[34,35]. Nevertheless, irrespective of the specific red blood cells used, our designer inhibitor **10** had significantly higher potency when compared with the benchmark compound **6**. Finally, we have also determined (Supplementary Methods) a K_m value for MUN of 5.1 mM and K_i values of 1.3 and 16 μM for inhibitors **10** and **6**, respectively.

Cell-based assays. Following initial enzymatic screening, the most potent inhibitor **10** and the reference hPIV inhibitor (BCX 2798, **6**) were then evaluated in a growth inhibition assay to compare their capacity to inhibit hPIV-3 virus infection and propagation in LLC-MK2 cells (Supplementary Fig. 6). Compound **6** was chosen as a reference inhibitor as it is the most documented hPIV-3 Neu5Ac2en-based inhibitor to date and has reasonable *in vitro* hPIV-3 antiviral potency[18,21]. In an initial assay, at an inhibitor concentration of 2 μM, the virus was propagated for 48 h in the presence of **6** or **10** and virus titres were determined. At this inhibitor concentration, a reduction of 14 and 94% in virus titre by **6** and **10,** respectively, was calculated (Supplementary Fig. 6b). Virus growth inhibition IC_{50} values were then determined for the two inhibitors in a well-established *in situ* enzyme-linked immunosorbent assay (ELISA) technique[11] using three different cell lines. We chose LLC-MK2 (monkey kidney epithelial cells) cell line as it is extensively used in hPIV-3 cell-based infection studies[1] as well as the hPIV-3 susceptible human respiratory cell lines A549 (lung adenocarcinoma epithelial cells)[36] and normal human bronchial epithelial primary cells to investigate virus growth inhibition in natural tissue-related cells. The method itself has useful advantages over the virus titration method as it is a faster, one-step, non-subjective technique that correlates non-immobilized virus growth to HN expression levels of a low multiplicity of infection-infected cell monolayer. Interestingly, slightly lower virus growth inhibition IC_{50} values were determined for **10** and **6** with the laboratory-established cell line LLC-MK2 in relation to the human cell lines. Overall, the same trend is observed for all the three cell lines in that a significantly stronger antiviral effect of inhibitor **10** (IC_{50} = 2.1–13.9 μM) is determined compared with inhibitor **6** (IC_{50} = 54.6–130.6 μM) (Fig. 5).

Structural biology. Saturation Transfer Difference (STD) NMR experiments of **8** in complex with recombinantly expressed hPIV-3 HN (Supplementary Fig. 7) and the most potent inhibitor **10** in complex with either recombinantly expressed hPIV-3 HN (Fig. 6) or intact hPIV-3 virus (Supplementary Fig. 8) were undertaken to further support our computational and biological studies that demonstrated specific binding and inhibition.

STD NMR signal intensities for all protons associated with **8** or **10** were clearly observed, to varying extents, when the inhibitor is in complex with either intact virus or recombinant hPIV-3 HN and clearly demonstrated that the ligand binds in both instances. The minor signals visible at 3.25, 3.5 and 4.0 p.p.m. in the ^1H NMR spectrum of **10** acquired in the presence of intact virus particles were a consequence of impurities from the virus purification process and belong to neither the virus particles nor **10**. As anticipated, none of these signals were observed in the STD NMR spectrum and clearly demonstrate that the impurities do not bind to the virus (Supplementary Fig. 8).

These experiments clearly demonstrate the specific binding of **10** to both intact hPIV-3 virus and hPIV-3 HN, further substantiating the inhibitor's biological relevance and potential.

Importantly, an overlay of the aromatic phenyl protons signals observed at 7.1–7.6 p.p.m. in the STD NMR spectra for both the intact virus and recombinant HN protein also reveals that the binding epitope of inhibitor **10** is similar, if not identical, when bound either to intact hPIV-3 virus or to recombinant hPIV-3 HN protein (Supplementary Fig. 9).

Epitope mapping of inhibitor 10. A complete ligand-binding epitope was determined by the analysis of STD NMR spectra (Fig. 6) of hPIV-3 HN protein in complex with **10**. All STD NMR signals of **10** were normalized to the strongest STD NMR signal observed, the inhibitor's H4′ proton at 7.18 p.p.m. Relative STD NMR effects for all protons of the inhibitor were then calculated (Supplementary Table 3). The extent of the STD NMR signal intensity strongly depends on the proton's proximity to the protein surface and reveals how the designed inhibitor **10** engages the HN protein's binding site.

Notably, very strong relative STD NMR effects were observed for the phenyl group protons H2′, H3′, H4′, H5′and H6′ between 7.1 and 7.6 p.p.m. revealing a close contact in that region of the molecule to the protein surface. Moreover, a significant STD NMR effect was likewise detected for the CH of the triazole moiety. In contrast, the C5 isobutyramido moiety's protons of the inhibitor showed less effect (relative STD NMR signal intensities in the range of 42–54%).

Interestingly, the protons associated with the Neu5Ac2en core structure of **10** displayed variable relative STD NMR effects. A significant H3-relative STD NMR signal intensity (80%) suggests a strong interaction of this part of the molecule with hPIV-3 HN. Furthermore, relative STD NMR signal intensities for H4, H5 and H6 of 59, 50 and 49%, respectively, demonstrate that the ring protons of the Neu5Ac2en core structure are also involved in inhibitor engagement to the protein.

Finally, weaker relative STD NMR effects of 36, 35, 24 and 21%, were observed for the glycerol side chain protons H7, H8, H9 and H9′, respectively, and suggest that the glycerol side chain makes less of a contribution to the inhibitor-binding event compared with the C4 triazolo functionality and the inhibitor's core ring structure (Fig. 6).

The inhibitor **8** epitope map (Supplementary Fig. 7) was for all intents and purposes identical to that of inhibitor **10**, with the C4 triazolo moiety clearly in close contact to the protein surface.

Discussion

We have utilized MD simulations to verify the possibility, and to design and study the effect, of accommodating a Neu5Ac2en-based inhibitor with a bulky C4 substituent in the binding pocket of hPIV-3 HN. Previous MD studies[24] on this protein have demonstrated the existence of a flexible loop, the 216 loop, which can adopt an open conformation creating a larger cavity in the region of the Neu5Ac2en C4 hydroxyl group. Our detailed MD simulations in the current study clearly demonstrate that substantially larger substituents at the C4 position of Neu5Ac2en

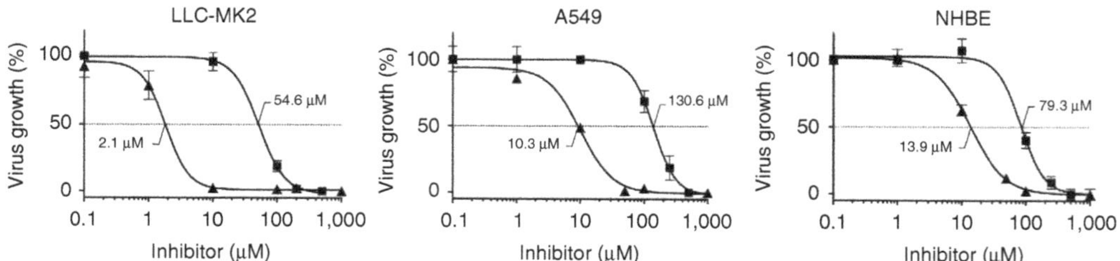

Figure 5 | Virus growth inhibition of the reference inhibitor 6 (■) and inhibitor 10 (▲) in various cell lines. Virus growth IC_{50} values of compounds **6** (■) and **10** (▲) were determined by an *in situ* ELISA technique against both human cell lines (A549 and NHBE) and a monkey kidney cell line (LLC-MK2). IC_{50} values of 54.6 ± 3.8 μM and 2.1 ± 0.6 μM (LLC-MK2); 130.6 ± 13.0 μM and 10.3 ± 0.3 μM (A549); 79.3 ± 1.0 μM and 13.9 ± 0.7 μM (NHBE) were determined for **6** and **10,** respectively. These values were determined from at least two independent experiments performed in triplicate and error bars correspond to the calculated s.d.

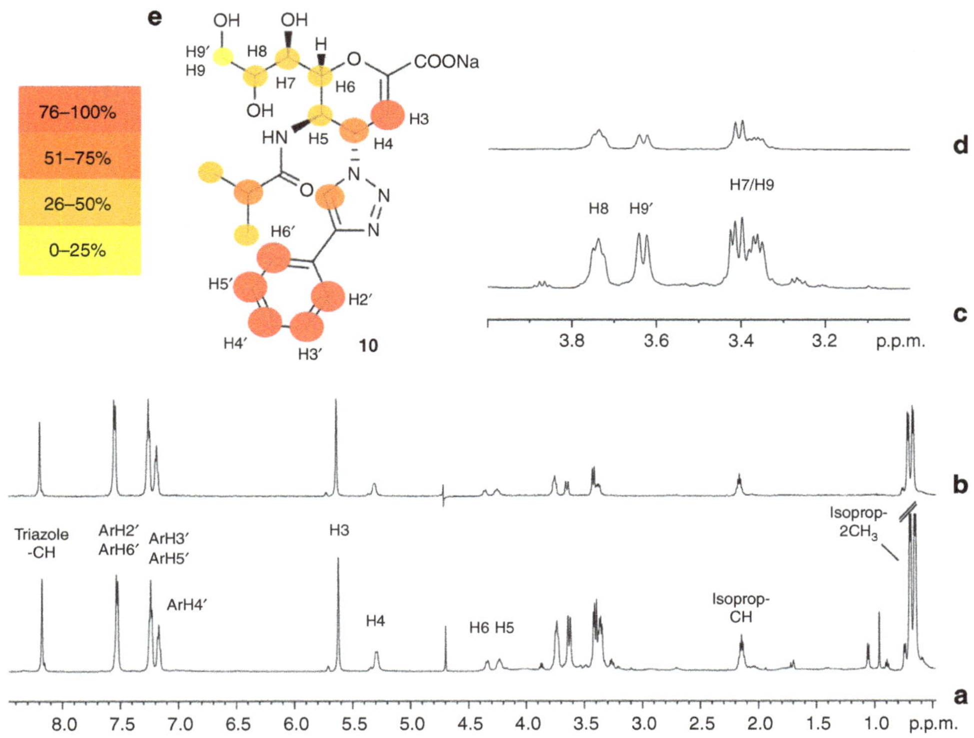

Figure 6 | ^{1}H and STD NMR spectra and epitope map of 10 in complex with hPIV-3 HN. (**a**) ^{1}H NMR spectrum of **10**. (**b**) STD NMR spectrum of **10** in the presence of 20 μM hPIV-3 HN at a protein:ligand ratio of 1:100 (2 mM of **10**). (**c**) ^{1}H NMR spectrum of the H7, H8, H9 and H9′ regions. (**d**) STD NMR spectrum of the H7, H8, H9 and H9′ regions. (**e**) Proposed binding epitope map of inhibitor **10**.

(**2**) may be accommodated in the hPIV-3 HN's active site. The accommodation of bulkier C4 substituents is achieved by the C4 functionality occupying the 216 cavity and locking open the 216 loop. Furthermore, our simulations predict that the binding of such C4-functionalized inhibitors is highly efficient and should result in potent inhibition of hPIV-3 HN. For example, a ΔE_{avI} of $-212.50\,\mathrm{kJ\,mol^{-1}}$ between **10** and the extensively studied neuraminidase inhibitor **2** in complex with hPIV-3 HN was calculated and confirms the positive influence on E_{avI} for the combined C4/C5 modification on the Neu5Ac2en template.

To experimentally validate our theoretical predictions, we successfully synthesized, in less than 10 steps, the designed C4- and C5-functionalized Neu5Ac2en inhibitors **8** and **10** from commercially available starting materials in very good overall yield. Our synthetic strategy towards these novel inhibitors provides great versatility for additional functionalization and enables further exploration of the Neu5Ac2en template in inhibitor optimization studies.

The biological evaluation of the reference and novel designer C4- and C5-functionalized Neu5Ac2en inhibitors using protein-based inhibition assays (NI and HI) led to a number of conclusions concerning the influence of C4 and C5 substituents on inhibitor potency. Within each of the two screened groups, that is Group 1 (C5 acetamido) and Group 2 (C5 isobutyramido), the order of potency based on the substituent at C4 was found to be as follows: hydroxyl < azido ≤ 4-methoxymethyltriazole < 4-phenyltriazole. The weakest inhibition in both groups was observed for the 4-hydroxy derivatives **2** and **5**. This outcome supports the notion that the C4-binding domain, which accommodates the C4 hydroxyl group on Neu5Ac2en (**2**), has significant hydrophobic character and consequently does not favour the interaction with a polar, hydrophilic group including a hydroxyl group[25]. The hydrophobic nature of the pocket, combined with the large 216 cavity size created by the opening of the 216 loop, does favour inhibitors, including inhibitors **8** and **10**, which have the C4 hydroxyl group replaced with bulky hydrophobic substituents.

Comparison of both group's IC_{50} values (Fig. 4) revealed that replacement of the C5 acetamido group with an isobutyramido group in all of the prepared inhibitors led to overall enhanced potency. Typically, close to an order of magnitude improvement was observed, except for the most potent inhibitor **10**. Furthermore, analysis of the IC_{50} values (Fig. 4) supports the notion that the potency enhancement in the best inhibitors, **8** and **10**, results predominantly from the introduction of the C4 substituent, with the C5 substituent contributing to a much lesser extent. This notion is also substantiated by STD NMR data analysis (Fig. 6) that led to an epitope map of inhibitor **10** in which the protons of the 4-phenyltriazole moiety showed the strongest contribution to the binding event of **10** in complex with hPIV-3 HN, while the relative interactions observed for the isobutyramido group were significantly less (~50%).

Further comparison of the various groups of inhibitors provided relative IC_{50} improvement factors for both NI and HI as detailed (Supplementary Fig. 4). Interestingly, a comparison of the parent templates **2** and **5**, which contain a C4 hydroxyl group, with their corresponding C4-functionalized derivatives **8** and **10**, respectively, shows dramatic HI improvement on C4 functionalization. The trend in the increase in NI is similar to that observed for HI; for example, inhibitors **5**, **6** and **9** had a 5–20-fold enhancement in potency by increasing the size of the C5 substituent from an acetamido to an isobutyramido functionality. However, a comparison of the potential NI and HI improvement factors also suggests that when a bulky C4 substituent is present, as in **8** and **10**, the introduction of the bulkier C5 isobutyramido moiety (**10**) improves potency to a lesser extent, by only a factor of two to three compared with the acetamido moiety (**8**). The consequence of locking the 216 cavity open by the bulky

C4-functionalized derivative is positional changes of amino acid side chains associated with the active site domains that recognize the C4 and C5 functionalities on *N*-acetylneuraminic acid (**1**) and its various unsaturated derivatives. These changes appear to equally accommodate the smaller C5 acetamido substituent and the bulkier C5 isobutyramido functionality.

The potent inhibition of both HN functions (NI and HI) by inhibitor **10** demonstrates that the compound exerts its antiviral effect against hPIV-3 by action on the virus' key HN protein. These findings are further supported by STD NMR experiments of **10** in complex with either the intact virus or the recombinant HN protein, which clearly show identical STD NMR signal intensities for the inhibitor's C4 triazole aromatic moiety (Supplementary Figs 8 and 9). Moreover, the calculated binding epitope for **10** in complex with hPIV-3 HN (Supplementary Table 3) is in excellent agreement with our MD simulations that clearly predict the close contact of the Neu5Ac2en derivative's H3 and the C4 triazolo moiety's phenyl protons to the protein surface (Fig. 3c). Furthermore, the *in situ* ELISA results (Fig. 5) were in good agreement with the NI and HI assay data. Interestingly, the LLC-MK2 cell-based assays demonstrated that **10** is even more potent at the cellular level compared with NI and HI protein-based assays. In this cell-based assay, **10** was found to be ~26 times more potent than **6**, whereas protein inhibition assays showed only ~8 and 11-fold improvement in NI and HI assays, respectively (Supplementary Fig. 4). This strongly suggests that **10** is a potent dual-acting inhibitor that derives efficient synergism from the inhibition of both the protein's neuraminidase and haemagglutinin activities. This is in contrast to the previously reported inhibitor **6**, which derives less synergistic effect as a result of its significantly poorer inhibition of the haemagglutinin activity. Finally, the extent of virus growth inhibition in both human cell lines for inhibitor **10** compared with **6** clearly demonstrates the superiority of the designer ligand **10** (Fig. 5).

In conclusion, we have taken advantage of the hPIV-3 HN 216 loop flexibility[24]. On the basis of the notion that the 216 cavity, created by loop movement, is of sufficient size to accommodate larger functionalities at C4 on the Neu5Ac2en-based template, we designed and synthesized inhibitors **7–10** that incorporate a bulky substituted triazolo substituent at C4. Our predicted efficient occupation of the HN active site and the proposed 216 cavity by these new bulky inhibitors translated to potent inhibition of both HN functions, as well as significant blockade of virus propagation. Moreover, our predicted trend in overall interaction energies of inhibitors **2**, **8** and **10** with hPIV-3 HN is confirmed by experimentally determined IC_{50} values and further demonstrates the power of structure-guided inhibitor design. The novel designer potent inhibitor **10** efficiently locks open the 216 loop and provides an exciting template for further hPIV-3 HN dual-acting inhibitor development. Finally, we have found that these inhibitors efficiently block both virus cell entry and virion progeny release and provide new direction towards anti-parainfluenza drug development.

Methods

MD simulations. MD simulations were performed with GROMOS software[37,38] using the force-field parameter set 54A4 (ref. 39). Initial coordinates were taken from the X-ray structure (PDB accession code 1V3E) (ref. 25) of hPIV-3 HN in complex with **4**. Compound **8** has been superimposed on zanamivir (**4**) ring atoms from the crystal structure. Parameters for **8** were generated in an analogous manner[40] to existing parameters in the GROMOS force field (Supplementary Table 1a–e). The number of atoms in the final composite system for 1V3E–**4** and IV3E–**8** was 78,253 and 78,084, respectively. Ionization states of amino acid residues were assigned at pH 7.0. The histidine side chains were protonated at the N_ε atom. Water molecules associated with the X-ray structure were removed, and replaced by explicit solvation using the simple point charge water model[41] and periodic boundary conditions, consistent with our previously published methodology[24]. In the simulations, water molecules were added around the protein within a truncated octahedron with a minimum distance of 1.4 nm between the protein atoms and the square walls of the periodic box. All bonds were constrained with a geometric tolerance of 10^{-4} using the SHAKE algorithm[42].

A steepest descent energy minimization of the system was performed to relax the solute–solvent contacts while positionally restraining the solute atoms using a harmonic interaction with a force constant of 2.5×10^4 kJ mol^{-1} nm^{-2}. Next, steepest descent energy minimization of the system without any restraints was performed to eliminate any residual strain. The energy minimizations were terminated when the energy change per step became smaller than 0.1 kJ mol^{-1}. For non-bonded interactions, a triple-range method with cutoff radii of 0.8/1.4 nm was used. Short-range van der Waals and electrostatic interactions were evaluated at each time step, based on a charge-group pair list. Medium-range van der Waals and electrostatic interactions, between (charge group) pairs at a distance longer than 0.8 nm and shorter than 1.4 nm, were evaluated every fifth time step, at which point the pair list was updated. Outside the longer cutoff radius, a reaction-field approximation[43] was used with a relative dielectric permittivity of 78.5. The centre of mass motion of the whole system was removed every 1,000 time steps. Solvent and solute were independently weakly coupled to a temperature bath of 295 K with a relaxation time of 0.1 ps (ref. 44).

The systems were also weakly coupled to a pressure bath of 1 atm with a relaxation time of 0.5 ps and an isothermal compressibility of 0.7513×10^{-3} (kJ mol^{-1} nm^{-3})$^{-1}$. MD simulations of 20 ps periods with harmonic position restraining of the solute atoms and force constants of 2.5×10^4, 2.5×10^3, 2.5×10^2 and 2.5×10^1 kJ mol^{-1} nm^{-2} were performed to further equilibrate the systems at 50, 120, 180, 240 and 300 K, respectively. The simulations were each carried out for 30 ns. The trajectory coordinates and energies were saved every 0.5 ps for analysis.

Simulation trajectories for hPIV-3 HN in complex with **4** were produced in an analogous manner to that described above[24] and were used for analysis and comparison of results obtained for hPIV-3 HN in complex with **8**.

Analyses were done with the analysis software GROMOS++ (ref. 45). Atom-positional r.m.s.d. between structures were calculated for the residues comprising the 216 loop (residues 210–221) by performing a rotational and translational atom-positional least-squares fit of one structure on the second (reference) structure using a given set of atoms (N, C_α, C).

Atom-positional r.m.s.f. were calculated as an average from a 30-ns period of simulation by performing a rotational and translational atom-positional least-squares fit of the C_α atoms of the trajectory structures on the reference. r.m.s.f. were calculated for all residues including the 216 loop (residues 210–221). To obtain reduced, representative structural ensembles for the simulations, r.m.s.d.-based conformational clustering was performed[46].

Structures extracted every 10 ps from simulations were superimposed on backbone-C_α atoms to remove overall rotation and translation. Clustering of all atoms of residues that line the binding site (residues 190–198, 210–221, 251–259, 274–280, 320–326, 334–339, 369–377, 407–413, 474–480 and 529–533) was performed to compare relative structural populations of hPIV-3 HN protein from the different simulation trajectories. The similarity criterion applied was the r.m.s.d. of all atoms of these residues with a cutoff of 0.13 nm. Final structures resulting from the 30 ns of MD simulations were extracted. Interaction energies between hPIV-3 HN and inhibitors **8** and **10** were calculated using GROMOS generated energies, free-energy λ derivatives and block averages as separate trajectory files, referred to as the energy trajectory[45]. The programme *ene_ana*[45] was used to extract individual interaction energy values such as non-bonded contributions, that is, van der Waals and Coulomb interactions from these files. Thus, these contributions between the ligand and the protein were extracted from the energy trajectory resulting from the simulation and interaction energies calculated. The error estimate was calculated from block averages of growing sizes extrapolating to infinite block size. Hydrophobic interactions were analysed and a map of interactions between inhibitor **10** and hPIV-3 HN was created using LIGPLOT[47]. To measure the extent of cavity opening for selected structures, the pocket volume was analysed using POVME[48]. Importantly, extended simulation times, up to 80 ns provided outcomes entirely consistent with the data presented.

Chemistry. *Synthesis of intermediates.* The synthesis of intermediates **11** (ref. 28), **12** (ref. 29) and **17–24** (ref. 29) and reference inhibitors **2** (ref. 49), **3** (ref. 50), **5** (ref. 29) and **6** (ref. 29) was achieved by the relevant literature procedure. General methods are described in the Supplementary Methods.

*General procedure for the synthesis of **18** and **19**.* A mixture of **17** or **11** (0.42 mmol), Boc_2O (275 mg, 1.27 mmol) and 4-Dimethylaminopyridine (50 mg, 0.42 mmol) in anhydrous tetrahydrofuran (5 ml) was stirred under argon atmosphere at 60 °C o/n (Supplementary Fig. 1). After cooling to RT, the solvent was evaporated under vacuum, and the residue was taken up in dichloromethane (DCM) for chromatographic separation on a silica gel column using ethyl acetate:hexane (1:2) as solvent to yield pure **18** (170 mg, 71%) or **19** (225 mg, 96%).

*General procedure for the synthesis of **20** and **21**.* To a methanolic solution of NaOMe, freshly prepared by dissolving sodium metal (0.39 mmol, 9 mg) in anhydrous MeOH (5 ml), was added compound **18** or **19** (0.26 mmol) (Supplementary Fig. 1). The mixture was stirred at RT for 1 h and then quenched with Amberlite IR-120 (H^+) resin (to pH=5). The resin was filtered off, washed with MeOH (5 ml × 3) and the combined filtrate and washings were evaporated under vacuum. The residue was redissolved in pyridine (2 ml), and acetic anhydride (0.5 ml) added. The reaction mixture was stirred at RT under argon atmosphere o/n and the solvent and excess Ac_2O were then removed under vacuum. Finally, the residue was taken up in DCM for chromatographic separation on a silica gel column using ethyl acetate:hexane (1:2) as solvent to yield pure **20** (112 mg, 81%) or **21** (84 mg, 63%).

General procedure for the synthesis of 22 and 23. To a solution of **20** or **21** (0.15 mmol) in anhydrous DCM (2 ml) was added TFA (230 µl, 3.0 mmol) and the mixture was stirred at RT under argon o/n (Supplementary Fig. 1). The reaction was diluted with DCM (20 ml) and quenched with saturated aqueous $NaHCO_3$ solution (20 ml). The DCM layer was washed with water and brine and then dried over anhydrous Na_2SO_4. The dried organic solvent was concentrated under vacuum, and purified by silica gel chromatography using the suitable solvent system to yield pure **22** (58 mg, 90%) or **23** (53 mg, 85%).

General procedure for the synthesis of 24 and 12. To a solution of **22** or **23** (0.116 mmol) in DCM (2 ml) under argon was added Et_3N (82 µl, 0.58 mmol) and isobutyryl chloride (18 µl, 0.17 mmol; Supplementary Fig. 1). The mixture was stirred at RT for 4 h and then loaded on a silica gel column for chromatographic separation using ethyl acetate:hexane (1:1) as solvent to yield pure **24** (50 mg, 84%) or **12** (51 mg, 91%).

General procedure for the synthesis of 5 and 6. To a suspension of compound **24** or **12** (0.08 mmol) in a 1:1 mixture of MeOH:H_2O (2 ml) at 0 °C was added dropwise a NaOH solution (1.0 M) until pH ~14 (Supplementary Fig. 1). The temperature was raised gradually to RT and the mixture was stirred at RT overnight. The solution was then acidified with Amberlite IR-120 (H^+) resin (to pH=5), filtered and washed with MeOH (10 ml) and H_2O (10 ml). The combined filtrate and washings were then concentrated under vacuum and the residue was diluted with distilled water (5 ml) and adjusted to pH=8.0 using 0.05 M NaOH to convert the compound to its sodium salt. The compounds were then purified on a C18-GracePure cartridge using 2% acetonitrile/water as solvent to yield pure **5** (26 mg, 94%) or **6** (24 mg, 82%) as fluffy white powders.

General procedure for the synthesis of 13–16. The appropriate 4-azido-4-deoxy-Neu5Ac2en derivative (**11** or **12**, 0.22 mmol) and the corresponding ethynyl derivative (0.33 mmol) were dissolved in a 1:1 mixture of *tert*-butanol:H_2O (4 ml; Supplementary Fig. 2). Copper(II) sulfate pentahydrate (4 mg, 0.015 mmol) was added to the mixture followed by sodium ascorbate (0.1 ml of freshly prepared 1 M solution in H_2O). The mixture was stirred at 45 °C for 6 h and then left to cool at RT. The mixture was then diluted with DCM (100 ml), washed with 10% NH_4OH (50 ml), followed by brine (50 ml). The organic layer was dried over anhydrous Na_2SO_4 and concentrated under vacuum to give the crude products **13–16**, which were purified by silica gel chromatography using an appropriate solvent system (Supplementary Methods).

General procedure for the synthesis of 7–10. To a suspension of the protected triazole derivative **13–16** in a 1:1 mixture of MeOH:H_2O (2 ml) at 0 °C was added dropwise a NaOH solution (1.0 M) until pH ~14 (Supplementary Fig. 2). The temperature was gradually raised to RT and the mixture was stirred at RT overnight. The solution was then acidified with Amberlite IR-120 (H^+) resin (to pH=5), filtered and washed with MeOH (10 ml) and H_2O (10 ml). The combined filtrate and washings were then concentrated under vacuum, then diluted with distilled water (5 ml) and adjusted to pH=8.0 using 0.05 M NaOH to convert the compound to its sodium salt. Finally, the compound was purified on a C18-GracePure cartridge using 2% acetonitrile/water as solvent to yield the pure products **7–10**.

All novel compounds were appropriately characterized and were of high purity (Supplementary Methods and Supplementary Fig. 3a–t).

Biology. *Cells and virus.* A549 cells (adenocarcinomic human alveolar basal epithelial cells) were provided by the European Collection of Cell Cultures (86012804-1VL, Sigma-Aldrich). Cells were propagated in Dulbecco's Modified Eagle Medium (Lonza, Basel, Switzerland) supplemented with 1% Glutamine (200 mM) and 5% fetal bovine serum. For infection and post-infection procedures, A549 cells were maintained in Dulbecco's Modified Eagle Medium supplemented with 1% Glutamine only. Normal human bronchial/tracheal epithelial cells (CC-2540, lot 313831, Lonza) were amplified in B-ALI growth medium (Lonza) and the same medium was used for infection and post-infection studies. LLC-MK2 cells (Rhesus monkey kidney, ATCC CCL-7) were cultured in Eagle's minimal essential medium (EMEM) (Lonza) supplemented with 1% Glutamine (200 mM) and 2% of heat-inactivated fetal bovine serum. During hPIV-3 infection and post-infection incubation, LLC-MK2 cells were maintained in EMEM supplemented with 1% glutamine. All cell lines were incubated at 37 °C in a humidified atmosphere of 5% CO_2.

hPIV-3 (strain C-243) was obtained from the American Type Culture Collection (ATCC, Manassas, VA). The virus was propagated in LLC-MK2 cells with EMEM supplemented with glutamine ($EMEM_{inf}$) at 35 °C in a humidified atmosphere of 5% CO_2. Virus-containing culture supernatant was collected 3 to 4 days post infection, while monitoring cytopathic effects, and clarified from cell debris by centrifugation (3,000 r.c.f. for 15 min). Virus was concentrated at least 10 times using 30 kDa Amicon Ultra filter unit (Millipore, Billerica, MA) for use in HI assays. NI assays and STD NMR experiments used virus that was polyethylene glycol (PEG)-precipitated and then purified as described below.

Clarified hPIV-3 supernatant was mixed with PEG6000 (8% final concentration) and NaCl (0.4 M final concentration) and then incubated overnight at 4 °C under gentle agitation. PEG6000/hPIV-3 complex was pelleted by centrifugation at 3,000 r.c.f. for 30 min at 4 °C. The supernatant was discarded and a volume of GNTE buffer (glycine, 200 mM, NaCl, 200 mM, Tris-HCl, 20 mM, EDTA, 2 mM, pH 7.4) corresponding to at least 1:40 of the initial virus suspension volume was used to resuspend the pellet overnight at 4 °C. The virus suspension was homogenized by up and down pipetting followed by a mechanical disruption of the remaining virus aggregates using a douncer with 'tight' pestle. The hPIV-3 homogenate was loaded on top of a 30–60% non-linear sucrose gradient prepared in GNTE buffer and centrifuged at 100,000 r.c.f. for 2 h 30 min at 4 °C without brake for deceleration. The virus was concentrated at the 30–60% sucrose interface and then collected and stored at −80 °C for NI assays or at 4 °C for STD NMR experiments.

Recombinant HN expression and purification. The peptide sequence of hPIV-3 prototype strain C-243 was used as a reference to design a secreted and soluble recombinant HN protein based on a substantially modified (Supplementary Methods) literature procedure[25].

HI assay. Both human (h RBC) and guinea pig red blood cells (gp RBC) were used in the HI assay[18,33] and had high agglutination efficiency (Supplementary Methods).

NI assay. The purified hPIV-3 NA was assayed using a method adapted[50] (Supplementary Methods) from Potier *et al.*[30] and measured the relative fluorescence of 4-methylumbelliferone, the product of the enzymatic hydrolysis of MUN (Sigma-Aldrich, St Louis, MO).

Virus growth inhibition assay. Before assessing the best inhibitors in cell-based assays, an MTT (3-(4,5-dimethylthiazol-2-yl)-2,5-diphenyltetrazolium bromide) assay was performed to evaluate the compound cytotoxicity. No cytotoxic effect was observed after incubation for 48 h of LLC-MK2 cells with **6**, **8** and **10** at 303 µM, the highest concentration tested. Virus growth inhibition was assessed using a focus-forming assay[51] by titration of progeny in the presence of 2 µM of **6**, **8** and **10** in $EMEM_{inf}$ from a low multiplicity of infection-infected confluent LLC-MK2 monolayer in a 48-well plate format. Virus inoculum (100 focus-forming units per well) was preincubated with **6**, **8** and **10** for 20 min. Infection was performed in duplicate and continued for 1 h at 37 °C with gentle agitation every 15 min. Inocula were removed and replaced with 500 µl per well of each respective 2 µM compound dilution (in $EMEM_{inf}$). A positive control for infection was included using the same conditions minus the compound. Virus proliferation on infected cell monolayers were maintained for 48 h at 37 °C, 5% CO_2. Culture supernatants from duplicates were collected, pooled and clarified at 15,000 r.c.f. for 10 min and stored at −80 °C. Supernatants were diluted in $EMEM_{inf}$ by 10^{-3}, 10^{-4} and 10^{-5} to avoid any remaining compound effect on the subsequent virus titration. Virus titrations were done in duplicate using the previously described conditions for virus infection. After 1 h, Avicel (FMC BioPolymer, Philadelphia, PA) in $EMEM_{inf}$ was directly added to the inoculum (1% final concentration) to restrict and localize virus proliferation. The plate was incubated for 36 to 40 h at 37 °C, 5% CO_2 to allow focus formation. Avicel was gently removed and replaced with 3.7% paraformaldehyde/PBS and the plate was then kept for 15 min at RT for virus inactivation and cell fixation. Cell monolayers were washed three times for 5 min each with PBS and then endogenous peroxidase inactivated with 0.3% H_2O_2/PBS for 30 min at 37 °C. The plate was washed again three times for 5 min each with PBS and incubated with mouse monoclonal IgG anti-hPIV-3 HN (Fitzgerald, clone# M02122321, 2.0 mg ml^{-1}) at 1 µg ml^{-1} in 5% milk/PBS for 1 h at 37 °C. Cell monolayers were washed three times for 5 min with 0.02% Tween20/PBS. Goat anti-Mouse-IgG(H+L)-HRP conjugate (BioRad, ref# 170-6516) diluted at 1:1,000 in 5% milk/PBS was added to each well and incubated for 1 h at 37 °C. Cell monolayers were washed as previously described with 0.02% Tween20/PBS and then rinsed twice with PBS. Foci were revealed by adding TrueBlue solution (HRP substrate) on each well and incubating the plate for 1 h at 37 °C. The TrueBlue solution was discarded and the plate rinsed twice with water then dried before being scanned (Supplementary Fig. 5) and foci counted. The IC_{50} value was considered as the concentration of inhibitor that reduced the progeny virus titre by 50% compared with a non-treated infected LLC-MK2 monolayer.

In situ ELISA. In situ ELISA is another technique used in drug discovery to evaluate virus growth inhibition[11,52–55]. This technique is highly sensitive and reliable as it measures, in one step, the expression level of hPIV-3 HN at the cell surface of an infected cell monolayer. The expression level is directly correlated to the ability of a non-immobilized virus to infect and reinfect target cells. Infection was performed on a confluent cell monolayer seeded in a 96-well plate. Virus (40 focus-forming units per well) was preincubated for 20 min with compound **6** and **10** at a final concentration from 1,000 µM to 0.001 µM as a 10-fold dilution series. Infection was done in triplicate and continued for 1 h at 37 °C with gentle agitation every 15 min. Inocula were removed and replaced with 200 µl per well of each respective compound dilution. A positive control for infection was incorporated by the use of identical experimental conditions, minus inhibitor. Infected cell monolayers were kept for 36–40 h at 37 °C, 5% CO_2 for virus proliferation. Virus was inactivated and cells fixed by the direct addition of 100 µl of 11.1% paraformaldehyde/PBS. The plate was maintained at RT for 15 min and then washed 3 times for 5 min with PBS and then endogenous peroxidases were inactivated by treatment with 0.3% H_2O_2/PBS for 30 min at 37 °C.
The cell monolayers were washed and incubated with mouse monoclonal IgG

anti-hPIV-3 HN (Fitzgerald, clone# M02122321, 2.0 mg ml^{-1}) at 1 µg ml^{-1} in 5% milk/PBS for 1 h at 37 °C. The wells were washed three times for 5 min with 0.02% Tween20/PBS. Goat anti-Mouse-IgG(H+L)-HRP conjugate (BioRad, ref# 170-6516), diluted at 1:2,000 in 5% milk/PBS, was added to each well and incubated for 1 h at 37 °C. Cell monolayers were washed with 0.02% Tween20/PBS and then rinsed twice with PBS. BD OptEIA TMB substrate (BD Biosciences, San Jose, CA, 100 µl) was added to each well and the plate was then incubated at 37 °C. The enzymatic reaction was stopped after 3–5 min by the addition of 50 µl of 0.6 M of H_2SO_4 per well. Raw data were obtained by reading the absorbance (OD) of each well at 450 nm for 0.1 s with a Victor 3 multilabel reader (PerkinElmer, Waltham, MA). Final ODs were obtained by subtraction of the negative control (non-infected cells) OD from the initial OD reading and the data analysed with GraphPadPrism4 (GraphPad Software, Inc., La Jolla, CA) to calculate IC_{50} values (non-linear regression (curve fit), Dose–response inhibition, four-parameter logistic). The IC_{50} value was considered as the concentration of inhibitor that reduced the absorbance at 450 nm by 50%, compared with a non-treated infected cell monolayer.

Standard deviation calculations. Standard deviations were calculated with GraphPadPrism4 (GraphPad Software, Inc., La Jolla, CA).

Structural biology. *Sample preparation and ^1H NMR experiments.* All NMR experiments were performed on a 600 MHz NMR spectrometer (Bruker) equipped with a 5-mm TXI probe with triple axis gradients. Intact virus suspension or recombinant hPIV-3 HN were buffer exchanged against 50 mM deuterated sodium acetate, 5 mM $CaCl_2$ in D_2O at pD 4.6 by ultrafiltration using an Amicon Filter Unit (Millipore) with a cutoff value of 30 or 10 kDa, respectively. For each experiment, 20 µM hPIV-3 HN protein and a protein:ligand molar ratio of 1:100 in a final volume of 200 µl was used.

^1H NMR spectra were acquired with 32 scans at 283 K, a 2-s relaxation delay over a spectral width of 6,000 Hz. An initial STD NMR experiment was performed on a complex between compound **10** and intact hPIV-3 virus and all subsequent STD NMR experiments were performed on compounds in complex with recombinant hPIV-3 HN protein.

STD NMR experiments. The protein was saturated on-resonance at − 1.0 p.p.m. and off-resonance at 300 p.p.m. with a cascade of 60 selective Gaussian-shaped pulses of 50 ms duration, resulting in a total saturation time of 3 s and the relaxation delay was set to 4 s. Each STD NMR experiment was acquired either with a total of 1,056 scans (recombinant hPIV-3 HN) or 1,512 scans (intact virus) and a WATERGATE sequence was used to suppress the residual HDO signal. A Spin-lock filter with 5 kHz strength and duration of 10 ms was applied to suppress protein background. Control STD NMR experiments were performed with an identical experimental setup and the same ligand concentration but in the absence of protein. On- and off-resonance spectra were stored and processed separately, and the final STD NMR spectra were obtained by subtracting the on- from the off-resonance spectra. All STD effects were quantified using the equation $A_{STD}=(I_0-I_{sat})/I_0=I_{STD}/I_0$. Therefore, signal intensities of the STD NMR spectrum (I_{STD}) were compared with the corresponding signal intensities of a reference spectrum (I_0). The strongest STD signal in the spectrum was assigned to a value of 100% and used as a reference to calculate relative STD effects accordingly[56–58].

References

1. Henrickson, K. J. Parainfluenza viruses. *Clin. Microbiol. Rev.* **16,** 242–264 (2003).
2. Glezen, W. P. & Denny, F. W. in *Viral Infection of Humans: Epidemiology and Control* 4th edn, Ch. 19 (eds Evans, A. S. & Kaslow, R. A.) 551–568 (Plenum Press, 1997).
3. Nichols, W. G., Peck Campbell, A. J. & Boeckh, M. Respiratory viruses other than influenza virus: impact and therapeutic advances. *Clin. Microbiol. Rev.* **21,** 274–290 (2008).
4. Reed, G., Jewett, P. H., Thompson, J., Tollefson, S. & Wright, P. F. Epidemiology and clinical impact of parainfluenza virus infections in otherwise healthy infants and young children <5 years old. *J. Infect. Dis.* **175,** 807–813 (1997).
5. Heilman, C. A. From the National Institute of Allergy and Infectious Diseases and the World Health Organization. Respiratory syncytial and parainfluenza viruses. *J. Infect. Dis.* **161,** 402–406 (1990).
6. Henrickson, K. J., Kuhn, S. M. & Savatski, L. L. Epidemiology and cost of infection with human parainfluenza virus types 1 and 2 in young children. *Clin. Infect. Dis.* **18,** 770–779 (1994).
7. Denny, F. W. & Clyde, W. A. J. Acute lower respiratory tract infections in non-hospitalized children. *J. Pediatr.* **108,** 635–646 (1986).
8. Sato, M. & Wright, P. F. Current status of vaccines for parainfluenza virus infections. *Pediatr. Infect. Dis. J.* **27,** S123–S125 (2008).
9. De La Mora, P. & Moscona, A. A daring treatment and a successful outcome: the need for targeted therapies for pediatric respiratory viruses. *Pediatr. Transplant.* **11,** 121–123 (2007).
10. Karron, R. A. *et al.* Evaluation of two chimeric bovine-human parainfluenza virus type 3 vaccines in infants and young children. *Vaccine* **30,** 3975–3981 (2012).
11. Moscona, A. *et al.* A recombinant sialidase fusion protein effectively inhibits human parainfluenza viral infection *in vitro* and *in vivo*. *J. Infect. Dis.* **202,** 234–241 (2010).
12. Porotto, M., Palmer, S. G., Palermo, L. M. & Moscona, A. Mechanism of fusion triggering by human parainfluenza virus type III: communication between viral glycoproteins during entry. *J. Biol. Chem.* **287,** 778–793 (2012).
13. Moscona, A. Entry of parainfluenza virus into cells as a target for interrupting childhood respiratory disease. *J. Clin. Invest.* **115,** 1688–1698 (2005).
14. Amonsen, M., Smith, D. F., Cummings, R. D. & Air, G. M. Human parainfluenza viruses hPIV1 and hPIV3 bind oligosaccharides with alpha2-3-linked sialic acids that are distinct from those bound by H5 avian influenza virus hemagglutinin. *J. Virol.* **81,** 8341–8345 (2007).
15. Song, X. *et al.* A sialylated glycan microarray reveals novel interactions of modified sialic acids with proteins and viruses. *J. Biol. Chem.* **286,** 31610–31622 (2011).
16. Alymova, I. V. *et al.* Receptor-binding specificity of the human parainfluenza virus type 1 hemagglutinin-neuraminidase glycoprotein. *Glycobiology* **22,** 174–180 (2012).
17. Palermo, L. M., Porotto, M., Greengard, O. & Moscona, A. Fusion promotion by a paramyxovirus hemagglutinin-neuraminidase protein: pH modulation of receptor avidity of binding sites I and II. *J. Virol.* **81,** 9152–9161 (2007).
18. Alymova, I. V. *et al.* Efficacy of novel hemagglutinin-neuraminidase inhibitors BCX 2798 and BCX 2855 against human parainfluenza viruses *in vitro* and *in vivo*. *Antimicrob. Agents Chemother.* **48,** 1495–1502 (2004).
19. Tindal, D. J. *et al.* Synthesis and evaluation of 4-*O*-alkylated 2-deoxy-2,3-didehydro-*N*-acetylneuraminic acid derivatives as inhibitors of human parainfluenza virus type-3 sialidase activity. *Bioorg. Med. Chem. Lett.* **17,** 1655–1658 (2007).
20. Alymova, I. V. *et al.* Efficacy of the novel parainfluenza virus haemagglutinin-neuraminidase inhibitor BCX 2798 in mice—further evaluation. *Antivir. Ther.* **14,** 891–898 (2009).
21. Watanabe, M. *et al.* Effect of hemagglutinin-neuraminidase inhibitors BCX 2798 and BCX 2855 on growth and pathogenicity of Sendai/human parainfluenza type 3 chimera virus in mice. *Antimicrob. Agents Chemother.* **53,** 3942–3951 (2009).
22. Nishino, R. *et al.* Syntheses of 2-deoxy-2,3-didehydro-*N*-acetylneuraminic acid analogues modified by *N*-sulfonylamidino groups at the C-4 position and biological evaluation as inhibitors of human parainfluenza virus type 1. *Bioorg. Med. Chem.* **19,** 2418–2427 (2011).
23. Nishino, R. *et al.* Syntheses of 2-deoxy-2,3-didehydro-*N*-acetylneuraminic acid analogues modified by α-acylaminoamido groups at the C-4 position using isocyanide-based four-component coupling and biological evaluation as inhibitors of human parainfluenza virus type 1. *Chem. Pharm. Bull. (Tokyo)* **61,** 69–74 (2013).
24. Winger, M. & von Itzstein, M. Exposing the flexibility of human parainfluenza virus hemagglutinin-neuraminidase. *J. Am. Chem. Soc.* **34,** 18447–18452 (2012).
25. Lawrence, M. C. *et al.* Structure of the haemagglutinin-neuraminidase from human parainfluenza virus type III. *J. Mol. Biol.* **335,** 1343–1357 (2004).
26. von Itzstein, M., Jin, B., Wu, W.-Y. & Chandler, M. A convenient method for the introduction of nitrogen and sulfur at C-4 on a sialic acid analogue. *Carbohydr. Res.* **244,** 181–185 (1993).
27. Lu, Y. & Gervay-Hague, J. Synthesis of C-4 and C-7 triazole analogs of zanamivir as multivalent sialic acid containing scaffolds. *Carbohydr. Res.* **342,** 1636–1650 (2007).
28. Li, J. *et al.* Syntheses of triazole-modified zanamivir analogues via click chemistry and anti-AIV activities. *Bioorg. Med. Chem. Lett.* **16,** 5009–5013 (2006).
29. Chand, P., Babu, Y. S., Rowland, S. R. & Lin, T.-H. Preparation of neuraminic acids and analogs useful for inhibiting paramyxovirus neuraminidase. PCT application WO2002076971 (2002).
30. Potier, M., Mameli, L., Bélisle, M., Dallaire, L. & Melançon, S. B. Fluorometric assay of neuraminidase with a sodium (4-methylumbelliferyl-alpha-D-*N*-acetylneuraminate) substrate. *Anal. Biochem.* **94,** 287–296 (1979).
31. Greengard, O., Poltoratskaia, N., Leikina, E., Zimmerberg, J. & Moscona, A. The anti-influenza virus agent 4-GU-DANA (zanamivir) inhibits cell fusion mediated by human parainfluenza virus and influenza virus HA. *J. Virol.* **74,** 11108–11114 (2000).
32. Suzuki, T. *et al.* Inhibition of human parainfluenza virus type 1 sialidase by analogs of 2-deoxy-2,3-didehydro-*N*-acetylneuraminic acid. *Glycoconj. J.* **18,** 331–337 (2001).
33. Suzuki, T. *et al.* Receptor specificities of human respiroviruses. *J. Virol.* **75,** 4604–4613 (2001).
34. Varki, A. Loss of *N*-glycolylneuraminic acid in humans: mechanisms, consequences, and implications for hominid evolution. *Am. J. Phys. Anthropol.* **116,** 54–69 (2001).
35. Bradley, K. C. *et al.* Analysis of influenza virus hemagglutinin receptor binding mutants with limited receptor recognition properties and conditional replication characteristics. *J. Virol.* **85,** 12387–12398 (2011).

36. Zhao, H., De, B. P., Das, T. & Banerjee, A. K. Inhibition of human parainfluenza virus-3 replication by interferon and human MxA. *Virology* **220,** 330–338 (1996).
37. van Gunsteren, W. F. *et al. Biomolecular Simulation: The GROMOS Manual and User Guide* (vdf Hochschulverlag, ETH Zürich, 1996).
38. Scott, W. R. P. *et al.* The GROMOS biomolecular simulation program package. *J. Phys. Chem. A* **103,** 3596–3607 (1999).
39. Schmid, N. *et al.* Definition and testing of the GROMOS force-field versions: 54A7 and 54B7. *Eur. Biophys. J.* **40,** 843–856 (2011).
40. Oostenbrink, C., Villa, A., Mark, A. E. & van Gunsteren, W. F. A biomolecular force field based on the free enthalpy of hydration and solvation: the GROMOS force-field parameter sets 53A5 and 53A6. *J. Comput. Chem.* **25,** 1656–1676 (2004).
41. Berendsen, H. J. C., Postma, J. P. M., van Gunsteren, W. F. & Hermans, J. in *Intermolecular Forces* (ed. Pullman, B.) 331–342 (Reidel, 1981).
42. Ryckaert, J.-P., Ciccotti, G. & Berendsen, H. J. C. Numerical integration of cartesian equations of motion of a system with constraints—molecular dynamics of n-alkanes. *J. Comput. Phys.* **23,** 327–341 (1977).
43. Tironi, I. G., Sperb, R., Smith, P. E. & van Gunsteren, W. F. A generalized reaction field method for molecular dynamics simulations. *J. Chem. Phys.* **102,** 5451–5459 (1995).
44. Berendsen, H. J. C., Postma, J. P. M., van Gunsteren, W. F., Di Nola, A. & Haak, J. R. Molecular dynamics with coupling to an external bath. *J. Chem. Phys.* **81,** 3684–3690 (1984).
45. Christen, M. *et al.* The GROMOS software for biomolecular simulation: GROMOS05. *J. Comput. Chem.* **26,** 1719–1751 (2005).
46. Daura, X., Jaun, B., Seebach, D., van Gunsteren, W. F. & Mark, A. E. Reversible peptide folding in solution by molecular dynamics simulation. *J. Mol. Biol.* **280,** 925–932 (1998).
47. Wallace, A. C., Laskowski, R. A. & Thornton, J. M. LIGPLOT: a program to generate schematic diagrams of protein-ligand interactions. *Protein Eng.* **8,** 127–134 (1996).
48. Durrant, J. D., de Oliveira, C. A. F. & McCammon, J. A. POVME: an algorithm for measuring binding-pocket volumes. *J. Mol. Graphics Modell.* **29,** 773–776 (2011).
49. Furuhata, K., Sato, S., Goto, M., Takayanagi, H. & Ogura, H. Studies on sialic acids. VII. The crystal and molecular structure of *N*-acetyl-2,3-dehydro-2-deoxyneuraminic acid. *Chem. Pharm. Bull.* **36,** 1872–1876 (1988).
50. Holzer, C. T. *et al.* Inhibition of sialidases from viral, bacterial and mammalian sources by analogues of 2-deoxy-2,3-didehydro-*N*-acetylneuraminic acid modified at the C-4 position. *Glycoconj. J.* **10,** 40–44 (1993).
51. Matrosovich, M., Matrosovich, T., Garten, W. & Klenk, H.-D. New low-viscosity overlay medium for viral plaque assays. *Virol. J.* **3,** 63 (2006).
52. Berkowitz, F. E. & Levin, M. J. Use of an enzyme-linked immunosorbent assay performed directly on fixed infected cell monolayers for evaluating drugs against varicella-zoster virus. *Antimicrob. Agents Chemother.* **28,** 207–210 (1985).
53. Ståhle, E. L. *et al.* Solid phase ELISA for determination of the virus dose dependent sensitivity of human cytomegalovirus to antiviral drugs in vitro. *Antiviral Res.* **40,** 105–112 (1998).
54. Myc, A., Anderson, M. J. & Baker, Jr J. R. Optimization of in situ cellular ELISA performed on influenza A virus-infected monolayers for screening of antiviral agents. *J. Virol. Methods* **77,** 165–177 (1999).
55. Koishi, A. C., Zanello, P. R., Bianco, É. M., Bordignon, J. & Nunes Duarte dos Santos, C. Screening of dengue virus antiviral activity of marine seaweeds by an *in situ* enzyme-linked immunosorbent assay. *PLoS ONE* **7,** e51089 (2012).
56. Mayer, M. & Meyer, B. Characterization of ligand binding by saturation transfer difference NMR spectroscopy. *Angew. Chem. Int. Ed.* **38,** 1784–1788 (1999).
57. Mayer, M. & Meyer, B. Group epitope mapping by saturation transfer difference NMR to identify segments of a ligand in direct contact with a protein receptor. *J. Am. Chem. Soc.* **123,** 6108–6117 (2001).
58. Haselhorst, T. *et al.* Recognition of the GM3 ganglioside glycan by Rhesus rotavirus particles. *Angew. Chem. Int. Ed.* **50,** 1055–1058 (2011).

Acknowledgements

The Australian Research Council (DP 1094549) is gratefully acknowledged for its financial support (M.v.I.) and for the award of an Australian Postdoctoral Award (P.G.). The National Health and Medical Research Council (ID 1047824) is thanked for its financial support (M.v.I.). Griffith University is gratefully acknowledged for the award of a Griffith University Postdoctoral Award (I.M.E.-D.). Finally, we are grateful for access to the Griffith University Gowonda High Performance Computing Cluster.

Author contributions

M.v.I. conceived and oversaw the project. I.M.E.-D. performed all of the described chemistry. M.W. performed all of the molecular dynamics simulation studies. P.G., L.D. and B.B. performed the biological experiments. J.C.D. contributed to the molecular modelling studies. P.G. and L.D. performed the STD NMR studies and T.H. provided advice and assisted in the analysis of these studies. All of the authors contributed to the design, analysis and discussion of the research and writing of the manuscript.

Additional information

Competing financial interests: The authors declare no competing financial interests.

5

An antioxidant nanozyme that uncovers the cytoprotective potential of vanadia nanowires

Amit A. Vernekar[1,*], Devanjan Sinha[2,*], Shubhi Srivastava[2], Prasath U. Paramasivam[1], Patrick D'Silva[2] & Govindasamy Mugesh[1]

Nanomaterials with enzyme-like properties has attracted significant interest, although limited information is available on their biological activities in cells. Here we show that V_2O_5 nanowires (Vn) functionally mimic the antioxidant enzyme glutathione peroxidase by using cellular glutathione. Although bulk V_2O_5 is known to be toxic to the cells, the property is altered when converted into a nanomaterial form. The Vn nanozymes readily internalize into mammalian cells of multiple origin (kidney, neuronal, prostate, cervical) and exhibit robust enzyme-like activity by scavenging the reactive oxygen species when challenged against intrinsic and extrinsic oxidative stress. The Vn nanozymes fully restore the redox balance without perturbing the cellular antioxidant defense, thus providing an important cytoprotection for biomolecules against harmful oxidative damage. Based on our findings, we envision that biocompatible Vn nanowires can provide future therapeutic potential to prevent ageing, cardiac disorders and several neurological conditions, including Parkinson's and Alzheimer's disease.

[1] Department of Inorganic and Physical Chemistry, Indian Institute of Science, Bangalore 560012, India. [2] Department of Biochemistry, Indian Institute of Science, Bangalore 560012, India. * These authors contributed equally to this work. Correspondence and requests for materials should be addressed to P.D. (email: patrick@biochem.iisc.ernet.in) or to G.M. (email: mugesh@ipc.iisc.ernet.in).

Reactive oxygen species (ROS), such as superoxide, hydroxyl radicals and hydrogen peroxide, are generated as byproducts of cellular metabolism and from the Nox/Duox family of membrane-bound NADPH-dependent oxidases[1,2]. At lower concentrations, ROS serve as critical second messengers in various signalling pathways, whereas at higher concentrations, they exhibit detrimental effects[3,4]. Enhanced ROS levels are associated with oxidative damage to lipid, protein, DNA and activation of apoptotic pathways through induction of caspases[5–7]. It is also responsible for several pathological conditions such as neurodegeneration, cancer, diabetes, atherosclerosis, arthritis, kidney disorders and ageing[8–13]. Thus, regulation of ROS is crucial for the maintenance of cellular homeostasis. Cells produce several antioxidant enzymes, such as catalase, superoxide dismutase, glutathione peroxidase (GPx) and so on, to sustain the redox equilibrium[14]. Glutathione (GSH) acts as an electron donor to replenish the active form of enzyme and maintain cells' reservoir of antioxidants[15]. The GSH-dependent GPx has a pancellular distribution with isoforms present in both cytosol and mitochondria, highlighting its significance in the maintenance of redox homeostasis[16]. Recently, organoselenium compounds having GPx-like antioxidant activity attracted considerable attention[17,18].

Nanomaterials with intrinsic enzyme-like activity attract significant current interest due to their ability to replace specific enzymes in enzyme-based applications[19]. A few nanostructured materials have been shown to mimic the activity of peroxidases[20,21], oxidase[22] and superoxide dismutase[23]. Very recently, we reported the peroxynitrite isomerase and reductase activities of graphene–hemin hybrid nanosheets[24]. During our investigations on novel materials with interesting biological activities, we observed that V_2O_5, largely known as an oxidant[25,26], can exhibit antioxidant activity at nanoscale.

In this paper, we demonstrate that V_2O_5 nanowires (Vn) exhibit remarkable antioxidant activity at physiologically relevant conditions. The internalization of Vn restores the ROS balance and controls the oxidative stress in the cell by catalytically reducing H_2O_2 in the presence of GSH. Furthermore, Vn prevents oxidative damage to cellular components such as lipids, proteins and DNA, and thus plays a cytoprotective role in the cells.

Results

Synthesis and antioxidant activity. Synthesis of Vn was carried out by a hydrothermal method as described earlier[27]. The nanomaterial was thoroughly characterized by various methods. Vn shows an absorption band at ~420 nm in the ultraviolet-visible spectrum (Supplementary Fig. 1a) corresponding to the bandgap of nano-V_2O_5, which is in agreement with the value reported earlier[28]. Scanning electron microscopy (SEM) and transmission electron microscopy (TEM) images indicate the nanowires of different sizes with width of ~100 nm and varying length (Fig. 1a,b, respectively). High-resolution TEM image and selected area electron diffraction pattern confirm the formation of monocrystalline and orthorhombic V_2O_5 (Fig. 1c). Electron dispersive X-ray (EDX) analysis shows the presence of V and O (Supplementary Fig. 1b). The formation of orthorhombic V_2O_5 is also confirmed from the X-ray diffraction pattern (JCPDS # 001-0359) (Fig. 1d).

To study the antioxidant activity of the water dispersible Vn, the glutathione reductase (GR) coupled assay was employed and the decrease of NADPH concentration was monitored spectrophotometrically at 340 nm[29]. Figure 1e shows the schematic representation of the GPx-like activity of Vn. In the absence of at least one of the components in the reaction mixture, Vn did not show GPx activity (Fig. 1f,g and Supplementary Fig. 2a). Although the reduction of vanadate (V) by GR in the presence of NADPH has been shown to represent a new pathway for vanadate metabolism[30], such reduction by GR was not observed for Vn. The initial rates determined for the reactions of Vn with GR and H_2O_2 in the presence of NADPH were very similar to that of the control reactions without H_2O_2 (Supplementary Fig. 2c,d). Interestingly, none of the peroxidase or oxidase nanozymes reported earlier exhibit the unique activity of Vn under similar reaction conditions (Fig. 1h). The reactivity of Vn appears to be different from that of the other peroxidase nanomimetics, where •OH mediates the oxidation of organic substrates in the presence of metal ions. The remarkable selectivity of Vn towards H_2O_2 is probably due to the activation of H_2O_2 by Vn to produce a polar peroxido species instead of OH radical[27,31]. The peroxido species reacts further with the nucleophile (GSH cofactor) to form glutathione disulfide (GSSG) (*vide infra*). The supernatant liquid obtained after incubation of Vn for 15 min in the assay buffer did not show any noticeable antioxidant activity, indicating that the reaction occurs on the surface of Vn (Supplementary Fig. 2b).

When the concentration of Vn was varied from 0 to 0.02 mg ml^{-1} in the presence of other required reagents, a proportional dependence of initial rate was observed for the reduction of H_2O_2 (Fig. 2a) with first-order reaction kinetics (Fig. 2a, inset). The apparent steady-state kinetic parameters were determined by independently varying the concentrations of H_2O_2 (0–480 μM) and GSH (0–6.0 mM) in the presence of GR (1.7 units) and NADPH (400 μM). A typical Michaelis–Menten kinetics was observed for both the reactions (Fig. 2b,c). The Michaelis constant K_M values, obtained from the corresponding Lineweaver–Burk plots (Supplementary Fig. 3a,b), for H_2O_2 and GSH are ~0.11 and ~2.22 mM, respectively. These values are different from those obtained for GPx1 enzyme isoform (K_M for H_2O_2 ~0.025 mM and GSH ~10 mM)[32,33], indicating different binding affinity for the substrates. Vn catalyses the reaction at the maximal reaction velocity V_{max} of ~0.43 and 0.83 mM min^{-1} for H_2O_2 and GSH, respectively, with $k_{cat} = 0.065\ s^{-1}$. Although GSSG is produced in the overall reaction, the Michaelis–Menten and Lineweaver–Burk profiles indicate that one GSH molecule is involved in the rate-determining step (Supplementary Fig. 3c–e).

As V_2O_5 nanoparticles generally exhibit vanadium haloperoxidase mimetic activity[27], we monitored the reaction of Vn with H_2O_2 in the presence of vanadium haloperoxidase substrates, that is, tyrosine/iodide or dopamine/iodide. However, the rate of the reactions was unaffected (Fig. 2d) on introduction of the haloperoxidase substrates into the reaction mixture. This is probably due to the greater nucleophilic character of GS^- over halide, which helps in a facile attack of GS^- at the polarized oxygen atoms of the vanadium peroxido species formed on the surface of Vn on reaction with H_2O_2. The observed difference can also be attributed to the differential binding affinity of the two substrates for the catalyst. A comparison of the reaction rates for various peroxides H_2O_2, *t*-butyl hydroperoxide and cumene hydroperoxide indicates that the antioxidant activity of Vn is specific to H_2O_2 (Fig. 2e). Although nanozymes are known to have incompatibility with a cascade of other enzymes[19], we found that Vn has an excellent compatibility with galactose oxidase (GO) and GR in series (Fig. 2f,g). As GO can work efficiently with Vn, the decrease in the concentration of NADPH during the catalysis directly correlates with the galactose levels. Therefore, Vn can be used for sensing galactose when coupled with GO and GR. It is known that the quantitative measurement of galactose is important in food industry and in medical monitoring and treatment of patients. To understand the reactivity of Vn towards other biologically relevant oxidants, such as peroxynitrite

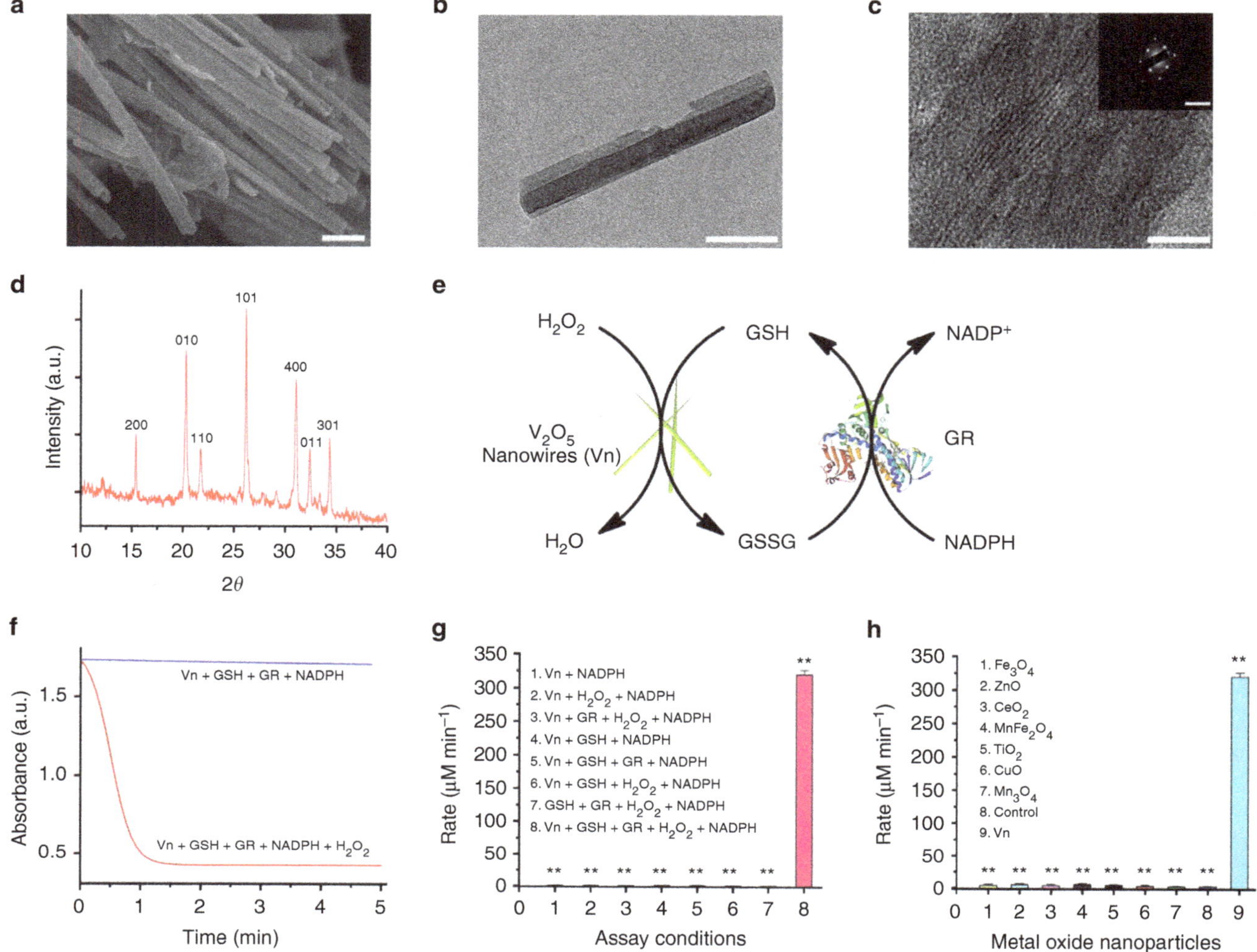

Figure 1 | Characterization and GPx-like activity of Vn. (**a**) SEM image of Vn showing the bunch of nanowires together. Scale bar, 200 nm. (**b**) TEM image of Vn. Scale bar, 100 nm (**c**) High-resolution TEM (HRTEM) image of Vn showing the planes and inset reveals the crystallinity and orthorhombic crystal structure of Vn. Scale bar, 10 nm (HRTEM), 10 nm^{-1} (SAED). (**d**) Powder X-ray diffraction (XRD) of Vn where all the reflections are indexed to orthorhombic structure. (**e**) Schematic diagram depicting the GPx-like antioxidant activity of Vn and GSH recycling by GR. (**f**) Plot of absorbance versus time (min) revealing the activity of Vn in the presence of Vn (0.020 mg ml^{-1}), GSH (2 mM), NADPH (0.4 mM), GR (1.7 units), H_2O_2 (240 μM) in phosphate buffer (100 mM, pH 7.4) at 25 °C. When H_2O_2 was absent in control, no reactivity was obtained. (**g**) Bar diagram showing the initial rates at different assay conditions. (**h**) Comparison of the GPx-like activity of various metal oxides that have been shown earlier as peroxidase and oxidase mimetics and Vn. Data represented as ± s.e.m., $n = 3$, $^{**}P$ (*t*-test) < 0.001.

($ONOO^-$, PN), we carried out the PN-mediated nitration of L-tyrosine and bovine serum albumin in the presence and absence of Vn. Although GSH and small molecule GPx mimetics such as ebselen have been shown to scavenge PN efficiently[17,18], Vn does not react with PN as the nitration reactions were not affected by different concentrations of Vn (Supplementary Fig. 4).

Internalization of Vn in mammalian cells. To understand the antioxidant activity of Vn nanozyme in cellular environment, we carried out cell-based studies. The cellular uptake of Vn was studied through three different approaches. First, the internalization of Vn in HEK293T (human embryonic kidney) cells was observed by SEM. Vn-treated cells showed the formation of depressions on the surface, which was absent in the untreated controls. However, the cells recovered after 2 h post treatment showed diminished indentation and restoration of surface morphology. This shows that the uptake of Vn probably occurs through endocytosis (Fig. 3a,b and Supplementary Fig. 5). To further ascertain that the endocytotic depressions were due to uptake of Vn, we carried out an EDX analysis on the concavity. The specific peak corresponding to the vanadium was observed in the Vn-treated cells (Fig. 3c,d). Second, the internalization and presence of Vn were verified by observing the alterations in scattering pattern of a laser beam by the intracellular nanowires[34,35]. The concomitant increase in the Vn concentration caused a comparable variation in the scatter pattern, indicating an enhanced intracellular presence of Vn (Fig. 3f,g). Lastly, we assessed quantitatively the percentage uptake of Vn in the cells by inductively coupled plasma atomic emission spectroscopy (ICP-AES) by analysing the amount of vanadium in the cells. In comparison with the untreated control, we found a significant increase of vanadium levels in the treated cells, which corresponds to ~2.5% of the total Vn added to the cell population (Fig. 3h). These observations indicate that Vn is efficiently internalized into the cell albeit in lower amounts, probably through endocytotic mechanism.

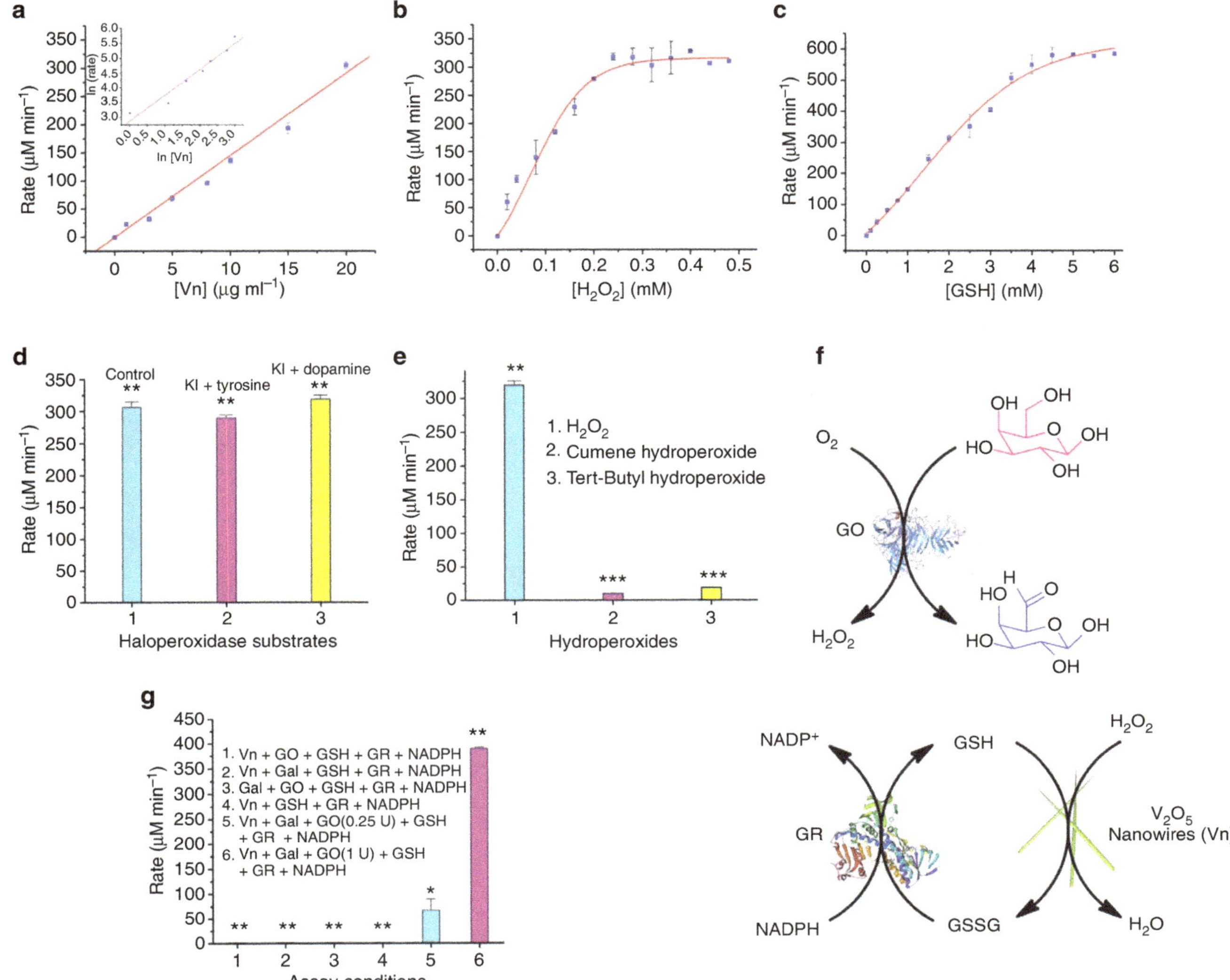

Figure 2 | Kinetic parameters and cooperativity studies. (**a**) Effect of concentration of Vn on the GPx-like activity showing the first-order kinetics as found in the enzyme catalysed reactions. Inset represents the plot of ln (rate) versus concentration of Vn. (**b**) Michaelis-Menten plot for the variation of the concentration of H_2O_2 (0-0.48 mM) and in the presence of Vn (0.020 mg ml^{-1}), GSH (2 mM), NADPH (0.4 mM), GR (1.7 units) in phosphate buffer (100 mM, pH 7.4) at 25 °C. (**c**) Michaelis-Menten plot for the variation of the concentration of GSH (0-6.0 mM) and in the presence of Vn (0.020 mg ml^{-1}), NADPH (0.4 mM), GR (1.7 units), H_2O_2 (240 μM) in phosphate buffer (100 mM, pH 7.4) at 25 °C. (**d**) Effect of the haloperoxidase substrate KI (2 mM), tyrosine or dopamine (2 mM) on the GPx-activity of Vn, showing that Vn preferably exhibits GPx-like activity and not haloperoxidase activity at pH 7.4. (**e**) Comparison of the reactivity of three different peroxides, H_2O_2, *t*-BuOOH and Cum-OOH. It shows that Vn is very selective to H_2O_2 as substrate. (**f**) Schematic diagram of coupling GO with Vn nanozyme. The H_2O_2 produced *in situ* by GO was directly used by Vn for its GPx activity. This proves that the Vn shows cooperativity with other enzymes. (**g**) Bar diagram showing the initial rates, which are directly related to the cooperativity of Vn with different concentrations of GO (0.25 and 1 unit). The reaction occurs only when all the components are present. Data represented as ± s.e.m., $n=3$, $^{**}P$ (*t*-test) <0.001.

Intracellular ROS scavenging activity of Vn. To test the ability of Vn to combat oxidative stress in the cells, we used two different approaches. The HEK293T cells pretreated with the nanoparticles were either treated exogenously by H_2O_2 or the intrinsic cellular levels of peroxides were elevated by inhibiting the antioxidant enzyme catalase using either Cu^{2+} ions[36] or 3-amino,1,2,4 triazole (3-AT)[37]. For the selection of appropriate concentrations of H_2O_2 and Vn, the cells were treated with increasing concentration of H_2O_2 and Vn for 15 min followed by measurement of cell viability and levels of cellular ROS using dihydrodichloro-fluoresceindiacetate (DCFDA-H2) probe (Supplementary Fig. 6b–d). Based on the relative fluorescence and cellular viability observed, 200 μM H_2O_2 and 50 ng μl^{-1} of Vn were used for further experiments. Inhibiting the intracellular catalase in the presence of Vn highlights the ability of Vn to act as GPx enzyme mimetic by restoring the redox state and viability of the cells. To measure the scavenging of H_2O_2 by Vn under stress conditions, we expressed a genetically encoded H_2O_2-specific probe HyPer and analysed the intracellular peroxide levels. The level of H_2O_2 was found to decrease in the cells pretreated with Vn, whereas the cells treated either with only H_2O_2 or Cu^{2+}, or 3-AT showed enhanced levels of H_2O_2 (Fig. 4a,c). Similarly, staining the cells with H_2O_2-specific dye Amplex Red and ROS-sensitive fluorescent dye DCFDA-H2 resulted in the detection of relatively lower ROS levels in Vn-pretreated cells under normal and oxidative stress conditions as compared with that of controls. Consistently, a substantial increase in the ROS levels was observed in the cells treated with either H_2O_2 or Cu^{2+}, or 3-

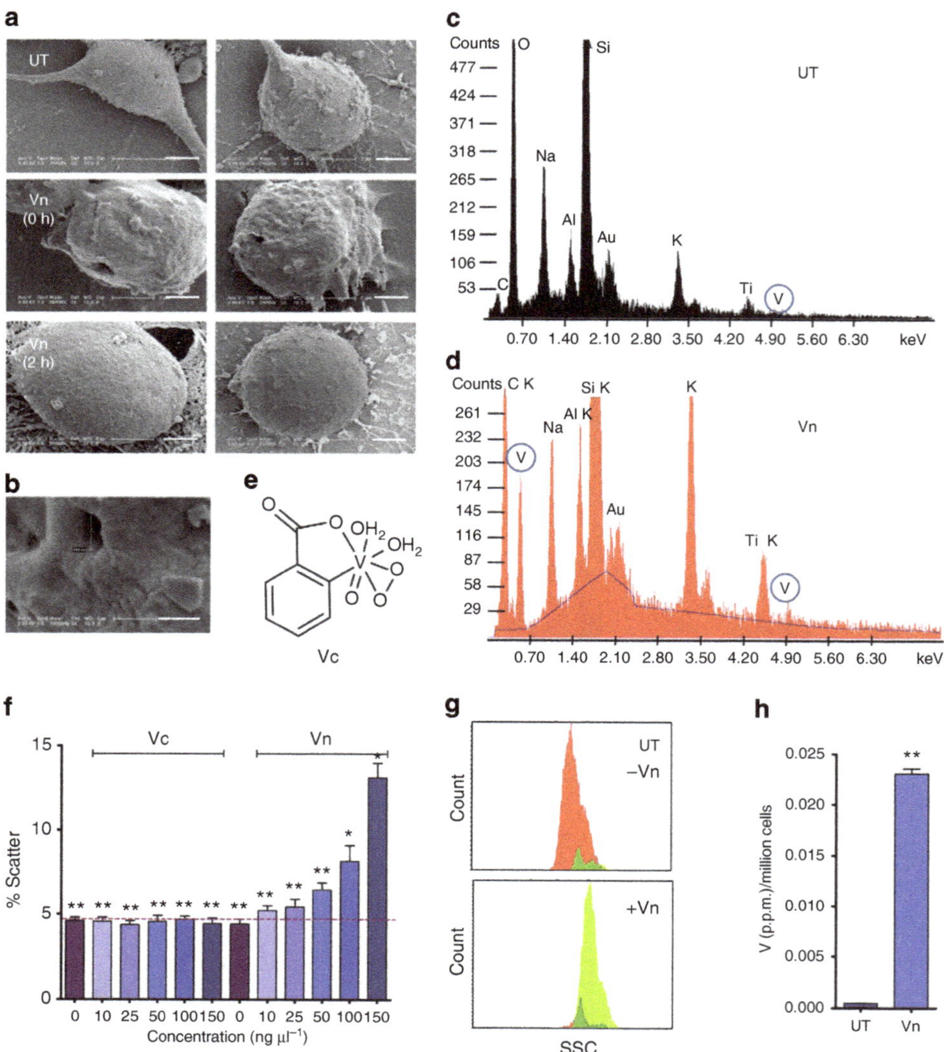

Figure 3 | Internalization of Vn in the cell. (**a**,**b**) HEK293T (human embryonic kidney) cells were either left untreated (UT), treated with Vn and immediately harvested (0 h) or recovered for 2 h post Vn exposure, before fixation, dehydration and imaging by scanning electron microscope; **b** represents the zoomed image of the middle panel to highlight the depression. Scale bars, 2 μm (**a**) and 500 nm (**b**). (**c**,**d**) The cell surface depressions resulting due to Vn internalization was verified by EDX analysis on the depressed regions. Representative EDX plots depicting the absence and presence of vanadium peak in untreated (UT) and Vn-treated cells, respectively. (**e**) Structure of Peroxido vanadium picolinate complex (Vc). (**f**,**g**) The presence of Vn in the cells were assessed by flow cytometric analysis of altered side scatter intensity (SSC) resulting due to differential density of the intracellular Vn accumulation. HEK293T cells were treated with increasing concentrations of Vn and subjected to flow cytometric analysis. Soluble Vc-treated cells were used as negative controls. (**g**) Representative SSC histograms of cells kept either untreated (UT) or treated with 100 ng μl^{-1} Vn. Data represented as mean ± s.e.m. $n = 3$, $^{**}P$ (*t*-test) < 0.001, $^{*}P$ (*t*-test) < 0.01. (**h**) The relative uptake of Vn by the cells was measured by ICP-AES and represented as amount of vanadium uptake per million cells with respect to untreated controls.

AT alone as measured by flow cytometric analysis (Fig. 4b,d and Supplementary Fig. 7a,b). To test the utilization of GSH as a cofactor by Vn, the intracellular GSH was depleted by allyl alcohol (AA)[38] or buthionine sulfoximine (BSO)[39], which resulted in loss of antioxidant function and an increase in the ROS. The antioxidant function was, however, restored on exogenous addition of GSH (Fig. 4a–d and Supplementary Fig. 7a,b). The broader effect of Vn was analysed using cells of diverse origin such as HeLa cells (cervical cancer), LNCaP (prostate cancer) and SH-SY5Y cells (neuroblastoma). In congruence to HEK293T cells, Vn showed similar H_2O_2 scavenging ability in other cells as observed through microscopic analysis and flow cytometry (Fig. 4e,f and Supplementary Fig. 8). This indicates that Vn nanozyme possesses intracellular ROS scavenging activity and its antioxidant function is mediated by GPx-like activity. In contrast, treatment of the cells with peroxido-vanadium-picolinate complex (Vc) (Fig. 3e), other similar complexes Vc_2 and Vc_3 (Supplementary Fig. 7i), and different forms of V_2O_5 such as bulk-V_2O_5 (Vb) and V_2O_5-foam (Vf) caused an increment in the cellular peroxides, which were further elevated on additional H_2O_2 or Cu^{2+} treatment (Supplementary Fig. 7f). These observations are in agreement with the fact that vanadium complexes can undergo redox reaction and generate ROS in cells[40–42]. Although V_2O_5 is known to cause severe oxidative stress in cells[25,26], in nano-form, it shows remarkable antioxidant GPx activity. It should be noted that complex Vc undergoes redox reactions without changing the ligand environment. Complex Vc exhibited a signal at −598 p.p.m. in the ^{51}V NMR spectrum, which disappeared completely on treatment with GSH. The

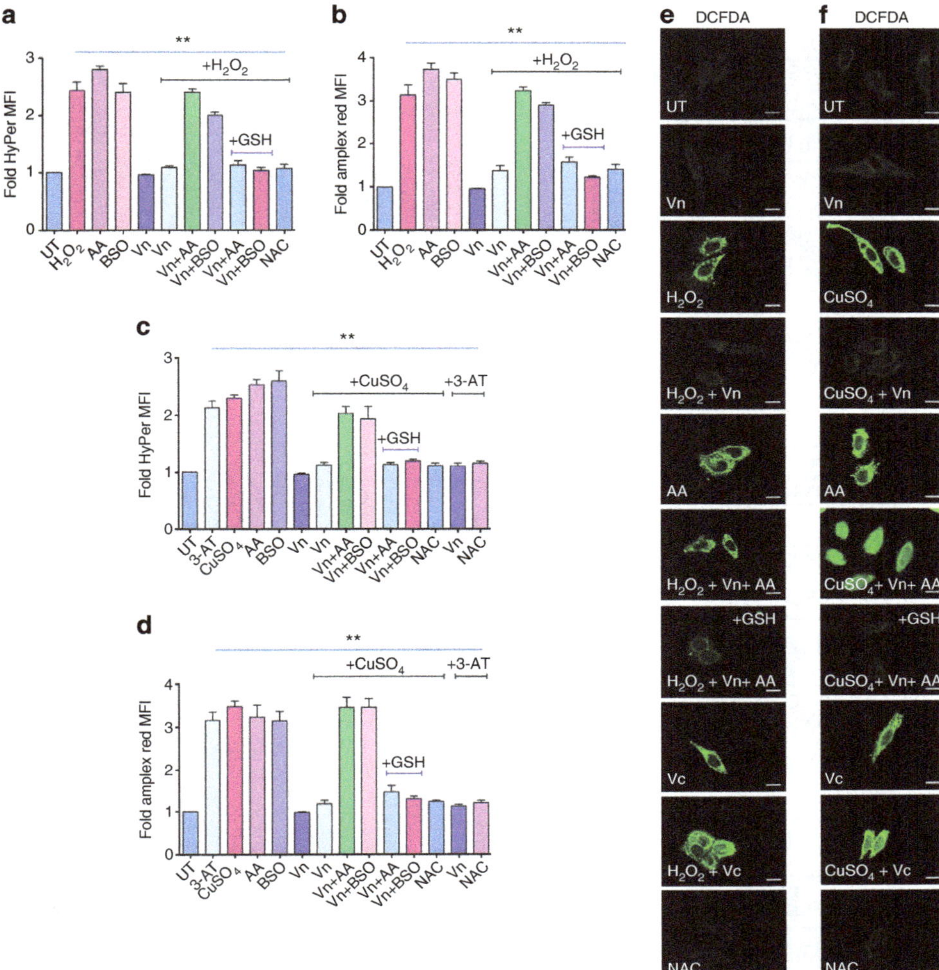

Figure 4 | Ability of Vn to scavenge intracellular ROS. (**a**,**b**) H_2O_2 scavenging activity of Vn was measured using genetically encoded H_2O_2-specific probe HyPer in HEK293T cells. Cells were either left untreated or pretreated with 50 ng μl^{-1} of nano-V_2O_5 (Vn) prior exposure to 200 μM H_2O_2 or 500 μM $CuSO_4$, or 20 mM 3-amino-1,2,4-triazole (3-AT). AA (0.1 mM) or 50 μM BSO was used to deplete cellular GSH level. GSH (100 μM) was used to replenish the GSH level to show the requirement of GSH as a cofactor for Vn. To measure the ROS scavenging ability of vanadium complex (Vc), 50 ng μl^{-1} Vc was used to treat the cells in the presence or absence of oxidative stress. N-acetyl cysteine-treated cells (NAC) (100 μM) were used as positive control. Data represented as mean ± s.e.m. $n = 3$, $^{**}P$ (*t*-test) < 0.001. (**c**,**d**) To further confirm, the H_2O_2 scavenging ability of Vn, HEK293T cells were subjected to various treatments as mentioned earlier and stained with H_2O_2-specific dye Amplex Red (50 μM). The fluorescence was measured at 590 nm using spectrofluorometer and data were represented as fold change in mean fluorescent intensity (MFI) of Amplex Red over untreated cells. Data represented as mean ± s.e.m. $n = 3$, $^{**}P$ (*t*-test) < 0.001. (**e**,**f**) HeLa cells were treated with Vn before the treatment with H_2O_2 (**e**) or $CuSO_4$ (**f**) (as mentioned earlier) and then stained with 15 μM DCFDA-H2 dye. The change in fluorescent intensity was observed through microscopic analysis (scale bar, 10 μm).

product is a V(IV) complex and, hence, electron paramagnetic resonance active. However, when the reaction mixture was treated with H_2O_2, the signal at −598 p.p.m. reappeared (Supplementary Fig. 6e).

The adaptability of the cells to nanowire treatment, the cytotoxicity of Vn and its ability to suppress ROS-induced apoptosis was analysed by MTT (3-(4,5-dimethylthiazol-2-yl)-2,5-diphenyltetrazolium bromide) assay, caspase 3/7 activation and propidium iodide staining. Treatment of cells with Vn alone did not alter the overall viability of the cells as compared with controls. However, it had a significant cell protective role and inhibited apoptosis under H_2O_2 or Cu^{2+} or 3-AT treatment. Consistent to the loss of antioxidant properties of Vn on GSH depletion, AA and BSO caused a decrease in the cell viability, which was reverted on addition of exogenous GSH (Fig. 5a–d and Supplementary Fig. 7c,d). This supports the idea that Vn possesses a GPx-like activity and uses GSH as a co-factor. To further confirm the cofactor requirement for the catalysis, the cellular GSH and GSSG levels were measured after treatment with Vn. Although no significant changes in GSH and GSSG levels were observed in the presence of Vn alone, an increase in the GSSG level (by ~1.5-fold) and a slight decrease in the GSH level (by ~0.8-fold) was observed when the cells pretreated with Vn were exposed to H_2O_2 (Fig. 5e,f and Supplementary Fig. 9a). Although two molecules of GSH are oxidized to form one GSSG molecule, the observed increase in the GSSG level did not result in a significant reduction in GSH level. This confirms that Vn uses GSH as a cofactor to scavenge H_2O_2, without compromising the recycling of GSSG to GSH.

In agreement with our previous ROS data, exposure of cells to the metal complex (Vc) resulted in higher cell death under both treated or untreated conditions. In contrast to Vn, the bulk material (Vb), the foam form (Vf) and the complexes (Vc, Vc_2 and Vc_3) lacked the ROS scavenging ability and had deleterious

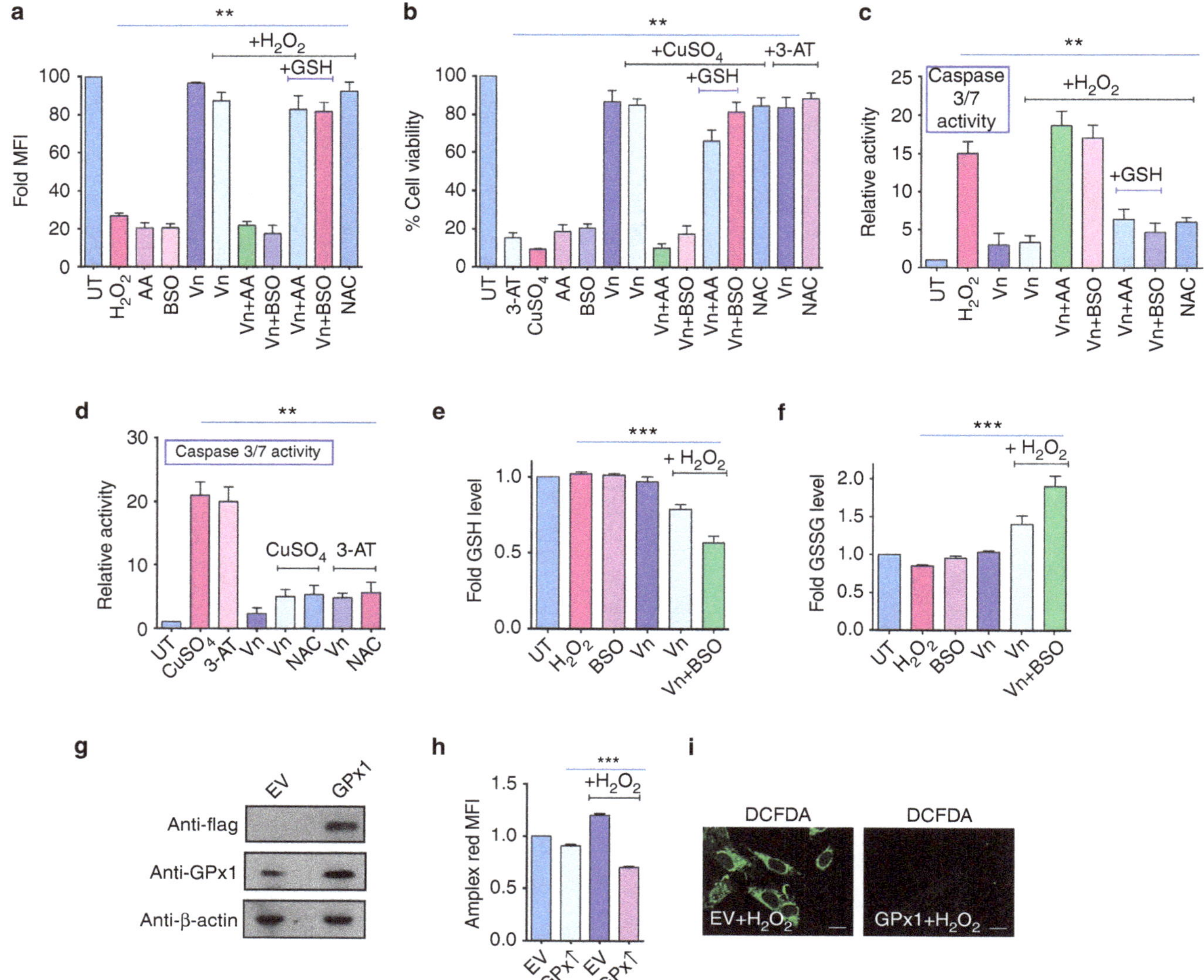

Figure 5 | Rescue of cell viability by Vn. **(a,b)** The viability of HEK293T cells under H_2O_2- or $CuSO_4$-treated conditions along with other ROS modulators was observed through MTT assay and represented as mean ± s.e.m.; $n = 8$, $^{**}P$ (*t*-test) < 0.001. **(c,d)** Prevention of ROS-mediated apoptosis induction by nano-V_2O_5 was analysed through the effector caspase-3/7 activity by measuring cleavage of specific substrate, resulting in the increase in fluorescence intensity. Bars denote the fold intensity over untreated cells as mean ± s.e.m.; $n = 3$, $^{***}P$ (*t*-test) < 0.0001. **(e,f)** The level of cellular GSH or GSSG was quantified in HEK293T cells treated with Vn and GSH inhibitor (BSO) using GSH/GSSG-Glo kit (Promega). Data are represented as mean ± s.e.m.; $n = 3$, $^{***}P$ (*t*-test) < 0.0001. **(g-i)** The GPx mimetic nature of Vn was confirmed by overexpressing GPx1 in HEK293T cells. Cells were transfected with pCDNA3.1a empty vector (EV) or vector containing GPx1. GPx1 overexpression was analysed in whole-cell lysate using the anti-GPx1 antibody **(g)**. Anti-Flag tag antibody and anti-β-actin antibodies were used as transfection control and loading control, respectively. The cellular H_2O_2 level was measured by staining the cells with Amplex Red after 48 h of transfection **(h)**. Results are presented as fold change in MFI over empty vector-transfected cells. Data are represented as mean ± s.e.m.; $n = 3$, $^{***}P$ (*t*-test) < 0.0001. HeLa cells overexpressing GPx1 were stained with DCFDA-H2 and the change in fluorescence was observed by microscopy **(i)**. Scale bar, 10 μm.

consequences for the cell viability (Supplementary Fig. 7g,h). Although Vb showed relatively lower antioxidant activity under *in vitro* conditions (Supplementary Fig. 6a), treatment of cells with Vb caused an intrinsic increase in the cellular free radical levels, which was further elevated on oxidative insult. Concurrently, the Vb-treated cells showed a sharp decrease in cell viability (Supplementary Fig. 7g). These data are in agreement with the EPR data that the metal ion in Vb undergoes reduction in the presence of GSH, which may lead to the generation of free radical species on reaction with H_2O_2 (*vide infra* and Supplementary Fig. 14b). Lastly, we addressed the overall retention ability and toxicity of the Vn on longer time scale. We found that Vn did not have any detrimental effect on the cell viability and retained a significant degree of ROS scavenging activity even after 24 h post treatment (Supplementary Figs 7e and 9b,c).

To rule out the possible involvement of cellular antioxidant machinery in Vn-mediated ROS scavenging through activation of oxidative stress-responsive transcription factors, we measured the expression level of downstream antioxidant enzymes in HEK293T cells. Analysis of the expression of Mn-superoxide dismutase (SOD-2), GPx1 and catalase in cells treated with Vn indicated no changes in the expression levels of these enzymes after Vn treatment. An increase in the expression of GPx1 after H_2O_2 and

3-AT treatment was observed, which is probably due to the cellular defense mechanism in response to oxidative stress. The increase in GPx1 level was, however, restored in cells treated with Vn along with H_2O_2 (Supplementary Fig. 9d). These results indicate that Vn itself acts as H_2O_2 scavenger without involving cellular antioxidant machinery for the antioxidant effect. To test the effect of Vn on the redox signalling pathways in the cells, we analysed the expression of genes regulated by the major stress-responsive factor Nrf2 (ref. 43). The suppression of Nrf2 target genes' expression was not observed when the cells were treated with Vn (Supplementary Fig. 9e), indicating that Vn does not interfere with the cellular redox sensing pathways, but it supplements the antioxidant system of the cell. Interestingly, although an upregulation of certain Nrf2 target genes such as

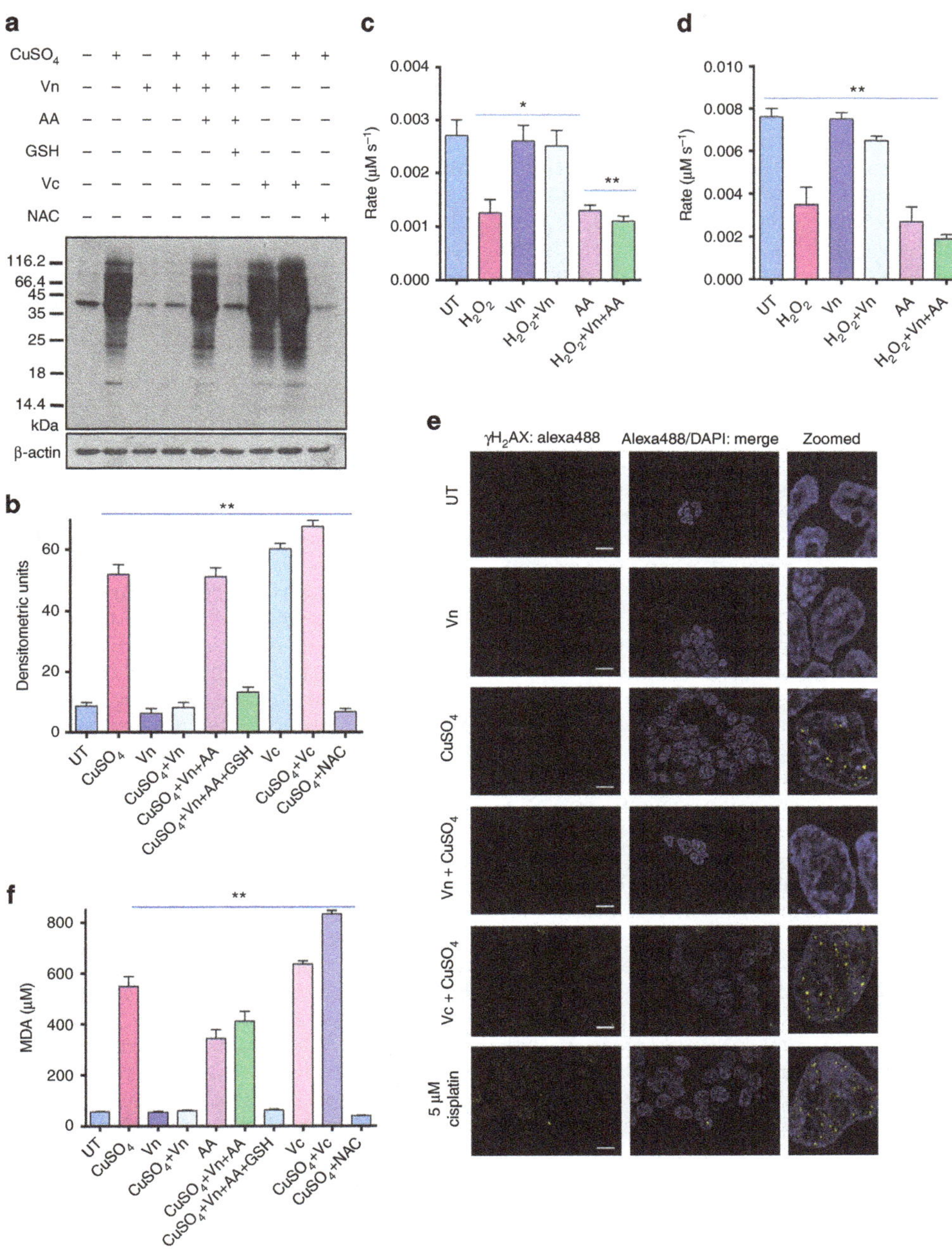

Figure 6 | Protection of cellular components from ROS-induced damage by Vn. (**a**,**b**) HEK293T cells subjected to treatment as indicated, were lysed and derivatized using 2,4-DNPH before SDS-PAGE and immunoblot analysis using anti-DNP antibodies. *N*-acetyl cysteine treated cells (NAC) (100 μM) were used as positive control. (**b**) The lanes were quantified and represented as fold densitometric values over untreated cells (**c**) The aconitase activity was quantified by recording an increase in absorbance at 240 nm for the production of *cis*-aconitate. (**d**) Succinate dehydogenase activity was measured by coupling the reduction of ubiquinone to 2,6-dichlorophenolindophenol (DCPIP). The loss in blue colour due to reduction of DCPIP was monitored at 600 nm. (**e**) The amount of DNA double-strand break was analysed by detecting the foci formation by phosphorylated form of γH_2AX through immunofluorescence microscopy. Data are represented as mean ± s.e.m.; $n=3$, $^{**}P$ (*t*-test) <0.001, $^{*}P$ ((*t*-test) <0.01. Scale bar,10 μm. (**f**) The amount of lipid peroxidation was measured by quantifying the levels of malondialdehyde (MDA) in the cell lysate through thiobarbituric acid reactive substances assay. The extent of lipid peroxidation was represented as fold changes in absorbance recorded at 532 nm.

glutamate–cysteine ligase catalytic (GCLC) and modifier (GCLM) subunits, and haem oxygenase-1 (HO-1) was observed under oxidative stress conditions (that is, in the presence of H_2O_2), these protein expression levels were found to be normal in the presence of Vn (Supplementary Fig. 9e). This is presumably due to scavenging of H_2O_2 by Vn that may prevent the stimulation of Nrf2 response.

To further prove the intracellular GPx mimetic nature of Vn, we overexpressed the most abundant isoform of GPx, GPx1, in HEK293T cells and exposed the cells to H_2O_2 treatment. We found through Amplex Red and DCFDA-H2 staining a decrease in total peroxide levels similar to that of Vn-pretreated cells, as analysed by flow cytometry and microscopy experiments (Fig. 5g–i and Supplementary Fig. 19). The overexpression of GPx1 did not alter the expression pattern of different Nrf2 target genes. However, an upregulation of GCLC, GCLM and HO-1, observed after treatment with H_2O_2, was restored back to normal levels similar to Vn treatment (Supplementary Fig. 9f). In summary, our results prove that nano-V_2O_5 (Vn) possess the unique property of scavenging intracellular ROS, prevents apoptotic trigger and protects cell viability by acting as a GPx enzyme mimetic by using GSH as a cofactor. The abundance of H_2O_2 in the cell is more as compared with other ROS species and hence plays a critical role in cellular damage[44]. Therefore, cells have evolved a variety of peroxide metabolizing systems to maintain the ROS balance. However, under pathogenic conditions deregulated, ROS levels become the causative agent of pleiotropic defects giving rise to disease conditions. The robust ROS scavenging activity of Vn nanozyme even in the absence of catalase, one of the most potent H_2O_2 degrading enzymes, underlines its applicability as an artificial enzyme to control ROS imbalance in the cells.

Protection of ROS-induced damage of intracellular components. The excess of free radicals generated in the cell mainly damage three major biomolecules, namely lipids, proteins and DNA[5–7]. Therefore, the cytoprotective role of Vn was analysed by measuring three parameters of intracellular damage such as lipid peroxidation, protein carbonylation and DNA strand breaks. The amount of lipid peroxides in the cell was quantified by measuring the levels of their decomposed highly reactive carbonyl product malondialdehyde[45]. We observed an increase in the amounts of lipid peroxides in the cells treated with Cu^{2+} alone as compared with those pretreated with Vn (Fig. 6f). Similarly, cells left unexposed to Vn showed higher levels of protein carbonyls in comparison with Vn-containing cells in the presence or absence of Cu^{2+} (Fig. 6a,b and Supplementary Fig. 19). The level of protection against DNA damage by Vn was addressed by quantifying the number of phosphorylated γH_2AX foci formed as a consequence of DNA double-strand breaks[5]. We found that Vn exerted a significant protective effect on DNA integrity and the cells accumulated lower amounts of intrastrand breaks than the nanowire-untreated cells (Fig. 6e). This is suggested by increased formation of γH_2AX foci in the absence of Vn than in cells pretreated with nanowires, on oxidative insult. A similar effect was observed for calf thymus DNA *in vitro* in the presence of H_2O_2 (Supplementary Fig. 10). Depletion of intracellular GSH by AA or exposure of cells to Vc resulted in increased levels of lipid peroxides, protein carbonyls and γH_2AX foci (Fig. 6a,b,e,f). As demonstrated above, in the latter case, redox reactions of Vc in cells cause these oxidative damages. These results underline that GSH is essential for the GPx-like activity of Vn nanozymes for their cytoprotective function.

It is known that mitochondria are the primary source of ROS via electron channelling through the respiratory complexes. An increase in the mitochondrial free-radical levels causes oxidation of the central Fe^{2+} moiety of Fe–S cluster protein, resulting in loss of tetrahedral geometry and loss of enzyme function[46,47]. Therefore, we attempted to address the ability of Vn to protect the Fe–S cluster enzyme function from free-radical damage. These experiments were carried out by using two model Fe–S cluster enzymes, membrane-associated succinate dehydrogenase and matrix-localized aconitase. The activities of these enzymes under oxidative stress conditions in the presence of Vn were found to be comparable to that of controls (Fig. 6c,d), suggesting that Vn in the presence of GSH effectively protect the function of Fe–S cluster proteins and activities of the enzymes.

Mechanistic details. As mentioned earlier, the reaction follows enzyme-like mechanism as inferred from the Michaelis–Menten plots. The surface-exposed 010 planes (Fig. 7a,b) may act as catalytic sites, which are similar to the ones shown for the vanadium haloperoxidase activity of Vn[27]. To understand the interactions of GSH on the Vn surface, we carried out elemental X-ray mapping of sulfur and vanadium (Supplementary Fig. 11a–c), which indicates that GSH molecules are bound to the surface of Vn. Further, appearance of S2p signal in XPS of Vn-treated GSH confirms such interactions (Supplementary Fig. 11d). When the decrease in the concentration of NADPH was monitored at 340 nm, a complete reduction of H_2O_2 was observed in the first cycle. However, subsequent addition of H_2O_2 (240 μM) led to a further decrease in the NADPH concentration, indicating the stability and catalytic nature of Vn during the reduction (Fig. 7c). A similar profile was observed when the formation of GSSG was monitored by high-performance liquid chromatography (HPLC) (Fig. 7d). Treatment of Vn with H_2O_2 alone led to the disappearance of a band at ~420 nm (Fig. 7f), which is probably due to the change in the functional groups on the surface by the formation of vanadium peroxido species **1** (Fig. 8). Addition of an excess amount of GSH to **1** did not reproduce the band at 420 nm (Fig. 7f), indicating that the reaction follows a shunt pathway and regeneration of vanadium oxo is not necessary for the GPx-like activity (Fig. 8). These observations were further supported by infrared analysis (Supplementary Fig. 12a). The ultraviolet–visible (Fig. 7f) and EPR (Fig. 7g) spectral analyses indicated that the oxidation state of vanadium in Vn was not affected by the addition of GSH. However, a partial reduction of vanadium(V) by H_2O_2 leading to the formation of V(IV) and •OOH was observed at liquid nitrogen temperature (Supplementary Fig. 13a)[31]. When the EPR was recorded at room temperature, the main unstructured signal almost disappeared, indicating a recombination of V(IV) and •OOH to produce the peroxido species in which the vanadium is in the +5 oxidation state (Fig. 7g). The formation of peroxido species was also confirmed by Raman spectroscopic studies, which showed a sharp peak at 591 cm^{-1} with another peak at 1,200 cm^{-1} corresponding to the overtone[48,49] (Supplementary Fig. 12b). The small signal in the EPR spectrum of Vn + H_2O_2 also suggests that the O–O bond in the peroxide complex is polarized. However, this small EPR signal disappeared completely after the treatment with an excess amount of GSH, suggesting that the GSH attacks on the polarized oxygen atoms of **1** (Fig. 8). According to the mechanism (Supplementary Fig. 13b), the protonation (H^+ originating from GSH) and nucleophilic attack of GS^- take place simultaneously at the oxygen atom that carries a partial negative charge (δ-) and positive charge ($\delta+$), respectively. In contrast to Vn, the eight line patterns in EPR spectra suggest that the vanadium in Vc and Vb is reduced from +5 to +4 oxidation state on treatment with GSH (Fig. 7g and Supplementary Fig. 14b), which is probably responsible for the

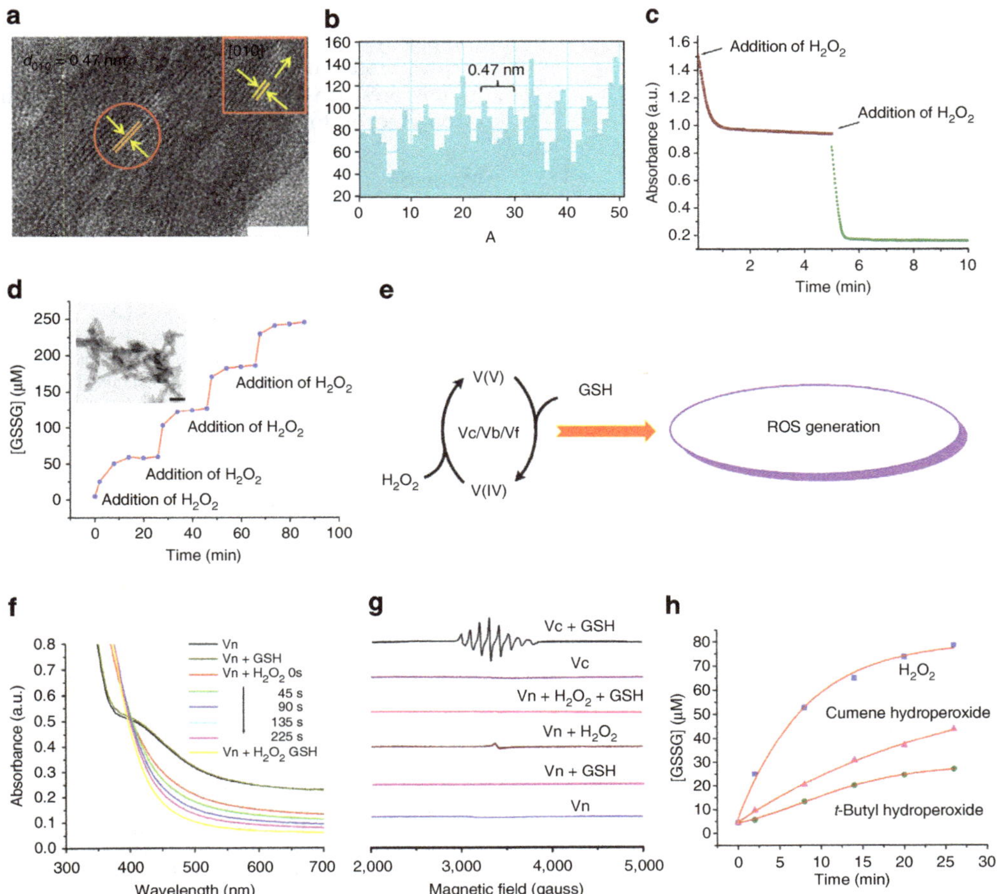

Figure 7 | Mechanistic investigation. (**a**) High-resolution TEM (HRTEM) images of the exposed plane 010 with $d=0.47$ nm, where the catalysis is known to take place. Inset is the magnified image of the highlighted part in HRTEM. Scale bar, 10 nm (**b**) The distance between the planes calculated by the software, Digital Micrograph. (**c**,**d**) The plots represent the mechanism is cyclic/catalytic. The activity was studied for two cycles in ultraviolet-visible spectroscopy by addition of H_2O_2 (240 μM) and then following the decrease of NADPH at 340 nm. Similarly, GSSG was followed by HPLC for four cycles by the addition of H_2O_2 (240 μM) at the end of each cycle. Inset shows the TEM image of the used Vn. Scale bar, 0.2 μm. (**e**) The redox recycling of vanadium in Vc and Vb. (**f**) Ultraviolet-visible spectra showing the band at ~420 nm (corresponding to the band gap of Vn) for Vn. The addition of GSH alone does not alter this band. However, the addition of H_2O_2 leads to the disappearance of this band, which may indicate the formation of peroxido species on the surface of Vn. Reappearance of the band at ~420 nm was not observed after addition of excess GSH to the produced vanadium peroxido species. (**g**) EPR spectra shows that the vanadium in Vn does not undergo reduction after the addition of GSH. The appearance of a signal at 3,200 Gauss at liquid nitrogen temperature (Supplementary Fig. 13) due to (•OOH) almost disappeared at room temperature, indicating the recombination of •OOH and V(IV) and the formation of peroxido species. Further, addition of GSH to the peroxido species does not result in the generation of V(IV), indicating the attack of thiolate (GS^-) at the peroxido species. However, GSH reduces vanadium centre V(V) to V(IV) in Vc. (**h**) Selectivity studies between H_2O_2, Cum-OOH and *t*-BuOOH by HPLC analysis. The reaction of H_2O_2 with Vn is much faster than that of Cum-OOH or *t*-BuOOH.

increase in the ROS level. The XPS data also confirm that the +5 oxidation state of vanadium centre in Vn is unaffected by GSH treatment (Supplementary Fig. 14a). Interestingly, the cyclic voltammograms show a significant difference in the redox potential of Vn as compared with that of Vb (Supplementary Fig. 14c)[50,51]. These observations confirm that the quantum size confinement of Vn alters the redox potential and enhances the stability of the +5 oxidation state of vanadium during the entire catalytic cycle. When a stronger reducing agent such as $NaBH_4$ is used, the vanadium centre does undergo a reduction as evidenced by a colour change from yellow (+5) to blue (+4) (Supplementary Fig. 14d). In the nanostructure, the surface of Vn acts as a template for the reduction of H_2O_2 by GSH. The nucleophilic attack of GS^- at the peroxide bond in complex **1** leads to the formation of an unstable sulfenate-bound intermediate **2**, which on hydrolysis generates glutathione sulfenic acid (**3**, GSOH) and the dihydroxo intermediate **4** (Fig. 8). The hydrolysis of **2** to produce GSOH is probably similar to the elimination of HOBr from V-OBr intermediate in vanadium haloperoxidase[27]. The formation of **3** was confirmed by HPLC and mass spectral analysis (Supplementary Fig. 15a,b). The reaction of **4** with H_2O_2 regenerates the peroxido species **1** (Fig. 8). This is similar to one of the steps proposed in the mechanism of vanadium chloroperoxidase[52]. The protonation of one of the hydroxyl units (HO^-) at vanadium centre by H_2O_2 produces a water molecule and HOO^-. The weakly bound water molecule then dissociates from the vanadium ion, which facilitates the attack of HOO^- at vanadium, leading to the formation of a hydroperoxido species. A spontaneous elimination of another water molecule then generates the vanadium peroxido species (Supplementary Fig. 16). The reaction of GSOH with GSH produces GSSG, which could be reduced to GSH by GR/NADPH. The formation of GSSG was also observed with Cum-OOH and *t*-BuOOH (Fig. 7h), although the antioxidant activity of Vn is

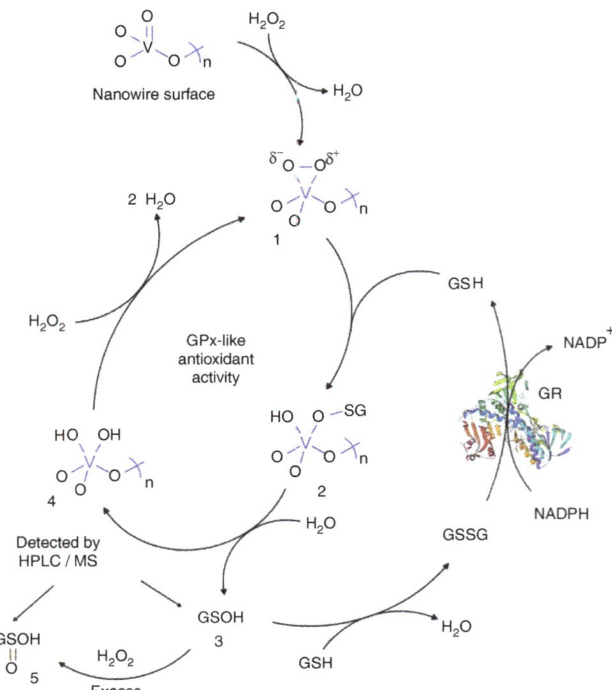

Figure 8 | Mechanism of GPx activity of Vn. Schematic diagram showing the molecular details of the mechanism of Vn nanozyme's activity. The formation of peroxido species **1** was confirmed by Raman spectroscopic studies.

more specific to H_2O_2. This is probably due to the formation of vanadium peroxido species, which were not produced when Vn was treated with Cum-OOH and *t*-BuOOH as seen from the Raman spectral data (Supplementary Fig. 12b). It should be noted that GSOH (**3**) undergoes further oxidation to produce the corresponding sulfinic acid (**5**, GSO_2H) at higher concentrations of H_2O_2 (Supplementary Fig. 17a,b). In addition to GSH, other thiol-containing small molecules such as cysteine, cysteamine and mercaptoethanol can also be used as thiol cofactor. Vn exhibited significant thiol peroxidase activity by catalytically reducing H_2O_2 in the presence of these thiols (Supplementary Fig. 18).

In conclusion, this study suggests that Vn nanowires have the potential to be used as an antioxidant therapeutic agent for the host defense against ROS-mediated cellular damage under pathological conditions. ROS such as H_2O_2 are generated as byproducts of the normal metabolism, but their levels are subdued due to a well-defined cellular antioxidant system. At the elevated ROS levels, the antioxidant defense mechanism fails to circumvent the detrimental effect of the free radicals, resulting in irreparable damage to biomolecules thereby causing severe oxidative stress. Organisms exposed to constant oxidative stress age quickly and are susceptible to multiple pathological conditions, including neurodegenerative diseases and neoplastic transformation. The deleterious effect of ROS-mediated cellular damages can be suppressed in several pathological conditions by synthetic compounds with potential antioxidant activity. Strikingly, the vanadia nanowires reported in this paper internalize in different cell types and display robust GPx mimetic activity under physiological conditions. The biocompatible Vn nanozyme exhibits significant cytoprotective effects against oxidative stress. Vn does not downregulate the endogenous antioxidant response, but rather, supplements the antioxidant system in mammalian cells. The Vn nanowires are able to completely suppress the ROS-mediated critical cellular damages such as protein oxidation, lipid peroxidation and DNA damages in the presence of glutathione, thus providing an important cytoprotection to the cell.

Methods

Synthesis of Vn. Vn were prepared by a hydrothermal method as described in the earlier report[27]. The mixture of $VOSO_4.H_2O$ (8 mmol) and $KBrO_3$ (5 mmol) were stirred for 30 min in 30 ml of distilled water. The pH of the solution was adjusted to 2 by addition of nitric acid and transferred to a teflon-lined stainless steel autoclave. After the reaction period of 24 h at 180 °C, the autoclave was allowed to cool to room temperature and the precipitate was washed several times with water. As this material contains traces of V(IV) species, the precipitate was treated with small amount of t-butyl hydroperoxide. The resulting nanomaterial was washed several times with ultrapure water followed by ethanol and dried at 80 °C overnight under vacuum to get high-quality Vn. The Vn was well characterized by various methods. Absorption spectrum was acquired on Perkin-Elmer Lambda 35 ultraviolet-visible spectrophotometer. SEM images and EDX spectra were recorded on Fei Sirion UHR SEM and ESEM-Quanta instruments. TEM images, high-resolution TEM images and selected area electron diffraction pattern were recorded on JEOL 2100 instrument operating at 200 KV. Powder X-ray diffraction of Vn was obtained by PANalytical Xpert pro theta-two theta diffractometer using a CuKα (1.5406 Å) radiation.

GPx-like activity of Vn. The GPx-like catalytic activity of Vn was studied using the GR-coupled assay by following the decrease in the concentration of NADPH spectrophotometrically at 340 nm on a Perkin-Elmer Lambda 35 ultraviolet-visible spectrophotometer under time drive mode. In a typical assay (1 ml), the reactants were added in the following order, Vn (0.02 mg ml^{-1}), GSH (2 mM), NADPH (0.4 mM), GR (1.7 units), H_2O_2 (240 μM) in 100 mM, pH 7.4 phosphate buffer and reaction rate was followed for 30 s at 25 °C. The control reactions were performed in the absence of at least one of the reactants. The steady-state kinetics of Vn were studied by varying the concentration of Vn (0–0.02 mg ml^{-1}), H_2O_2 (0–480 μM) and GSH (0–6.0 mM) at a time and at the fixed concentration of GR and NADPH in 100 mM phosphate buffer (pH 7.4). Michaelis–Menten curves and Lineweaver–Burk plots were obtained by using origin 6.1 software. To understand the effect of haloperoxidase substrates on the GPx-like activity of Vn, the GPx-like activity of Vn was followed in the presence of KI (2 mM) and tyrosine or dopamine (2 mM) with GR-coupled assay in 100 mM phosphate buffer (pH 7.4).

Cooperativity of Vn to work in a cascade. To study the cooperativity of Vn with other enzymes, we employed GO in an assay to generate H_2O_2 *in situ* using galactose as a substrate. Briefly, the GO (0.25 or 1 unit) was incubated with galactose (245 mM) for 1 min and then other reagents required for the GPx-like activity were added to the reaction mixture. The decrease in the concentration of NADPH was monitored at 340 nm by ultraviolet-visible spectrophotometry.

Cell lines and cell culture. HEK293T (Human Embryonic kidney cells ATCC Number: CRL-3216) and HeLa cells (ATCC Number: CCL-2) were grown in DMEM and Eagle's minimum essential medium (Invitrogen), respectively, containing 10% fetal bovine serum (Gibco) and 1% penicillin–streptomycin (Gibco) at 37 °C in 5% CO_2. LNCaP (ATCC Number: CRL-1740) and SH-SY5Y (ATCC Number: CRL-2266) cells were cultured in DMEM/F12 and RPMI 1640 (Invitrogen) medium, respectively, containing the above mentioned growth supplements. Cells were maintained at 60% confluency before measurement of ROS.

Plasmids. For the overexpression of GPx1, the ORF encoding GPx1 was amplified from HeLa cells complementary DNA library and cloned in pCDNA3.1a (+) vector under cytomegalovirus promoter. The GPx1 construct was transfected in HEK293T cells using Lipofectamine 2000 (Invitrogen). Empty pCDNA3.1a vector was transfected as a control for comparison.

Measurement of ROS. The cells were either left untreated or pretreated with 50 ng μl^{-1} of Vn (sonicated by probe sonicator for 5 min) before oxidative insult. The cellular monolayer was washed thoroughly by 1 × phosphate-buffered saline to remove the unincorporated nanoparticles. Oxidative stress was induced by exposing the cells to 200 μM H_2O_2, 500 μM $CuSO_4$ or 20 mM 3-amino-1,2,4-triazole for 15 min at 37 °C. AA (0.1 mM) and 50 μM BSO were used (for 15 min) to deplete the cellular GSH levels[38]. Replenishment of GSH was done by extensively washing the cells with 1 × phosphate-buffered saline to remove the AA or BSO, followed by addition of 100 μM GSH for 5 min. The effect of vanadium complexes was assessed by exposing the cells to 50 ng μl^{-1} of complexes for 15 min. After treatment, cells were trypsinized, washed with 1 × phosphate-buffered saline and stained with 15 μM DCFDA-H2 for 10 min at 30 °C. Ten thousand events were analysed by flow cytometry and the respective mean fluorescence intensity values were co-related with the ROS levels. For fluorescence microscopy, 5,000 cells were seeded and treated with ROS-modulating agents as stated above. Post treatment, the cells were stained with 5 μM DCFDA-H2. Images were acquired by Zeiss AxioObserver Z1 Apotome 2.0 63 x numerical aperture 1.45, Zeiss AxioCam MRm camera at a constant exposure of 300 ms and processed using Zeiss Axiovision Rel.4.8 software. For measurement of ROS using HyPer probe, the cells were transfected with the plasmid encoding HyPer (Evrogen) using Lipofectamine 2000 (Invitrogen). Post 48 h incubation, the cells were similarly treated as mentioned above and the relative HyPer fluorescence intensity was analysed using Tecan infinite Pro-200 spectrofluorometer. Amplex Red (Molecular Probes; Invitrogen) staining was performed following the manufacturer's instructions.

Cell viability and apoptosis. The relative viability of cells was determined by MTT assay kit (Invitrogen) according to manufacturer's instructions. The induction of apoptosis was measured by analysing caspase 3/7 activity as per the manufacturer's protocol supplied in caspase-activity detection kit (Promega). The treatment of the cells was carried out similar to the protocol followed for ROS measurement.

Measurement of cellular GSH and GSSG levels. To measure the cellular level of GSH and GSSG, HEK293T cells were treated with Vn, H_2O_2 and BSO as mentioned previously, followed by GSH/GSSG quantification using GSH/GSSH-Glo kit (Promega) as per the manufacturer's instructions.

Internalization of Vn in mammalian cells. Approximately 20,000 HEK293T cells were seeded and allowed to grow overnight. The cells were treated with the vanadium nanowires for 15 min and then subjected to 3% paraformaldehyde fixation for 2 h. The fixed cells were dehydrated through alcohol gradient and allowed to air dry at room temperature. Further, the dried cells were sputtered with gold and images were recorded by SEM. The vanadium content was analysed by EDX spectroscopy.

For the flow cytometry analysis, 1×10^5 HEK293T cells were treated with increasing concentrations (10, 25, 50, 100 and 150 ng μl^{-1}) of Vn for 15 min. The cells were harvested by trypsinization and the change in the side scatter due to uptake of nanowires was analysed by flow cytometry[34,35]. As a control, equivalent concentrations of a soluble vanadium complex were used.

For the quantification, ~60 million HEK293T cells were exposed to Vn, followed by cell lysis and ionization by addition of the concentrated nitric acid for 20 h. The samples were analysed by ICP-AES.

Protein carbonylation. Approximately 12 million cells were treated essentially as mentioned for the detection of ROS. Post treatment, the cells were harvested and lysed in RIPA buffer (50 mM Tris-HCl pH 7.6, 150 mM NaCl, 1% deoxycholate, 0.1% SDS, 1 mM phenylmethylsulfonyl fluoride). Equivalent amount of proteins was analysed for carbonylation through OxyBlot Protein Oxidation Detection Kit (Millipore), following the manufacturer's instructions.

Lipid peroxidation. Treated or untreated HEK293T cells were harvested and sonicated at 30% amplitude for 3 pulses of 20 s. The cell lysate was incubated with 1% thiobarbituric acid for 1 h at 90 °C. The samples were centrifuged at 16,000*g* for 3 min and the colour developed in the supernatant fraction was quantified spectrophotometrically at 530 nm.

Assessment of DNA damage. Approximately 20,000 cells were incubated with Vn for 15 min. Cells were fixed with 3% formaldehyde followed by a treatment with 90% methanol. The samples were washed with 1 × phosphate-buffered saline and blocked with 0.05% IgG-free BSA with 0.05% TritonX-100 for 30 min. After washing two times with 1 × phosphate-buffered saline, cells were incubated with anti- γH_2AX antibody for 1 h. Secondary antibody detection was performed by Alexa488-conjugated antibody. Images were acquired using Zeiss AxioObserver Z1 Apotome 2.0 63 × numerical aperture 1.45. Images were digitally zoomed by Adobe Photoshop 7.0.

Measurement of Fe–S cluster enzyme activity. Measurement of Fe–S cluster enzyme activity was performed as described[53,54]. Briefly, succinate dehydrogenase activity was measured after activation of the complex by incubation with 20 mM succinate for 10 min at 30 °C. After the inhibition of other three respiratory complexes, 65 μM ubiquinone was added as an electron acceptor. The reduction of ubiquinone was coupled to formation of reduced 2,6-dichlorophenolindophenol. The loss in blue colour of 2,6-dichlorophenolindophenol was measured at 600 nm. Aconitase activity was carried out according to the procedure described[53].

Electron paramagnetic spectroscopy. The formation of vanadium peroxido species and change in oxidation states were performed on Bruker ER 041X Microwave Bridge X-band EPR spectrometer. The spectrum was recorded by addition of H_2O_2 (7%, 30 μl) to the capillary tube containing Vn (4 mg), followed by quenching in liquid N_2 and at room temperature. Control experiments were carried out in the same condition, with addition of GSH (25 mM, 30 μl) to Vn alone and vanadium peroxido species formed on Vn. Similarly, Vc (4 mg) and bulk V_2O_5 (4 mg) in the presence of GSH was also analysed.

HPLC analysis of GSH to GSSG conversion. The reaction mixture was produced in such a way that it contained 0.02 mg Vn, 2 mM GSH, 240 μM H_2O_2 in 1 ml H_2O. This mixture was incubated in the auto sampler and injected automatically using 10 μl each at the appropriate time. The formation of GSSG was followed at 220 nm using Waters 2695 HPLC instrument having automatic injection system equipped with photodiode array detector. Intermediates such as GSOH and GSO_2H were also detected by HPLC analysis and confirmed by mass spectroscopy using Bruker esquire 6000 mass spectrometer working in electron spray ionization mode.

Antibodies and immunoblotting. Immunodetection of catalase, GPx1 and SOD2 was performed using the antibodies, anti-catalase (Calbiochem, 1:4,000), anti-GPx1 (Pierce Thermo Scientific, 1:2,000) and anti-SOD2 (Pierce Thermo Scientific, 1:500), respectively. The other specific antibodies, anti-Prx3 (Pierce Thermo Scientific, 1:5,000), anti-FTH1 (Pierce Thermo Scientific, 1:500), anti-FLT1 (Pierce Thermo Scientific, 1:1,000), anti-TrxR1 (Pierce Thermo Scientific, 1:1,000), anti-Trx (Pierce Thermo Scientific, 1:1,000), anti-GCLM (Pierce Thermo Scientific, 1:1,000), anti-GCLC (Pierce Thermo Scientific, 1:500) and anti-HO-1 (Pierce Thermo Scientific, 1:500) were used to detect the expression profile of respective proteins. Anti-β-actin (Sigma, 1:20,000) was used as a loading control. The secondary detection was performed using horseradish peroxidase-conjugated anti-rabbit IgG (GE Amersham 1:20,000) or anti-mouse IgG (GE Amersham 1:10,000), and visualized by ECL chemiluminescent reagent (GE Amersham).

Electrode preparation and cyclic voltammetric analysis. For electrochemical studies, Vn and Vb electrodes were fabricated on stainless steel (SS) disks as the current collectors. Briefly, a commercial-grade SS foil disk (diameter 16 mm) was dipped in 30% dilute HNO_3 for about 5 min, washed several times with ultrapure water followed by acetone and dried in air. A mixture of Vn/Vb (90 wt %), acetylene carbon black (Alfa Aesar) (5 wt %) and polyvinylidene difluoride (5 wt %) was ground and a few drops of *N*-Methyl-2-pyrrolidone were added to get an ink, which was applied on the pre-treated SS disk of area 2.0 cm^2. The disk was dried at 100 °C for about 30 min. The coating and drying steps were repeated to achieve a loading level of 6.0 mg cm^{-2}. Finally, the electrodes were dried at 110 °C under vacuum for 12 h. Coin-type cells (CR 2025) were assembled using a Li foil for the counter electrode in coin cell containers purchased from Hohsen Corporation, Japan. Before the cell assembly, the surface of Li ribbon was scraped to remove surface film. A microporous polypropylene film (Celgard model 2400) was used as the separator and the electrolyte was 1 M $LiPF_6$ in 1:1 (v/v) mixed solvents of dry ethylene carbonate and dimethyl carbonate. All the manipulations such as preparation of the mixed solvent, its purification, electrolyte preparation and cell assembly were carried out in an Ar atmosphere using a glove box (MBraun model UNILAB). The cyclic voltammetry was performed in a potential range from 2.00 to 4.00 V at 0.1 mV s^{-1} scan rate.

References

1. Brand, M. D. The sites and topology of mitochondrial superoxide production. *Exp. Gerontol.* **45,** 466–472 (2010).
2. Lambeth, J. D. NOX enzymes and the biology of reactive oxygen. *Nat. Rev. Immunol.* **4,** 181–189 (2004).
3. Finkel, T. Signal transduction by reactive oxygen species. *J. Cell Biol.* **194,** 7–15 (2011).
4. Finkel, T. Signal transduction by mitochondrial oxidants. *J. Biol. Chem.* **287,** 4434–4440 (2012).
5. Kuo, L. J. & Yang, L. X. Gamma-H2AX—a novel biomarker for DNA double-strand breaks. *In Vivo* **22,** 305–309 (2008).
6. Ray, G. *et al.* Lipid peroxidation, free radical production and antioxidant status in breast cancer. *Breast Cancer Res. Treat.* **59,** 163–170 (2000).
7. Dalle-Donne, I. *et al.* Protein carbonylation, cellular dysfunction, and disease progression. *J. Cell. Mol. Med.* **10,** 389–406 (2006).
8. Baynes, J. W. Role of oxidative stress in development of complications in diabetes. *Diabetes* **40,** 405–412 (1991).
9. Ceccarelli, J. *et al.* The redox state of the lung cancer microenvironment depends on the levels of thioredoxin expressed by tumor cells and affects tumor progression and response to prooxidants. *Int. J. Cancer* **123,** 1770–1778 (2008).
10. Le Bras, M., Clement, M. V., Pervaiz, S. & Brenner, C. Reactive oxygen species and the mitochondrial signaling pathway of cell death. *Histol. Histopathol.* **20,** 205–219 (2005).
11. Nishikawa, T. *et al.* Normalizing mitochondrial superoxide production blocks three pathways of hyperglycaemic damage. *Nature* **404,** 787–790 (2000).
12. Oberley, L. W. & Buettner, G. R. Role of superoxide dismutase in cancer: a review. *Cancer Res.* **39,** 1141–1149 (1979).

13. Oberley, T. D. & Oberley, L. W. Antioxidant enzyme levels in cancer. *Histol. Histopathol.* **12,** 525–535 (1997).
14. Sena, L. A. & Chandel, N. S. Physiological roles of mitochondrial reactive oxygen species. *Mol. Cell* **48,** 158–167 (2012).
15. Sies, H. Glutathione and its role in cellular functions. *Free Radic. Biol. Med.* **27,** 916–921 (1999).
16. Arthur, J. R. The glutathione peroxidases. *Cell Mol. Life Sci.* **57,** 1825–1835 (2000).
17. Mugesh, G. & Singh, H. B. Synthetic organoselenium compounds as antioxidants: glutathione peroxidase activity. *Chem. Soc. Rev.* **29,** 347–357 (2000).
18. Bhabak, K. P. & Mugesh, G. Functional mimics of glutathione peroxidase: bioinspired synthetic antioxidants. *Acc. Chem. Res.* **43,** 1408–1419 (2010).
19. Wei, H. & Wang, E. Nanomaterials with enzyme-like characteristics (nanozymes): next-generation artificial enzymes. *Chem. Soc. Rev.* **42,** 6060–6093 (2013).
20. Gao, L. *et al.* Intrinsic peroxidase-like activity of ferromagnetic nanoparticles. *Nat. Nanotechnol.* **2,** 577–583 (2007).
21. Hou, C. *et al.* Construction of GPx active centers on natural protein nanodisk/nanotube: a new way to develop artificial nanoenzyme. *ACS Nano* **6,** 8692–8701 (2012).
22. Asati, A., Santra, S., Kaittanis, C., Nath, S. & Perez, J. M. Oxidase-like activity of polymer-coated cerium oxide nanoparticles. *Angew. Chem. Int. Ed. Engl.* **48,** 2308–2312 (2009).
23. Korsvik, C., Patil, S., Seal, S. & Self, W. T. Superoxide dismutase mimetic properties exhibited by vacancy engineered ceria nanoparticles. *Chem. Commun.* **10,** 1056–1058 (2007).
24. Vernekar, A. A. & Mugesh, G. Hemin-functionalized reduced graphene oxide nanosheets reveal peroxynitrite reduction and isomerization activity. *Chem. Eur. J.* **18,** 15122–15132 (2012).
25. Montiel-Davalos, A. *et al.* Vanadium pentoxide induces activation and death of endothelial cells. *J. Appl. Toxicol.* **32,** 26–33 (2012).
26. Rondini, E. A., Walters, D. M. & Bauer, A. K. Vanadium pentoxide induces pulmonary inflammation and tumor promotion in a strain-dependent manner. *Part. Fibre Toxicol.* **7,** 9 (2010).
27. Natalio, F. *et al.* Vanadium pentoxide nanoparticles mimic vanadium haloperoxidases and thwart biofilm formation. *Nat. Nanotechnol.* **7,** 530–535 (2012).
28. Liu, J. & Xue, D. Cation-Induced Coiling of Vanadium Pentoxide Nanobelts. *Nanoscale Res. Lett.* **5,** 1619–1626 (2010).
29. Bhabak, K. P. & Mugesh, G. Synthesis, characterization, and antioxidant activity of some ebselen analogues. *Chem. Eur. J.* **13,** 4594–4601 (2007).
30. Shi, X. L. & Dalal, N. S. Glutathione-reductase functions as vanadate (V) reductase. *Arch. Biochem. Biophys.* **278,** 288–290 (1990).
31. Andre, R. *et al.* V_2O_5 nanowires with an intrinsic peroxidase-like activity. *Adv. Funct. Mater.* **21,** 501–509 (2011).
32. Flohe, L. & Brand, I. Kinetics of glutathione peroxidase. *Biochim. Biophys. Acta* **191,** 541–549 (1969).
33. Paglia, D. E. & Valentine, W. N. Studies on the quantitative and qualitative characterization of erythrocyte glutathione peroxidase. *J. Lab. Clin. Med.* **70,** 158–169 (1967).
34. Ibuki, Y. & Toyooka, T. Nanoparticle uptake measured by flow cytometry. *Methods Mol. Biol.* **926,** 157–166 (2012).
35. Greulich, C. *et al.* Uptake and intracellular distribution of silver nanoparticles in human mesenchymal stem cells. *Acta Biomater.* **7,** 347–354 (2011).
36. Gutteridge, J. M. & Wilkins, S. Copper salt-dependent hydroxyl radical formation. Damage to proteins acting as antioxidants. *Biochim. Biophys. Acta* **759,** 38–41 (1983).
37. Ueda, M. *et al.* Effect of catalase-specific inhibitor 3-amino-1,2,4-triazole on yeast peroxisomal catalase in vivo *FEMS Microbiol. Lett.* **219,** 93–98 (2003).
38. Penttila, K. E. Allyl alcohol cytotoxicity and glutathione depletion in isolated periportal and perivenous rat hepatocytes. *Chem. Biol. Interact.* **65,** 107–121 (1988).
39. Martensson, J. *et al.* Inhibition of glutathione synthesis in the newborn rat: a model for endogenously produced oxidative stress. *Proc. Natl Acad. Sci. USA* **88,** 9360–9364 (1991).
40. Crans, D. C., Trujillo, A. M., Pharazyn, P. S. & Cohen, M. D. How environment affects drug activity: localization, compartmentalization and reactions of a vanadium insulin-enhancing compound, dipicolinatooxovanadium(V). *Coord. Chem. Rev.* **255,** 2178–2192 (2011).
41. Shi, X., Jiang, H., Mao, Y., Ye, J. & Saffiotti, U. Vanadium(IV)-mediated free radical generation and related 2'-deoxyguanosine hydroxylation and DNA damage. *Toxicology* **106,** 27–38 (1996).
42. Zhang, Z. *et al.* Vanadate-induced cell growth regulation and the role of reactive oxygen species. *Arch. Biochem. Biophys.* **392,** 311–320 (2001).
43. Hayes, J. D. & Dinkova-Kostova, A. T. The Nrf2 regulatory network provides an interface between redox and intermediary metabolism. *Trends Biochem. Sci.* **39,** 199–218 (2014).
44. D'Autreaux, B. & Toledano, M. B. ROS as signalling molecules: mechanisms that generate specificity in ROS homeostasis. *Nat. Rev. Mol. Cell Biol.* **8,** 813–824 (2007).
45. Rael, L. T. *et al.* Lipid peroxidation and the thiobarbituric acid assay: standardization of the assay when using saturated and unsaturated fatty acids. *J. Biochem. Mol. Biol.* **37,** 749–752 (2004).
46. Imlay, J. A. Pathways of oxidative damage. *Annu. Rev. Microbiol.* **57,** 395–418 (2003).
47. Vaubel, R. A. & Isaya, G. Iron-sulfur cluster synthesis, iron homeostasis and oxidative stress in Friedreich ataxia. *Mol. Cell Neurosci.* **55,** 50–61 (2013).
48. Wachs, I. E. & Roberts, C. A. Monitoring surface metal oxide catalytic active sites with Raman spectroscopy. *Chem. Soc. Rev.* **39,** 5002–5017 (2010).
49. Molinari, J. E. & Wachs, I. E. Presence of surface vanadium peroxo-oxo umbrella structures in supported vanadium oxide catalysts: fact or fiction? *J. Am. Chem. Soc.* **132,** 12559–12561 (2010).
50. Światowska-Mrowiecka, J., Maurice, V., Zanna, S., Klein, L. & Marcus, P. XPS study of Li ion intercalation in V_2O_5 thin films prepared by thermal oxidation of vanadium metal. *Electrochim. Acta* **52,** 5644–5653 (2007).
51. Perera, S. D. *et al.* Vanadium oxide nanowire—Graphene binder free nanocomposite paper electrodes for supercapacitors: A facile green approach. *J. Power Sources* **230,** 130–137 (2013).
52. Ligtenbarg, A. G. J., Hage, R. & Feringa, B. L. Catalytic oxidations by vanadium complexes. *Coord. Chem. Rev.* **237,** 89–101 (2003).
53. Pierik, A. J., Netz, D. J. & Lill, R. Analysis of iron-sulfur protein maturation in eukaryotes. *Nat. Protoc.* **4,** 753–766 (2009).
54. Spinazzi, M., Casarin, A., Pertegato, V., Salviati, L. & Angelini, C. Assessment of mitochondrial respiratory chain enzymatic activities on tissues and cultured cells. *Nat. Protoc.* **7,** 1235–1246 (2012).

Acknowledgements

This work was supported by the Department of Science and Technology (DST) and Department of Biotechnology (DBT), New Delhi. G.M. and P.D. thank the DST for the award of Swarnajayanti Fellowship. A.A.V. and D.S. thank the Council for Scientific and Industrial Research (CSIR) for a research fellowship. S.S. acknowledges the DST for INSPIRE fellowship. P.D. also thanks Lady Tata Memorial Research Award. We acknowledge Professor S.V. Bhat, K.S. Bhagyashree and L.R. Goveas for providing the EPR facility, B.L. Prahlada for Raman spectroscopic analysis and Professor N. Munichandraiah, S. Kumar and T.R. Penki for cyclic voltammetric studies. We also thank Sophisticated Analytical Instrumentation Facility (SAIF), Indian Institute of Technology, Bombay (IITB) for the ICP-AES facility and Indian Institute of Science for the FACS facility, fluorescence microscopy, TEM and SEM facilities.

Author contributions

A.A.V. and G.M. conceived the study and designed the project. D.S. and P.D. conceptualized the experiments on biological systems. P.U.P. carried out the synthesis and characterization of nanoparticles. A.A.V. and P.U.P. explored the reaction kinetics and mechanism of Vn activity. D.S. and S.S. designed and performed experiments on biological systems. A.A.V., D.S. and S.S. performed electron microscopic analysis in cells. A.A.V. interpreted data on chemical characterization of Vn and D.S. its biological properties. All the authors prepared the manuscript.

Additional information

Competing financial interests: The authors declare no competing financial interests.

6

Virus-like glycodendrinanoparticles displaying quasi-equivalent nested polyvalency upon glycoprotein platforms potently block viral infection

Renato Ribeiro-Viana[1,2], Macarena Sánchez-Navarro[1], Joanna Luczkowiak[3], Julia R. Koeppe[1], Rafael Delgado[3], Javier Rojo[2] & Benjamin G. Davis[1]

Ligand polyvalency is a powerful modulator of protein-receptor interactions. Host-pathogen infection interactions are often mediated by glycan ligand-protein interactions, yet its interrogation with very high copy number ligands has been limited to heterogenous systems. Here we report that through the use of nested layers of multivalency we are able to assemble the most highly valent glycodendrimeric constructs yet seen (bearing up to 1,620 glycans). These constructs are pure and well-defined single entities that at diameters of up to 32 nm are capable of mimicking pathogens both in size and in their highly glycosylated surfaces. Through this mimicry these glyco-dendri-protein-nano-particles are capable of blocking (at picomolar concentrations) a model of the infection of T-lymphocytes and human dendritic cells by Ebola virus. The high associated polyvalency effects ($\beta > 10^6$, $\beta/N \sim 10^2$-10^3) displayed on an unprecedented surface area by precise clusters suggest a general strategy for modulation of such interactions.

[1] Department of Chemistry, University of Oxford, Chemistry Research Laboratory, 12 Mansfield Road, Oxford OX1 3TA, UK. [2] Glycosystems Laboratory, Instituto de Investigaciones Químicas (IIQ), CSIC—Universidad de Sevilla, Américo Vespucio 49, Seville 41092, Spain. [3] Laboratorio de Microbiología Molecular, Instituto de Investigación Hospital 12 de Octubre (imas12), Madrid 28041, Spain. Correspondence and requests for materials should be addressed to R.D. (email: rdelgado.hdoc@salud.madrid.org) or to J.R. (email: javier.rojo@iiq.csic.es) or to B.G.D. (email: ben.davis@chem.ox.ac.uk).

The initial stages of an infectious process are crucial for subsequent immune response and elimination of pathogens[1]. The innate immune system comprises mechanisms and specialized cells responsible for first contact with external biological agents[2]. Detection of invaders via pathogen recognition receptors and subsequent activation of antimicrobial defences triggers specific antigen responses[3]. DC-SIGN (dendritic cell-specific intercellular adhesion molecule-3-grabbing nonintegrin) receptor is one of the most important pathogen recognition receptor. It is expressed mainly on the surface of dendritic cells (DCs), and some subtypes of macrophages[4]. DC-SIGN recognizes in a multivalent manner mannose and fucose containing glycoproteins[5], such as ICAM-3 (intercellular adhesion molecule 3) present in T cells, and envelope glycoproteins found on pathogens[6]. By using DC-SIGN as an entry point some viruses are capable of escaping from the processing and degradation events carried out by the immune defence machinery at antigen-presenting cells[7]. Therefore, the inhibition of pathogen entry through the blockade of this receptor at early stages of infection is one strategy for new antiviral agents.

Several studies have been directed towards the preparation of synthetic carbohydrate systems able to block or stimulate DC-SIGN[8–21]. Despite their elegant design, one of the problems that these artificial systems face is achieving adequate size and multivalency to sufficiently mimic natural systems such as viruses or other pathogens while maintaining full control of shape and structure[16]. Indeed, ligand valencies beyond 32 (refs 9,18) have not been possible before with full control (Indeed, valencies >100 are rare in any glycodendrimeric structure. See the following references André *et al.*[22] and Camponovo *et al.*[23] for examples of 128-mer lactoside and 243-mer xyloside display, respectively.)[22,23].

We have previously demonstrated that symmetrically multivalent glycan ligands mounted on protein platforms (glycodendriproteins) are useful tools to study carbohydrate–protein interactions and are able to control or modulate a desired response[24–27]. Other dendrimeric displays on proteins have also been explored subsequently[28–30]. However, to date, this approach has provided only limited carbohydrate valency levels on single protein platforms. We envisaged that a controlled design for a highly polyvalent protein display of sugars might be achieved through a novel strategy of 'nested polyvalency' (polyvalent display of polyvalency) (Fig. 1a).

We describe here the realization of this approach through the multivalent assembly of protein monomers themselves carrying polyvalent glycan display motifs (glycodendrons). The resulting glycodendriprotein homomultimers display many glycans in a precise manner. Consistent with associated guiding physical principles[31–33], these constructs therefore display symmetry and pseudosymmetry at both the level of protein assembly and glycodendron. These synthetic glycoprotein assemblies display the highest known number of glycans ($n = 1{,}620$) yet presented in a homogeneous manner. We have applied this idea (Fig. 1) here to the inhibitory immunomodulation of a DC-SIGN-pathogen glycoprotein interaction (Fig. 1b).

Results

Construction of glyco-dendri-protein-nano-particles. We reasoned that assembly of an entity with similar dimensions (in the form of a self-assembled protein sphere-like icosahedron Qβ[34], $\sim$28 nm in diameter) might mimic the display in target pathogens (Ebola pseudotyped virus particles have $\sim$90 nm in diameter). Using a tag-and-modify[27] strategy, we chose to selectively introduce a non-natural amino acid (tag) on the protein that could be used for the attachment (modify) of the selected glycodendrons appropriately functionalized at the focal position. As a stringent test of this approach we chose to mimic the highly glycosylated pathogen envelopes of Ebola virus. We selected a monomer Qβ[34,35] protein as carrier, which assembles into a 180-copy multimer. Qβ multimer has been used by us and others to display glycans for other purposes but in these prior experiments only partial levels of nonspecific modification were achieved (see Supplementary Discussion). The result of these prior incomplete reactions was a formation of mixtures and not the desired homogeneous and (pseudo)symmetrical display required for this study[36,37]. This proteic platform provided the necessary viral mimic scaffold (core diameter, $\sim$28 nm)[34] to construct the desired multivalent systems.

The designed glycodendrons were prepared in a straightforward manner by the Cu(I)-catalysed modification[38,39] of the Huisgen cycloaddition as depicted in Fig. 2. α-D-Mannose was chosen to be introduced onto the dendritic scaffolds as a relevant ligand that is recognized by DC-SIGN[5]. Synthesis of glycodendron **4** was accomplished using a modular strategy that advantageously avoided the need for carbohydrate protection. First, unprotected azidoethyl mannoside **3** (see Supplementary Methods)[8] was coupled to the trialkynyl pentaerythritol core **2** using $CuSO_4$ and sodium ascorbate in a 1:1 mixture of water:THF (tetrahydrofuran) at room temperature (RT)[40]. The focal azido group required for subsequent site-specific conjugation to the protein tag, was introduced by reaction with sodium azide to give **5**. The designed modular strategy also allowed use of **5** in the construction of higher generation glycodendron **8**. Thus, coupling of **5** with the trialkynyl core **6** gave **7** (Fig. 2), which was similarly converted to an azide **8** for protein modification.

Unnatural alkyne-containing amino acid L-homopropargylglycine (Hpg) was site-specifically introduced into the protein that would make up the proteic scaffold (Qβ) to serve as an alkyne 'tag' through the expression of corresponding gene sequences in an auxotrophic strain of *E. coli* (B834(DE3))[41]. Gene sequences were designed to create a protein displaying alkyne at a site on the outer surface of the eventual icosahedral platform (Hpg16) for which the position could simply be controlled by the 'Met' triplet codon ATG. Replacement of wildtype methionine (Met) residues, with near-isosteric amino acid isoleucine allows reassignment of the codons in the gene sequence to allow incorporation instead of Hpg as a 'tag' (see Supplementary Methods for full details). The resulting Qβ-$(Hpg16)_{180}$ was characterized, including by mass spectrometry and dynamic light scattering (Fig. 3 and see Supplementary Methods and Supplementary Fig. S1), demonstrating the introduction of the Hpg amino acid into the sequence. On the basis of previous results[42,43], Qβ-$(Hpg16)_{180}$ was modified using a reaction mixture of Cu(I)Br complexed by tris[(1-ethylacetate-1*H*-1,2,3-triazol-4-yl) methyl]amine in acetonitrile (Fig. 3a). It should be noted that the presence of Hpg on the protein results in slower Huisgen cycloaddition reaction rates in comparison with those obtained when azide in the form of azidohomoalanine (Aha) is present in the protein[42,43]. Optimization of the reaction conditions by varying catalyst loading and stepwise addition, afforded the desired glycodendron-bearing virus-like particles. Thus, reaction of Qβ-$(Hpg16)_{180}$ with trivalent glycodendron **5** afforded Qβ-$(Man_3)_{180}$ bearing 540 terminal mannosyl residues and reaction with second-generation nonavalent glycodendron **8** gave Qβ -$(Man_9)_{180}$. Both reactions proceeded with $>95\%$ conversion; consistent with greater bulk a longer reaction time (up to 7.5 h) was required for reaction of **8** to form 1,620-mer Qβ- $(Man_9)_{180}$. Increasing particle diameter was observed, Qβ (27.6 nm)$\rightarrow$Qβ-$(Man_3)_{180}$ (29.8)$\rightarrow$Qβ-$(Man_9)_{180}$ (32.0), consistent with the controlled introduction of 'shells' of glycosylation $\sim$1.1 nm thick (Fig. 3b and see Supplementary Table S1 for rough estimate of dendron length)

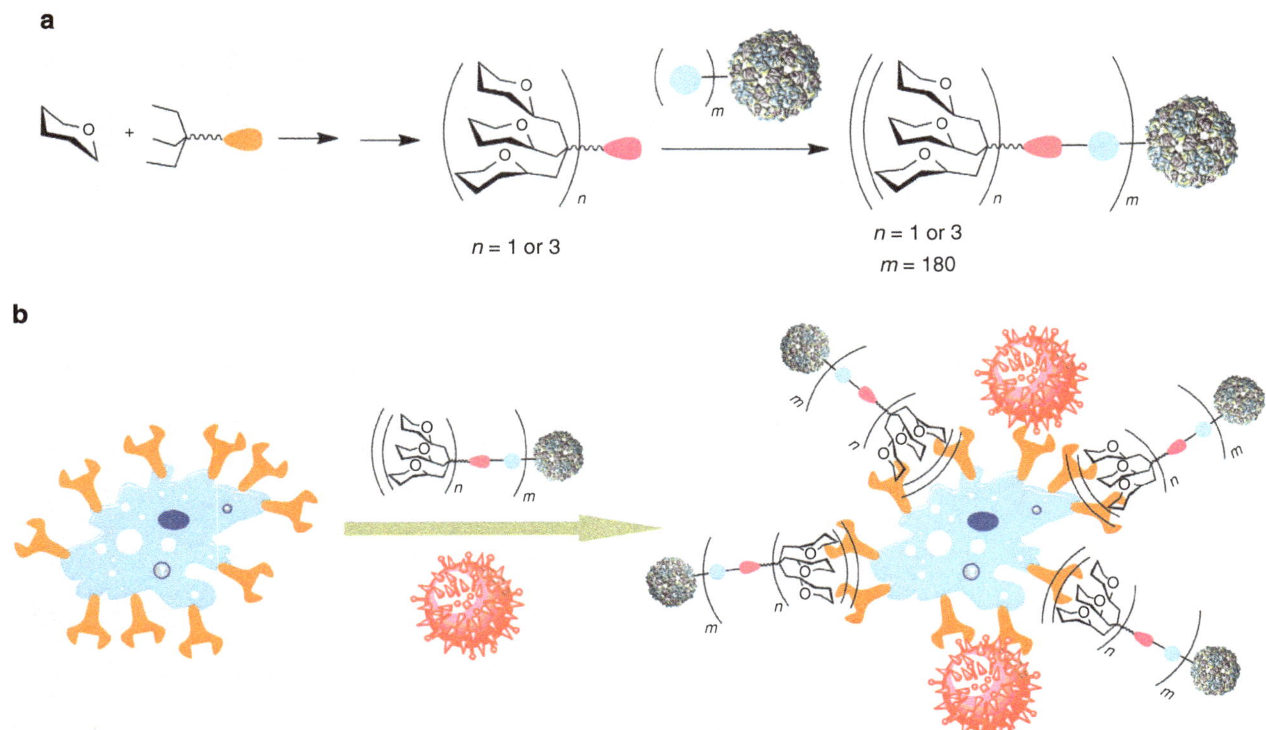

Figure 1 | Schematic representation of the nested polyvalency strategy. (**a**) Nested symmetrical assembly of virus-like glycodendrinanoparticles using a tag-and-modify strategy. Glycodendrons are created through iterative multivalent assembly and then attached to multiple tags, each in a monomer protein. (**b**) Ebola (shown in red) infection model and its competitive inhibition with virus-like glycodendrinanoparticles.

for each dendron generation. To the best of our knowledge, this is the first synthesis reported of such highly functionalized monodisperse glycodendriproteins (bearing up to 1,620 terminal sugar moieties) using a convergent approach.

Inhibition of DC-SIGN *in vitro* and on T lymphocytes. The inhibitory function of these glycodendriprotein particles was tested in several ways. Competition ELISA assay (See Supplementary Methods and Supplementary Figs S2 and S3) revealed that Qβ-$(Man_3)_{180}$ could completely inhibit the binding of DC-SIGN (as an Fc chimera) to a synthetically mannosylated glycoprotein (albumin bearing Manα1–3(Manα1–6)Man) with an estimated IC_{50} ~35–40 nM. A complete lack of inhibition by control, non-glycosylated Qβ confirmed dependence of this promisingly potent inhibition upon glycan.

Next, an Ebola viral infection model[44], was explored using mammalian T-lymphocyte (Jurkat) cells displaying DC-SIGN. Recombinant viruses were produced in HEK 293 T cells; the viral construction was pseudotyped with Ebola virus envelope GP (EboGP) or the vesicular stomatitis virus envelope glycoprotein (VSV-G) and expressed luciferase as a reporter of the infection[45]. The inhibition of DC-SIGN-dependent infection of T-lymphocyte Jurkat cells (examined in at least three independent experiments) demonstrated that unglycosylated Qβ reduced infection minimally (Fig. 4a). In contrast, Qβ-$(Man_3)_{180}$ and Qβ-$(Man_9)_{180}$ showed strong dose-dependent inhibition of the infection process (Fig. 4a–c). Indeed, Qβ-$(Man_9)_{180}$ presented a notable antiviral activity, inhibiting infection by ~80% at 5 nM; estimated IC_{50}s = 9.62 nM for β-$(Man_3)_{180}$ and = 910 pM for Qβ-$(Man_9)_{180}$.

VSV-G is able to infect T-lymphocyte Jurkat cells independently of DC-SIGN[44] and provided a positive control in infection experiments; consistent with the proposed model of inhibition (Fig. 1) this glycan-independent pathway for VSV-G was completely uninhibited (Fig. 4b,c). In this model, the Ebola infection process is absolutely dependent on the presence of DC-SIGN on the cell surface. Jurkat cells not expressing DC-SIGN were used as a negative control in the infection studies and showed no infection by Ebola pseudovirus (See Supplementary Fig. S4). The ratio of infection *in cis* between Jurkat DC-SIGN+ and Jurkat cells was ~2,600 for Ebola virus infection and 0.96 for VSV infection.

Blocking of DC infection by pseudotyped Ebola. Having shown such potent inhibition of infection of a stable cell line that displays DC-SIGN, we next evaluated inhibition in the perhaps more relevant and more demanding context of inhibition of primary cells. DCs are a primary target of Ebola infection; these display multiple C-type lectins that could provide a different or modulated route for infection with potentially higher affinty for virus. Accordingly, DCs were generated from isolated human peripheral blood mononuclear cells (PBMCs) and tested. We were pleased to find that as for the stable Jurkat cell line presenting DC-SIGN alone, Qβ-$(Man_9)_{180}$ displayed potent activity (Fig. 4d), inhibiting infection by >80% at 5 nM and >95% at 25 nM (estimated IC_{50} ~2 nM for Qβ-$(Man_9)_{180}$). Excitingly, these data indicate that the mode of inhibition of these synthetic glycodendrinanoparticles translates into cellular contexts relevant to human infection and are consistent with the mode of action suggested in Fig. 1.

Discussion

Although the evaluation of the number of monomer units interacting during these inhibitory processes is complicated by quasi-equivalence[32], the data obtained indicate that these systems afford a clear polyvalency effect (β)[46] when compared with the

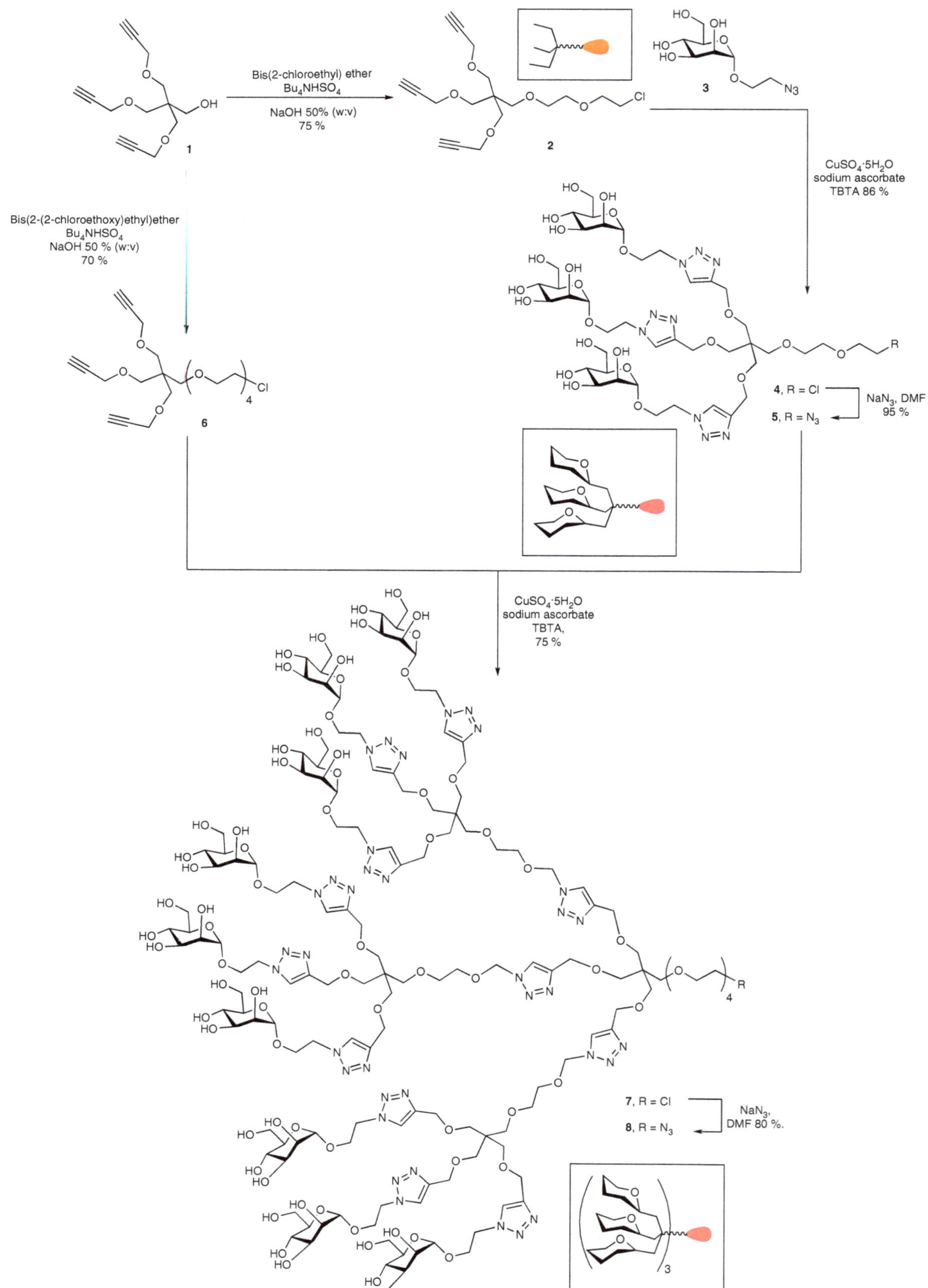

Figure 2 | Creation of polyvalent mannose-terminated glycodendrons. Synthesis of the glycondendron reagents **5** and **8** used in the assembly of virus-like glycodendri-nano-particles (see Fig. 3). TBTA, tribenzyl(tris)triazoylamine; DMF, *N,N*-dimethylformamide.

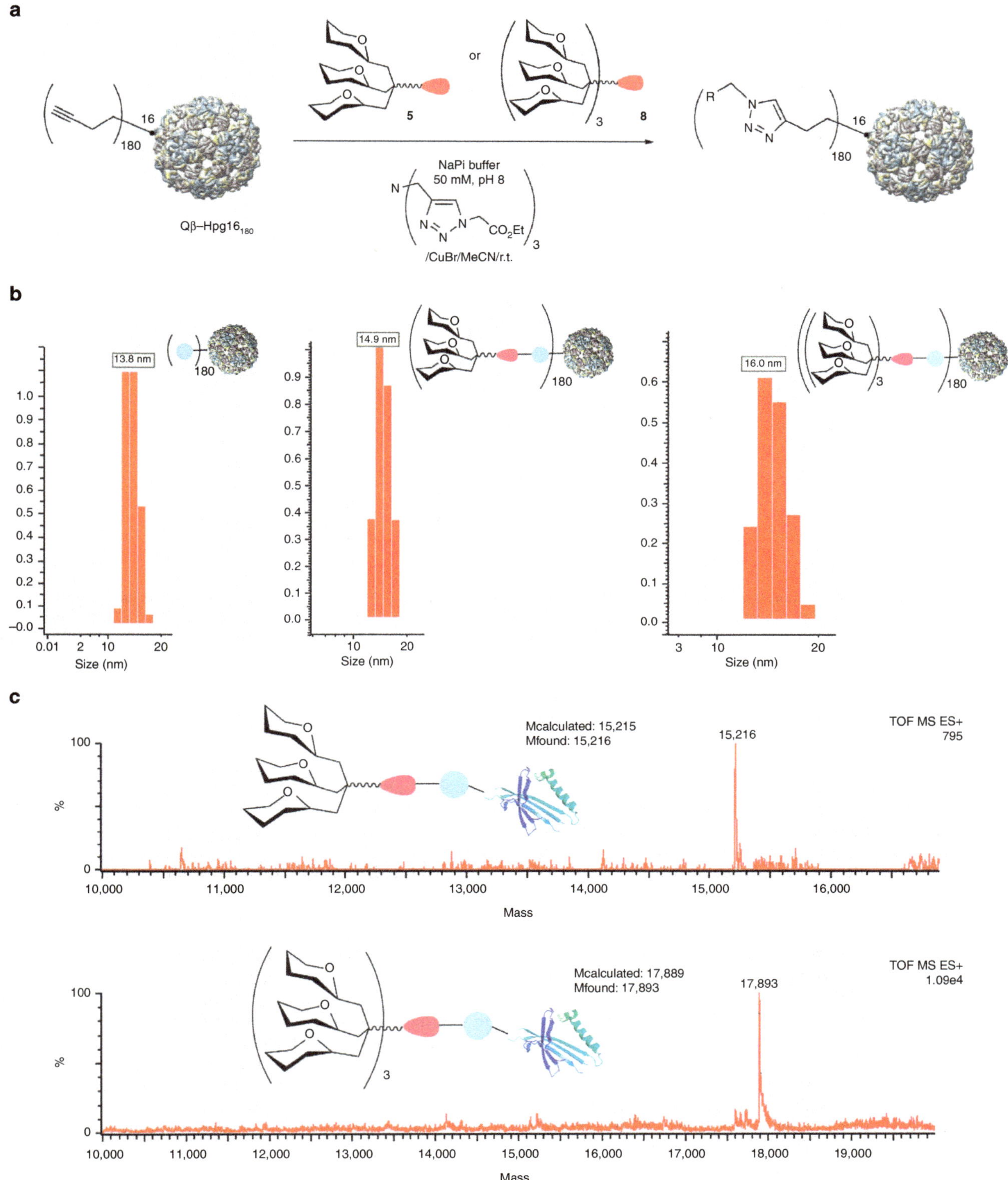

Figure 3 | Controlled assembly and characterization of virus-like glycodendri-nano-particles. (**a**) A tag-and-modify strategy allowed the generation of the second nested layer of multivalency from Qβ-(Hpg16)$_{180}$ using glycondendron reagents **5** and **8**. R = corresponding glycodendron. (**b**) Dynamic light scattering histograms showing the hydrodynamic radius of Qβ (radius 13.8 nm), Qβ-(Man$_3$)$_{180}$ (radius 14.9) and Qβ-(Man$_9$)$_{180}$ (radius 16.0). (**c**) Mass spectrometric analysis of monomer proteins of the particles. P$_i$, phosphate.

monomer methyl α-D-mannopyranoside) (see Supplementary Table S2). The inhibitory properties of each mannoside monomer unit can therefore be considered[46] to be ~250-fold and ~860-fold (as judged by β/N, see Supplementary Table S2) more potent when displayed in Qβ(Man$_3$)$_{180}$ and Qβ-(Man$_9$)$_{180}$, respectively, than when displayed alone. The efficiency of this system therefore

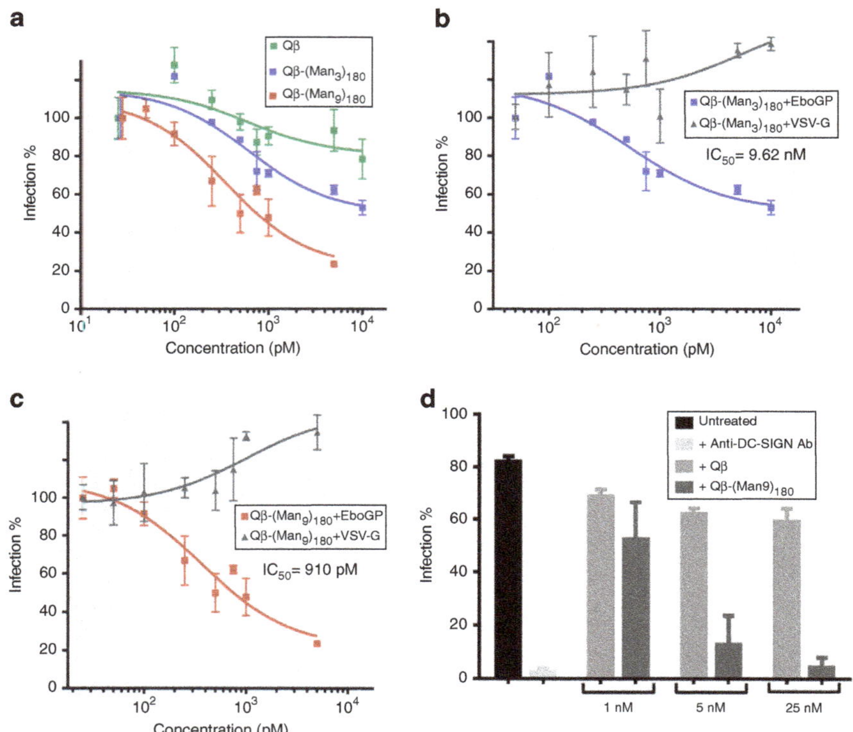

Figure 4 | Inhibition of viral infection of mammalian cells. (**a**) Comparison of infection rates of T-lymphocyte (Jurkat) cells displaying DC-SIGN by EboGP pseudovirus in the presence of Qβ, Qβ-$(Man_3)_{180}$, Qβ-$(Man_9)_{180}$; (**b**) Inhibition by Qβ-$(Man_3)_{180}$ of EBOV-GP (EboG) pseudovirus and vesicular stomatitis psuedovirus (VSV-G) in the infection (% infection)of T-lymphocyte (Jurkat) cells displaying DC-SIGN; (**c**) as for (**b**) using Qβ-$(Man_9)_{180}$. Values correspond to means of three experiments with s.e.m. shown; the IC_{50}s were estimated using Graphpad Prism v4.0 at 95% with a 95% confidence interval (4.43–20.9 nM for Qβ-$(Man_3)_{180}$ and 651 pM-1.3 nM for Qβ-$(Man_9)_{180}$) and settings for normalized dose-response curves. See the Supplementary Fig. S5 for duplicated inhibition assays. (**d**) Inhibition of infection in *cis* of human DCs by EBOV-GP (EboG) using Qβ-$(Man_9)_{180}$. Anti-DC-SIGN Ab is an antibody that blocks DC-SIGN. Immature DCs were generated from isolated human PBMCs. Blockade with anti-DC-sign antibody was used as a positive control.

relies upon a vital combination of not only a high number of displayed ligands but also display size and geometry. To date, no homogeneous polyvalent systems have been described that can generate such a large surface area (solvent-accessible surface area ~725,000 Å[247]) as the systems we have described here. The system we describe here is based on an icosahedral scaffold ($T = 3$, triakis iscosahedral) that generates several underlying quasi-symmetry elements including those that relate the displayed glycodendrons in a two-fold, three-fold and six-fold manner (see Supplementary Movie 1). It is tempting to speculate that this, in turn, allows the simultaneous display of many distinct putative global glycan clusters where the glycan 'tips' are also quasi-equivalent (for example, 6-fold-related faces displaying a resultant 54-mer in Qβ-$(Man_9)_{180}$ or a 3-fold-related 9-mer in Qβ-$(Man_3)_{180}$, see Supplementary Movie 1). In this way, the nested glycan polyvalency that we have developed here may allow many subtly varying polyvalent combinations to be displayed, each of which (or even a combination of which) might give rise to optimal biological function (here inhibition of Ebola binding). These constructs are therefore not 'balls of sugar' but homogenous constructs that array varying faces with different polyvalent glycan arrangements. Thus, their most relevant structural features may well not be simply their average glycan-to-glycan distance (as estimated, say, from Cα-to-Cα residue distances of ~28–40 Å for 2-fold up to 6-fold quasi-symmetry) but instead the specific topology of glycan display and how that relates to both the inter-domain distances in the DC-SIGN tetramer[48] as well as its organization on cell surfaces.[49] Moreover, initial inspection of other viral surfaces suggests that such topologies might effectively out-compete not only Ebola but also other human pathogens. The striking β values that we have discovered here may well arise from such specific 'optimal' faces (see Supplementary Movie 1 for illustrative examples of these quasi-symmetrical faces). Indeed, although direct comparison with non-viral systems is not possible, non-viral particles displaying multiple mannosyl residues in a less ordered manner are notably less potent and show much lower multivalency effects ($\beta \leq 20$, see Supplementary Table S2).

In summary, a novel nested polyvalency approach combined with tag-and-modify site-selective protein synthesis has allowed the creation of homogeneous protein platforms bearing glycodendrons. These well-defined polyvalent glycoprotein assemblies present on their surface up to 1,620 copies of glycan, a remarkably high valency never obtained before using a fully controlled strategy. These glycodendriprotein particles show exciting antiviral activity, preventing mammalian cell infection by Ebola pseudotyped virus through competitive blockade of the DC-SIGN receptor in the nanomolar to picomolar range. These results clearly indicate the efficiency of these systems to interact with this pattern recognition receptor and to compete with pathogens during their entry into target cells. Their *in vivo* activity remains to be tested and it is possible that such constructs, if used in this context, could elicit humoral responses that might potentially neutralize some of the interactions studied here. The high activity and fascinating (quasi)symmetric, high surface area morphology of these new glycoconjugates provides promising candidates for the development of both new antiviral agents as well as probes of larger-scale biological events.

Methods

Synthesis of glycodendrons. *Glycodendron 4*: 2-Azidoethyl α-D-mannopyranoside (306 mg, 1.2 mmol), 2-(2-chloroethoxy)ethoxymethyl trikis(2-propynyloxymethyl)methane (128 mg. 0.37 mmol), $CuSO_4 \cdot 5H_2O$ (9 mg, 0.04 mmol), tribenzyl(tris)triazoylamine (39 mg, 0.07 mmol) and sodium ascorbate (29 mg, 0.15 mmol) were dissolved in 2 ml of THF/H_2O (1:1). After consumption of the starting material (3 h), the solvent was evaporated and the crude was purified by size-exclusion chromatography (Sephadex LH-20 MeOH 100%), furnishing the glycondendron **4** as a white foam (347 mg, 86%).

Glycodendron 5: Glycodendron **4** (80 mg, 0.07 mmol) and sodium azide (47 mg, 0.7 mmol) were dissolved in *N,N*-dimethylformamide (2 ml). The mixture was stirred at 60 °C for 4 days. After consumption of the starting material, the solvent was concentrated and the crude was purified by size-exclusion chromatography (Sephadex G-25 H_2O/MeOH 9:1), furnishing glycondendron **5** (76 mg, 95%) as a white foam.

Glycodendron 7: Glycodendron **5** (30 mg, 0.03 mmol), [2-[2-(2-chloroethoxy)ethoxy]ethoxy]ethoxymethyl tris(2-propynyloxymethyl)methane (3.6 mg, 0.008 mmol), $CuSO_4 \cdot 5H_2O$ (0.5 mg, 0.002 mmol), tribenzyl(tris)triazoylamine (1.7 mg, 0.003 mmol) and sodium ascorbate (1.3 mg, 0.006 mmol) were dissolved in THF/H_2O (1:1, 1 ml). After consumption of the starting material, the solvent was evaporated and the crude was purified by size-exclusion chromatography (Sephadex LH-20 MeOH 100%), furnishing glycondendron **7** (22 mg, 75%) as a white foam.

Glycodendron 8: Glycodendron **7** (25 mg, 0.007 mmol) and sodium azide (4 mg, 0.07 mmol) were dissolved in *N,N*-dimethylformamide (1 ml). The mixture was stirred at 60 °C for 4 days. After that, the solvent was concentrated and the crude was purified by size-exclusion chromatography (Sephadex G-25 H_2O/MeOH 9:1), furnishing glycondendron **8** (20 mg, 80%) as a white foam.

Synthesis of virus-like glycodendrinanoparticles. *Glycoprotein Qβ-(Man$_3$)$_{180}$*: Glycodendron **5** (2.84 mg, 0.002 mmol) was dissolved in sodium phosphate buffer (50 mM, pH = 8, 200 µl). Protein solution (180 µg, 100 µl) was added to the above solution and mixed thoroughly. A freshly prepared solution of copper (I) bromide (99.999%) in acetonitrile (32.6 µl of 10 mg ml^{-1}) was premixed with an acetonitrile solution of tris[(1-ethylacetate-1*H*-1,2,3- triazol-4-yl)methyl] amine (12.6 µl of 100 mg ml^{-1}). The preformed Cu-complex solution (25 µl) was added to the mixture and the reaction was agitated on a rotator for at RT. After 4 h, 150 µl of buffer and 50 µl of fresh Cu-complex solution were added to the mixture again and the reaction was agitated for a further 1.5 h. The resulting mixture was purified in PD-MiniTrap (G-25) twice and concentrated on a vivaspin membrane concentrator (30 KDa molecular weight cut off) to 400 µl. To a virus-like particle aliquot (20 µl) was added 1 µl of TCEP (1 M) to allow the protein to denature before analysis by liquid chromatography–mass spectrometry. Electrospray Ionization Mass Spectrometry (TOF ES+) (*m/z*): calc. 15,215; found 15,216.

Glycoprotein Qβ-(Man$_9$)$_{180}$: Glycodendron **8** (4.8 mg, 0.001 mmol) was dissolved in sodium phosphate buffer (50 mM, pH = 8, 50 µl). Protein solution (90 µg, 50 µl) was added to the above solution and mixed thoroughly. A freshly prepared solution of copper (I) bromide (99.999%) in acetonitrile (32.6 µl of 10 mg ml^{-1}) was premixed with an acetonitrile solution tris[(1-ethylacetate-1*H*-1,2,3- triazol-4-yl)methyl] amine, (12.6 µl of 100 mg ml^{-1}). The preformed Cu-complex solution (25 µl) was added to the mixture and the reaction was agitated on a rotator at RT. After 3 and 6 h, 50 µl of buffer and 12.5 µl of fresh Cu-complex solution were added to the mixture again (each time) and the reaction was agitated for further 1.5 h. The resulting mixture was purified in PD-MiniTrap (G-25) twice and concentrated on a vivaspin membrane concentrator (30 KDa molecular weight cut off) to 400 µl. To a virus-like particle aliquot (20 µl) was added 1 µl of TCEP (1M) to allow the protein to denature before analysis by liquid chromatography–mass spectrometry. ESI-MS (TOF ES+) (*m/z*): calc. 17,889; found 17,893.

Production of recombinant viruses. Recombinant viruses were produced in 293T cells. The viral construction was pseudotyped with EboGP or VSV-G and expressed luciferase as a reporter of the infection[45]. One day (18–24 h) before transfection, 6×10^6 293T were seeded onto 10 cm plates. Cells were cultured in DMEM medium supplemented with 10% heat-inactivated FBS, 25 mg gentamycin, 2 mM L-glutamine. A few minutes before transfection, the medium on transfection plates was changed to 9 ml DMEM and chloroquine was added to 25 µM final concentration. Transfection reaction with all reagents at RT was prepared in 15 ml tubes: 183 µl of 2M $CaCl_2$, 450 ng of Ebola virus envelope, 21 µg of pNL4-3 luc[50], 1,300 µl of water. Next, 1.5 ml of 2xHBS (hepes buffer saline) pH 7.0 was added quickly to the tubes and bubbled for 30 s. HBS/DNA solution was gently dropped onto medium. After 8 h of incubation at 37 °C with 5% CO_2, medium on transfection plates was changed to 10 ml DMEM and once again 1 day after transfection to 7 ml DMEM. Transfection supernatants were collected after 48 h, centrifuged at 1,200 rpm for 10 min at RT to remove cell debris, and stored frozen at −80 °C (ref. 51).

Infection of Jurkat cells displaying DC-SIGN in cis. Infection was performed on Jurkat cells (T-lymphocyte cell line) expressing receptor DC-SIGN on their surface. One day before infection, 5×10^4 of Jurkat DC-SIGN cells were plated into each well of 96-well plate. Cells were incubated at RT for 20 min with the carbohydrate-based compounds and then challenged with 5000 Tissue Culture Infective Dose of recombinant viruses. After 48 h of incubation cells were washed twice with PBS and lysed for luciferase assay. The range of concentrations tested for compounds Qβ and Qβ-(Man$_3$)$_{180}$ was 100 pM–50 nM and for compound Qβ-(Man$_9$)$_{180}$ was 50 pM–50 nM. As a control, an experiment of infection with VSV-G pseudoviruses was performed under the same conditions. Infection with VSV-G is independent of the presence of DC-SIGN receptor.

Generation of monocyte-derived DCs (DCs). PBMCs were isolated from buffy coats from healthy human donors (Hospital 12 de Octubre, Madrid, Spain) by Ficoll-Paque (Pharmacia, Uppsala, Sweden) density-gradient centrifugation. Following the centrifugation of 40 ml of whole blood samples on Ficoll-Paque at 2,000 rpm for 30 min, the cells from interface were collected and washed five times with PBS at 1,500 rpm for 5 min at RT. PBMCs were then resuspended in RPMI medium supplemented with 10% heat-inactivated FBS, 25 mg gentamycin, 2 mM L-glutamine at concentration 2×10^6 cells per ml and placed onto 24-well plate for 1 h at 37 °C with 5% CO_2. The adherent monolayer of monocytes were then washed twice with PBS and resuspended in RPMI medium supplemented with cytokines granulocyte–macrophage colony-stimulating factor (200 ng ml^{-1}) and IL-4 (10 ng ml^{-1}). For the differentiation of immature monocyte-derived DCs, cells were incubated at 37 °C with 5% CO_2 for 7 days and subsequently activated with cytokines on day 2 and 5 (refs 44,52,53).

Infection of immature monocyte-derived DCs in cis. Immature monocyte-derived DCs were incubated at RT for 20 min with the carbohydrate-based compounds and then challenged with 5000 TCID of EBOV-GP recombinant pseudoviruses. After 48 h of incubation cells were washed twice with PBS and lysed for luciferase assay. The range of concentrations tested for Qβ-(Man$_9$)$_{180}$ was 1, 5 and 25 nM. As a control, experiment of inhibition of infection of EBOV-GP was performed in the presence of antibody anti-DC-SIGN and mannan at concentration of 25 µg ml^{-1}.

Statistical methods. *Dynamic light scattering*: Dynamic light scattering values represent the average of 10 independent measurements, where 10 individual acquisitions were taken per measurement the results analysed using OmniSIZE software.

Infection assays: Statistical analysis was performed using GraphPad Prism v6.0.

Infection of mammalian Jurkat cells displaying DC-SIGN by EboV-GP pseudotyped viruses: The values of percentage of infection presented on the graph correspond to the mean of six independent experiments with error bars corresponding to the s.e.m. The IC_{50} values were estimated using GraphPad Prism v6.0 with a 95% confidence interval and settings to normalize dose-response curves.

Infection of primary monocyte-derived DC by EboV-GP pseudotyped viruses: The values of percentage of infection correspond to the mean of two independent experiments (error bars describe the range between the two values obtained).

References

1. Neyrolles, O., Gicquel, B. & Quintana-Murci, L. Towards a crucial role for DC-SIGN in tuberculosis and beyond. *Trends Microbiol.* **14,** 383–387 (2006).
2. Gordon, S. Pattern recognition receptors: doubling up for the innate immune response. *Cell* **111,** 927–930 (2002).
3. Medzhitov, R. Recognition of microorganisms and activation of the immune response. *Nature* **449,** 819–826 (2007).
4. Geijtenbeek, T. B. H. *et al.* Identification of DC-SIGN, a novel dendritic cell specific ICAM-3 receptor that supports primary immune responses. *Cell* **100,** 575–585 (2000).
5. Guo, Y. *et al.* Structural basis for distinct ligand-binding and targeting properties of the receptors DC-SIGN and DC-SIGNR. *Nat. Struct. Mol. Biol.* **11,** 591–598 (2004).
6. Steinman, R. M. DC-SIGN: a guide to some mysteries of dendritic cells. *Cell* **100,** 491–494 (2000).
7. van, K. Y. & Geijtenbeek, T. B. H. DC-SIGN: escape mechanism for pathogens. *Nat. Rev. Immunol.* **3,** 697–709 (2003).
8. Arce, E. *et al.* Glycodendritic structures based on Boltorn hyperbranched polymers and their interactions with Lens culinaris lectin. *Bioconjugate Chem.* **14,** 817–823 (2003).
9. Lasala, F., Arce, E., Otero, J. R., Rojo, J. & Delgado, R. Mannosyl glycodendritic structure inhibits DC-SIGN-mediated ebola virus infection in cis and in trans. *Antimicrob. Agents Chemother.* **47,** 3970–3972 (2003).
10. Borrok, M. J. & Kiessling, L. L. Non-carbohydrate inhibitors of the lectin DC-SIGN. *J. Am. Chem. Soc.* **129,** 12780–12785 (2007).
11. Reina, J. J. *et al.* 1,2-Mannobioside mimic: synthesis, DC-SIGN interaction by NMR and docking, and antiviral activity. *ChemMedChem* **2,** 1030–1036 (2007).
12. Mitchell, D. A. *et al.* Synthesis 2-C-branched derivatives of D-mannose: 2-C-aminomethyl-D-mannose binds to the human C-type lectin DC-SIGN with affinity greater than an order of magnitude compared to that of D-mannose. *Tetrahedron Asymmetry* **18,** 1502–1510 (2007).

13. Martínez-Ávila, O. *et al.* Multivalent manno-glyconanoparticles inhibit DC-SIGN-mediated HIV-1 trans-infection of human T cells. *ChemBioChem* **10**, 1806–1809 (2009).
14. Martínez-Ávila, O. *et al.* Gold manno-glyconanoparticles: multivalent systems to block HIV-1 gp120 binding to the lectin DC-SIGN. *Chem. Eur. J.* **15**, 9874–9888 (2009).
15. Sattin, S. *et al.* Inhibition of DC-SIGN-mediated HIV infection by a linear trimannoside mimic in a tetravalent presentation. *ACS Chem. Biol.* **5**, 301–312 (2010).
16. Sanchez-Navarro, M. & Rojo, J. Targeting DC-SIGN wih carbohydrate multivalent systems. *Drug News Perspect.* **23**, 557–572 (2010).
17. Wang, S.-K. *et al.* Targeting the carbohydrates on HIV-1: interaction of oligomannose dendrons with human monoclonal antibody 2G12 and DC-SIGN. *Proc. Natl Acad. Sci. USA* **105**, 3690–3695 (2008).
18. Greatrex, B. W. *et al.* The synthesis and immune stimulating action of mannose-capped lysine-based dendrimers. *Tetrahedron* **65**, 2939–2950 (2009).
19. Luczkowiak, J. *et al.* Pseudosaccharide functionalized dendrimers as potent inhibitors of DC-SIGN dependent Ebola pseudotyped viral infection. *Bioconjugate Chem.* **22**, 1354–1365 (2011).
20. Andreini, M. *et al.* Second generation of fucose-based DC-SIGN ligands: affinity improvement and specificity versus Langerin. *Org. Biomol. Chem.* **9**, 5778–5786 (2011).
21. Prost, L. R., Grim, J. C., Tonelli, M. & Kiessling, L. L. Noncarbohydrate glycomimetics and glycoprotein surrogates as DC-SIGN antagonists and agonists. *ACS Chem. Biol.* **7**, 1603–1608 (2012).
22. André, S., Ortega, P. J. C., Perez, M. A., Roy, R. & Gabius, H.-J. Lactose-containing starburst dendrimers: influence of dendrimer generation and binding-site orientation of receptors (plant/animal lectins and immunoglobulins) on binding properties. *Glycobiology* **9**, 1253–1261 (1999).
23. Camponovo, J. *et al.* 'Click' glycodendrimers containing 27, 81, and 243 modified xylopyranoside termini. *J. Org. Chem.* **74**, 5071–5074 (2009).
24. Davis, B. G. The controlled glycosylation of a protein with a bivalent glycan: towards a new class of glycoconjugates, glycodendriproteins. *Chem. Commun.* 351–352 (2001).
25. Rendle, P. M. *et al.* Glycodendriproteins: a synthetic glycoprotein mimic enzyme with branched sugar-display potently inhibits bacterial aggregation. *J. Am. Chem. Soc.* **126**, 4750–4751 (2004).
26. Robinson, M. A. *et al.* LEAPT: lectin-directed enzyme-activated prodrug therapy. *Proc. Natl Acad. Sci. USA* **101**, 14527–14532 (2004).
27. Chalker, J. M., Bernardes, G. J. L. & Davis, B. G. A 'tag-and-modify' approach to site-selective protein modification. *Acc. Chem. Res.* **44**, 730–741 (2011).
28. Sato, M. *et al.* Glycoinsulins: dendritic sialyloligosaccharide-displaying insulins showing a prolonged blood-sugar-lowering activity. *J. Am. Chem. Soc.* **126**, 14013–14022 (2004).
29. Ni, J., Song, H., Wang, Y., Stamatos, N. M. & Wang, L. -X. Toward a carbohydrate-based HIV-1 vaccine: synthesis and immunological studies of oligomannose-containing glycoconjugates. *Bioconjugate Chem.* **17**, 493–500 (2006).
30. Kostiainen, M. A., Szilvay, G. R., Smith, D. K., Linder, M. B. & Ikkala, O. Multivalent dendrons for high-affinity adhesion of proteins to DNA. *Angew. Chem. Int. Ed.* **45**, 3538–3542 (2006).
31. Crick, F. H. C. & Watson, J. D. The structure of small viruses. *Nature* **177**, 473–475 (1956).
32. Caspar, D. L. D. & Klug, A. Physical principles in the construction of regular viruses. *Cold Spring Harbor Symp. Quant. Biol.* **27**, 1–24 (1962).
33. Johnson, J. E. & Speir, J. A. Quasi-equivalent viruses: a paradigm for protein assemblies. *J. Mol. Biol.* **269**, 665–675 (1997).
34. Kozlovska, T. M. *et al.* Recombinant RNA phage Qβ capsid particles synthesized and self-assembled in *Escherichia coli. Gene* **137**, 133–137 (1993).
35. Strable, E. *et al.* Unnatural amino acid incorporation into virus-like particles. *Bioconjugate Chem.* **19**, 866–875 (2008).
36. Astronomo, R. *et al.* Defining criteria for oligomannose immunogens for HIV using icosahedral virus capsid scaffolds. *Chem. Biol.* **17**, 357–370 (2010).
37. Doores, K. J. *et al.* A nonself sugar mimic of the HIV glycan shield shows enhanced antigenicity. *Proc. Natl Acad. Sci. USA* **107**, 17107–17112 (2010).
38. Tornøe, C. W., Christensen, C. & Meldal, M. Peptidotriazoles on solid phase: [1,2,3]-triazoles by regiospecific copper(I)-catalyzed 1,3-dipolar cycloadditions of terminal alkynes to azides. *J. Org. Chem.* **67**, 3057–3064 (2002).
39. Rostovtsev, V. V., Green, L. G., Fokin, V. V. & Sharpless, K. B. A stepwise huisgen cycloaddition process: copper(I)-catalyzed regioselective 'ligation' of azides and terminal alkynes. *Angew. Chem. Int. Ed.* **41**, 2596–2599 (2002).
40. Ortega-Muñoz, M., Lopez-Jaramillo, J., Hernandez-Mateo, F. & Santoyo-Gonzalez, F. Synthesis of glyco-silicas by Cu(I)-catalyzed 'click-chemistry' and their applications in affinity chromatography. *Adv. Synth. Catal.* **348**, 2410–2420 (2006).
41. Van, H. J. C. M., Kiick, K. L. & Tirrell, D. A. Efficient incorporation of unsaturated methionine analogues into proteins *in vivo*. *J. Am. Chem. Soc.* **122**, 1282–1288 (2000).
42. van Kasteren, S. I., Kramer, H. B., Gamblin, D. P. & Davis, B. G. Site-selective glycosylation of proteins: creating synthetic glycoproteins. *Nat. Protoc.* **2**, 3185–3194 (2007).
43. van Kasteren, S. I. *et al.* Expanding the diversity of chemical protein modification allows post-translational mimicry. *Nature* **446**, 1105–1109 (2007).
44. Alvarez, C. P. *et al.* C-type lectins DC-SIGN and L-SIGN mediate cellular entry by Ebola virus in cis and in trans. *J. Virol.* **76**, 6841–6844 (2002).
45. Yang, Z.-y. *et al.* Distinct cellular interactions of secreted and transmembrane Ebola virus glycoproteins. *Science* **279**, 1034–1037 (1998).
46. Mammen, M., Choi, S.-K. & Whitesides, G. M. Polyvalent interactions in biological systems: implications for design and use of multivalent ligands and inhibitors. *Angew. Chem. Int. Ed.* **37** **(1998).**
47. Golmohammadi, R., Fridborg, K., Bundule, M., Valegard, K. & Liljas, L. The crystal structure of bacteriophage Q beta at 3.5 A resolution. *Structure* **4**, 543 (1996).
48. Tabarani, G. *et al.* DC-SIGN neck domain is a pH-sensor controlling oligomerization. *J. Biol. Chem.* **284**, 21229–21240 (2009).
49. de Bakker, B. I. *et al.* Nanoscale organization of the pathogen receptor DC-SIGN mapped by single-molecule high-resolution fluorescence microscopy. *ChemPhysChem* **8**, 1473–1480 (2007).
50. He, J. *et al.* Human immunodeficiency virus type 1 viral protein R (Vpr) arrests cells in the G2 phase of the cell cycle by inhibiting p34cdc2 activity. *J. Virol.* **69**, 6705–6711 (1995).
51. Yang, S. *et al.* Generation of retroviral vector for clinical studies using transient transfection. *Hum. Gene Ther.* **10**, 123–132 (1999).
52. Puig-Kroger, A. *et al.* Maturation-dependent expression and function of the CD49d integrin on monocyte-derived human dendritic cells. *J. Immunol.* **165**, 4338–4345 (2000).
53. Relloso, M. *et al.* DC-SIGN (CD209) expression is IL-4 dependent and is negatively regulated by IFN, TGF-β, and anti-inflammatory agents. *J. Immunol.* **168**, 2634–2643 (2002).

Acknowledgements

We acknowledge the financial support by the MICINN of Spain CTQ2008-01694 and CTQ2011-23410, the EU RTN CARMUSYS (PITN-GA-2008-213592), Instituto de Salud Carlos III (FIS PI080806 and PI1101580) and Fundación para la Investigación y Prevención del SIDA (FIPSE 36749) and the European FEDER funds. We thank Professors A. Sánchez (Centers for Disease Control and Prevention, Atlanta, GA) and M.G. Finn (TSRI, La Jolla, CA) for providing Zaire Ebola Virus glycoprotein and p75m/Qβ plasmids, respectively. MSN thanks Fundación Ramón Areces for funding, BGD is a Royal Society Wolfson Research Merit Award recipient and is supported by an EPSRC LSI Platform grant.

Author contributions

R.R.-V. and M.S.N. synthesized the glycodendrons and the glycodendriproteins, J.L. carried out the Ebola infection experiments. J.R.K. expressed and purified Qβ. M.S.N., R.D., J.R. and B.G.D. designed the experiments. All the authors discussed results and analysed the data. M.S.N. and B.G.D. wrote the manuscript. Correspondence and requests for materials should be addressed to R.D., J.R. and B.G.D.

Additional information

Competing financial interests: The authors declare no competing financial interests.

7

Total synthesis of tetraacylated phosphatidylinositol hexamannoside and evaluation of its immunomodulatory activity

Pratap S. Patil[1], Ting-Jen Rachel Cheng[1], Medel Manuel L. Zulueta[1], Shih-Ting Yang[1], Larry S. Lico[1] & Shang-Cheng Hung[1]

Tuberculosis, aggravated by drug-resistant strains and HIV co-infection of the causative agent *Mycobacterium tuberculosis*, is a global problem that affects millions of people. With essential immunoregulatory roles, phosphatidylinositol mannosides are among the cell-envelope components critical to the pathogenesis and survival of *M. tuberculosis* inside its host. Here we report the first synthesis of the highly complex tetraacylated phosphatidylinositol hexamannoside (Ac_2PIM_6), having stearic and tuberculostearic acids as lipid components. Our effort makes use of stereoelectronic and steric effects to control the regioselective and stereoselective outcomes and minimize the synthetic steps, particularly in the key desymmetrization and functionalization of *myo*-inositol. A short synthesis of tuberculostearic acid in six steps from the Roche ester is also described. Mice exposed to the synthesized Ac_2PIM_6 exhibit increased production of interleukin-4 and interferon-γ, and the corresponding adjuvant effect is shown by the induction of ovalbumin- and tetanus toxoid-specific antibodies.

[1]Genomics Research Center, Academia Sinica, No. 128, Section 2, Academia Road, Taipei 115, Taiwan. Correspondence and requests for materials should be addressed to S.-C.H. (email: schung@gate.sinica.edu.tw).

Mycobacterium tuberculosis is a dreaded pathogen that causes tuberculosis, one of the leading causes of death in the world. Although the disease becomes active for only 5–10% of infected individuals, 1.5 million people died of tuberculosis in 2013 alone despite progress in the global effort for diagnosis, treatment and prevention[1]. Moreover, it is estimated that one-third of the human population is latently infected with *M. tuberculosis* and is highly vulnerable if immunocompromised. The antituberculosis vaccine bacillus Calmette-Guérin, made by using an attenuated strain of *M. bovis*, only gives protection to children but is highly variable in adults[2]. Co-infection with HIV and the rising cases of multidrug and extensive drug resistance also add to the high morbidity and mortality of the disease[3]. Clearly, fresh insights on the character of the causative agent and its pathogenesis are needed to help alleviate this human condition[4].

The thick glycolipid-containing cell envelope[5] of *M. tuberculosis* is critical for bacterial survival and growth. It is involved in sabotaging immunoregulatory responses[6–8] and it forms a protective barrier for various drugs[9,10]. Among the vital cell-envelope components, phosphatidylinositol mannosides (PIMs) and their hypermannosylated structural relatives (lipomannans and lipoarabinomannans) are found noncovalently anchored to the plasma membrane and the outer capsule through palmitate, stearate and tuberculostearate lipid chains[11]. PIMs, in particular, dictate the intercellular fate of mycobacteria by binding to macrophages[12], regulate cytokines and reactive radical species and stimulate early endosomal fusion by acting as ligands to Toll-like receptors, C-type lectins and DC-SIGN[13]. PIMs can also act as CD1d antigen to activate natural killer T cells for the production of interferon-γ (ref. 14), indicating their potential as vaccine or adjuvant candidates. In addition, PIMs interact with $\alpha_5\beta_1$ integrin on $CD4^+$ lymphocytes, which can either promote granuloma formation and enhance host immune response or help in bacterial survival[15].

Structurally, *myo*-inositol is the central support unit of PIMs with a diacylated glycerophospholipid moiety at O1 and α-mannosylation sites at O2 and O6 (ref. 16). Additional lipid chains may be linked at the primary hydroxyl of the 2-*O*-mannosyl unit and at the O3 position of *myo*-inositol to form triacylated PIMs (AcPIMs) and tetraacylated PIMs (Ac_2PIMs), respectively. Higher PIMs (for example, $Ac_nPIM_3 - Ac_nPIM_6$) are formed by elongation at the mannose residue linked at O6 of *myo*-inositol. The number of mannose residues and the degree and type of the fatty acyl groups present in the PIM molecules determine their unique role in immunoregulation[11]. As a result, elegant synthetic strategies have been developed for PIMs and their related compounds[17–34]. Nevertheless, the synthesis of a tetraacylated phosphatidylinositol hexamannoside (Ac_2PIM_6), the most complex among this class of compounds, is yet to be reported. Thus far, previous disclosures explored the synthesis of Ac_2PIM_2 (ref. 34), PIM_4 (ref. 24), PIM_6 (ref. 32) and $AcPIM_6$ (ref. 25) to name a few.

We describe herein the first synthesis of Ac_2PIM_6, using stearic and tuberculostearic acids as the lipid components. The immunomodulatory activity of the synthesized Ac_2PIM_6 was also evaluated.

Results

Synthetic strategy. Compound **1** possesses multiple components and functionalizations. To arrive at this molecule, one rational synthetic design would be to fragment this sizeable structure into separate segments, which could later be assembled in a convergent manner. For this purpose, we conceived the pseudo-trisaccharide **2**, tetramannoside donor **3** and phosphonate **4** as the primary targets (Fig. 1). The readily perceptible synthetic issues include the transformation of the ordinarily meso *myo*-inositol into the unsymmetrical counterpart in **2** as well as the regioselective protection to afford the mannosyl-building blocks useful enough to deliver the necessary $\alpha1\rightarrow2$ and $\alpha1\rightarrow6$ linkages and the acylation of one mannosyl unit. Accordingly, along with benzyl groups for the global protection of hydroxyls that would be free in the desired product, we selected two additional orthogonal protecting groups for the primary positions of the mannosyl residues in intermediates leading to compound **2**. The *tert*-butyldiphenylsilyl (TBDPS) group should allow, on deprotection, the subsequent coupling with the tetramannoside **3**, whereas the 2-naphthylmethyl (2-NAP) group protects the position that would later be acylated. Being a core constituent of inositol phosphates and other phosphatidyl lipoglycans, various methods have been published for the *myo*-inositol resolution and

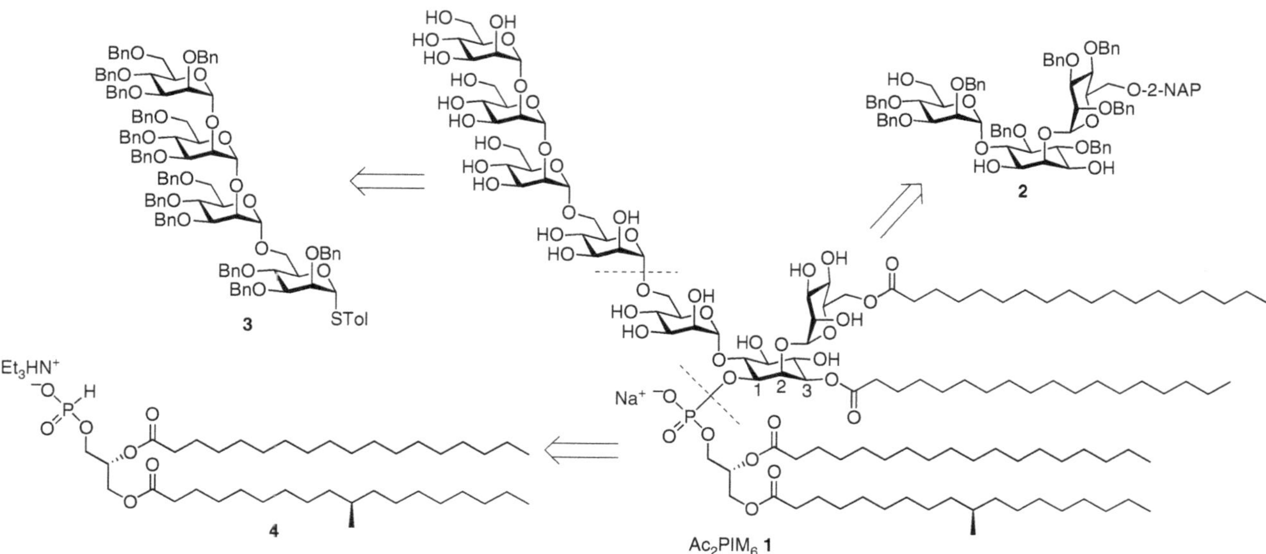

Figure 1 | Our target tetraacylated phosphatidylinositol hexamannoside (Ac_2PIM_6) and the main blocks designed to represent each segment. 2-NAP, 2-naphthylmethyl; Bn, benzyl; Tol, *p*-tolyl.

desymmetrization[35,36]. However, the suitably protected chiral *myo*-inositol derivative required for PIMs and glycosyl phosphatidylinositide synthesis were mainly achieved through multistep synthesis from D-glucose via the Ferrier reaction[37]. Recently, we have shown that a mannosyl donor can directly act as chiral auxiliary to differentiate the enantiotopic hydroxyls of meso *myo*-inositol derivatives[30,31]. This direct approach bypasses many transformation steps in affording an appropriately mannosylated and desymmetrized *myo*-inositol. We intend to apply this capacity towards diol **2** while also relying on the steric hindrance created by the installed mannosyl residues to strategically position the 4,5-di-*O*-benzyl moieties on the *myo*-inositol unit and sufficiently favour regioselective acylation at the free 3-OH. An extra temporary protecting group and participating moiety is also needed to permit the construction of the tetramannoside **3**, in which case we chose a 2-*O*-benzoyl group. We planned to assemble **3** through linear glycosylation from the reducing end to the nonreducing end using a single elongation unit. For the phosphonate **4**, access to the rare tuberculostearic acid is the main concern, and this fatty acid should be synthesized to complete the desired phospholipid moiety.

Mannosyl-building blocks. Considering the stability of the thiotolyl leaving group on various functional group interconversions, we selected the thiomannoside **5** (ref. 38) as a starting point in our transformations towards several mannosyl building blocks (Fig. 2). In general, the building blocks needed for the assembly of our target structure required differentiation at either O6 or O2. With a bulky functionality such as the TBDPS group, the protection sequence aimed regioselectively at the primary O6 position seems clear-cut. Thus, the 6-*O*-silylation of **5** using *tert*-butyldiphenylchlorosilane, triethylamine and 4-(*N*,*N*-dimethylamino)pyridine gave compound **6** in excellent yield. Subsequent benzylation under Williamson condition supplied the necessary thioglycoside **7**. The 6-alcohol **8**, intended as the starting acceptor in generating the tetramannoside **3**, was also readily acquired from **7** by acidic desilylation.

In contrast to the route above, traditional approaches concerning the effective acquisitions of the 6-*O*-naphthylmethylated thiomannoside **13** and the 2-benzoate **14** do not appear to be straightforward. The complexity arises from the desire to carry out the fully regioselective installations of the vital ether groups. Apparently, the regioselective one-pot protection strategy that we introduced[39,40] and further expanded to other sugars[41–44] could simplify such preparations. Our recent work on the stereoselective dioxolane-type benzylidene formation on thiomannosides[43] should provide a convenient gateway to the 2,6-diol **11**, a potential common intermediate towards compounds **13** and **14**. It was envisioned that, with benzyl groups permanently protecting O3 and O4, the

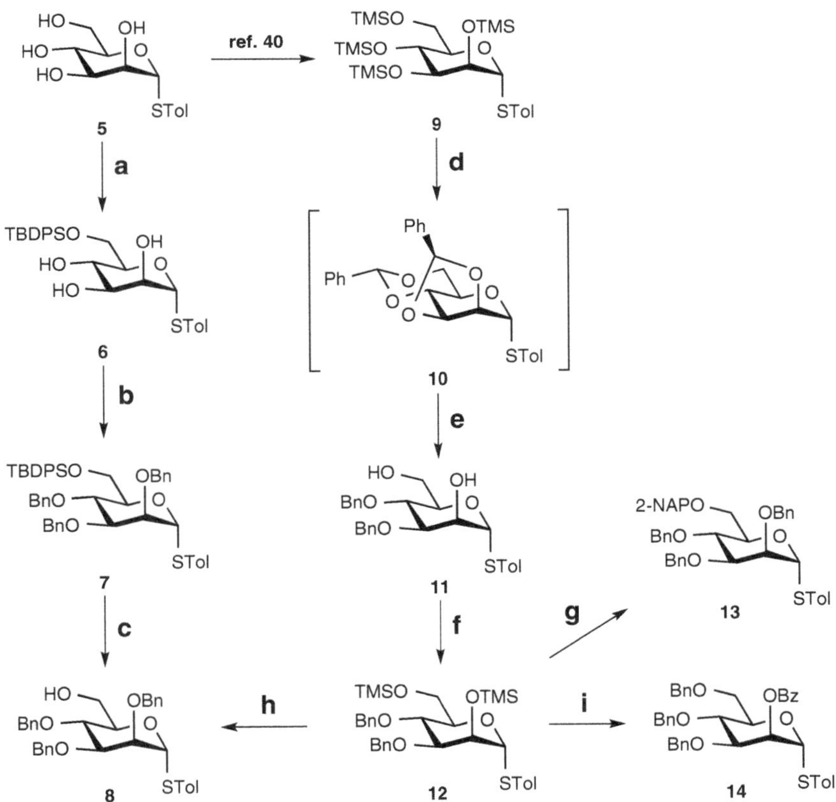

Figure 2 | Preparations of the mannosyl-building blocks. Reagents and conditions: (**a**) *tert*-butyldiphenylchlorosilane, Et_3N, DMAP, 93%; (**b**) NaH, BnBr, DMF, 94%; (**c**) PTSA, MeOH, CH_2Cl_2, 92%; (**d**) benzaldehyde (2.1 equivalents), TMSOTf, MeCN, 0 °C, 30 min; (**e**) $BH_3 \cdot THF$, $Cu(OTf)_2$, CH_2Cl_2, 87% (one pot from **9**); (**f**) trimethylchlorosilane, Et_3N, quantitative; (**g**) 2-naphthaldehyde, Et_3SiH, TMSOTf, CH_2Cl_2, −78 to −40 °C, 2 h, then, NaH, BnBr, DMF, 81% (one pot); (**h**) 2-naphthaldehyde, Et_3SiH, TMSOTf, CH_2Cl_2, −78 to −40 °C, 2 h, then, NaH, BnBr, DMF, then, DDQ, H_2O, 73% (one pot); (**i**) benzaldehyde, Et_3SiH, TMSOTf, −78 °C, 1.5 h, then, $BF_3 \cdot Et_2O$, MeCN, −78 to −20 °C, 30 min, then, Bz_2O, Et_3N, 93% (one pot). Bz, benzoyl; Bz_2O, benzoic anhydride; $Cu(OTf)_2$, copper(II) trifluoromethanesulfonate; DDQ, 2,3-dichloro-5,6-dicyano-1,4-benzoquinone; DMAP, 4-(*N*,*N*-dimethylamino)pyridine; DMF, *N*,*N*-dimethylformamide; Ph, phenyl; PTSA, *p*-toluenesulfonic acid; TBDPS, *tert*-butyldiphenylsilyl; THF, tetrahydrofuran; TMS, trimethylsilyl, TMSOTf, trimethylsilyl trifluoromethanesulfonate.

primary 6-hydroxyl could be easily differentiated from the secondary and axial 2-hydroxyl. We were also keen to check whether stereoselective dibenzylidenation and simultaneous regioselective ring opening could be achieved in one pot.

Starting from the tetrakis-trimethylsilyl ether **9** acquired in one step from **5** (ref. 43), treatment with 2.1 equivalents of benzaldehyde along with catalytic trimethylsilyl trifluoromethanesulfonate (TMSOTf) in acetonitrile at 0 °C exclusively delivered the *exo*-product **10** as evidenced by NMR spectroscopy and X-ray crystallography (Supplementary Fig. 1, Supplementary Data 1). This fully stereoselective transformation is beneficial because unlike the regioselectivity in the 4,6-*O*-benzylidene ring opening, which is determined by the choice of reducing agent[45], the opening of the dioxolane-type 2,3-*O*-benzylidine moiety is guided by the orientation of the phenyl group (that is, *exo*-isomers generally open at the axial position). Delightfully, the subsequent exposure of **10** to $BH_3 \cdot$tetrahydrofuran in the same vessel provided the diol **11** in a two-stage one-pot yield of 87%. Anticipating a smooth regioselective reductive etherification at O6 (ref. 46), we subjected the diol **11** to trimethylsilylation. Consequently, treatment of the so-formed **12** with 2-naphthaldehyde, triethylsilane and TMSOTf in subzero temperature supplied the intermediate that was benzylated in one pot using the typical etherification method to afford compound **13**. An X-ray single crystal analysis fully supported the desired structure (Supplementary Fig. 1, Supplementary Data 2). Continuing further, addition of 2,3-dichloro-5,6-dicyano-1,4-benzoquinone to the *in situ*-generated **13** successfully delivered the same acceptor **8**, thus providing an alternative pathway for its acquisition. Similarly, the corresponding reductive 6-O-benzylation of **12** was carried out, followed by desilylation at O2 with tetrabutylammonium fluoride (TBAF) and basic benzoylation in the same flask. Unfortunately, the yield for compound **14** was less than satisfactory even when benzoic acid and TBAF were used together[41] to perform the desilylation, probably due to the interference of TBAF to the benzoylation stage. Desilylation with $BF_3 \cdot Et_2O$ apparently solved this issue and furnished **14** in an excellent 93% yield from **12**.

Synthesis of the pseudotrisaccharide 2. For the desymmetrization of *myo*-inositol, we evaluated the coupling of the mannosyl donor **7** with the meso diol **16** (Fig. 3), which can be easily prepared in one step[30] from the commercially available Kishi's triol. The asymmetric nature of the mannosyl donor itself should provide certain preferences between the axial hydroxyls of **16** as we have demonstrated previously[30] but without the TBDPS group on the sugar. Because of the wider opening available for a nucleophilic attack on the half-chair mannosyl oxocarbenium ion intermediate by O6 as compared with O4 (Supplementary Fig. 2), it is expected that the required 6-*O*-mannosylation would be more favoured. Our attempts at coupling of **7** and **16** using

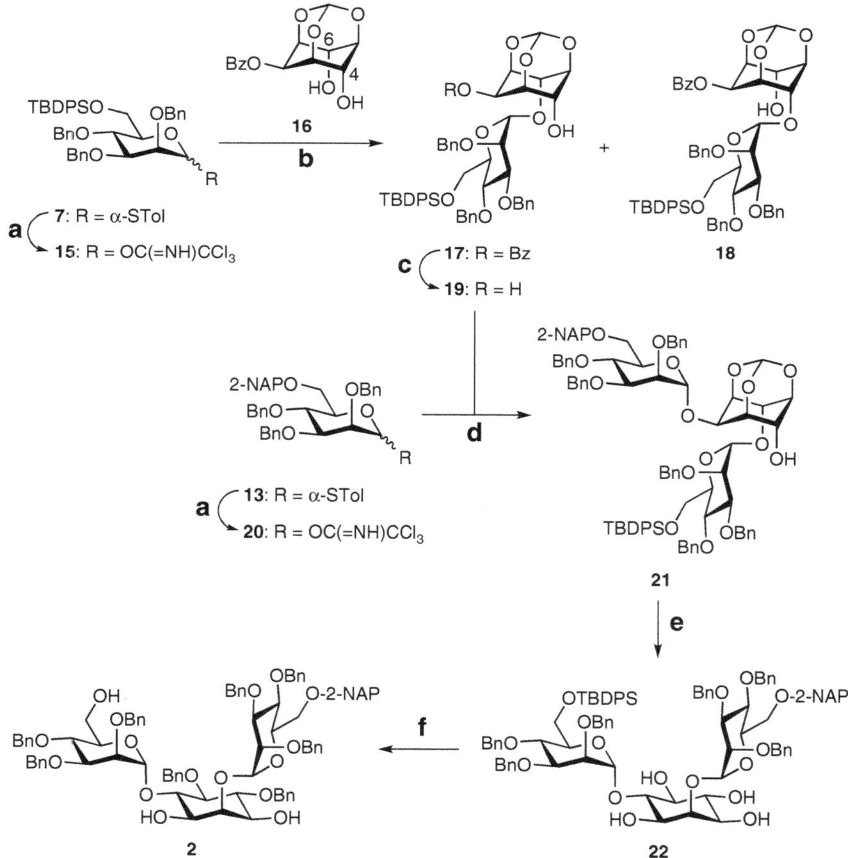

Figure 3 | Preparation of the pseudotrisaccharide 2. Reagents and conditions: (**a**) (1) NBS, acetone, H_2O; (2) K_2CO_3, CCl_3CN, **15**: 94% (two steps), **20**: 90% (two steps); (**b**) silver trif uoromethanesulfonate, 1,4-dioxane, CH_2Cl_2, **17**: 68%, **18**: 20%; (**c**) NaOMe, MeOH, CH_2Cl_2, quantitative; (**d**) $BF_3 \cdot Et_2O$, CH_2Cl_2, −60 to −20 °C, 72%; (**e**) (1) PTSA, MeOH, CH_2Cl_2, 84%; (2) *tert*-butyldiphenylchlorosilane, Et_3N, DMAP, 82%; (**f**) (1) trimethylchlorosilane, Et_3N, quantitative; (2) benzaldehyde (3 equivalent), Et_3SiH, TMSOTf, CH_2Cl_2, −40 °C, then, tetrabutylammonium fluoride, 72%. NBS, *N*-bromosuccinimide.

N-iodosuccinimide and TMSOTf in CH_2Cl_2 and 1,4-dioxane to improve the solubility of diol **16**, unfortunately, led only to donor hydrolysis and full recovery of the acceptor. We suspected that the axial hydroxyls are too unreactive for mannosyl thioglycoside to foster productive couplings. With strong activators avoided to maintain the acid-sensitive orthoformate group, focus was shifted to the imidate versions of the donor. After some optimization (see the Supplementary Table 1), silver trifluoromethanesulfonate promoted the glycosylation step at room temperature, supplying the desired pseudodisaccharide **17** at 68% yield, along with its regioisomer **18** (20%). Here and in the succeeding glycosylations, we verified the α-orientations of the mannosidic bonds through the coupling constants of the anomeric carbons and protons (~170 Hz, see Supplementary Methods)[47,48]. Distinguishing the structures of **17** and **18** with confidence is not possible with NMR analysis alone. We, therefore, resorted to exchange the primary TBDPS with benzyl group (Supplementary Fig. 3) and compare agreement with the NMR spectra from previously published data[30].

For the preparation of the key intermediate **21**, the pseudodisaccharide **17** was subjected to Zemplén deacylation to generate the diol **19**. Regioselective mannosylation at the equatorial hydroxy group should be more likely because of steric reasons. A thorough evaluation of the subsequent coupling also made us consider the application of the imidate **20** over the thioglycoside **13**. Under $BF_3 \cdot Et_2O$ promotion, compound **21** was, therefore, acquired in 72% yield with complete regioselectivity and stereoselectivity. The orthoformate group was cleaved using *p*-toluenesulfonic acid, which also removed the TBDPS group. The tetraol **22** was obtained after re-installation of the silyl group. With **22** in hand, regioselective benzylation at O4 and O5 of the inositol unit is the next challenge. Williamson condition and acidic benzylation using benzyl imidate are not sufficiently selective, whereas the reductive benzylation of the trimethylsilylated substrate showed greater promise. True enough, excellent selectivity was achieved by using 3 equivalents of benzaldehyde, furnishing, after further full desilylation with TBAF, the desired compound **2** in 72% yield from **22**.

It should be stated that other less successful means in acquiring the pseudotrisaccharide backbone have been studied. Our effort at condensation of the imidate donor **20** with the diol **16** led to mixtures of inseparable regioisomers and stereoisomers, a demonstration of the known potential of the bulky 6-*O*-TBDPS group at enhancing α-selectivity[49]. A participating moiety at O2 of the mannosyl donor was ruled out to avoid complications that may be encountered in later reactions. Sequential dimannosylation of Kishi's triol also seemed feasible under our synthetic design, with glycosylation at the more reactive O2 using donor **20** followed by asymmetric 6-*O*-mannosylation with donor **15**. Unfortunately, poor yields for both couplings were observed. Another procedure we have tried included the 2-*O*-mannosylation of **19** with a donor already carrying the fatty acyl functionality at the primary position. While the glycosylation step worked as intended, the acyl moiety was also removed along with the TBDPS group on acid treatment intended to cleave the orthoformate function.

Synthesis of tuberculostearic acid and the *H*-phosphonate 4. Tuberculostearic acid was first isolated from *M. tuberculosis* in 1927 (ref. 50) and several methods for its synthesis have been reported[25,26,51–53]. Nevertheless, an updated, shorter and more effective method for accessing this important fatty acid is still desirable. We decided to acquire the chiral carbon of tuberculostearic acid from the commercially available Roche ester (**23**). Tosylation of **23** to afford compound **24**, followed by reduction with diisobutylaluminium hydride and methylene insertion by Wittig reaction furnished the olefin **25** (ref. 54; Fig. 4). The first long-chain elongation of **25** towards compound **26** was achieved by Grignard reaction under catalytic Li_2CuCl_2. Grubbs metathesis of olefin **26** with the olefinic acid **27** provided the *E*/*Z* olefin mixture, which was exposed to palladium-catalysed hydrogenation to finally secure tuberculostearic acid (**28**). Accomplished in just six steps, this acquisition is the shortest synthetic preparation reported, thus far, for this compound.

Elaborations of the commercially available 3-*O*-benzyl-*sn*-glycerol were performed next. Under dicyclohexylcarbodiimide and 4-(*N*,*N*-dimethylamino)pyridine, the fatty acid **28** was first condensed with the primary hydroxyl followed by stearic acid esterification at the secondary position in good yields. Cleavage of the benzyl group was achieved through hydrogenolysis and the generated alcohol was phosphorylated using PCl_3, imidazole and Et_3N to afford the *H*-phosphonate **2**.

Ac_2PIM_6 assembly and final transformations. Our planned sugar assembly towards the tetramannoside **3** hinges on the chemoselective activation of a trichloroacetimidate donor in the presence of a thioglycoside acceptor[55] (Fig. 5). Accordingly,

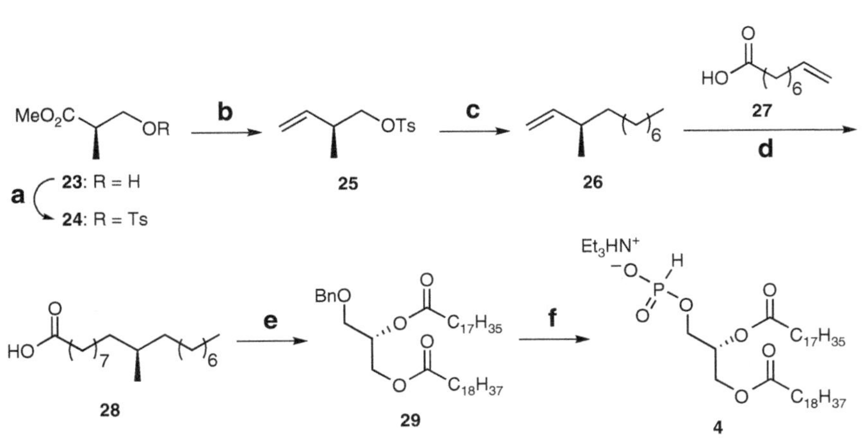

Figure 4 | Preparation of tuberculostearic acid (28) and the *H*-phosphonate 4. Reagents and conditions: (**a**) TsCl, Et_3N, DMAP, 94%; (**b**) (1) diisobutylaluminium hydride, −78 °C; (2) $Ph_3P{=}CH_2$, 72% (two steps); (**c**) $C_7H_{15}MgBr$, Li_2CuCl_4, −78 to 0 °C, 92%; (**d**) (1) Grubbs second-generation catalyst, CH_2Cl_2, reflux; (2) H_2, Pd/C, 75% (two steps); (**e**) (1) 3-*O*-benzyl-*sn*-glycerol, DCC, DMAP, 75%; (2) stearic acid, DCC, DMAP, 88%; (**f**) (1) H_2, Pd/C, 92%; (2) PCl_3, imidazole, Et_3N, −10 °C, 69%. DCC, dicyclohexylcarbodiimide; Ts, Tosyl.

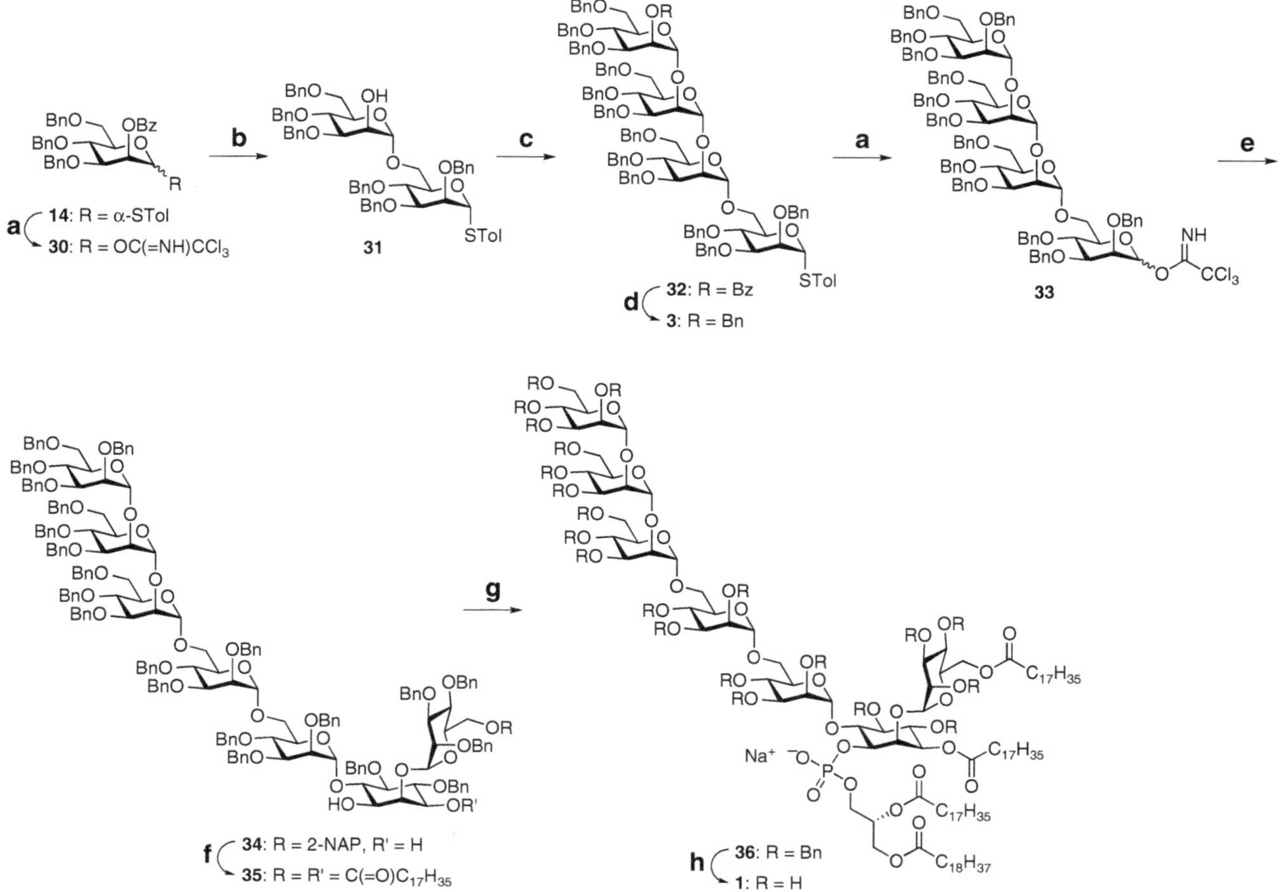

Figure 5 | Synthesis of compound 1. Reagents and conditions: (**a**) (1) NBS, acetone, H_2O; (2) CCl_3CN, 1,8-diazabicyclo[5.4.0]undec-7-ene, **30**: 96% (two steps), **33**: 86% (two steps); (**b**) **8**, TMSOTf, CH_2Cl_2, −78 °C, then, NaOMe, MeOH, 87% (one pot); (**c**) (1) **30**, TfOH, CH_2Cl_2, −60 to −40 °C, then, NaOMe, MeOH, 70% (one pot); (2) **30**, TfOH, CH_2Cl_2, −60 to −40 °C, 74%; (**d**) BnBr, NaH, 98%; (**e**) **2**, TMSOTf, Et_2O, −40 °C, 52% (89% yield based on the recovered **2**); (**f**) (1) DDQ, CH_2Cl_2, H_2O, 71%; (2) stearic acid, DCC, DMAP, 86%; (**g**) (1) **4**, pivaloyl chloride, pyridine; (2) I_2, pyridine, H_2O; (3) DOWEX 50WX8 Na^+ form, 77% from **35**; (**h**) H_2, Pd/C, 88%. TfOH, trifluoromethanesulfonic acid.

the elongation unit is formed by converting compound **14** to **30** under the usual procedures. Glycosylation of the thioglycoside **8** with **30** followed by debenzoylation in the same flask supplied the disaccharide acceptor **31** in 87% yield. Two more elongation cycles easily formed the tetramannoside **32**. Knowing that the benzoate group is base-sensitive, the benzoyl-to-benzyl exchange was achieved in one step by NaH and benzyl bromide treatment, smoothly offering the target compound **3** in 98% yield.

With all segment backbones available, we moved forward in putting all these pieces together. The glycosylation of the pseudotrisaccharide acceptor **2** by the thioglycoside **3**, however, produced only a meager 10% yield for compound **34** despite our best efforts, prompting us to use the more reactive imidate counterpart **33** instead (see Supplementary Table 2). With Et_2O as solvent and TMSOTf as activator, we eventually obtained the desired **34** in 52% yield (89%, if the recovered acceptor is considered). The 2-NAP ether was then cleaved, which paved the way for the concurrent installation of two stearate esters at the mannosyl and the inositol units, leading to the alcohol **35**. This reaction exhibited no regioselectivity issues, with O1 of the inositol unit spared because it experiences the highest steric hindrance among the three free hydroxyls. The attachment of the *H*-phosphonate **4** and the pseudo-heptasaccharide **35** was carried out by using pivaloyl chloride, followed by iodine-mediated *in situ* oxidation and cation exchange, delivering the derivative **36**. Global hydrogenolysis of the benzyl ethers provided the Ac_2PIM_6 construct **1** in 82% yield.

Evaluation of immunomodulatory activity. The adjuvant effects of compound **1** were examined through co-administration with ovalbumin (Fig. 6a) or tetanus toxoid (Fig. 6b) antigen in BALB/c mice. PIMs isolated from *M. tuberculosis* strain H37Rv ($iPIM_{1,2}$ and $iPIM_6$) and alum were also investigated in parallel for comparison. It was observed that compound **1** induced an approximately two to fourfold increase in the level of antigen-specific antibodies. The adjuvant activity of **1** is similar to the bacteria-derived PIMs and slightly lower than alum.

Furthermore, we evaluated the cytokine-producing activity of compound **1** as well as $iPIM_{1,2}$ and $iPIM_6$ (Fig. 6c,d). The level of interleukin-4 and interferon-γ was not detectable in mouse sera at 1 h after injection of Ac_2PIM **1** and the bacteria-derived PIMs. At 18 h after injection, the cytokine levels increased. Lipid and glycolipid molecules derived from *M. tuberculosis* are presented to T cells by CD1 antigen-presenting molecules, specifically CD1d[14,56]. Compared with the well-known CD1d-targeting α-galactosylceramide, which can activate the invariant natural killer T cells and induce high levels of interleukin-4 and

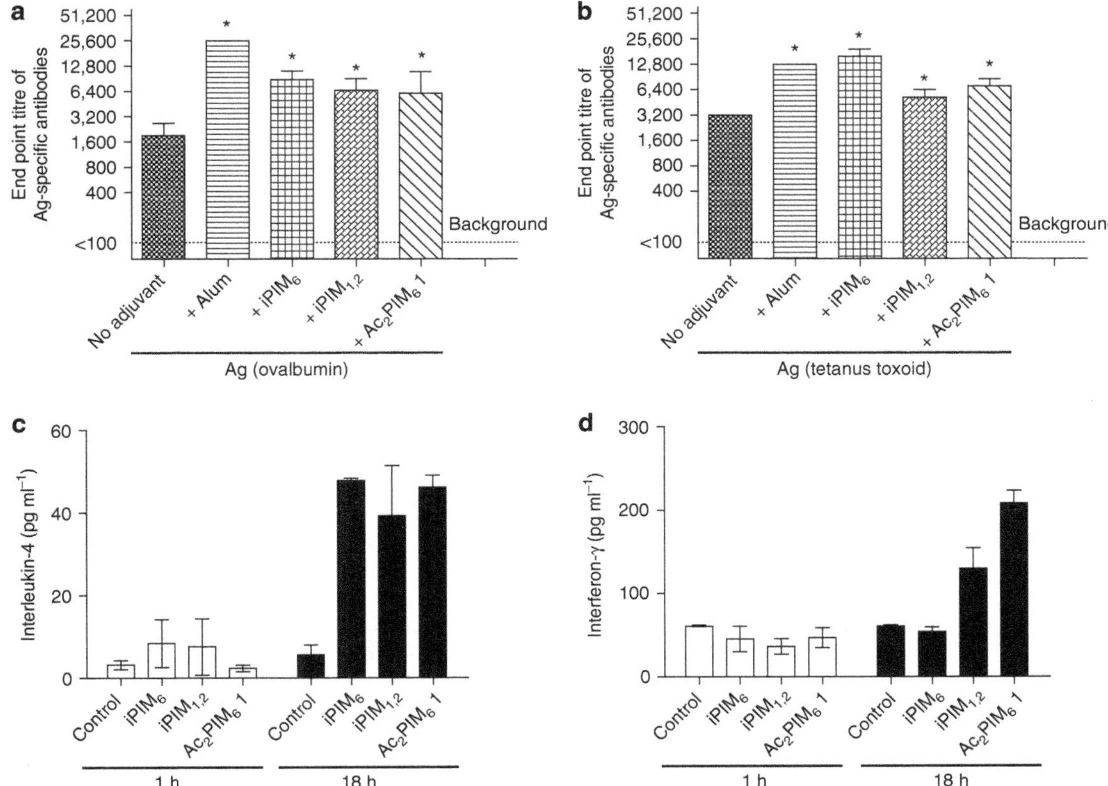

Figure 6 | Immunological evaluation in BALB/c mice. (**a**,**b**) Induction of antigen (Ag)-specific antibodies in mice immunized with ovalbumin or tetanus toxoid adjuvanted with alum or various PIMs; (**c**,**d**) secreted cytokines (interleukin-4 and interferon-γ) in mice 1 and 18 h after injection with various PIMs (control represents injection only with PBS). Both end point antibody titres and the cytokine levels were measured by using enzyme-linked immunosorbent assay. The results displayed represent the mean + s.d.'s ($n = 5$). Data were analysed by using one-way analysis of variance, and differences were considered significant at $^*P < 0.05$. $iPIM_6$ and $iPIM_{1,2}$, isolated PIM_6 and mixture of PIM_1 and PIM_2, respectively, from *M. tuberculosis* strain H37Rv.

interferon-γ within 24 h (ref. 57), Ac_2PIM_6 **1** appeared to have moderate effects.

Discussion

We have successfully developed a convenient route to synthesize an Ac_2PIM_6 construct in the form of compound **1** containing tuberculostearic acid and stearic acid as the fatty acid components. This is the first time that an Ac_2PIM_6 molecule was synthesized. Further, a novel and short synthetic route towards tuberculostearic acid was developed, with only six synthetic steps from the commercially available Roche ester and four purification stages. Our synthetic approach benefitted from the use of shared mannoside-building blocks, the carefully chosen orthogonal protecting groups and the features of the regioselective one-pot transformations from trimethylsilylated starting materials previously developed by us. The trichloroacetimidate donor types[58] are vital factors in achieving the successful assembly processes. Regioselectivity and stereoselectivity were achieved through the aid of steric and stereoelectronic effects. Steric effects were also exploited in the direct desymmetrization of *myo*-inositol by mannosyl donors and in minimizing the number of protecting groups used in the synthesis. With practical access and functional group flexibility, the key intermediates such as the pseudotrisaccharide **2** possess good potential in supplying PIMs of different mannosylation and lipidation patterns as well. Our synthesized Ac_2PIM_6 has comparable adjuvant activity with the natural PIMs against ovalbumin and tetanus toxoid antigens and induced the production of interleukin-4 and interferon-γ, thus, validating the immunological qualities of PIM molecules and its value in vaccine research.

Methods

Chemical synthesis. The complete experimental details and compound characterization data can be found in the Supplementary Methods. For the NMR spectra of the compounds in this article, see Supplementary Figs 4–120. The mass spectrum of the synthesized Ac_2PIM_6 **1** is shown in Supplementary Fig. 121.

Materials for immunological evaluation. All BALB/c mice were housed at the animal facility in the Institute of Cell Biology, Academia Sinica, Taiwan in accordance with the Institutional Animal Care Committee guidelines. Purified $iPIM_{1,2}$ (NR-14846) and $iPIM_6$ (NR-14847) were obtained through BEI Resources, National Institute of Allergy and Infectious Diseases, National Institutes of Health (USA). Ovalbumin and tetanus toxoid were purchased from InvivoGen (San Diego, CA, USA) and Adimmune Inc. (Taichung, Taiwan), respectively.

Evaluation of adjuvant activity. Five- to six-week-old female BALB/c mice were immunized with ovalbumin (100 µg) or tetanus toxoid (2 µg) adjuvanted with 10 µg of PIM compounds (Ac_2PIM_6 **1**, $iPIM_{1,2}$ or $iPIM_6$) or alum in PBS for three times at 2-week intervals by intramuscular injection. Two weeks after the third immunization, the immunized mice were bled for antigen-specific antibody analysis.

Ovalbumin- and tetanus toxoid-specific antibodies in heat-inactivated serum were monitored with direct enzyme-linked immunosorbent assay (ELISA). The ovalbumin- or tetanus toxoid-coated plates were incubated with mouse serum in twofold serial dilutions for 1 h. Antigen-specific IgG was monitored by using horseradish peroxidase-conjugated anti-mouse antibodies and 3,3′,5,5′-tetramethylbenzidine substrate (Thermo Scientific Inc). After colour development, absorbance at 450 nm was recorded by using a plate reader (SpectraMax M5, Molecular Device). The end point antibody titre was defined as the highest dilution of serum to produce an absorbance 2.5 times higher than the optical absorbance produced by the pre-immune serum. The background end point antibody titre was assigned as < 1:100.

Evaluation of cytokine-producing activity. Five- to six-week-old female BALB/c mice were intramuscularly injected with 10 μg of the PIM compounds (Ac_2PIM_6 **1**, $iPIM_{1,2}$ or $iPIM_6$) in PBS and bled at 1 or 18 h after injection (five mice per group). The cytokines in the sera were measured with sandwich ELISA using paired anti-interleukin-4 and anti-interferon-γ monoclonal antibodies (R&D Systems).

Statistical analysis. The response of each mouse was counted as an individual data point for statistical analysis. Data obtained from animal studies were analysed by using one-way analysis of variance from Graphpad and differences were considered significant at $P < 0.05$.

References

1. WHO. Tuberculosis factsheet N°1C4 http://www.who.int/mediacentre/factsheets/fs104/en/ (2014).
2. Orme, I. M. The search for new vaccines against tuberculosis. *J. Leukoc. Biol.* **70,** 1–10 (2001).
3. Zumla, A. I. *et al.* New antituberculosis drugs, regimens, and adjunct therapies: needs, advances, and future prospects. *Lancet Infect. Dis.* **14,** 327–340 (2014).
4. Dye, C. & Williams, B. G. The population dynamics and control of tuberculosis. *Science* **328,** 856–861 (2010).
5. Karakousis, P. C., Bishai, W. R. & Dorman, S. E. *Mycobacterium tuberculosis* cell envelope lipids and the host immune response. *Cell Microbiol.* **6,** 105–116 (2004).
6. Flynn, J. L. & Chan, J. What's good for the host is good for the bug. *Trends Microbiol.* **13,** 98–102 (2005).
7. Russell, D. G. Who puts the tubercle in tuberculosis? *Nat. Rev. Microbiol.* **5,** 39–47 (2007).
8. Hestvik, A. L. K., Hmama, Z. & Av-Gay, Y. Mycobacterial manipulation of the host cell. *FEMS Microbiol. Rev.* **29,** 1041–1050 (2005).
9. Bhowruth, V., Alderwick, L. J., Brown, A. K., Bhatt, A. & Besra, G. S. Tuberculosis: a balanced diet of lipids and carbohydrates. *Biochem. Soc. Trans.* **36,** 555–565 (2008).
10. Józefowski, S., Sobota, A. & Kwiatkowska, K. How *Mycobacterium tuberculosis* subverts host immune responses. *BioEssays* **30,** 943–954 (2008).
11. Cao, B. & Williams, S. J. Chemical approaches for the study of the mycobacterial glycolipids phosphatidylinositol mannosides, lipomannan and lipoarabinomannan. *Nat. Prod. Rep.* **27,** 919–947 (2010).
12. Gilleron, M. *et al.* Acylation state of the phosphatidylinositol mannosides from *Mycobacterium bovis* Bacillus Calmette Guérin and ability to induce granuloma and recruit natural killer T cells. *J. Biol. Chem.* **276,** 34896–34904 (2001).
13. Torrelles, J. B., Azad, A. K. & Schlesinger, L. S. Fine discrimination in the recognition of individual species of phosphatidyl-*myo*-inositol mannosides from *Mycobacterium tuberculosis* by C-type lectin pattern recognition receptors. *J. Immunol.* **177,** 1805–1816 (2006).
14. Fischer, K. *et al.* Mycobacterial phosphatidylinositol mannoside is a natural antigen for CD1d-restricted T cells. *Proc. Natl Acad. Sci. USA* **101,** 10685–10690 (2004).
15. Rojas, R. E. *et al.* Phosphatidylinositol mannoside from *Mycobacterium tuberculosis* binds $\alpha_5\beta_1$ integrin (VLA-5) on $CD4^+$ T cells and induces adhesion to fibronectin. *J. Immunol.* **177,** 2959–2968 (2006).
16. Guerin, M. E., Kordulàková, J., Alzari, P. M., Brennan, P. J. & Jackson, M. Molecular basis of phosphatidyl-*myo*-inositol mannoside biosynthesis and regulation in mycobacteria. *J. Biol. Chem.* **285,** 33577–33583 (2010).
17. Elie, C. J. J., Verduyn, R., Dreef, C. E., van der Marel, G. A. & van Boom, J. H. Iodinium ion-mediated mannosylations of *myo*-inositol: synthesis of a mycobacteria phospholipid fragment. *J. Carbohydr. Chem.* **11,** 715–739 (1992).
18. Watanabe, Y., Yamamoto, T. & Okazaki, T. Synthesis of 2,6-di-*O*-α-D-mannopyranosylphosphatidyl-D-*myo*-inositol. Utilization of glycosylation and phosphorylation based on phosphite chemistry. *Tetrahedron* **53,** 903–918 (1997).
19. Stadelmaier, A. & Schmidt, R. R. Synthesis of phosphatidylinositol mannosides (PIMs). *Carbohydr. Res.* **338,** 2557–2569 (2003).
20. Stadelmaier, A., Biskup, M. B. & Schmidt, R. R. Synthesis of serine-linked phosphatidylinositol mannosides (PIMs). *Eur. J. Org. Chem.* **2004,** 3292–3303 (2004).
21. Jayaprakash, K. N., Lu, J. & Fraser-Reid, B. Synthesis of a key *Mycobacterium tuberculosis* biosynthetic phosphoinositide intermediate. *Bioorg. Med. Chem. Lett.* **14,** 3815–3819 (2004).
22. Jayaprakash, K. N., Lu, J. & Fraser-Reid, B. Synthesis of a lipomannan component of the cell-wall complex of *Mycobacterium tuberculosis* is based on Paulsen's concept of donor/acceptor "match". *Angew. Chem. Int. Ed.* **44,** 5894–5898 (2005).
23. Ainge, G. D. *et al.* Phosphatidylinositol mannosides: synthesis and suppression of allergic airway disease. *Bioorg. Med. Chem.* **14,** 5632–5642 (2006).
24. Ainge, G. D. *et al.* Phosphatidylinositol mannosides: synthesis and adjuvant properties of phosphatidylinositol di- and tetramannosides. *Bioorg. Med. Chem.* **14,** 7615–7624 (2006).
25. Liu, X., Stocker, B. L. & Seeberger, P. H. Total synthesis of phosphatidylinositol mannosides of *Mycobacterium tuberculosis*. *J. Am. Chem. Soc.* **128,** 3638–3648 (2006).
26. Dyer, B. S. *et al.* Synthesis and structure of phosphatidylinositol dimannoside. *J. Org. Chem.* **72,** 3282–3288 (2007).
27. Ainge, G. D. *et al.* Phosphatidylinositol mannoside ether analogues: syntheses and interleukin-12-inducing properties. *J. Org. Chem.* **72,** 5291–5296 (2007).
28. Boonyarattanakalin, S., Liu, X., Michieletti, M., Lepenies, B. & Seeberger, P. H. Chemical synthesis of all phosphatidylinositol mannoside (PIM) glycans from *Mycobacterium tuberculosis*. *J. Am. Chem. Soc.* **130,** 16791–16799 (2008).
29. Ali, A., Wenk, M. R. & Lear, M. J. Total synthesis of a fully lipidated form of phosphatidyl-*myo*-inositol dimannoside (PIM-2) of *Mycobacterium tuberculosis*. *Tetrahedron Lett.* **50,** 5664–5666 (2009).
30. Patil, P. S. & Hung, S.-C. Total synthesis of phosphatidylinositol dimannoside: a cell-envelope component of *Mycobacterium tuberculosis*. *Chem. Eur. J.* **15,** 1091–1094 (2009).
31. Patil, P. S. & Hung, S.-C. Synthesis of mycobacterial triacylated phosphatidylinositol dimannoside containing an acyl lipid chain at 3-O of inositol. *Org. Lett.* **12,** 2618–2621 (2010).
32. Ainge, G. D. *et al.* Chemical synthesis and immunosuppressive activity of dipalmitoyl phosphatidylinositol hexamannoside. *J. Org. Chem.* **76,** 4941–4951 (2011).
33. Ainge, G. D. *et al.* Synthesis and Toll-like receptor 4 (TLR4) activity of phosphatidylinositol dimannoside analogues. *J. Med. Chem.* **54,** 7268–7279 (2011).
34. Rankin, G. M. *et al.* Synthesis and mass spectral characterization of mycobacterial phosphatidylinositol and its dimannosides. *J. Org. Chem.* **77,** 6743–6759 (2012).
35. Sureshan, K. M., Shashidhar, M. S., Praveen, T. & Das, T. Regioselective protection and deprotection of inositol hydroxyl groups. *Chem. Rev.* **103,** 4477–4504 (2003).
36. Patil, P. S., Zulueta, M. M. L. & Hung, S.-C. Synthesis of phosphatidylinositol mannosides. *J. Chin. Chem. Soc.* **61,** 151–162 (2014).
37. Takahashi, H., Kittaka, H. & Ikegami, S. Novel synthesis of enantiomerically pure natural inositols and their diastereoisomers. *J. Org. Chem.* **66,** 2705–2716 (2001).
38. Watt, J. A. & Williams, S. J. Rapid, iterative assembly of octyl α-1,6-oligomannosides and their 6-deoxy equivalents. *Org. Biomol. Chem.* **3,** 1982–1992 (2005).
39. Wang, C.-C. *et al.* Regioselective one-pot protection of carbohydrates. *Nature* **446,** 896–899 (2007).
40. Wang, C.-C., Kulkarni, S. S., Lee, J.-C., Luo, S.-Y. & Hung, S.-C. Regioselective one-pot protection of glucose. *Nat. Protoc.* **3,** 97–113 (2008).
41. Chang, K.-L., Zulueta, M. M. L., Lu, X.-A., Zhong, Y.-Q. & Hung, S.-C. Regioselective one-pot protection of D-glucosamine. *J. Org. Chem.* **75,** 7424–7427 (2010).
42. Huang, T.-Y., Zulueta, M. M. L. & Hung, S.-C. One-pot strategies for the synthesis of the tetrasaccharide linkage region of proteoglycans. *Org. Lett.* **13,** 1506–1509 (2011).
43. Patil, P. S., Lee, C.-C., Huang, Y.-W., Zulueta, M. M. L. & Hung, S.-C. Regioselective and stereoselective benzylidene installation and one-pot protection of D-mannose. *Org. Biomol. Chem.* **11,** 2605–2612 (2013).
44. Huang, T.-Y., Zulueta, M. M. L. & Hung, S.-C. Regioselective one-pot protection, protection-glycosylation and protection-glycosylation-glycosylation of carbohydrates: a case study with D-glucose. *Org. Biomol. Chem.* **12,** 376–382 (2014).
45. Shie, C.-R. *et al.* $Cu(OTf)_2$ as an efficient and dual-purpose catalyst in the regioselective reductive ring opening of benzylidene acetals. *Angew. Chem. Int. Ed.* **44,** 1665–1668 (2005).
46. Wang, C.-C. *et al.* Synthesis of biologically potent α1→2-linked disaccharide derivatives via regioselective one-pot protection-glycosylation. *Angew. Chem. Int. Ed.* **41,** 2360–2362 (2002).
47. Bock, K. & Pedersen, C. A study of ^{13}CH coupling constants in hexopyranoses. *J. Chem. Soc. Perkin. Trans.* **2,** 293–297 (1974).
48. Duus, J. Ø., Gotfredsen, C. H. & Bock, K. Carbohydrate structural determination by NMR spectroscopy: modern methods and limitations. *Chem. Rev.* **100,** 4589–4614 (2000).
49. Zulueta, M. M. L. *et al.* α-Glycosylation by D-glucosamine-derived donors: synthesis of heparosan and heparin analogues that interact with mycobacterial heparin-binding hemagglutinin. *J. Am. Chem. Soc.* **134,** 8988–8995 (2012).
50. French, G. L. *et al.* Diagnosis of tuberculous meningitis by detection of tuberculostearic acid in cerebrospinal fluid. *Lancet* **330,** 117–119 (1987).
51. Prout, F. S., Cason, J. & Ingersoll, A. W. The synthesis of tuberculostearic acid. *J. Am. Chem. Soc.* **69,** 1233–1233 (1947).

52. Schmidt, G. A. & Shirley, D. A. A new synthesis of tuberculostearic acid. *J. Am. Chem. Soc.* **71,** 3804–3806 (1949).
53. Roberts, I. O. & Baird, M. S. A new short synthesis of 10-(*R*)-tuberculostearic acid and its enantiomer. *Chem. Phys. Lipids* **142,** 111–117 (2006).
54. Li, H., Wu, J., Luo, J. & Dai, W.-M. A concise total synthesis of amphidinolide T2. *Chem. Eur. J.* **16,** 11530–11534 (2010).
55. Kaeothip, S. & Demchenko, A. V. Expeditious oligosaccharide synthesis via selective, semi-orthogonal, and orthogonal activation. *Carbohydr. Res.* **346,** 1371–1388 (2011).
56. De Libero, G. & Mori, L. The T-Cell response to lipid antigens of *Mycobacterium tuberculosis*. *Front. Immunol.* **5,** 219 (2014).
57. Shiozaki, M. *et al.* Synthesis of RCAI-172 (C6 epimer of RCAI-147) and its biological activity. *Bioorg. Med. Chem.* **22,** 827–833 (2014).
58. Schmidt, R. R. & Kinzy, W. Anomeric-oxygen activation for glycoside synthesis: the trichloroacetimidate method. *Adv. Carbohydr. Chem. Biochem.* **50,** 21–123 (1994).

Acknowledgements

This work was supported by the Ministry of Science and Technology (MOST 100-2113-M-001-019-MY3 and MOST 102-2628-M-001-001), National Health Research Institute (NHRI-EX103-10146NI) and Academia Sinica.

Author contributions

S.-C.H. designed the study, supervised students and staffs, and finalized the manuscript preparation. P.S.P. performed the synthesis of Ac_2PIM_6 **1**. T.-J.R.C. and S.-T.Y. carried out the evaluation of immunological activity. M.M.L.Z. prepared the figures and wrote the manuscript. L.S.L. is involved in the early stages of manuscript preparation and assisted in compiling the Supplementary Information. All authors discussed the results and commented on the manuscript.

Additional information

Accession codes: The X-ray crystallographic coordinates for compounds **10** and **13** in this study have been deposited at the Cambridge Crystallographic Data Centre (CCDC), under deposition numbers CCDC 1040371 and CCDC 1040372, respectively. These data can be obtained free of charge from the CCDC via www.ccdc.cam.ac.uk/data_request/cif.

Competing financial interests: The authors declare no competing financial interests.

8

Translocation path of a substrate protein through its Omp85 transporter

Catherine Baud[1,2,3,4], Jérémy Guérin[1,2,3,4], Emmanuelle Petit[1,2,3,4], Elodie Lesne[1,2,3,4], Elian Dupré[1,2,3,4], Camille Locht[1,2,3,4] & Françoise Jacob-Dubuisson[1,2,3,4]

TpsB proteins are Omp85 superfamily members that mediate protein translocation across the outer membrane of Gram-negative bacteria. Omp85 transporters are composed of N-terminal POTRA domains and a C-terminal transmembrane β-barrel. In this work, we track the *in vivo* secretion path of the *Bordetella pertussis* filamentous haemagglutinin (FHA), the substrate of the model TpsB transporter FhaC, using site-specific crosslinking. The conserved secretion domain of FHA interacts with the POTRA domains, specific extracellular loops and strands of FhaC and the inner β-barrel surface. The interaction map indicates a funnel-like pathway, with conformationally flexible FHA entering the channel in a non-exclusive manner and exiting along a four-stranded β-sheet at the surface of the FhaC barrel. This sheet of FhaC guides the secretion domain of FHA along discrete steps of translocation and folding. This work demonstrates that the Omp85 barrel serves as a channel for translocation of substrate proteins.

[1]Center for Infection and Immunity of Lille, Institut Pasteur de Lille, 1 rue Calmette, Lille 59021, France. [2]CNRS UMR8204, Lille 59021, France. [3]INSERM U1019, Lille 59045, France. [4]University of Lille Nord de France, Lille 59044, France. Correspondence and requests for materials should be addressed to F.J.-D. (email: francoise.jacob@ibl.cnrs.fr).

The widespread 'two-partner secretion' (TPS) pathway mediates the translocation of large proteins, involved in adherence, cytolysis, iron acquisition or growth inhibition, across the outer membrane of both pathogenic and non-pathogenic Gram-negative bacteria[1]. TPS systems are composed of two proteins, collectively called 'TpsA' for the secretory proteins and 'TpsB' for their transporters[2]. The secreted TspA proteins share a conserved, 250-residue-long N-terminal 'TPS' domain essential for secretion and a β-helix fold[3–7]. TpsB transporters are integral outer membrane proteins of the Omp85 superfamily, which is found in all branches of the phylogenetic tree[8]. Omp85 transporters mediate the translocation of their protein substrate(s) across, or their assembly into, specific cellular membranes. They share a common architecture that consists of a transmembrane β-barrel domain preceded by one or several POTRA domain(s) located in the inter-membrane space[9–12]. The POTRA domains appear to mediate protein–protein interactions[13–16]. However, the molecular mechanisms of protein transport or integration and in particular the role of the β-barrel remain poorly understood[11,12,17–21].

The filamentous haemagglutinin (FHA)/FhaC system of the whooping cough agent, *Bordetella pertussis*, is a model for the TPS pathway. The TpsA protein FHA, a major adhesin of *B. pertussis*[22], is translocated to the bacterial surface by its TpsB partner, FhaC. The crystal structures of Fha30, a 30-kDa secretion-competent N-terminal FHA truncated fragment, and of FhaC have been determined[4,9]. Fha30 comprises the entire TPS domain of FHA, which forms a right-handed, parallel β-helix flanked by conserved anti-parallel β-structure elements, and a few additional β-helix coils after the TPS domain[4] (Fig. 1a). FhaC is composed of two periplasmic POTRA domains in tandem followed by a 16-stranded transmembrane β-barrel[9] (Fig. 1b). The pore of the barrel is obstructed by the N-terminal α-helix H1 and the extracellular loop L6 of FhaC. H1 is joined to the barrel-distal POTRA1 domain by a 25-residue-long periplasmic linker. We have recently shown that H1 is mobile within the pore and can move to the periplasm[23]. The extracellular loop L6, which folds back into the pore, harbours a conserved sequence motif characteristic of the Omp85 superfamily and is essential for function[9,24–26]. According to the current secretion model, FhaB, the FHA precursor, is exported across the cytoplasmic membrane by the Sec machinery and chaperoned by DegP in the periplasm[27–29]. The POTRA domains of FhaC recognize the TPS domain of FHA in an extended conformation, leading to the translocation of the secretory polypeptide across the outer membrane[14,30,31]. Whether FHA transport occurs through the pore of the FhaC β-barrel has not been shown. Upon secretion, FHA folds progressively into a long β-helix at the cell surface before undergoing a proteolytic maturation that partially releases it into the milieu[32].

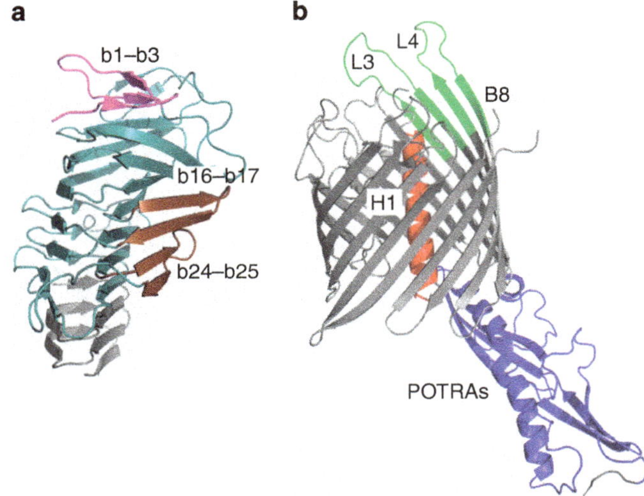

Figure 1 | Structures of Fha30 and FhaC. Cartoon representation of Fha30 (protein data bank: 1rwr, **a**) and FhaC (protein data bank: 2qdz, **b**). In Fha30, the TPS domain is coloured while the additional β-strands are in grey. The strands that form extra-β-helix elements in the TPS domain have been indicated with small 'b' letters to distinguish them from the FhaC strands (capital 'B' letters) discussed in the text. Note that in the X-ray structure of FhaC, the linker and L5 are not resolved. The figures were created with Pymol.

In this work, we track the translocation path of FHA across the outer membrane by performing *in vivo*, cysteine-directed crosslinking. We show that the β-barrel of FhaC serves as the protein-conducting channel. An extracellular β-sheet of FhaC is crucial for function, and translocation of the TPS domain proceeds by discrete steps.

Results

Mapping of FhaC regions that interact with FHA. To map the regions of FhaC that are in contact with FHA during secretion, we looked for a model substrate that crosses the outer membrane in an FhaC-dependent manner and folds independently of the rest of FHA[4,30], which is produced at good levels in *Escherichia coli*, and that interacts long enough with FhaC for detectable inter-protein crosslinking to occur. Although Fha30, a secretion-competent, N-terminal truncated fragment of FHA, met the first conditions[4], initial experiments with nonspecific crosslinkers indicated that it was secreted much too fast. Thus, to freeze the interactions between the two partners, we used the Fha30-BugE chimaera[23]. When co-produced with FhaC in *E. coli*, this chimaera stalls across the outer membrane, with its Fha30 moiety exposed to the cell surface and the globular BugE moiety in the periplasm. We have shown that such chimaeras mimic translocation intermediates and can thus be used as tools to probe the on-going secretion process[23].

Single Cys residues were introduced at >50 positions in FhaC by site-directed mutagenesis (Fig. 2a). The substitutions did not affect the production of FhaC, its location in the outer membrane or its ability to secrete Fha30 (Supplementary Fig. 1). We co-produced Fha30-BugE with each $FhaC_{Cys}$ variant in *E. coli*. In this system, the expression of FhaC is under the control of a weak constitutive promoter, while that of the chimaera is induced with isopropyl-β-D-thiogalactoside (IPTG) for a short period of time at the exponential growth phase of the culture, so that the chimaera is presented to preformed FhaC in the outer membrane. The bacteria were treated with the heterofunctional sulfhydryl-to-amine crosslinkers SPDP (succinimidyl 3-(2-pyridyl-dithio) propionate), LC-SPDP (long chain SPDP)or SMCC (succinimidyl 4-(N-maleimidomethyl)cyclohexane-1-carboxylate), and following disruption of the bacterial membranes, FhaC- or FhaC-containing complexes were isolated by taking advantage of the property of FhaC to bind to Ni^{++} beads irrespective of a 6-His tag. The material eluted from the beads was analysed by immunoblotting using anti-Fha30 and anti-FhaC antibodies (Fig. 2b and Supplementary Fig. 2). Complexes between the two proteins were detected for FhaC derivatives harbouring Cys residues in the POTRA domains, a periplasmic loop, the barrel interior (B9–B11), the extracellular portions of β-strands B5, B7 and B8, and the extracellular loops L3, L4 and L5, but not in H1, the linker, other extracellular loops or in a lipid-facing position of the β-barrel (Cys468). Low amounts of crosslinked species were

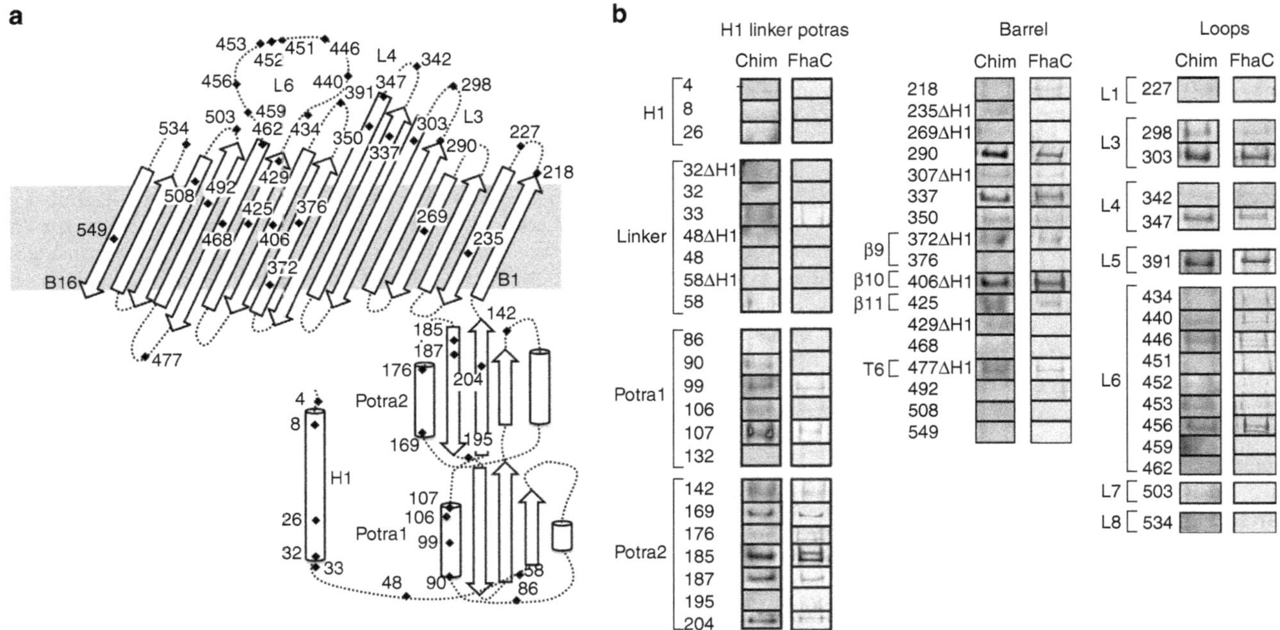

Figure 2 | Crosslinking analyses with FhaC Cys variants. (**a**) Schematic representation of the FhaC topology, with the positions of the Cys residues introduced for crosslinking experiments indicated as black diamonds. The topology is based on a slightly revised version of the FhaC structure (protein data bank: 4qky). (**b**) Immunoblot analyses of the SMCC-crosslinked complexes or the SPDP-crosslinked complexes for the FhaCΔH1$_{Cys429}$ and FhaCΔH1$_{Cys372}$ variants following precipitation of FhaC. The membranes were probed successively with anti-Fha30 antibodies followed by chemiluminescence detection, and with anti-FhaC antibodies followed by alkaline phosphatase detection. The crosslinked complex migrates slightly under the 150-kDa band of the molecular mass markers that is indicated by a small horizontal dash at the left of the first subpanel. Note the presence of two FhaC-containing bands in some cases, the upper one corresponding to the complex and the other to an FhaC dimer that most likely formed upon cell lysis. Some FhaC variants with Cys in the barrel were devoid of H1 to facilitate crosslinker access (denoted as ΔH1), since H1 is not essential for activity[37] and moves to the periplasm for FHA translocation[23]. We checked for one such variant, FhaC$_{C406}$, that similar results were obtained with or without H1. In the β-barrel, we mainly selected residues oriented towards the pore based on the crystal structure of FhaC. Lipid-oriented residue 468 was used as a control.

also found for some FhaC variants with Cys residues in the conserved L6 loop.

Thus, three regions of FhaC principally interact with the stalled Fha30-BugE chimaera: the surface of the POTRA domains oriented towards the β-barrel, the inner wall of the barrel, and specific extracellular loops and strands. Detection of crosslinks between the chimaera and inward-facing residues of the FhaC β-barrel strands B9–B11 located halfway into the pore (Fig. 2) provides the first direct evidence that the TpsA protein crosses the outer membrane through the proteinaceous channel formed by its TpsB partner. In addition, most FhaC–chimaera crosslinks involving extracellular portions of FhaC are localized in an extracellular β-sheet formed by the longest β-barrel strands (B5–B8) and in nearby surface loops L3, L4 and L5. As for the interactions of the POTRA domains with the chimaera, they involve the same regions of the POTRA domains as those identified to interact with Fha30 *in vitro*[14]. The topology of the chimaera suggests that BugE, rather than Fha30, is in contact with the POTRA domains in these stalled complexes.

To confirm the pathway observed with Fha30-BugE and to ascertain that it was not affected by the presence of the BugE cargo, we performed a limited number of crosslinking experiments with another model substrate harbouring a different cargo, Fha30-calmo. Of note, we have shown that this chimaera could be released into the milieu from the stalled complex after unfolding its calmodulin cargo[23]. The Fha30-calmo chimaera was found to crosslink with FhaC in a similar manner as the Fha30-BugE model substrate, although the amounts of complex were weaker (Supplementary Fig. 3).

Regions of FHA that interact with FhaC. To identify regions of the TPS domain that are close to FhaC in the course of translocation, we introduced Cys residues at various positions of the Fha30 moiety of the Fha30-BugE chimaera (Fig. 3a and Supplementary Table 1 for the list of positions tested). In addition to a few β-helix positions, we particularly targeted segments that form extra-β-helix elements conserved in the TpsA family[4–6]. Most substitutions do not affect the secretion of Fha30 alone, enabling us to use the corresponding chimaeras for crosslinking, while those that abolish secretion or cause intracellular proteolytic degradation of the chimaera were discarded (Supplementary Table 1). *In vivo* crosslinking experiments showed that Cys residues in two major discrete regions of the TPS domain mediate the formation of complexes between the chimaera and FhaC: the N-terminal region up to b8, and the region encompassing residues 176–200 in the second part of the TPS domain, that is, in the less conserved 'LC2' region[4] (Fig. 3b and Supplementary Fig. 4).

Tracking the FHA path in FhaC. Next, we combined single Cys variants of FhaC with those of Fha30-BugE, and looked for spontaneous formation of inter-protein disulfide (S–S) bonds in the course of translocation in order to obtain a site-specific interaction map. N-ethyl maleimide was added before cell lysis to avoid extraneous bonds. A number of specific FhaC–chimaera complexes were detected (Fig. 4, Supplementary Table 2 and Supplementary Fig. 5). Positions up to b16–b17 in Fha30 formed S–S bonds with the POTRA domains of FhaC, as well as with the linker. In addition, several regions of FHA including the b7, b8,

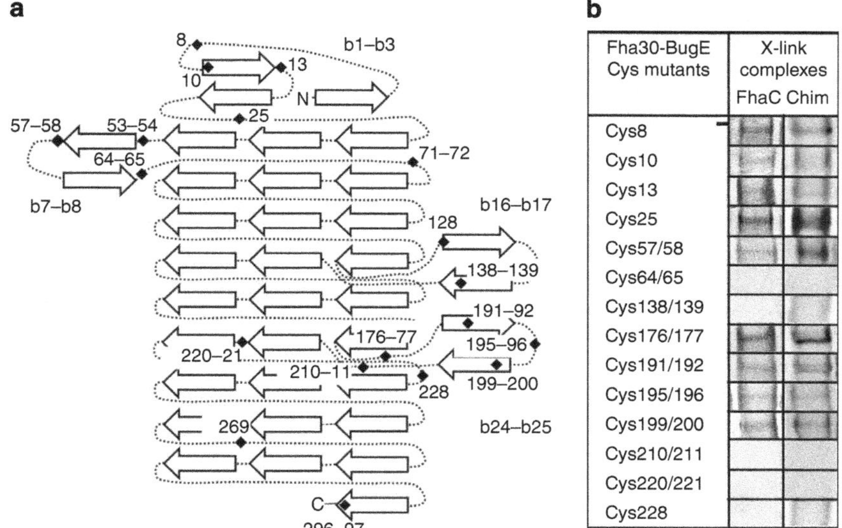

Figure 3 | Crosslinking analyses with Fha30-BugE Cys variants. (**a**) Schematic representation of the Fha30 topology, with the positions of the Cys residues introduced for crosslinking experiments indicated as black diamonds. (**b**) Immunoblot analyses of the SMCC-crosslinked complexes or the LC-SPDP-crosslinked complexes for the chimaera Cys13, Cys191/192 and Cys199/200 variants following precipitation of FhaC. The membranes were probed successively with anti-Fha30 antibodies and with anti-FhaC antibodies as above. The crosslinked complex migrates slightly under the 150-kDa band of the markers that is indicated by a short horizontal dash at the left of the first subpanel.

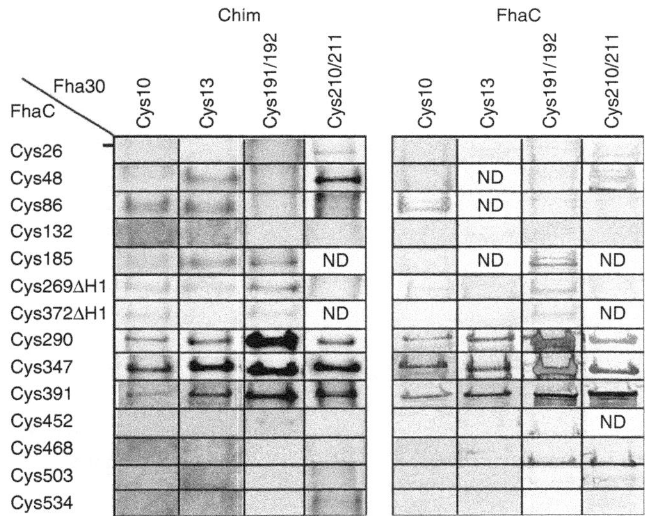

Figure 4 | Spontaneous formation of S-S bonds between FhaC and Fha30-BugE. The membranes were successively probed with anti-Fha30 antibodies followed by chemiluminescence detection (left panel), and with anti-FhaC antibodies followed by alkaline phosphatase detection (right panel). The crosslinked complex migrates slightly under the 150-kDa band of the markers that is indicated by a short horizontal dash at the left of the first subpanel. ND, not determined.

b24 and b25 strands formed S–S bonds with the barrel interior. Finally, the N-terminal cap (b1–b3) and a central region of the TPS domain (residues 191–221) both formed crosslinks with the extracellular sheet of FhaC (Fig. 4, Supplementary Table 2). Altogether, there is a good agreement between the chemical crosslinks and the spontaneous S–S bonds.

In many cases, a given Cys in Fha30 was involved in S–S bonds with several Cys residues located in non-contiguous regions of FhaC (Supplementary Table 2), indicating sequential or alternative interactions of the secretory polypeptide with its transporter. In particular, each of the three N-proximal Cys of Fha30 crosslinked with the POTRA domains, the inner barrel surface, the extracellular β-strands B5–B8 and the L5 loop. These interactions thus track possible paths of the Fha30 N terminus through FhaC.

The observation that some Fha30 Cys residues (for example, Cys8 or Cys190/191) formed S–S bonds with opposite sites in the first half of the barrel (Cys269 in B4 and Cys372 in B9) indicates that the chimaera does not enter the FhaC channel along a strictly defined path. Instead, it appears to interact by >1 manner with the entrance of the FhaC channel. In contrast, interactions at the exit of the channel involved principally one side of the barrel, with intense S–S-bonded complexes involving B5–B8 (Cys290, Cys337 and Cys347) and L5 (Cys391) of FhaC, and N-terminal (Cys8 and Cys25) and central (residues 190–221) regions of Fha30. Interestingly, these two regions harbour non-β-helix, anti-parallel structural elements in the native TPS domain, including the b1–b3 cap of the β-helix and the b24–b25 β-hairpin (Fig. 1a).

Identification of putative translocation intermediates. Two regions that are not spatially close to each other in Fha30—that is, the N-terminal region and a central region of the TPS domain—both interact with the extracellular B5–B8 β sheet of FhaC. Therefore, we hypothesized that these interactions reflect sequential intermediates of translocation captured by crosslinking because they correspond to translocation pauses. This was tested by treating bacteria that co-produce Fha30-BugE and FhaC with proteinase K without any crosslinking. This was done on intact or outer membrane-permeabilized bacteria. BugE in the chimaera was tagged with a C-terminal myc epitope for detection (Fig. 5). Cell samples were precipitated with trichloroacetic acid (TCA), and the chimaera fragments were detected by immunoblotting with anti-Fha30 or anti-myc antibodies.

Treatment of intact cells yielded species of ~60, 50 and 45 kDa that reacted with both antibodies (denoted I–IV) and shorter species ~22–23 kDa (V and VI) detected only with anti-Fha30

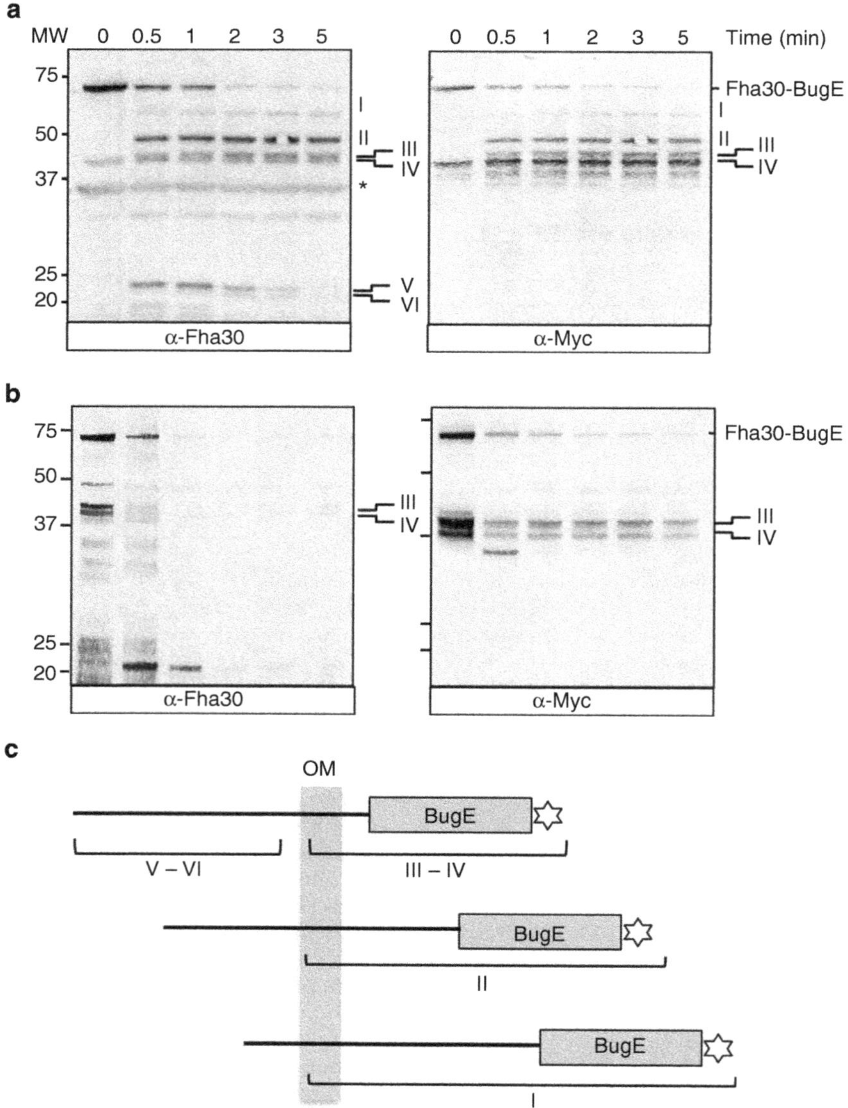

Figure 5 | Identification of translocation intermediates by proteolysis. Intact (**a**) or permeabilized (**b**) cells co-expressing Fha30-BugE with a C-terminal myc tag and FhaC were treated with proteinase K for the indicated times. Neither protein harboured a Cys residue and no chemical cross-linker was added. After TCA precipitation, total cellular proteins were analysed by immunoblotting using anti-Fha30 (left panels) or anti-myc (right panels) antibodies. The asterisk indicates a nonspecific band. A schematic representation of the chimaera and its proteolytic fragments is shown in **c**. OM and the grey rectangle denote the outer membrane.

antibodies (Fig. 5a,c). In permeabilized cells, bands I and II disappeared, and species slightly smaller than III and IV were only detected with the anti-myc antibodies (Fig. 5b,c). This indicated that BugE is resistant to proteolysis, while Fha30 portions in species I and II are protected from degradation by the outer membrane in intact cells but mostly degraded after permeabilization. Species V and VI most likely encompass surface-exposed Fha30 fragments fairly resistant to protease treatment.

The low-abundance species detected by immunoblotting could not be identified by mass fingerprinting analyses from total cell lysates. To confirm the identity of species V and VI, we treated purified Fha30 with proteinase K and analysed the polypeptides by mass fingerprinting (Supplementary Fig. 6). The major proteolytic product of native Fha30 that most likely corresponds to species V or VI encompasses the N-terminal two-thirds of Fha30.

Altogether, thus, the presence of species I–IV confirms the occurrence of intermediates of translocation, which is consistent with the idea that secretion proceeds by steps.

Role of extracellular β-sheet of FhaC. Finally, to probe the importance of the extracellular B5–B8 β-sheet for FhaC secretion activity, we deleted the L3 and L4 loops and shortened the extracellular portions of the B5–B8 β-strands. The FhaC variants were detected in normal amounts in the cells, but secretion was affected or abolished by these deletions, unlike for the L1 or L2 deletion variants used as controls (Fig. 6a). Consistent with this secretion defect, low amounts of cell-associated Fha30-BugE were found, indicating significant intracellular degradation of the chimaera. Integrity of the extracellular B5–B8 sheet and of the L3 and L4 loops is thus important for FhaC function.

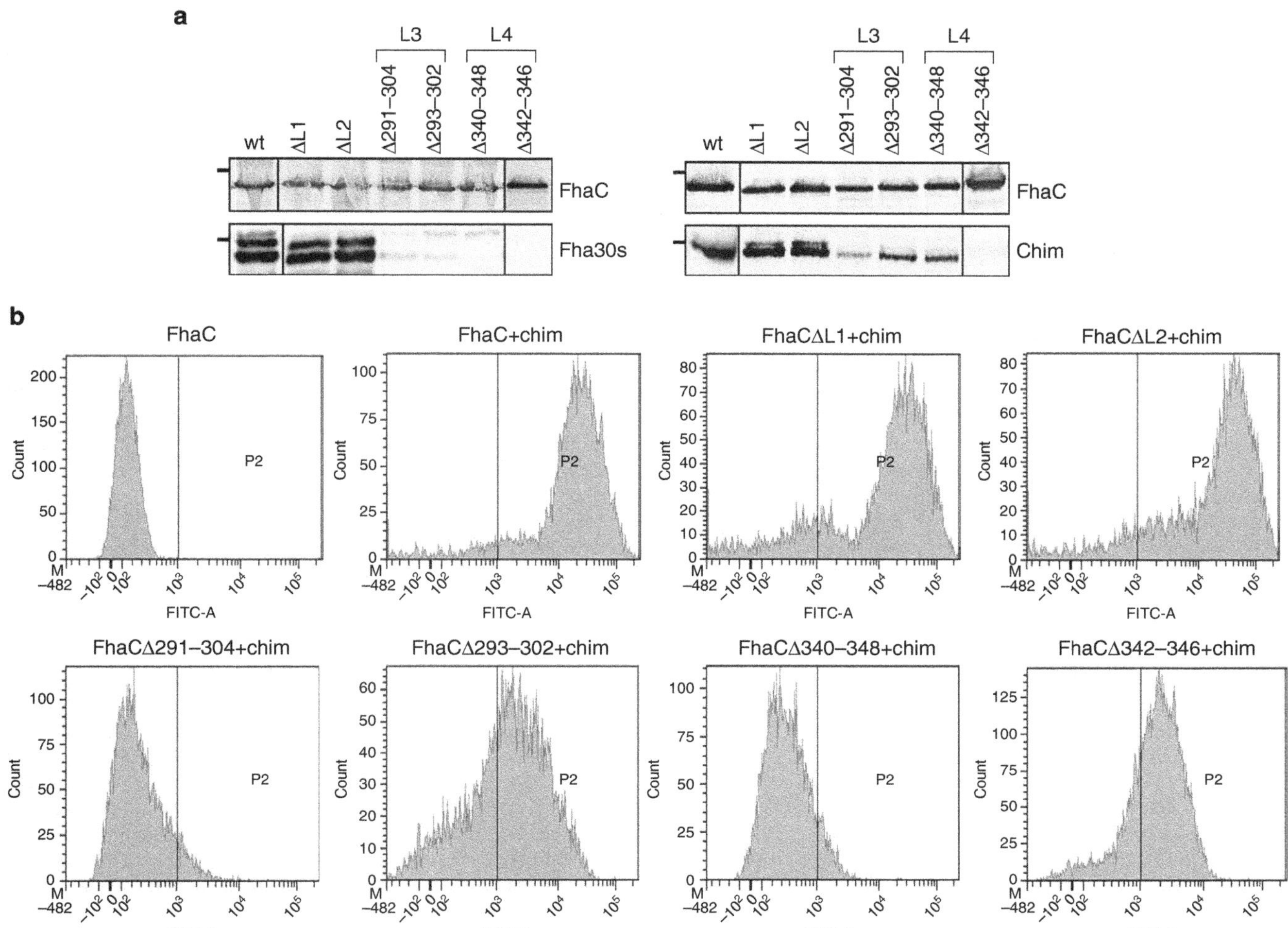

Figure 6 | Importance of the extracellular β sheet B5–B8 for FhaC activity. (**a**) Effects of deletions in the L3 and L4 loops on Fha30 secretion (denoted as Fha30s) and on the presence of cell-associated FhaC and Fha30-BugE (denoted as chim). Culture supernatants of cells co-producing FhaC and Fha30 (left panel), or lysates of cells co-producing FhaC and Fha30-BugE (right panel) were analysed by immunoblotting with anti-FhaC and anti-Fha30 antibodies. FhaC, Fha30 and Fha30-BugE chimaera migrate below the 75-kDa band of the markers, slightly below the 37-kDa band and slightly below the 75-kDa band, respectively, as indicated by short horizontal dashes at the left of the respective panels. (**b**) Flow cytometry analyses of *E. coli* co-expressing Fha30-BugE with an N-terminal myc tag and selected FhaC variants. Exposure of the Fha30 moiety of the chimaera at the cell surface was revealed using an anti-myc fluorescein isothiocyanate (FITC)-conjugated antibody. Wt, wild type.

Flow cytometry analyses were performed on cells co-producing Fha30-BugE that harbours an N-terminal myc tag and the FhaC variants (Fig. 6b). The bacteria were treated with an anti-myc fluorescein isothiocyanate conjugate for detection of the chimaera at the surface. Cells that produced the FhaC variants with the longer deletions showed no labelling at all, indicating that they could not translocate the chimaera, consistent with its intracellular degradation. The other bacteria were labelled by the antibody at lower levels than controls (Fig. 6b). Alterations of the B5–B8 β sheet thus prevent the chimaera from engaging properly into the channel and/or from stably reaching the cell surface, which strongly compromises secretion. Thus, the extracellular β-sheet of FhaC is a critical determinant for activity.

Discussion

In this work, we use the model FHA/FhaC TPS system to define the pathway of the secreted TpsA protein across its outer membrane transporter TpsB. By freezing the interactions between the partners, we characterize them during translocation and provide here the first evidence of an Omp85 substrate using the β-barrel of its transporter as a channel. Spontaneous S–S bond formation between the two proteins in the course of secretion also provides a dynamic view with snapshots of the transport process. We uncover the critical role of an extracellular β-sheet for FhaC secretion activity. Interestingly, corresponding surface regions of the *E. coli* Omp85 transporter BamA were also found to be essential for function[33,34].

In the crystal structure, the FhaC channel is mostly obstructed by the N-terminal α-helix H1 (ref. 9). Our findings that FHA threads its way through the FhaC pore is consistent with our findings that H1 plugs the resting barrel and moves to the periplasm for FHA translocation[23]. L6 is also located in the β-barrel pore of Omp85 transporters[9,11,12]. Unlike H1, however, we do not know whether it fully moves out of the FhaC pore in the course of secretion. The drastic effects of deletions, amino-acid substitutions and the observation of conformational changes have suggested that L6 participates in the transport mechanism of Omp85 proteins[11,21,26,35,36]. Our findings that L6 of FhaC weakly interacts with the substrate in the course of translocation argue against its playing a direct role to pull the secretory polypeptide towards the surface. How it contributes to activity remains a major unanswered question for Omp85 transporters.

The four-stranded B5–B8 surface β-sheet of FhaC strongly interacts with FHA in the course of translocation. Its structural integrity is critical for FhaC function, as shown by the drastic effects of deletions. In support of this, we showed earlier that insertions in B5, B6 and L4 inactivated FhaC[35,37]. Notably, B5–B8 are generally long, and B9 is short in TpsB proteins (Supplementary Fig. 7). In addition, the available Omp85 structures show that the B5–B8 β sheet is a conserved structural feature of the β-barrel[9,11,12,34]. These observations support a specific role for this sheet in the transport mechanism. In FhaC, B5–B8 appears to serve as a guide to which specific portions of the TPS domain bind in the course of translocation. This binding might involve β-augmentation of the edge strand of the FhaC β-sheet. In BamA, the extracellular loops L3 and L4 that join B5 to B6 and B7 to B8 form a dome over the barrel together with two other surface loops, thus limiting the opening of the channel to the milieu[11,34]. In the *E. coli* BamA, L3 also delineates with other loops a hydrophilic surface cavity proposed to facilitate the transport of soluble loops or domains of the substrate proteins[34]. Thus, the distinct conformations of these extracellular regions in FhaC and BamA are in good agreement with the respective functions of the two types of transporters.

The preferential crosslinks of two non-contiguous regions of the TPS domain to the extracellular β-sheet and loops, and the occurrence of protected species comprising large portions of Fha30 in the proteolysis experiments both support the hypothesis of discrete translocation intermediates. *In vitro* translocation experiments have also suggested the existence of intermediates[31]. We thus propose that translocation of the TPS domain proceeds by steps of binding, pause and release. The TPS regions that bind strongly to the extracellular sheet in these putative translocation intermediates mainly form extra-β-helix, anti-parallel β-structures in the native TPS domain. Their binding to the FhaC extracellular sheet is thus compatible with the progressive folding of β-helical segments at the surface.

The Cys–Cys bonds approach provides a dynamic picture of the FhaC–Fha30 interactions and indicates a funnel-like route for the FHA polypeptide through it transporter. Several crosslinks of a given Fha30 residue with spatially distant residues of FhaC in the POTRA domains and at the barrel entrance indicate >1 possible path(s) as FHA initiates translocation. A major site for POTRA–TPS domain interactions is a hydrophobic groove formed by the edge strand of the β-sheet of the POTRA2 domain and its flanking α-helix, which could accommodate extended, amphipathic segments of the substrate[14]. The highly repetitive, amphipathic structure of the TPS domain[4,38] makes it likely that its initial positioning along the POTRA domains is not univocal, and these initial interactions might then determine the entry path of FHA into the channel. As the TPS domain moves through the pore and starts to fold at the surface, it becomes more constrained, and its pathway becomes more defined, as shown by the contacts between the two proteins at the extracellular side of the pore involving exclusively one face of the barrel.

We thus propose the following model for the mechanism of secretion. In the absence of its substrate, FhaC transitions from a closed conformation with H1 inside the pore to an open conformation with H1 in the periplasm[23]. The binding of extended amphipathic FHA segments to the POTRA domains of FhaC stabilizes that open conformation and enables the N terminus of FHA to enter and thread its way into the pore. At the exit, specific anti-parallel β-hairpins of the TPS domain of FHA bind to the extracellular β-sheet of FhaC, transiently anchoring the polypeptide at the cell surface and facilitating its folding. Once a sufficient portion of the β-helix is stably formed, backsliding can no longer occur and the rest of the FHA polypeptide progressively emerges and prolongs the β-helix in the extracellular milieu. This scenario is likely to apply to other TPS systems given the good conservation of critical features in both the transporters and the secreted proteins.

In the Omp85 superfamily, some members mediate the translocation of their protein substrate across the membrane, whereas others mediate protein insertion into a membrane. However, this distinction is more blurred than generally assumed, and some Omp85 transporters may combine both functions. This is probably the case for TamA and BamA when they secrete autotransporters, which harbour both a transmembrane β-barrel domain and a soluble, extracellular passenger domain[39–42]. Thus, we believe that some features of the transport process uncovered in this work will be relevant for the other superfamily members. In particular and most importantly, we propose that the direct role for the β-barrel evidenced in this work applies to all Omp85 transporters. This model indeed concurs with mechanisms proposed for BamA and TamA based on recent X-ray structures[11,12,34]. A lateral opening of the Omp85 β-barrel to enable the transfer of the substrate into the lipid bilayer has been proposed, and evidence supporting such a mechanism was recently obtained[43]. A lateral opening implies that the soluble, surface loop regions of the substrate proteins transit through the barrel while the transmembrane segments are integrated in the bilayer, as discussed in ref. 34. Those authors have even proposed that the extracellular dome of BamA might function as a lid that restrains misrouting of the substrate membrane strands that might otherwise be secreted[34]. Indeed, the β-strands of these β-barrel substrate proteins are amphipathic, similar to the β-helix-forming segments of TpsA proteins. Unlike the BamA proteins, TamA has no extracellular dome. It has been proposed that the passenger domain of its substrate passes through an enlarged barrel combining those of TamA and the autotransporter, after which the composite barrel splits to release the autotransporter's barrel into the membrane[12]. The fact that two features of the barrel, L6 and a specific sequence motif in the β-barrel strand B13 are conserved and essential for function[10,11,25,26] corroborates the essential role of the β barrel in the transport process for the entire superfamily.

Methods

Plasmids. pFc3 is the expression plasmid for FhaC[35]. It was modified by site-directed mutagenesis to introduce Cys codons at specific positions using the QuikChange II Xl kit (Agilent Technologies). All mutated fragments were fully verified by sequencing. Deletions were introduced by generating EcoRI–BamHI and BglII–HindIII PCR fragments that encompass the 5′ and 3′ portions of *fhaC* and ligating them together in EcoRI–HindIII restricted pFc3. Cys codons were introduced into *fha30* by site-directed mutagenesis on a modified version of pEC138b (ref. 44), harbouring the 3′ NotI–BamHI portion of *fha30* made as a synthetic gene fragment (GeneCust) without the PstI site and with codon optimization. To enhance crosslinking, two consecutive Cys codons were introduced together in several Fha30 variants. The relevant restriction fragments were then exchanged for their parent fragments in pEC141bis, which codes for Fha30-BugE (ref. 23). The final expression plasmids are based on pBBItac[44] harbouring the EcoRI–HindIII fragments from the corresponding pEC138 and pEC141 variants. pBBItac141b, pBBItac141b-Cmyc and pBBItac-Nmyc for the expression of the Fha30-BugE chimaera and its myc-tagged versions, as well as pBBitac140-calm for the expression of Fha30-calmo were described earlier[23].

***In vivo* crosslinking.** *E. coli* UT5600 cells harbouring both a pFC3 derivative and a pBBItac141b derivative were grown to an OD_{600} of 0.8 in 25 ml of LB medium with gentamycin (10 μg ml^{-1}) and ampicillin (150 μg ml^{-1}) and then treated for 2.5 h with 1 mM IPTG. Cells (4 ml) were harvested by centrifugation, washed once and concentrated 10 times in crosslinking buffer (20 mM HEPES, pH 7.4, 150 mM NaCl and 1 mM EDTA). DMSO or 0.2 mM SPDP, LC-SPDP or SMCC (Thermo Scientific) dissolved in DMSO was added, and the samples were incubated for 1 h at 37 °C under rotation. After quenching for 10 min on ice with 100 mM Tris-HCl (pH 7.5), cells were washed with the crosslinking buffer and lysed by freezing and thawing. The membranes were solubilized in 8 M urea, 1% Triton X-100, 20 mM HEPES (pH 7.4) and 150 mM NaCl. Urea concentration was adjusted to 6 M and the complexes were affinity-purified by incubation with 50 µl of Ni-NTA magnetic beads (Millipore), taking advantage of the natural affinity of FhaC for Ni-NTA. Beads were washed twice in 0.5% Triton X-100, 20 mM HEPES (pH 7.4), 150 mM NaCl containing 6 M urea (washing buffer) and then 2 M urea. The complexes were eluted with 400 mM imidazole in washing buffer. They were resolved by electrophoresis using 3–8% Tris acetate gels (Nu-PAGE—Invitrogen) without reducing agent in the sample buffer and analysed by immunoblotting with polyclonal anti-Fha30 antibodies (dilution 1: 3,000; ref. 23) and horseradish peroxidase-coupled anti-guinea pigs antibodies (Jackson ImmunoResearch, catalogue no. 706-035-148; dilution 1:10,000), and the complexes were detected by chemiluminescence. The same blots were then revealed using anti-FhaC antibodies[14] (dilution 1:2,500) and anti-rat alcaline phosphate-conjugated antibodies (Promega, catalogue no. S3831; dilution 1:7,500), followed by colorimetric detection. The contrast of the blot scans for the chemical crosslinking experiments with the chimaera Cys variants was emphasized for better visualization of the complex bands.

Cys-Cys crosslinking. Cultures were performed as above. Samples of 4 ml were harvested by centrifugation, resuspended in 1 ml PBS containing 5 mM N-ethylmaleimide (Sigma) and incubated for 30 min at room temperature. Cells were then washed in PBS, and membranes were solubilized in 8 M urea, 1% Triton X-100, 20 mM HEPES (pH 7.4), 300 mM NaCl and 1 mM N-ethylmaleimide. Complexes were purified and analysed as described above except that all washing and elution steps were performed in 6 M urea, 0.5% Triton X-100, 20 mM HEPES (pH 7.4) and 300 mM NaCl. The protocol was standardized so that a relative quantification of the complexes could be performed by densitometry scanning of the corresponding bands on the immunoblots using the ImageJ software.

Proteolysis. Cultures were carried out as above, and 0.7-ml aliquots were centrifuged, washed in PBS and resuspended in 0.6 ml of PBS for intact cells or in 50 mM Tris–HCl (pH 7.5), 10 mM EDTA, 0.1 mg ml^{-1} lysozyme for outer membrane permeabilization. After 20 min of incubation on ice, proteinase K was added to a final concentration of 500 µg ml^{-1}, and proteolysis was carried out at 37 °C. Samples of 100 µl were precipitated with TCA after various times, and the proteins were analysed using 12% Tris-glycine gels (Novex, Invitrogen) and immunoblotting with polyclonal anti-Fha30 antibodies[23] or a Myc epitope tag monoclonal antibody (Thermo Scientific, catalogue no. MA1-21316; dilution 1:1,500), followed by secondary horseradish peroxidase-conjugated antibodies as above. For the mass fingerprinting analyses, native Fha30 was purified from culture supernatants[4] and used at a concentration of 20 µg ml^{-1}. Following proteinase K treatment and electrophoresis, the gel was coloured with Coomassie blue (SimplyBlue Safe Stain, Invitrogen), and the bands of interest were cut and subjected to mass fingerprinting using an Auto Speed TOF/TOF mass spectrometer (Bruker).

Flow cytometry analyses. Cultures were performed as above, and 1-ml aliquots were harvested at 7,000 r.p.m. for 3 min in a tabletop centrifuge. The cells were washed with ice-cold PBS, 3% BSA, 1% sodium azide and resuspended in 400 µl PBS, 3% BSA, 1% sodium azide containing fluorescein isothiocyanate-conjugated anti-Myc tag antibody (Abcam, catalogue no. 1263; dilution 1:100). After 1 h incubation at room temperature in the dark, cells were pelleted as described above, washed twice in ice-cold PBS with 3% BSA and resuspended in 500 µl of PBS with 3% BSA. Flow cytometry data were acquired on a LSR Fortessa using a photomultiplicator to increase the forward scatter (FSC) signal and analysed with the FACS Diva software (Becton Dickinson).

Sequence alignments. TpsB proteins were aligned with the Jalview software[45].

References

1. Jacob-Dubuisson, F., Guerin, J., Baelen, S. & Clantin, B. Two-partner secretion: as simple as it sounds? *Res. Microbiol.* **164,** 583–595 (2013).
2. Jacob-Dubuisson, F., Locht, C. & Antoine, R. Two-partner secretion in Gram-negative bacteria: a thrifty, specific pathway for large virulence proteins. *Mol. Microbiol.* **40,** 306–313 (2001).
3. Kajava, A. V. & Steven, A. C. The turn of the screw: variations of the abundant beta-solenoid motif in passenger domains of Type V secretory proteins. *J. Struct. Biol.* **155,** 306–315 (2006).
4. Clantin, B. *et al.* The crystal structure of filamentous hemagglutinin secretion domain and its implications for the two-partner secretion pathway. *Proc. Natl Acad. Sci. USA* **101,** 6194–6199 (2004).
5. Yeo, H. J. *et al.* The structure of the *Haemophilus influenzae* HMW1 pro-piece reveals a structural domain essential for bacterial two-partner secretion. *J. Biol. Chem.* **282,** 31076–31084 (2007).
6. Weaver, T. M. *et al.* Structural and functional studies of truncated hemolysin a from *Proteus mirabilis*. *J. Biol. Chem.* **284,** 22297–22309 (2009).
7. Baelen, S., Dewitte, F., Clantin, B. & Villeret, V. Structure of the secretion domain of HxuA from Haemophilus influenzae. *Acta. Crystallogr. Sect. F. Struct. Biol. Cryst. Commun.* **69,** 1322–1327 (2013).
8. Gentle, I. E., Burri, L. & Lithgow, T. Molecular architecture and function of the Omp85 family of proteins. *Mol. Microbiol.* **58,** 1216–1225 (2005).
9. Clantin, B. *et al.* Structure of the membrane protein FhaC: a member of the Omp85-TpsB transporter superfamily. *Science* **317,** 957–961 (2007).
10. Jacob-Dubuisson, F., Villeret, V., Clantin, B., Delattre, A. S. & Saint, N. First structural insights into the TpsB/Omp85 superfamily. *Biol. Chem.* **390,** 675–684 (2009).
11. Noinaj, N. *et al.* Structural insight into the biogenesis of beta-barrel membrane proteins. *Nature* **501,** 385–390 (2013).
12. Gruss, F. *et al.* The structural basis of autotransporter translocation by TamA. *Nat. Struct. Mol. Biol.* **20,** 1318–1320 (2013).
13. Kim, S. *et al.* Structure and function of an essential component of the outer membrane protein assembly machine. *Science* **317,** 961–964 (2007).
14. Delattre, A. S. *et al.* Substrate recognition by the POTRA domains of TpsB transporter FhaC. *Mol. Microbiol.* **81,** 99–112 (2011).
15. Knowles, T. J. *et al.* Fold and function of polypeptide transport-associated domains responsible for delivering unfolded proteins to membranes. *Mol. Microbiol.* **68,** 1216–1227 (2008).
16. Ricci, D. P., Hagan, C. L., Kahne, D. & Silhavy, T. J. Activation of the *Escherichia coli* beta-barrel assembly machine (Bam) is required for essential components to interact properly with substrate. *Proc. Natl Acad. Sci. USA* **109,** 3487–3491 (2012).
17. Robert, V. *et al.* Assembly factor Omp85 recognizes its outer membrane protein substrates by a species-specific C-terminal motif. *PLoS Biol.* **4,** e377 (2006).
18. Bos, M. P., Robert, V. & Tommassen, J. Biogenesis of the gram-negative bacterial outer membrane. *Annu. Rev. Microbiol.* **61,** 191–214 (2007).
19. Stegmeier, J. F. & Andersen, C. Characterization of pores formed by YaeT (Omp85) from *Escherichia coli*. *J. Biochem.* **140,** 275–283 (2006).
20. Knowles, T. J., Scott-Tucker, A., Overduin, M. & Henderson, I. R. Membrane protein architects: the role of the BAM complex in outer membrane protein assembly. *Nat. Rev. Microbiol.* **7,** 206–214 (2009).
21. Rigel, N. W., Ricci, D. P. & Silhavy, T. J. Conformation-specific labeling of BamA and suppressor analysis suggest a cyclic mechanism for beta-barrel assembly in *Escherichia coli*. *Proc. Natl Acad. Sci. USA* **110,** 5151–5156 (2013).
22. Jacob-Dubuisson, F. & Locht, C. in *Bordetella Molecular Microbiology* (ed. Locht, C.) 69–95 (Horizon Bioscience, 2007).
23. Guerin, J. *et al.* Conformational dynamics of protein transporter FhaC: large-scale motions of plug helix. *Mol. Microbiol.* **92,** 1164–1176 (2014).
24. Moslavac, S. *et al.* Conserved pore-forming regions in polypeptide-transporting proteins. *FEBS J.* **272,** 1367–1378 (2005).
25. Delattre, A. S. *et al.* Functional importance of a conserved sequence motif in FhaC, a prototypic member of the TpsB/Omp85 superfamily. *FEBS J.* **277,** 4755–4765 (2010).
26. Leonard-Rivera, M. & Misra, R. Conserved residues of the putative L6 loop of *Escherichia coli* BamA play a critical role in the assembly of beta-barrel outer membrane proteins, including that of BamA itself. *J. Bacteriol.* **194,** 4662–4668 (2012).
27. Chevalier, N. *et al.* Membrane targeting of a bacterial virulence factor harbouring an extended signal peptide. *J. Mol. Microbiol. Biotechnol.* **8,** 7–18 (2004).
28. Baud, C. *et al.* Membrane-associated DegP in *Bordetella* chaperones a repeat-rich secretory protein. *Mol. Microbiol.* **80,** 1625–1636 (2011).
29. Baud, C. *et al.* Role of DegP for two-partner secretion in *Bordetella*. *Mol. Microbiol.* **74,** 315–329 (2009).
30. Hodak, H. *et al.* Secretion signal of the filamentous haemagglutinin, a model two-partner secretion substrate. *Mol. Microbiol.* **61,** 368–382 (2006).
31. Fan, E., Fiedler, S., Jacob-Dubuisson, F. & Muller, M. Two-partner secretion of gram-negative bacteria: a single beta-barrel protein enables transport across the outer membrane. *J. Biol. Chem.* **287,** 2591–2599 (2012).
32. Coutte, L., Antoine, R., Drobecq, H., Locht, C. & Jacob-Dubuisson, F. Subtilisin-like autotransporter serves as maturation protease in a bacterial secretion pathway. *EMBO J.* **20,** 5040–5048 (2001).
33. Browning, D. F. *et al.* Mutational and topological analysis of the *Escherichia coli* BamA protein. *PLoS ONE* **8,** e84512 (2013).
34. Ni, D. *et al.* Structural and functional analysis of the beta-barrel domain of BamA from *Escherichia coli*. *FASEB J.* **28,** 2677–2685 (2014).
35. Guédin, S. *et al.* Novel topological features of FhaC, the outer membrane transporter involved in the secretion of the *Bordetella pertussis* filamentous hemagglutinin. *J. Biol. Chem.* **275,** 30202–30210 (2000).
36. Tellez, Jr R. & Misra, R. Substitutions in the BamA beta-barrel domain overcome the conditional lethal phenotype of a DeltabamB DeltabamE strain of *Escherichia coli*. *J. Bacteriol.* **194,** 317–324 (2012).

37. Méli, A. C. *et al.* Channel properties of TpsB transporter FhaC point to two functional domains with a C-terminal protein-conducting pore. *J. Biol. Chem.* **281,** 158–166 (2006).
38. Kajava, A. V. *et al.* Beta-helix model for the filamentous haemagglutinin adhesin of *Bordetella pertussis* and related bacterial secretory proteins. *Mol. Microbiol.* **42,** 279–292 (2001).
39. Ieva, R. & Bernstein, H. D. Interaction of an autotransporter passenger domain with BamA during its translocation across the bacterial outer membrane. *Proc. Natl Acad. Sci. USA* **106,** 19120–19125 (2009).
40. Sauri, A. *et al.* The Bam (Omp85) complex is involved in secretion of the autotransporter haemoglobin protease. *Microbiology* **155,** 3982–3991 (2009).
41. Jain, S. & Goldberg, M. B. Requirement for YaeT in the outer membrane assembly of autotransporter proteins. *J. Bacteriol.* **189,** 5393–5398 (2007).
42. Selkrig, J. *et al.* Discovery of an archetypal protein transport system in bacterial outer membranes. *Nat. Struct. Mol. Biol.* **19,** 506–510 (2012).
43. Noinaj, N., Kuszak, A. J., Balusek, C., Gumbart, J. C. & Buchanan, S. K. Lateral opening and exit pore formation are required for BamA function. *Structure* **22,** 1055–1062 (2014).
44. Alsteens, D., Martinez, N., Jamin, M. & Jacob-Dubuisson, F. Sequential unfolding of Beta helical protein by single-molecule atomic force microscopy. *PLoS ONE* **8,** e73572 (2013).
45. Waterhouse, A. M., Procter, J. B., Martin, D. M. A., Clamp, M. & Barton, G. J. Jalview Version 2-a multiple sequence alignment editor and analysis workbench. *Bioinformatics* **25,** 1189–1191 (2009).

Acknowledgements

We thank M. Müller and E. Fan for their fruitful discussions, H. Drobecq for mass spectrometry analyses, A.S. Delattre, E. Willery and S. Lecher for their help with some experiments, and B. Clantin for comments on the manuscript. J. Guérin acknowledges the receipt of a predoctoral fellowship from the Institut Pasteur de Lille and the Region Nord-Pas de Calais. This work was supported by the grant ANR-10-BLAN-1306 'DYN FHAC' to F.J.-D.

Author contributions

C.B. and F.J.-D. conceived the project; C.B., J.G., E.P., E.L. and E.D. conducted the experiments; C.B., J.G. and F.J.-D. analysed the data; and C.B., J.G., C.L. and F.J.-D. contributed to writing the manuscript.

Additional information

Competing financial interests: The authors declare no competing financial interests.

Caenorhabditis elegans is a useful model for anthelmintic discovery

Andrew R. Burns[1,*], Genna M. Luciani[1,2,*], Gabriel Musso[3,4], Rachel Bagg[1], May Yeo[1], Yuqian Zhang[1], Luckshika Rajendran[1], John Glavin[1], Robert Hunter[1], Elizabeth Redman[5], Susan Stasiuk[5], Michael Schertzberg[1], G. Angus McQuibban[6], Conor R. Caffrey[7], Sean R. Cutler[8], Mike Tyers[9], Guri Giaever[10], Corey Nislow[10], Andy G. Fraser[1,2], Calum A. MacRae[3,4], John Gilleard[5] & Peter J. Roy[1,2,11]

Parasitic nematodes infect one quarter of the world's population and impact all humans through widespread infection of crops and livestock. Resistance to current anthelmintics has prompted the search for new drugs. Traditional screens that rely on parasitic worms are costly and labour intensive and target-based approaches have failed to yield novel anthelmintics. Here, we present our screen of 67,012 compounds to identify those that kill the non-parasitic nematode *Caenorhabditis elegans*. We then rescreen our hits in two parasitic nematode species and two vertebrate models (HEK293 cells and zebrafish), and identify 30 structurally distinct anthelmintic lead molecules. Genetic screens of 19 million *C. elegans* mutants reveal those nematicides for which the generation of resistance is and is not likely. We identify the target of one lead with nematode specificity and nanomolar potency as complex II of the electron transport chain. This work establishes *C. elegans* as an effective and cost-efficient model system for anthelmintic discovery.

[1] The Donnelly Centre for Cellular and Biomolecular Research, University of Toronto, Toronto, Ontario, Canada M5S 3E1. [2] Department of Molecular Genetics, University of Toronto, Toronto, Ontario, Canada M5S 1A8. [3] Cardiovascular Division, Brigham and Women's Hospital, Harvard Medical School, and Harvard Stem Cell Institute, Boston, Massachusetts 02115, USA. [4] Department of Medicine, Harvard Medical School, Boston, Massachusetts 02115, USA. [5] Department of Comparative Biology and Experimental Medicine, Faculty of Veterinary Medicine, University of Calgary, Calgary, Alberta, Canada T2N 4Z6. [6] Department of Biochemistry, University of Toronto, 1 King's College Circle, Toronto, Ontario, Canada M5S 1A8. [7] Center for Discovery and Innovation in Parasitic Diseases and Department of Pathology, University of California, San Francisco, California 94158, USA. [8] Center for Plant Cell Biology, Department of Botany and Plant Sciences, University of California, Riverside, California 92521, USA. [9] Institute for Research in Immunology and Cancer, University of Montreal, Montreal, Quebec, Canada H3T 1J4. [10] Department of Pharmaceutical Sciences, University of British Columbia, Vancouver, British Columbia, Canada V6T 1Z3. [11] Department of Pharmacology and Toxicology, University of Toronto, Toronto, Ontario, Canada M5S 1A8. * These authors contributed equally to this work. Correspondence and requests for materials should be addressed to P.J.R. (email: peter.roy@utoronto.ca).

Parasitic nematodes are estimated to infect about one quarter of all humans and have a dramatic negative impact on human health and productivity in developing nations[1,2]. Nematode infections of agriculturally important plants and animals also result in huge economic losses worldwide[3,4]. Despite this, only a handful of anthelmintic families are currently available. These include the benzimidazoles, macrocyclic lactones (for example, ivermectin), imidazothiazoles (for example, levamisole) and cyclic octadepsipeptides (for example, emodepside), most of which were introduced decades ago. Nematode resistance has been reported for each class of compound, with some natural isolates showing multidrug resistance[3,5]. Anthelmintic resistance is a global issue; although some regions, such as New Zealand, have a particularly high prevalence of resistant parasites[5]. Amino-acetonitrile derivatives (AADs) such as monepantel have recently been introduced to the market; however, resistance to this class of compounds has already been reported[6–8]. While combinatorial strategies may prolong an anthelmitic's utility, growing resistance poses significant challenges for the management of parasitic infections.

One reason for the limited number of available anthelmintics may be related to the difficulty in identifying lead compounds at high throughput. The complex life cycle of parasitic nematodes, which rely on a host for propagation, make it challenging to examine a small molecule's impact on these animals with the throughput required to identify large numbers of candidate molecules for further development. The free-living nematode *Caenorhabditis elegans* may offer a convenient alternative model system to search for new compounds that specifically kill nematodes. *C. elegans*, which is $\sim$1 mm in length as an adult, can be cultured in high-throughput format for multiple generations, allowing the identification of molecules that perturb the worm at any point during its life cycle[9–12].

The majority of marketed anthelmintics are active against *C. elegans*[6,13], and the use of this model system has been instrumental in improving the understanding of the mechanism of action of several anthelmintic compounds, including levamisole, benzimidazole and the amino-acetonitrile derivatives[6,13,14]. Notably, the targets of each of these compounds have been elucidated through forward genetic screens for *C. elegans* mutants that resist their effects. In these screens, *C. elegans* parents are randomly mutagenized and their progeny are subsequently screened for individuals that can resist the effects of a given bioactive molecule. 'Drug'-resistant strains are analysed genetically to identify the resistance-conferring mutant gene. The most frequent resistance-conferring mutant gene within the collection of resistant strains has been shown to encode either the target or the targeted pathway/complex of these bioactive molecules[6,9,14].

Clearly, *C. elegans* is a useful model system to study anthelmintics and offers throughput that is not possible with parasitic species. It therefore follows that it might also be a powerful system with which to screen for anthelmintic lead compounds, as has been suggested over 30 years ago[15]. However, there have only been anecdotal references to the use of *C. elegans* in the anthelmintic screening programs of the pharmaceutical industry[16–20], the details of which have not been publically described. Thus, whether bioactivity in *C. elegans* is generally predictive of bioactivity in parasitic nematode species remains unknown.

Here, we describe our screen for anthelmintic lead compounds using whole *C. elegans* nematodes as the primary model system. We screened 67,012 distinct small molecules for their ability to kill *C. elegans* and re-screened our hits in two widely studied parasitic nematode models: *Cooperia onchophora*, a parasite of cattle, and *Haemonchus contortus*, a parasite of sheep[5,21]. We counter-screened the nematicidal molecules in two vertebrate models of development (HEK293 cells and zebrafish) and identified a set of molecules that kills nematodes but may be inactive in vertebrates. In an effort to identify the protein targets for 39 nematicides, we screened more than 19 million mutant *C. elegans* for resistance. We identified the target of one family of these lethal molecules that is closely related to nematicides that have recently been introduced to the market[22,23], demonstrating the value of *C. elegans* as a model system for the discovery of useful nematicidal molecules.

Results

Molecules that kill *C. elegans* are likely to kill parasites. To identify nematicidal compounds, we screened 67,012 commercially available small drug-like molecules for those that induce obvious phenotypes in *C. elegans* at a concentration of 60 μM or less (see Fig. 1a and Supplementary Data 1). From our preliminary screens, we identified 627 bioactive molecules that we call 'worm actives' or 'wactives'. Rescreening revealed 275 wactives that kill *C. elegans* at a concentration of 60 μM or less (see Supplementary Data 1). By contrast, none of the 182 molecules chosen at random from the set of 67,012 compounds killed *C. elegans* (see Supplementary Data 1).

We next screened the wactive library against the nematode parasites *C. onchophora* and *H. contortus* (Fig. 1a). We chose these two species, both of which are from the same phylogenetic clade as *C. elegans* (clade V), because we could screen them using similar methods that we used to screen *C. elegans* and because many important parasites of humans and domestic livestock are from clade V. We collected nematode eggs from infected animals and tested whether the wactives could kill the eggs or hatched animals (see Methods). Of the 275 wactives that killed *C. elegans*, 129 and 116 killed at least 90% of the *C. onchophora* and *H. contortus* animals, respectively, and 103 killed all three nematode species (Fig. 1b). Of the 182 randomly chosen molecules, none killed *C. onchophora* and five killed *H. contortus*. Hence, molecules that kill *C. elegans* are more than 15 times more likely to kill these parasitic nematodes compared with randomly chosen molecules (Fig. 1c).

We counter-screened the wactive and random control libraries for activity against two vertebrate models: *Danio rerio* (zebrafish) and HEK293 cells (Fig. 1a). Fifty-nine of the 275 wactives that kill *C. elegans* and 28 of the random molecules either kill or cause substantial morbidity in zebrafish (see Methods), representing an enrichment of $<$1.4-fold (Fig. 1c). Similarly, 76 of the 275 wactives that kill *C. elegans* and 40 of the random molecules caused substantial growth defects in HEK293 cells (see Methods), representing an enrichment of $<$1.3-fold (Fig. 1c). These results suggest that *C. elegans* is a useful model system with which to identify molecules that are lethal in parasitic nematodes, without generally being cytotoxic in vertebrates.

On analysis of chemical properties, we found that nematicidal compounds had a higher average computed octanol/water partition coefficient (logP; 3.9 versus 3.2, $P<10^{-13}$; Student's *t*-test) and lower average molecular weight (273 versus 328, $P<10^{-20}$; Student's *t*-test) when compared against the complete set of 67,012 compounds (Supplementary Fig. 1). This suggests that molecules that are smaller and with greater lipid-solubility might be more effective nematicides.

Structure analyses reveal 30 classes of anthelmintic leads. To further characterize our 275 *C. elegans*-lethal molecules, we organized them into three separate groups based on their phylogenetic bioactivity profiles (Fig. 2a). Group 1 contains 102 molecules that are lethal to only one or two of the three nematode species tested, but are non-lethal to zebrafish and HEK cells.

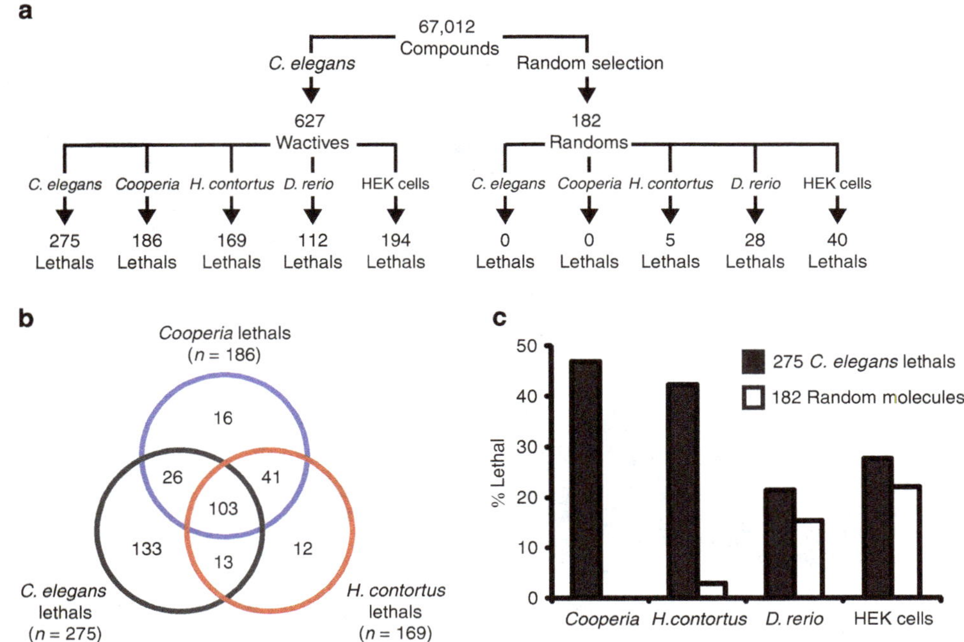

Figure 1 | Molecules that kill *C. elegans* are enriched for those that are lethal to parasitic nematodes. (**a**) Flow chart outlining the multi-organism small-molecule screening pipeline. (**b**) Venn diagram showing the overlap of wactive library molecules that kill *C. elegans*, *Cooperia oncophora* and *H. contortus*. (**c**) Chart showing the enrichment of molecules that kill *Cooperia*, *H. contortus*, zebrafish, and HEK cells in the set of 275 *C. elegans*-lethals, relative to a randomly selected set of 182 compounds.

Group 2 contains 67 compounds that are lethal to all three nematode species, but are non-lethal to zebrafish and human cells. Group 3 contains the remaining 106 compounds that are lethal to fish or HEK cells, and have varied bioactivity in different nematode species. In particular, the 67 molecules in group 2 represent potentially ideal anthelmintic leads; they have activity across multiple nematode species, and appear not to affect vertebrates.

To better understand the structural relationships that exist among our *C. elegans*-lethal compounds, we constructed a structure similarity network that connects molecules if they have a pairwise Tanimoto/FP2 similarity >0.55 (Fig. 2b; see Methods). This network contains 19 isolated clusters composed of three molecules or more, leaving 72 unconnected singletons or pairs. Each cluster represents a unique structural family that could, in principle, target a single protein, although the larger C1 and C2 clusters may contain multiple subfamilies of structures. The 67 group 2 molecules are distributed across 12 clusters, two pairs and 16 singletons, representing 30 structurally unique classes of anthelmintic leads that may target 30 or more distinct protein targets.

To estimate our ability to improve upon the biological activity of the 67 group 2 molecules through medicinal chemistry, we compared the structural similarity of each of these wactives with the 67,012 molecules that we screened (see Methods; Supplementary Data 1). We reasoned that the fraction of molecules within a family of structural analogues that are bioactive may be predictive of the ability to create novel analogues that are bioactive, some of which may have improved bioactivity. We found that 38 (57%) of the 67 wactives are members of a structural analogue family (based on a pairwise Tanimoto/FP2 similarity score of 0.55 or greater) for which more than 10% are lethal to *C. elegans* (Supplementary Fig. 3). Considering only the 18 group 2 wactives that are excluded from the 19 structural clusters in Fig. 2b, we found that 10 (56%) are members of a structural analogue family for which more than 10% are lethal to *C. elegans*. These results suggest that many of the group 2 wactives have the potential for improvement through medicinal chemistry efforts.

Modest structural changes impact phylogenetic specificity. The C3, C13 and C14 clusters in Fig. 2b are composed exclusively of molecules that selectively kill nematodes, suggesting that these families may be targeting nematode-specific proteins. The remaining 16 structural families contain at least one molecule that is lethal to either fish or human cells, suggesting that if the compounds in a cluster target a single protein, the target might be conserved in vertebrates. At the very least, these 16 clusters suggest that relatively modest structural changes can alter the species selectivity of the molecules in a family. To further explore the divergence of species selectivity within these 16 structural families, we focused on pairs of molecules that have a Tanimoto/FP2 pairwise similarity score of 80% or more, and for which one molecule in the pair specifically kills nematodes (group 2 molecules) and the other kills both nematodes and a vertebrate model (group 3 molecules). Seventeen pairs of molecules satisfy these criteria (Supplementary Fig. 2). Inspection of the structural differences of the individual molecules within each pair reveals that very small structural changes can restrict a molecule's bioactivity to nematodes. For example, wact-1, wact-433 and wact-434 in cluster 18 are identical except that an ethyl group in wact-434 replaces the halogen of wact-1 and wact-433. The halogen substitution destroys the core molecule's bioactivity in fish and restricts its activity to nematodes. Medicinal chemistry often yields structural analogues that have reduced or abolished bioactivity. However, our structure–activity analysis has revealed analogues that have not lost bioactivity but have instead become phylogenetically restricted.

Genetic resistance to most nematicides is not easily induced. Forward genetic screens with *C. elegans* have been previously

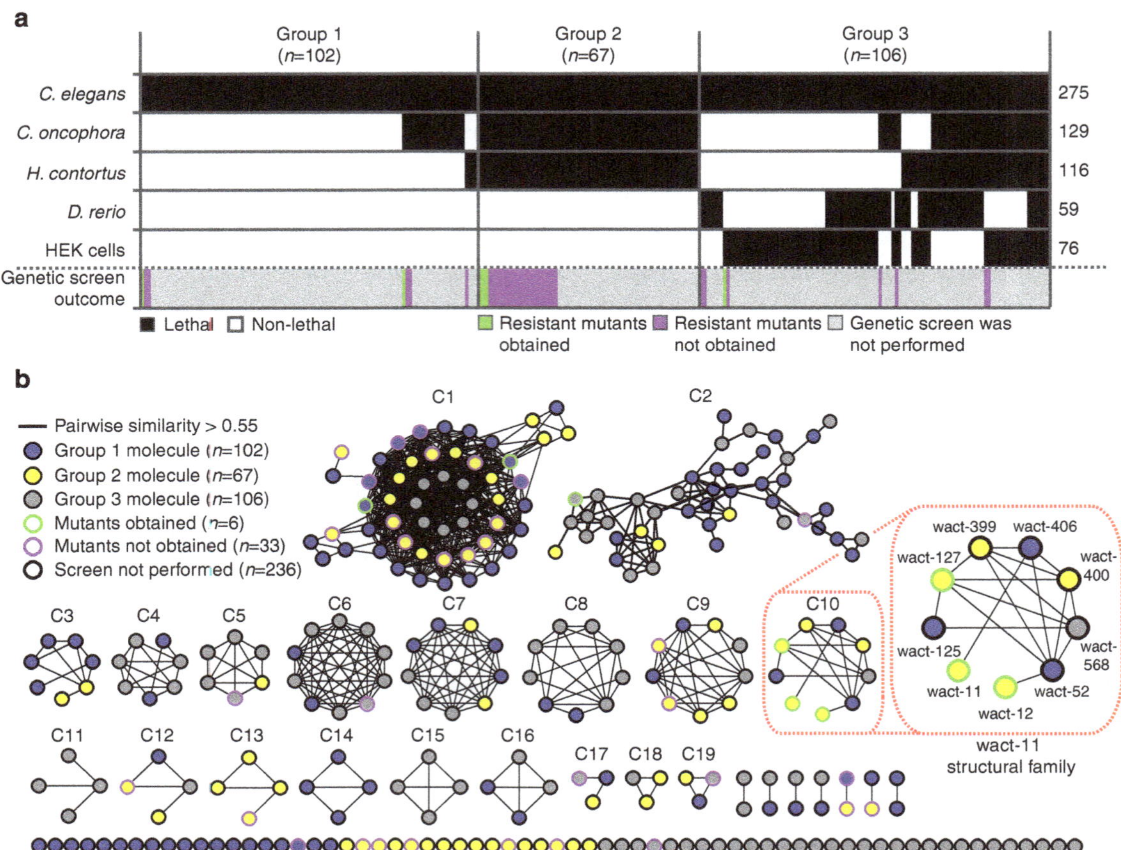

Figure 2 | Nematode selectivity and structural profiling of the 275 *C. elegans*-lethal molecules. (**a**) Heat map indicating the lethality (or lack thereof) induced by each of the 275 *C. elegans*-lethals in two species of parasitic nematode, as well as zebrafish embryos and human embryonic kidney (HEK) cells. For each species, the number of molecules that induce lethality is indicated to the right of the heat map. The molecules segregate into three groups based on their nematode selectivity and cross-species lethality. If a genetic screen for resistant mutants was performed for a given molecule, this is indicated, as well as the outcome of the screen. (**b**) Network based on the structural similarity of the 275 *C. elegans*-lethal molecules. Nodes represent molecules, and edges connect molecules with a pairwise Tanimoto/FP2 score >0.55 (see Methods). The group to which each molecule belongs is indicated by the node fill colour, whereas the genetic screen information is indicated by the node border colour. In the legend, the number of molecules is indicated in parentheses. The 19 clusters containing three or more molecules are named C1 to C19. The wact-11 structural family (cluster C10) is magnified, and the names of each molecule in the family are indicated.

used to identify the targets of bioactive compounds[6,9,14]. Here, we chose 39 compounds from the set of 275 *C. elegans*-lethal wactives to pursue their target genetically (see Methods; Supplementary Data 1; Fig. 2). These 39 molecules span 19 distinct structural classes (Fig. 2b), and the majority of these compounds are found in group 2, which are lethal to all three nematodes tested and non-lethal to zebrafish and HEK293 cells (Fig. 2a).

To identify mutants that are resistant to specific compounds, we randomly mutagenized wild-type *C. elegans* parental (P0) worms using chemical mutagens (see Methods) and screened for animals that resist lethality in either the first (F1) or second (F2) generation. Resistant mutants that arise in F1 screens are dominant and typically encode missense mutations that confer resistance against antagonists, while resistance-conferring mutations in F2 animals are typically recessive reduction-of-function mutations that confer resistance to agonists[24]. Molecules against which F1 screens did not yield resistant mutants were screened again for F2-resistant mutants. We performed F1 screens for all 39 lethal molecules, and F2 screens for 29 of the 39 compounds (Supplementary Table 1). In total, we screened over 19 million mutant genomes and we were able to isolate resistant mutants against only six of the 39 molecules (Supplementary Table 1).

Wact-11-resistant mutants show intra-family cross-resistance. Wact-11, wact-12 and wact-127 are three of the molecules against which we could generate resistant mutants (Supplementary Table 1). These three molecules are part of the C10 cluster (Fig. 2b), which we refer to as the 'wact-11 family', and share an ethyl benzamide moiety (Fig. 3). In total, we isolated 37 mutants that resist the wact-11 family members at a rate of one mutant per 100,000 genomes screened (Supplementary Table 1). Using a representative set of 21 mutants, we performed a detailed dose-response analysis of each mutant against wact-11 and the structurally unrelated nematicide wact-2 in liquid media (Supplementary Fig. 4). All of the tested mutants show at least some resistance to wact-11, but not to wact-2, indicating that they are specifically resistant to wact-11.

Given their structural similarity, we hypothesized that each compound within the wact-11 family may share the same mechanism of action. If true, then mutants that were isolated based on their resistance to one wact-11 family member will resist the lethality that is induced by other family members. To test this, we performed a dose-response analyses of two wact-11-family resistant mutants (isolated based on their respective resistance to wact-11 and wact-12) against all nine wact-11-family members. Both mutants were resistant to all nine wact-11-family members

a

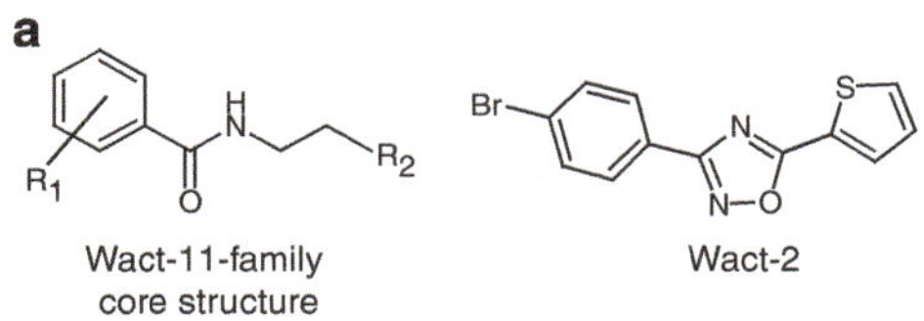

b

N2 dose-response (μM) | RP2674 dose-response (μM) | RP2698 dose-response (μM): 0, 0.03, 0.12, 0.47, 1.9, 7.5, 30, 60, 120

Compound	R_1	R_2
wact-11	2-CF_3	Ph (4′-Cl)
wact-12	2-I	OPh (4′-CH_2CH_3)
wact-127	2-SCH_3	$CH_2CH_2CH_3$
wact-52	2-I	CH_2CH_3
wact-125	2-SCH_3	SC_6H_{12}
wact-399	3-Br	CH_2CH_2Ph
wact-400	2-F	CH_2CH_2Ph
wact-406	2-CH3	Ph
wact-568	2-SCH3	CH_2Ph
wact-2	-	-

☐ More than 50 worms ☐ 12 to 50 worms ☐ 0 to 11 worms

Figure 3 | Wact-11 and wact-12 resistant mutants are cross-resistant to all nine wact-11-family members. (**a**) The wact-11-family core structure and the structure of an unrelated molecule, wact-2, which was used as a negative control throughout this work. (**b**) Heat maps of the wact-11-family dose-response experiments with wild-type worms (N2 strain), as well as two mutant strains, RP2674 and RP2698, isolated as being resistant to wact-12 and wact-11, respectively. The dose-response experiments were carried out using a 96-well plate liquid-based assay (see Methods). White indicates that there were more than 50 worms in three out of four replicate wells. Pink indicates that there were between 12 and 50 worms in three out of four replicate wells. Red indicates that there were between 0 and 11 worms in three out of four replicate wells. In the case of ties, the higher number prevailed (for example, at a given concentration, if two wells had 55 worms, and the other two wells had 20 worms, the chemical would be scored as having more than 50 worms). The R_1 and R_2 groups are indicated for each wact-11-family member. Wact-2 is used here as a negative control.

(Fig. 3), supporting the idea that all nine members of the wact-11 family act by the same mechanism.

The wact-11 family inhibits worm mitochondrial complex II. To identify candidate targets of the wact-11-family, we sequenced the genomes of 33 resistant mutants to identify mutated genes common to multiple strains (Supplementary Data 2 and 3). Ten strains had missense mutations in *sdhb-1*, a different set of 16 strains had a missense mutation in *sdhc-1* (otherwise known as *mev-1*), six other strains had missense mutations in *sdhd-1* and one remaining strain had no commonly mutated gene (Table 1). By contrast, no other gene is represented by distinct mutant alleles in more than four of the 33 strains, and none of the *sdh* genes are mutated in 36 strains that resist the effects of two other unrelated molecules (A.R.B., Houtan Moshiri and P.J.R., unpublished results). Consistent with the isolation of the majority of these mutants in F1 screens, none of the *sdh* mutations are nonsense, frame-shifts or deletions that would be indicative of loss-of-function. Instead, the missense mutations change four unique residues in SDHB-1, seven unique residues in SDHC-1 and three unique residues in SDHD-1 (Table 1).

Table 1 | Complex II residue changes for the wact-11-family-resistant strains.

Number of strains	*C. elegans* mutated gene	*C. elegans* residue change	*Ascaris suum* orthologous residue	Human orthologous residue
1	*sdhb-1*	P145L	P127	P131
2	*sdhb-1*	H146Y	H128	H132
6	*sdhb-1*	P211L	P193	P207
1	*sdhb-1*	I260N	I242	I246
3	*sdhc-1*	T66I	T81	P64
1	*sdhc-1*	G71E	G86	I69
8	*sdhc-1*	R74K	R89	R72
1	*sdhc-1*	G77D	G92	G75
1	*sdhc-1*	C78Y	C93	I76
1	*sdhc-1*	G133E	G148	G131
1	*sdhc-1*	F136S	F151	H134
1	*sdhd-1*	H84Q	H95	H98
4	*sdhd-1*	D95N	D106	D109
1	*sdhd-1*	A97T	G108	V111
1	?			
33 total				

SDHB-1, SDHC-1 and SDHD-1, along with SDHA-1, are the four protein subunits of *C. elegans* mitochondrial complex II[25] (otherwise known as succinate dehydrogenase or *sdh*), which couples the citric acid cycle to the electron transport chain and is highly conserved among eukaryotes[26]. Complex II couples the oxidation of succinate to fumarate, with the reduction of ubiquinone to ubiquinol[26]. Eukaryotic complex II has at least one ubiquinone-binding site, referred to as the Qp site or Q-site, that exists at the intersection of the SDHB, SDHC and SDHD subunits. In contrast, the succinate-binding site is found exclusively in the SDHA subunit.

A number of Q-site inhibitors are used as fungicides and interest in their use against nematodes is growing[27–29]. For example, flutolanil has been shown to inhibit complex II from the parasitic nematode *Ascaris suum in vitro*, and a co-crystal structure of flutolanil with this complex has been solved[30,31]. We rendered an image of this crystal structure and highlighted the corresponding 14 orthologous residues that are mutated in the wact-11-resistant *C. elegans* mutants (Fig. 4a). Despite residing in three distinct proteins, all the 14 residues cluster around the Q-site where flutolanil is bound. Furthermore, of the 12 residues that are within 4 angstroms of flutolanil's central mass, four are mutated in our wact-11-family resistant mutants (Fig. 4b). Finally, the most frequently mutated residue in our screen is in SDHC-1's R74, which corresponds to *Ascaris*' R89 of SDHC that likely makes electrostatic contacts with the benzene ring of flutolanil's 2-trifluoromethyl-benzamide group[30,31]. Like flutolanil, wact-11 also has a 2-trifluoromethyl-benzamide group, and all wact-11 family members have the benzamide

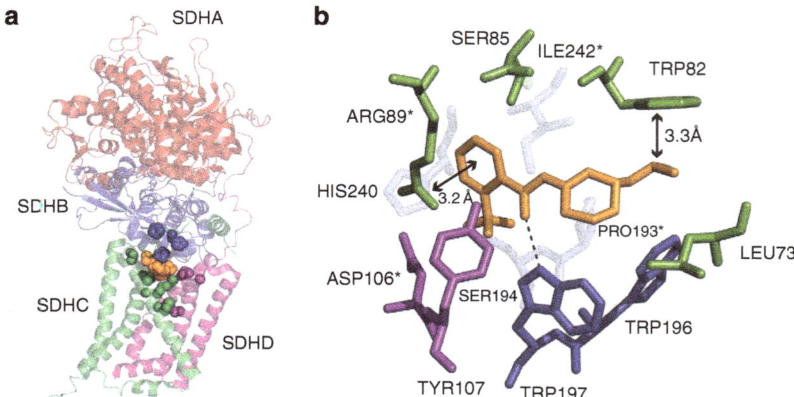

Figure 4 | Complex II residues that are mutated in the wact-11 family resistant mutants cluster near the ubiquinone-binding site (Q-site). (**a**) Rendering of the crystal structure of *Ascaris suum* Complex II bound to the Q-site inhibitor flutolanil (PDB: 3VRB). The side chains of the 14 orthologous residues that are mutated in the wact-11-family resistant mutants are shown as opaque spheres. The atoms of the bound flutolanil molecule are shown as orange-coloured opaque spheres. (**b**) Close-up view of flutolanil bound at the Q-site of Complex II from *Ascaris suum*. The 12 residues shown are no more than 4 Å away from flutolanil, and make up the flutolanil binding pocket. Intermolecular distances are indicated with bidirectional arrows. The dashed line represents a hydrogen bond (H-bond) interaction. Only those H-bonds that occur between Complex II residues and flutolanil are shown; H-bonds that occur between residues of Complex II were omitted for clarity. Bound cofactors, and a bound fumarate molecule, were also omitted for clarity.

moiety. Taken together, our observations suggest that the wact-11-family kills nematodes by binding the Q-site of complex II, and consequently disrupts the interaction of ubiquinone with the complex. Furthermore, the viability of the resistant mutants suggests that the missense mutations alter the Q-site in a way that preserves its function.

We directly tested whether wact-11 and wact-12 can inhibit the enzymatic activity of wild-type *C. elegans* complex II *in vitro* (see Methods). We found that both molecules could inhibit complex II activity with IC50s of 7.4 nM and 5.7 nM, respectively (Table 2, Supplementary Fig. 5). We also tested whether these molecules could inhibit complex II from two independently isolated wact-11-resistant mutants that each harbour the SDHC-1(R74K) missense mutation. We found that complex II from these mutants is insensitive to the molecules up to the highest concentration tested (10 μM; Table 2). As a control, we tested whether wild-type and mutant complex II activity could be inhibited by malonate, which inhibits SDHA-1's succinate-binding activity. We found that malonate inhibits the wild-type complex II to a similar extent as the mutant enzymes (Table 2, Supplementary Fig. 5). These results provide evidence that: (i) mutations in complex II confer resistance to the wact-11-family and (ii) wact-11-family members kill worms by specifically inhibiting complex II at the Q-site.

A SAR analysis reveals potent wact-11 analogues. We performed a focused structure–activity relationship (SAR) analysis with 16 purchasable analogues of the wact-11 family to better understand the structural elements that impact its bioactivity. We first tested the ability of the analogues to inhibit complex II activity *in vitro*. In general, the presence of an electron-withdrawing group at the 2' position of the benzamide benzene ring favours complex II inhibition because the absence of such a group decreases the inhibition by at least 86-fold relative to wact-11 (see wact-11b and wact-11k in Table 2). This observation is consistent with the proposed binding mechanism of flutolanil (see above). The position of the trifluoromethyl group is also important because relocating it to the 4' position (see wact-11 g in Table 2) decreases complex II inhibition by at least 1,300-fold. The R_2 phenyl ring of wact-11 promotes complex II inhibition because removing it (see wact-11i) decreases inhibition 44-fold. Finally, having chloride groups attached to the R_2 phenyl ring promotes complex II inhibition. For example, the two most potent analogues, wact-11 f and wact-11 m, have IC_{50} values of 1 nM, which is over 7-fold lower than that of wact-11, and both of these compounds have electron-withdrawing groups at the 2′ position of their benzamide benzene rings, as well as chloride groups at the 2′ and 4′ positions of their R_2 phenyl rings.

We next tested the *in vivo* potency of the analogues, and found a positive correlation between the *in vitro* IC_{50} and the *in vivo* LD_{100} (dose lethal to 100% of animals tested) values (Table 2; Pearson's correlation coefficient = 0.85), further strengthening the argument that complex II is the *in vivo* target of the wact-11-family. The difference between the *in vitro* and *in vivo* potencies reported in Table 2 is likely due to the resistance of intact *C. elegans* worms to the accumulation of exogenous small molecules[32]. Notably, the two most potent analogues, wact-11 f and wact-11 m, have LD_{100} values in *C. elegans* of 0.469 μM (Table 2). Thus, our SAR analysis revealed nematicides with submicromolar potency.

Few known complex II inhibitors kill *C. elegans*. In addition to flutolanil, we found other commercial complex II Q-site inhibitors that have structural similarity to the wact-11-family (Supplementary Fig. 6). In particular, fluopyram is structurally similar to wact-11 and has recently been developed as part of a crop spray used to kill parasitic nematodes of plants[22,23]. We tested fluopyram and the other structurally related compounds, along with established complex II inhibitors that are structurally unrelated to the wact-11-family (Supplementary Fig. 6), for their ability to kill *C. elegans*. None of these complex II inhibitors are nematicidal up to the highest concentrations tested (120 μM), except for fluopyram and benodanil, which have LD_{100} values of 0.469 μM and 120 μM, respectively (Table 2; Supplementary Fig 7). We found that the wact-11-resistant mutants also resist the lethality induced by fluopyram and benodanil (Supplementary Fig. 7), suggesting that these molecules also target complex II *in vivo*. We also tested the ability of the Q-site inhibitors to inhibit *C. elegans* complex II *in vitro*. Only fluopyram had a potent IC_{50} (1.8 nM), which is almost 2-fold less inhibiting than our two most potent wact-11-family analogues, wact-11 f and wact-11 m.

Table 2 | Complex II IC_{50} and *in vivo* LD_{100} values for wact-11-family molecules and known complex II inhibitors.

Compound	R_1*	R_2*	Species	Strain	SDHC residue change	*In vitro* Complex II IC_{50} (nM)†	*In vivo* LD_{100} (μM)‡
wact-11	2-CF_3	Ph (4′-Cl)	*C. elegans*	N2	None	7.4	7.5
				RP2674	R74K	>10,000	>120
				RP2698	R74K	>10,000	>120
			M. musculus	C57Bl/6	None	>10,000	ND
wact-12	2-I	OPh (4′-CH_2CH_3)	*C. elegans*	N2	None	5.7	7.5
				RP2674	R74K	>10,000	>120
				RP2698	R74K	>10,000	>120
			M. musculus	C57Bl/6	None	>10,000	ND
wact-11f	2-CF_3	Ph (2′-Cl, 4′-Cl)	*C. elegans*	N2	None	1.0	0.469
				RP2674	R74K	>10,000	>120
				RP2698	R74K	>10,000	>120
			M. musculus	C57Bl/6	None	>10,000	ND
wact-11a	2-CF_3	Ph	*C. elegans*	N2	None	26.1	60
wact-11i	2-CF_3	CH_2CH_3	*C. elegans*	N2	None	327.2	>120
wact-11g	4-CF_3	Ph (4′-Cl)	*C. elegans*	N2	None	>10,000	>120
wact-11p	2-I	Ph (4′-Cl)	*C. elegans*	N2	None	5.8	7.5
wact-11e	2-I	Ph (4′-F)	*C. elegans*	N2	None	15.3	60
wact-11d	2-Br	Ph (4′-Cl)	*C. elegans*	N2	None	7.5	1.875
wact-11m	2-Br	Ph (2′-Cl, 4′-Cl)	*C. elegans*	N2	None	1.0	0.469
wact-11j	2-Br	CH_2CH_3	*C. elegans*	N2	None	269.6	120
wact-11c	2-F	Ph (4′-Cl)	*C. elegans*	N2	None	170.1	60
wact-11b	-	Ph (4′-Cl)	*C. elegans*	N2	None	632.9	>120
wact-11k	-	CH_2CH_3	*C. elegans*	N2	None	>10,000	>120
wact-12b	2-I	OPh (4′-CH_3)	*C. elegans*	N2	None	7.7	7.5
wact-12c	2-I	SPh (4′-CH_3)	*C. elegans*	N2	None	132.9	>120
wact-12d	2-I	SPh (4′-Cl)	*C. elegans*	N2	None	128.5	>120
wact-12e	2-Br	OPh (4′-Cl)	*C. elegans*	N2	None	7.8	30
Benodanil			*C. elegans*	N2	None	186.2	120
Boscalid			*C. elegans*	N2	None	549.5	>120
Carboxine			*C. elegans*	N2	None	>10,000	>120
Diazoxide			*C. elegans*	N2	None	>10,000	>120
Fenfuran			*C. elegans*	N2	None	5,279.0	>120
Fluopyram			*C. elegans*	N2	None	1.8	0.469
Flutolanil			*C. elegans*	N2	None	311.2	>120
Harz			*C. elegans*	N2	None	>10,000	>120
Thifluzamide			*C. elegans*	N2	None	3,819	>120
TTFA			*C. elegans*	N2	None	>10,000	>120
Atpenin A5§			*C. elegans*	N2	None	1,678	>120
			M. musculus	C57Bl/6	None	593.3	ND
Malonate‖			*C. elegans*	N2	None	4.9×10^6	>120
				RP2674	R74K	4.2×10^6	ND
				RP2698	R74K	4.2×10^6	ND

Harz, harzianopyridone; ND, not determined; TTFA, thenoyltrifluoroacetone.
*The wact-11-family core structure, with the positions of the R_1 and R_2 groups indicated, is shown in Fig. 3
†The inhibitory curves used to generate the complex II IC_{50} values can be found in Supplementary Fig. 5.
‡The *in vivo* LD_{100} value is defined as the lowest concentration at which no viable animals are visible in four out of four replicate wells, 6 days after 20 first larval-stage worms are deposited. The LD_{100} was determined from a 4-fold dilution series from 120 to 0.00183 μM, and including 60 μM.
§For mouse complex II experiments, atpenin A5 was used as a positive control.
‖For the RP2698 and RP2674 complex II experiments, malonate was used as a positive control.

The wact-11 family fails to inhibit mammalian complex II. The evidence we have presented supports the idea that mitochondrial complex II is the *in vivo* target of the wact-11-family in nematodes. Because the wact-11 family kills nematodes but not human cells, we hypothesized that mammalian complex II is insensitive to these compounds. We tested this hypothesis by assaying the ability of wact-11, wact-12 and wact-11f to inhibit murine complex II *in vitro*. Mouse complex II was insensitive to the highest concentrations tested (10 μM) for all three of these compounds (Table 2; Supplementary Fig. 5).

To better understand the phylogenetic selectivity of the wact-11 family, we inspected the conservation among the SDH subunits in nematodes and vertebrates (Supplementary Fig. 8a). First, we found that 12 of the 14 resistance-conferring residues are conserved in all 10 nematode species examined. Of the two that diverge, SDHC-1's C78 diverges in only one of the 10 species and SDHD-1's A97 diverges in only two species. In each case, the substitutions are conservative. These observations suggest that nematodes may in general be sensitive to the wact-11-family of compounds. Second, we analysed the conservation of the 14 residues among seven vertebrate sequences and found that five of the 14 residues are divergent in all vertebrates examined with four of these substitutions being nonconservative (Supplementary Fig. 8b). Given that mutations of any single one of these residues is sufficient to confer resistance to the wact-11-family, it is reasonable to infer that the vertebrate substitutions at these positions will confer resistance to the wact-11 family of nematicides.

Discussion

Two factors may have discouraged the use of *C. elegans* as a primary high-throughput screening tool to identify novel anthelmintics. First, it is not a parasite and therefore lacks many of the adaptations required for parasitism and the potential anthelmintic targets associated with those processes[16]. Second, the rapid evolution of species within phylum nematoda suggests that *C. elegans* may have essential gene products that may function differently or not exist in some parasitic species[33]. Hence, many of the compounds that kill *C. elegans* may not be effective against parasitic nematodes. However, our work has revealed that molecules that do kill *C. elegans* are more than 15 times more likely to kill parasitic nematodes compared with randomly selected molecules. Given that parasitic nematodes are difficult to screen in high throughput, these results make pre-screening with *C. elegans* an attractive option to increase the throughput of future anthelmintic discovery campaigns.

As expected, not all molecules that kill *C. elegans* are effective against the parasitic models that we tested. In addition, by first screening in *C. elegans*, we have certainly missed molecules that are effective at killing parasitic nematodes but are ineffective in *C. elegans*. However, the speed and ease at which molecules can be screened using *C. elegans* may outweigh the disadvantages it carries as a primary screening system. In principle, *C. elegans* can be used to evaluate hundreds of thousands of molecules at multiple concentrations at a fraction of the cost and time that would be required with most parasitic nematode models.

The extent to which our hits have broad-spectrum activity against distantly-related nematodes is unknown. However, *C. elegans*, *C. oncophora* and *H. contortus* are all clade V nematodes and so molecules that are active against all three of these species are more likely to have broad activity against multiple species in this clade, which include many important parasites of humans and animals[34].

Using forward small molecule screens to identify anthelmintic leads is a powerful approach because it makes no assumptions about what kind of protein makes a good target. Furthermore, these screens have the potential to yield phylum-specific compounds with unexpected and conserved targets that may not have been considered in target-based searches. Our discovery of the activity and target of the wact-11 family provides a good proof-of-principle for the utility of *C. elegans* as a pre-screening model system.

Multiple lines of evidence show that the wact-11 family targets the conserved complex II of the electron transport chain *in vivo*. First, a good correlation exists between complex II *in vitro* inhibition and *in vivo* potency. Second, out of 33 mutants that resist the wact-11-family, 32 have missense mutations in residues that surround the ubiquinone-binding pocket of complex II. By contrast none of the 36 strains that resist unrelated molecules have mutations in complex II. Third, *in vitro* assays show that the wact-11-family can inhibit complex II from wild-type worms but not from worms that have a mutation in complex II that confers resistance to these molecules *in vivo*. Together, these results indicate that the wact-11 family kills *C. elegans* through its inhibition of complex II.

Our screens have revealed that phylogenetically selective bioactivity is highly dependent upon molecular structure. A systematic analysis of close structural analogues revealed 17 pairs of molecules whose phylogenetic bioactivity profile becomes restricted to nematodes with only small alterations in structure. In addition to the 30 groups of anthelmintic lead structures we describe above, the 275 *C. elegans*-lethals comprised 61 structural groups, 33 of which do not contain a single molecule that kills nematodes selectively. However, given the structure–bioactivity analyses presented above, it may be possible to identify structural analogues that specifically kill nematodes for at least some of these structural groups, raising the total number of potential anthelmintic lead structural classes beyond 30.

Of the 30 distinct groups of anthelmintic leads that we have uncovered, we have attempted to screen for resistance against 16 representative molecules and have failed to generate resistance against all but three. The reason behind this is unclear. Typically, we use ethyl methanesulfonate as a mutagen in our genetic screens, which is biased towards inducing G/C to A/T transitions[35] and therefore limits the type of non-synonymous mutations that are induced. This is unlikely to explain the lack of success, however, since we also carried out resistance screens using the *N*-ethyl-*N*-nitrosourea mutagen[35], which produces a variety of nucleotide transitions and transversions, but was equally unsuccessful in yielding resistant mutants (Supplementary Table 1). Instead, we think it more likely that for most lethal molecules, there is no single mutation in the respective target that is capable of conferring resistance. This explanation might be especially true for molecules that inhibit an essential target. It may be that only rare essential targets (like complex II) can be mutated to disrupt the efficacy of an inhibitor without disrupting the target's activity below a viable state. Alternatively, it is possible that many lethal molecules may have multiple essential targets. If true, the generation and isolation of a single mutant animal that has all of the targets mutated to confer resistance would be an exceptionally rare event.

The inability to generate resistant mutants against these molecules has two implications. The first is trivial in that approaches aside from genetics will have to be exploited to identify the target(s) of these molecules. The more important implication is that if the evolution of resistance in the lab can foretell evolution in the field, and there is good evidence for this[3,5–8,13,14], then perhaps the converse is true and that the set of anthelmintic leads for which we are unable to generate resistance should be high priority compounds for further development. Regardless, the evolution of parasitic resistance does not immediately negate the usefulness of an anthelmintic. For example, *C. elegans* mutants that resist the effects of benzimidazoles, imidazothiazoles and cyclooctadepsipeptides can be readily generated in the lab[14,36], yet these molecules have been effective in the field for many years despite the eventual emergence of resistance.

Materials and methods

Chemical sources. The sources for the chemicals and chemical libraries used in our preliminary screens are indicated in Supplementary Data 1. The wact-11-family and structural analogues were purchased from ChemBridge Corporation. The established complex II inhibitors were purchased from Sigma-Aldrich, with the exception of atpenin A5 and harzianopyridone, which were purchased from Enzo Life Sciences, and thifluzamide, which was purchased from AnGene.

***C. elegans* strains and culture methods.** All the animals were cultured using standard methods at 20 °C (ref. 37), unless otherwise indicated. The N2 (wild-type) strain of *Caenorhabditis elegans* was obtained from the *C. elegans* Genetics Center (University of Minnesota).

***C. elegans* liquid-based chemical screening.** The 96-well liquid-based chemical screening assay was adapted from an established RNAi screening protocol[38]. Briefly, saturated HB101 *Escherichia coli* culture was concentrated 2-fold using NGM (nematode growth media) containing 3 mg ml^{-1} NaCl, 2.5 mg ml^{-1} peptone, 5 μg ml^{-1} cholesterol, 1 mM $CaCl_2$, 1 mM $MgSO_4$ and 25 mM KH_2PO_4. A total of 40 μl of NGM + HB101 was dispensed into each well of a 96-well plate, and chemicals were pinned into the wells using a pinning tool with a 300 nl slot volume (V&P Scientific). Approximately 20 synchronized first larval-stage (L1) worms, in 10 μl of M9 buffer (see ref. 24 for the recipe), were then added to each well. The synchronized L1s were obtained from an embryo preparation (see ref. 24 for the protocol) performed the previous day. The final concentration of dimethyl sulfoxide (DMSO) in the wells was 0.6% v/v. A dissection microscope was used to visualize the wells either 5 or 6 days post worm deposition and any obvious chemical-induced phenotypes were noted.

For our preliminary screens, 50,596 out of 67,012 compounds were assayed in liquid at a 60 μM concentration, and the other 16,416 molecules were screened on solid media at 25 μM (see ref. 24 for a description of our solid-based screening method). From these screens, 672 compounds that induced at least a partially penetrant phenotype were re-ordered and arrayed into a 10-plate 'worm active' or 'wactive' library. One hundred and eighty-two molecules chosen at random from the 67,012 compounds were also included in the wactive library, along with many DMSO control wells distributed across the plates.

Using the liquid-based assay, the re-ordered wactive library was re-screened in worms at 7.5, 30 and 60 μM concentrations. Chemicals that induced an obvious phenotype were classified as follows: 'very strong' molecules induced 100% lethality at 7.5 μM, 'strong' molecules induced 100% lethality at 30 μM, 'medium' molecules induced 100% lethality at 60 μM, 'weak' molecules induced incompletely penetrant lethality at 60 μM and 'PEP' molecules induced a non-lethal post-embryonic phenotype such as dumpy (Dpy) or uncoordinated (Unc). The 275 *C. elegans*-lethals that are referred to in the text are made up of the 'very strong', 'strong' and 'medium' molecules.

The 96-well liquid-based assay was also used for all follow-up dose-response experiments in this work. These experiments were carried out in quadruplicate, and the total number of worms in each well was counted 6 days after worm deposition.

***C. oncophora* and *H. contortus* chemical screens.** Fresh cattle and sheep faeces containing eggs of an ivermectin-resistant strain of *C. onchophora*[39] and the MHco3(ISE) strain of *H. contortus*[40,41], respectively, were kindly supplied by Dr Doug Colwell and Dawn Gray (Lethbridge Research Station, Agriculture and Agri-Food Canada). Experimental infections used to generate this material were carried out using established methods[39,41], and were approved by the Lethbridge AAFC Animal Care committee and conducted under animal use license ACC1407. Cattle faeces containing *C. onchophora* eggs were stored anaerobically at 4 °C for a maximum of 3 weeks, whereas sheep faeces containing *H. contortus* eggs were stored at 20 °C for no more than 48 h before harvesting eggs for use. Eggs were isolated from faeces using a standard saturated salt flotation method[42] immediately before each egg hatch assay. Approximately 100 eggs suspended in 100 μl of water were added to each well of a 96-well plate, and the wactive library chemicals were screened at two different concentrations (7.5 and 60 μM, 0.6% DMSO v/v). Baseline egg hatch rates were determined in DMSO control wells ~48 h after the initial set-up of the assay by the addition of iodine tincture to stop development. Plates having DMSO control wells with hatch rates >70% were assayed on a semi-quantitative gradient of '–' to '+ + +', where '–' wells had a hatch rate of <10%, and '+ + +' wells had a hatch rate close to wild type (usually >80%). A dissection microscope was used for visualization purposes. Chemicals were considered bioactive if they consistently had a '–' in more than one trial, with 'very very strong' assigned to compounds that were 90–100% lethal at 7.5 μM in all replicates, 'very strong' if the same was true at 60 μM, 'strong' if replicates had a hatch rate between 10 and 50%, 'medium' if replicates had a 50–80% hatch rate and 'weak' if only one replicate was between 50 and 80% hatch rate. A molecule was considered 'lethal' if it exhibited 'very very strong' or 'very strong' bioactivity.

Zebrafish culture and chemical screening. Wild-type (AB) zebrafish embryos were collected in E3 solution (5 mM NaCl, 0.17 mM KCl, 0.33 mM CaCl2, 0.33 mM MgSO4) immediately after fertilization and arrayed at three embryos per well in 96-well plates, 200 μl per well. Wild-type (AB) zebrafish were originally obtained from Zebrafish International Resource Center (University of Oregon). Chemicals were added to each well at 6 h post fertilization at a final concentration of 10 μM (0.5% v/v DMSO), with each plate containing nine wells of DMSO controls. Embryos were examined for mortality and observable developmental phenotypes at 24 and 48 h post fertilization using an Olympus SZX10 Brightfield microscope. Phenotypes examined were death, developmental delay, reduced pigmentation, cranial oedema or cardiac defects (slow/absent heart rate, abnormal heart size). Each compound was screened in duplicate, with only phenotypes appearing in both replicates associated with a given compound. Any compound producing multiple, distinct phenotypes across replicates (for example, cardiac defects in one replicate, mortality in another) was labelled 'toxic'. A molecule was considered 'lethal' to zebrafish if it induced 'death' or 'toxicity'.

HEK293 cell culture and chemical screening. HEK293T cells (Attisano Lab, University of Toronto) were maintained in Dulbecco's Modified Eagle's Medium (Gibco) supplemented with 10% FBS (DMEM-10% FBS). Cells at a concentration of 50 cells μl^{-1} were seeded into 96-well plates at a final volume of 100 μl (~5,000 cells per well). Chemicals from the wactive library were added to the wells for a final concentration of 60 μM (0.6% DMSO v/v). The wactive library plates were screened at least in triplicate. Cell proliferation was determined using a bromodeoxyuridine (BrdU) assay kit (Exalpha Biologicals Inc.). The BrdU was added 2 days after chemical addition. Fixation and denaturation was performed ~16–18 h later. Anti-BrdU antibody was added, and incorporated BrdU was detected using a horseradish peroxidase-conjugated goat anti-mouse antibody. The BrdU incorporation signal was measured at 450/550 nm for the amount of conversion of tetramethylbenzidine that is proportional to the amount of BrdU incorporated. For each replicate of each plate, the average signal for the DMSO control wells was calculated. For each well in the plate (including the DMSO control wells), the signal was normalized by dividing by the average DMSO signal. The mean and standard deviation for the population of 960 normalized sample signals of the 10-plate wactive library were calculated and found to be 0.6 and 0.44, respectively. A molecule was considered 'lethal' if its normalized signal had a magnitude <0.16 (that is, a value less than the s.d. subtracted from the mean).

Cheminformatics. Chemical structures as supplied by the manufacturers were analysed using the ChemAxon calculator (http://www.chemaxon.com). Specifically, number of hydrogen bond donors, number of hydrogen bond acceptors, mass, atom count, rotatable bond count, logP (a measure of hydrophobicity), Van der Waals surface area, polar surface area, Van der Waals volume and refractivity were computed using default parameters. In the case of salts, all properties were calculated on the largest molecule. Pairwise similarity scores were calculated as the Tanimoto coefficient of shared FP2 fingerprints using OpenBabel (http://openbabel.org). An FP2 fingerprint is a linear fragment of a molecule, containing one to seven atoms. Each pair of compounds to be analysed for similarity were evaluated for presence or absence of any of thousands of possible FP2 fingerprints, and the Tanimoto coefficient represents the number of fingerprints in common between the two compounds divided by the total number of fingerprints present in both compounds. Network visualization for Fig. 2b was performed using Cytoscape[43].

Forward genetic screens for resistant mutants. Our forward genetic screens were carried out as previously described[9,24]. In brief, wild-type parental (P0) worms were mutagenized in 50 mM ethyl methanesulfonate for 4 h, or in 0.5 mM *N*-ethyl-*N*-nitrosourea for 4 h, as previously described. Tens of thousands of synchronized L1s from either the F1 (progeny) or F2 (grand-progeny) generations were dispensed onto 10 cm MYOB agar plates (see ref. 24 for how to prepare MYOB/agar media) containing an ~100% penetrant lethal dose of the nematicide. Candidate-resistant mutants are those worms that can grow in the presence of the chemical. Candidates were picked onto solid MYOB plates without any added chemical, and 12 of their progeny were individually re-tested on a 100%-penetrant lethal dose of the nematicide. Those candidates that re-tested were subsequently homozygosed as previously described[9,24].

Whole-genome sequencing of wact-11-family-resistant mutants. A total 100 μl of packed worms were harvested in a 15 ml conical tube and washed three times with M9 buffer. The worms were then incubated in 6 ml of M9 buffer for 1 h on a nutating shaker at 20 °C. The worms were then washed once with 1 × phosphate-buffered saline (PBS) buffer. The tube was centrifuged and the PBS buffer was aspirated without disturbing the worm pellet. The worms were flash frozen in liquid nitrogen and ground with a pestle until the pellet defrosted. The DNeasy Blood and Tissue Kit (Qiagen) was used to lyse the worm cells and purify the genomic DNA. The Nextera DNA Sample Preparation Kit (Illumina) was used to generate the genomic DNA libraries for sequencing. Individual libraries were quantified with quantitative PCR with reverse transcription using KAPA standards. Multiplexed libraries were sequenced on an Illumina HiSeq2500, paired end reads, 125 bp × 125 bp, using version 4 reagents and flow cells.

Sequence variants were identified using a BWA-GATK pipeline. Briefly, the 125-bp sequencing reads were examined for sequence quality using FastQC (http://www.bioinformatics.babraham.ac.uk/projects/fastqc/) and bases lower than a quality threshold of 30 were trimmed off using Trimmomatic[44]. Reads were aligned to the *C. elegans* N2 reference genome (release W220) using BWA-mem[45]. Alignments were sorted by coordinate order and duplicates removed using Picard (http://picard.sourceforge.net). Before variant calling, reads were processed in Genome Analysis Tool Kit (GATK) v2.5 (ref. 46) for indel realignment and base quality score recalibration, using known *C. elegans* variants from dbSNP build 138 (http://www.ncbi.nlm.nih.gov/SNP/). GATK HaplotypeCaller was used to call variants, and results were filtered for a phred-scaled Q score >30. Finally, called variants were annotated using Annovar[47] to obtain a list of exonic variants for each sample.

***Ascaris suum* complex II structure rendering.** PyMOL[48] was used to generate the images in Fig. 4a,b, using the crystal structure 3VRB (downloaded from the Protein Data Bank). H-bonds were identified by performing the 'find > polar contacts' action in PyMOL[48], using the default settings.

Mitochondria isolation from worms. HB101 *E. coli* cells (*C. elegans* Genetics Center, University of Minnesota) from a 1 l saturated culture were pelleted by centrifugation at 2,500*g* for 10 min, and then resuspended in 50 ml complete S-medium (see ref. 37 for recipe). In all, 450,000 synchronized first larval-stage worms, in M9 buffer, were added to the S-media/HB101 suspension and were grown to adulthood over 3.5 days at 20 °C with shaking at 200 r.p.m. Worms were collected in 6 × 15 ml conical tubes and washed eight times with M9 buffer. The worms from the six tubes were combined into one 15 ml conical tube, and resuspended in 15 ml M9 buffer. One millilitre aliquots of the worm suspension were distributed to each of the 15 × 1.5 ml Sarstedt microcentrifuge tubes. The worms were pelleted by centrifugation at 800*g*, and the M9 buffer was aspirated without disrupting the pellet. A total 600 μl of cold isolation buffer A (250 mM sucrose, 10 mM Tris (pH 7.5), 1 mM EDTA, 1 mM PMSF) was added to each tube. A total 300 µl of cold glass beads was added to each tube. The tubes were cooled on ice for 10 min, and the worms were disrupted by bead beating 6 × 30 s, with 1 min cooling intervals. The tubes were spun down at 1,000*g* for 10 min at 4 °C and the supernatants were transferred to a single 15 ml conical tube on ice. The homogenate was centrifuged at 1,000*g* for 10 min at 4 °C. The supernatant was transferred to a new cold tube, and centrifuged at 16,000*g* for 10 min at 4 °C. The pellet was washed twice by re-suspending gently in 5 ml of cold isolation buffer B (250 mM sucrose, 10 mM Tris (pH 7.5), 1 mM EDTA). After the final wash, 310 µl aliquots of the mitochondrial suspension were distributed across 16 microcentrifuge tubes and the tubes were centrifuged at 16,000*g* for 10 min at 4 °C. The supernatant was aspirated and the pellets were snap frozen in liquid nitrogen and stored at − 80 °C until needed.

Mitochondria isolation from mouse liver. The livers from three 8–10-week-old C57Bl/6 female mice (Charles River) were removed, collected in 1.5 ml micro-centrifuge tubes, flash frozen in liquid nitrogen and stored at − 80 °C until needed. Just before mitochondria isolation, the livers were weighed, placed into a 10-cm petri dish and 10 ml isolation buffer A was added per gram of liver tissue. The tissue was finely minced with a razor blade, transferred to a glass Dounce homo-genizer and homogenized by 10 strokes on ice. The homogenate was centrifuged at 1,000*g* for 10 min at 4 °C. The supernatant was collected and centrifuged at 1,000*g* for 10 min at 4 °C. The supernatant was again collected and centrifuged at 16,000*g* for 10 min at 4 °C. The pellet was resuspended in 20 ml of isolation buffer B and centrifuged at 16,000*g* for 10 min at 4 °C. The pellet was resuspended in 20 ml of isolation buffer B, and 1 ml aliquots of the resuspension were distributed into 20 × 1.5 ml microcentrifuge tubes. The aliquoted resuspensions were centrifuged at 16,000*g* for 10 min at 4 °C. The supernatant was aspirated, the pellet was flash frozen in liquid nitrogen and stored frozen at − 80 °C until needed. The mice used for experimentation were housed and used in accordance with 'the use and care of experimental animals' guidelines. The animal protocols were reviewed and approved by the Animal Care Committee of the University of Toronto.

Cell-free Complex II functional assay. Mitochondrial pellets were thawed on ice and resuspended in 300 µl of cold isolation buffer B. Using the BCA assay[49], the protein concentration of the mitochondria suspension was determined and was subsequently diluted to a concentration of 0.2 mg ml^{-1} with cold isolation buffer B. Complex II enzymatic assays were carried out in 96-well flat bottom plates. A total 150 µl of complex II assay buffer (1X PBS, 0.35% BSA, 20 mM succinate, 240 µM KCN, 60 µM DCIP, 70 µM decylubiquinone, 25 µM antimycin A, 2 µM rotenone) containing dissolved compounds at the desired concentration, or DMSO (2.4% v/v) alone for control purposes, was added to each well. All of the compounds tested were dissolved in DMSO, except malonate, which was dissolved in water, so DMSO was omitted from the malonate control wells. Five microlitres of the 0.2 mg ml^{-1} mitochondria suspension was added to each well and mixed by pipetting up and down five times. Absorbance for each well was measured at 600 nm using a SpectraMax Plus 384-well Microplate Reader, combined with SoftmaxPro software at 30-s intervals over a 35-min time period. Absorbance versus time was plotted for each well and enzyme activity was calculated as the slope of the line defined by the points ranging from 4 to 10 min. Per cent activity was calculated by dividing the enzyme activity of the chemical-treated wells by that of the DMSO control wells. The per cent activity plotted in Supplementary Fig. 5 is the average of four technical replicates.

References

1. *Parasitic Helminths. Targets, Screens, Drugs and Vaccines* (Wiley-VCH, 2012).
2. Keiser, J. & Utzinger, J. The drugs we have and the drugs we need against major helminth infections. *Adv. Parasitol.* **73,** 197–230 (2010).
3. Besier, B. New anthelmintics for livestock: the time is right. *Trends Parasitol.* **23,** 21–24 (2007).
4. Fuller, V. L., Lilley, C. J. & Urwin, P. E. Nematode resistance. *New Phytol.* **180,** 27–44 (2008).
5. Sutherland, I. A. & Leathwick, D. M. Anthelmintic resistance in nematode parasites of cattle: a global issue? *Trends Parasitol.* **27,** 176–181 (2011).
6. Kaminsky, R. *et al.* A new class of anthelmintics effective against drug-resistant nematodes. *Nature* **452,** 176–180 (2008).
7. Kaminsky, R., Mosimann, D., Sager, H., Stein, P. & Hosking, B. Determination of the effective dose rate for monepantel (AAD 1566) against adult gastro-intestinal nematodes in sheep. *Int. J. Parasitol.* **39,** 443–446 (2009).
8. Scott, I. *et al.* Lack of efficacy of monepantel against *Teladorsagia circumcincta* and *Trichostrongylus colubriformis*. *Vet. Parasitol.* **198,** 166–171 (2013).
9. Kwok, T. C. *et al.* A small-molecule screen in *C. elegans* yields a new calcium channel antagonist. *Nature* **441,** 91–95 (2006).
10. Lemieux, G. A. *et al.* A whole-organism screen identifies new regulators of fat storage. *Nat. Chem. Biol.* **7,** 206–213 (2011).
11. Petrascheck, M., Ye, X. & Buck, L. B. An antidepressant that extends lifespan in adult *Caenorhabditis elegans*. *Nature* **450,** 553–556 (2007).
12. Leung, C. K. *et al.* An ultra high-throughput, whole-animal screen for small molecule modulators of a specific genetic pathway in *Caenorhabditis elegans*. *PLoS ONE* **8,** e62166 (2013).
13. Holden-Dye, L. & Walker, R. J. in *WormBook* 1-13 (The C. elegans Research Community, 2007).
14. Jones, A. K., Buckingham, S. D. & Sattelle, D. B. Chemistry-to-gene screens in *Caenorhabditis elegans*. *Nat. Rev. Drug Discov.* **4,** 321–330 (2005).
15. Simpkin, K. G. & Coles, G. C. The use of *Caenorhabditis elegans* for anthelmintic screening. *J. Chem. Tech Biotechnol* **31,** 66–69 (1981).
16. Geary, T. G. & Thompson, D. P. *Caenorhabditis elegans*: how good a model for veterinary parasites? *Vet. Parasitol.* **101,** 371–386 (2001).
17. Gilleard, J. S. The use of *Caenorhabditis elegans* in parasitic nematode research. *Parasitology* **128**(Suppl 1): S49–S70 (2004).
18. Lee, B. H. *et al.* Marcfortine and paraherquamide class of anthelmintics: discovery of PNU-141962. *Curr. Top. Med. Chem.* **2,** 779–793 (2002).
19. Geary, T. G. in *Parasitic Helminths: Targets, Screens, Drugs and Vaccines (ed. Caffrey, C. R.) 123–134 (Wiley-VCH, 2012).*
20. Woods, D. J. *et al.*in *Parasitic Helminths: Targets, Screens, Drugs and Vaccines*. (ed. Caffrey, C. R.) 297–307 (Wiley-VCH, 2012).
21. Gilleard, J. S. *Haemonchus contortus* as a paradigm and model to study anthelmintic drug resistance. *Parasitology* **140,** 1506–1522 (2013).
22. Hungenberg, H., Fursch, H., Rieck, H. & Hellwege, E. Use of fluopyram for controlling nematodes in crops and for increasing yield. European patent EP2645856 (2013).
23. Broeksma, A., Puetzkuhl, K., Lamprecht, S. & Fuersch, H. VELUM—A evolutionary nematicide for efficient crop production. Presented at the 6th International Congress of NematologyCape Town, South Africa (2014).
24. Burns, A. R. *et al.* High-throughput screening of small molecules for bioactivity and target identification in Caenorhabditis elegans. *Nat. Protoc.* **1,** 1906–1914 (2006).
25. Ichimiya, H. *et al.* Complex II inactivation is lethal in the nematode *Caenorhabditis elegans*. *Mitochondrion* **2,** 191–198 (2002).
26. Sun, F. *et al.* Crystal structure of mitochondrial respiratory membrane protein complex II. *Cell* **121,** 1043–1057 (2005).
27. Sierotzki, H. & Scalliet, G. A review of current knowledge of resistance aspects for the next-generation succinate dehydrogenase inhibitor fungicides. *Phytopathology* **103,** 880–887 (2013).
28. Sakai, C., Tomitsuka, E., Esumi, H., Harada, S. & Kita, K. Mitochondrial fumarate reductase as a target of chemotherapy: from parasites to cancer cells. *Biochim. Biophys. Acta* **1820,** 643–651 (2012).
29. Ishii, H., Miyamoto, T., Ushio, S. & Kakishima, M. Lack of cross-resistance to a novel succinate dehydrogenase inhibitor, fluopyram, in highly boscalid-resistant isolates of *Corynespora cassiicola* and *Podosphaera xanthii*. *Pest Manag. Sci.* **67,** 474–482 (2011).
30. Osanai, A. *et al.* Crystallization of mitochondrial rhodoquinol-fumarate reductase from the parasitic nematode *Ascaris suum* with the specific inhibitor flutolanil. *Acta Crystallogr. Sect. F Struct. Biol. Cryst. Commun.* **65,** 941–944 (2009).
31. Harada, S., Inaoka, D. K., Ohmori, J. & Kita, K. Diversity of parasite complex II. *Biochim. Biophys. Acta* **1827,** 658–667 (2013).
32. Burns, A. R. *et al.* A predictive model for drug bioaccumulation and bioactivity in *Caenorhabditis elegans*. *Nat. Chem. Biol.* **6,** 549–557 (2010).
33. Wasmuth, J., Schmid, R., Hedley, A. & Blaxter, M. On the extent and origins of genic novelty in the phylum Nematoda. *PLoS Negl. Trop. Dis.* **2,** e258 (2008).
34. Holden-Dye, L. & Walker, R. J. in *Parasitic Helminths: Targets, Screens, Drugs and Vaccines*. (ed. Caffrey, C. R.) 23–41 (Wiley-VCH, 2012).
35. Anderson, P. in *Caenorhabditis: Modern Biological Analysis of an Organism*. (eds Epstein, H. F. & Shakes, D. C.) 31–58 (Academic, Inc., 1995).
36. Guest, M. *et al.* The calcium-activated potassium channel, SLO-1, is required for the action of the novel cyclo-octadepsipeptide anthelmintic, emodepside, in *Caenorhabditis elegans*. *Int. J. Parasitol.* **37,** 1577–1588 (2007).
37. Lewis, J. A. & Fleming, J. T. in *Caenorhabditis elegans: Modern Biological Analysis of an Organism*. (eds Epstein, H. F. & Shakes, D. C.) 4–29 (Academic, Inc., 1995).
38. Lehner, B., Tischler, J. & Fraser, A. G. RNAi screens in *Caenorhabditis elegans* in a 96-well liquid format and their application to the systematic identification of genetic interactions. *Nat. Protoc.* **1,** 1617–1620 (2006).
39. Demeler, J., Kuttler, U. & von Samson-Himmelstjerna, G. Adaptation and evaluation of three different *in vitro* tests for the detection of resistance to anthelmintics in gastro intestinal nematodes of cattle. *Vet. Parasitol.* **170,** 61–70 (2010).
40. Laing, R. *et al.* The genome and transcriptome of *Haemonchus contortus*, a key model parasite for drug and vaccine discovery. *Genome Biol.* **14,** R88 (2013).
41. Redman, E. *et al.* Microsatellite analysis reveals marked genetic differentiation between *Haemonchus contortus* laboratory isolates and provides a rapid system of genetic fingerprinting. *Int. J. Parasitol.* **38,** 111–122 (2008).

42. Bartley, D. J. *et al.* A survey of anthelmintic resistant nematode parasites in Scottish sheep flocks. *Vet. Parasitol.* **117,** 61–71 (2003).
43. Cline, M. S. *et al.* Integration of biological networks and gene expression data using Cytoscape. *Nat. Protoc.* **2,** 2366–2382 (2007).
44. Bolger, A. M., Lohse, M. & Usadel, B. Trimmomatic: a flexible trimmer for Illumina sequence data. *Bioinformatics* **30,** 2114–2120 (2014).
45. Li, H. & Durbin, R. Fast and accurate short read alignment with Burrows-Wheeler transform. *Bioinformatics* **25,** 1754–1760 (2009).
46. DePristo, M. A. *et al.* A framework for variation discovery and genotyping using next-generation DNA sequencing data. *Nat. Genet.* **43,** 491–498 (2011).
47. Wang, K., Li, M. & Hakonarson, H. ANNOVAR: functional annotation of genetic variants from high-throughput sequencing data. *Nucleic Acids Res.* **38,** e164 (2010).
48. The PyMOL Molecular Graphics System, Version 1.3r1, (Schrodinger, LLC, 2010).
49. Walker, J. M. The bicinchoninic acid (BCA) assay for protein quantitation. *Methods Mol. Biol.* **32,** 5–8 (1994).

Acknowledgements

We thank Dr Doug Colwell and Dawn Gray at the Lethbridge and Agri-Food Canada Research Centre for supplying faeces from infected sheep and calves for parasite egg collection. We thank Dr Liliana Attisano from the Donnelly CCBR at the University of Toronto for the HEK293T cells. We also thank Dr Derek van der Kooy, Brenda Takabe and Timothy Liao from the Donnelly CCBR at the University of Toronto for the mouse tissue. Whole-genome sequencing was carried out by The Donnelly Sequencing Centre at the University of Toronto. This work was supported by grants to G.M. and C.A.M. from the NIH (HL098938), Burroughs Welcome Foundation and the Harvard Stem Cell Institute; to A.G.F. from the CIHR (488367); to J.G. from the CIHR (230927) and the NSERC-CREATE HPI graduate training programme at the University of Calgary; and to P.J.R. from the CIHR (313296). P.J.R. is a Canada Research Chair in Chemical Genetics.

Author contributions

A.R.B. and G.M.L. performed the primary *C. elegans* chemical screens in P.J.R.'s lab. The chemical re-screens in *C. elegans* were performed by G.M.L. and R.B. in P.J.R.'s lab. G.M.L. performed the *C. oncophora* and *H. contortus* chemical screens, with the help of E.R. and S.S., in J.G.'s lab. G.M. performed the zebrafish chemical screens in C.A.M.'s lab. Y.Z. performed the HEK cell chemical screens in P.J.R.'s lab. A.R.B., G.M.L., G.M. and P.J.R. analysed the chemical screening data. C.R.C. helped perform some chemical screens. G.M. performed all cheminformatic analyses. R.B., L.R., J.G. and R.H. carried out the forward genetic screens in P.J.R.'s lab. Mutant genomic DNA libraries for sequencing were prepared by A.R.B. in P.J.R.'s lab, and sequence analysis was performed by M.S. in A.G.F.'s lab. The complex II functional assays were performed by A.R.B. with input from G.A.M. S.R.C., M.T., G.G., C.N. and P.J.R. contributed chemical libraries for screening. The project was conceived by P.J.R. and the paper was written by A.R.B. and P.J.R.

Additional information

Competing financial interests: The authors declare no competing financial interests.

10

Supramolecular high-aspect ratio assemblies with strong antifungal activity

Kazuki Fukushima[1,2,*], Shaoqiong Liu[3,*], Hong Wu[3], Amanda C. Engler[1], Daniel J. Coady[1], Hareem Maune[1], Jed Pitera[1], Alshakim Nelson[1], Nikken Wiradharma[3], Shrinivas Venkataraman[3], Yuan Huang[4], Weimin Fan[4], Jackie Y. Ying[3], Yi Yan Yang[3] & James L. Hedrick[1]

Efficient and pathogen-specific antifungal agents are required to mitigate drug resistance problems. Here we present cationic small molecules that exhibit excellent microbial selectivity with minimal host toxicity. Unlike typical cationic polymers possessing molecular weight distributions, these compounds have an absolute molecular weight aiding in isolation and characterization. However, their specific molecular recognition motif (terephthalamide-bisurea) facilitates spontaneous supramolecular self-assembly manifesting in several polymer-like properties. Computational modelling of the terephthalamide-bisurea structures predicts zig-zag or bent arrangements where distal benzyl urea groups stabilize the high-aspect ratio aqueous supramolecular assemblies. These nanostructures are confirmed by transmission electron microscopy and atomic force microscopy. Antifungal activity against drug-sensitive and drug-resistant strains with *in vitro* and *in vivo* biocompatibility is observed. Additionally, despite repeated sub-lethal exposures, drug resistance is not induced. Comparison with clinically used amphotericin B shows similar antifungal behaviour without any significant toxicity in a *C. albicans* biofilm-induced mouse keratitis model.

[1] IBM Almaden Research Center, 650 Harry Road, San Jose, California 95120, USA. [2] Department of Polymer Science and Engineering, Yamagata University, Yonezawa, Yamagata 992-8510, Japan. [3] Institute of Bioengineering and Nanotechnology, 31 Biopolis Way, The Nanos, Singapore 138669, Singapore. [4] State Key Laboratory for Diagnosis and Treatment of Infectious Diseases, First Affiliated Hospital, College of Medicine, Zhejiang University, Hangzhou 310003, China. * These authors contributed equally to this work. Correspondence and requests for materials should be addressed to Y.Y.Y. (email: yyyang@ibn.a-star.edu.sg) or to J.L.H. (email: hedrick@us.ibm.com).

The number of opportunistic fungal infection cases is increasing due to growing populations of immunocompromised patients[1]. These invasive infections are mainly caused by *Candida* and *Aspergillus* species as well as *Cryptococcus neoformans* (*C. neoformans*). It has been reported that candidiasis, a fungal infection caused by *Candida*, was the third most common blood stream infection in the United States[2,3]. Fungal infections resistant to conventional antifungal drugs have been increasingly documented[4,5], and many existing antifungal agents (for example, triazoles and polyenes) have witnessed resistance development in patients[1]. This is of huge concern within health-care and clinical settings due to the extremely limited selection of antifungal agents.

Another challenge in developing antifungal drugs is that fungi are metabolically similar to mammalian cells, providing limited fungi-specific targets. For example, amphotericin B has broad-spectrum antimicrobial activities by binding ergosterol, the key sterol in fungal membrane, to form aggregates[6]. These aggregates induce membrane pores resulting in cell lysis. In a similar fashion, amphotericin B can also bind cholesterol in mammalian cell membranes, leading to non-specific toxicity. Haemolysis and nephrotoxicity are commonly reported side-effects caused by this drug in patients[7]. In aggregate, all these issues have created a pressing need for the development of novel antifungal agents that are efficient and pathogen-specific.

Host defence peptides and synthetic polymers are two classes of macromolecules currently being studied as effective antimicrobials[8–11]. These materials are amphiphilic while also carrying cationic charge. They selectively interact and disintegrate negatively charged microbial walls or membranes via electrostatic interactions and insertion into membrane lipid domains. In addition, it is difficult for microbial cells to repair a physically damaged cell wall or membrane, hence avoiding potential microbial resistance development. Despite their efficacious antimicrobial activity, both peptides and synthetic polymers have seen limited clinical applications because of several inherent problems. For example, antimicrobial peptides generally have a short half-life *in vivo* due to enzymatic degradation, and suffer from high production costs. Bio-inspired synthetic polymers have been reported and have achieved considerable success in overcoming some of the drawbacks found with antimicrobial peptides, but many of them are cytotoxic to mammalian cells.

In this study, we describe the synthesis, self-assembly and therapeutic activity for a novel class of discrete low-molecular weight antifungal agents. Their chemical structures are designed to incorporate specific molecular recognition motifs that induce formation of high-aspect ratio supramolecular assemblies. The assembled structures have polymer-like properties including a glass transition temperature (T_g), and fibre-like morphologies in water. Compared with discrete molecules, fibre formation increases local concentration of cationic charges and compound mass, which facilitates the targeting and subsequent fungal membrane lysis with high efficiency and minimal haemolysis/cytotoxicity at concentrations far exceeding the therapeutic dosage. The nano-assemblies are effective against clinically isolated drug-resistant fungi and fungal biofilm, and prevent drug resistance development. In a fungal keratitis mouse model, these nanostructures decrease the severity of keratitis without causing any toxicity.

Results

Compound synthesis and characterization. A key design motif of these small molecules was the rigid terephthalamide diamine that was readily modified to generate cationic terephthalamide-bisurea amphipathic compounds. These monodisperse molecules were constructed in a one-pot synthesis by reaction of a diamine with bis(pentafluorophenyl)carbonate generating reactive carbamates (Fig. 1). Subsequent reaction with an alkyl diamine, where a single amine group was previously protected by *tert*-butyloxycarbonyl (^{t}Boc), generated the terephthalamide-bisurea compound readily isolated by precipitation into ether. These compounds were then dissolved in trifluoroacetic acid (TFA) (20 h) for removal of ^{t}Boc groups and generation of amine/TFA salts, again isolated by simple precipitation in ether. Four compounds were prepared having ethyl, butyl, hexyl and benzyl amine spacers between the urea and cationic charge, with absolute molecular weights ranging from 774.7 to 926.9 g mol^{-1} (Supplementary Figs S1–S4; Supplementary Table S1 and Supplementary Methods).

Interestingly, these compounds did not show a melting point, but rather manifested a T_g as confirmed by both differential scanning calorimetry (DSC) and dynamic mechanical analysis (DMA) performed on a solid support. For example, compound **3b** showed a T_g at $\sim$120 °C (DSC), and an associated modulus drop and tan δ increase via DMA (Fig. 2a,b). These findings indicated similarities to the amorphous glasses synthesized by Ober *et al.*[12], low molecular weight resist compounds that have a T_g, low viscosity and distinctive dissolution properties due to the lack of molecular weight distribution. Furthermore, the aforementioned compounds formed supramolecular structures with cationic surfaces (zeta potential: 32–45 mV) when dissolved in water above their critical micellar concentrations (CMCs) (12-100 mg l^{-1} in de-ionized water; 6–56 mg l^{-1} in the fungus culture medium) (Table 1). For example, **3b** and **3d** formed the nanofibers (several μm and several hundred nm in length, $\sim$5 nm and $\sim$10 nm in diameter, respectively) after dialysis against water, as seen by transmission electron microscopy (TEM) (Fig. 2d,e, respectively). Interestingly, **3b** self-assembled into nanofibers with high flexibility, while **3d** formed relatively rigid nanofibers presumably due to its rigid molecular structure. Solution atomic force microscopy (AFM) of **3b** (Fig. 2c) also shows anisotropic structures, although of considerably shorter lengths. Molecular mechanics conformational analysis of the terephthalamide-bisurea core structure revealed a zig-zag or bent structure with distal benzyl urea groups perpendicular to the terephthalamide core (Fig. 1 and Supplementary Fig. S5). These zig-zag structures pack together into planar sheets stabilized by urea–urea hydrogen bonds and aromatic stacking. As the amide and urea groups are perpendicular, planar sheets further stack against one another, stabilized by hydrophobic interactions and amide–amide hydrogen bonds, generating a multilayer nanorod (Fig. 1 and Supplementary Fig. S5). This cross-braced nanorod structure is mechanically stable and allows high-aspect ratio structures.

***In vitro* antifungal activity.** We evaluated these cationic assemblies for antifungal activity against clinically relevant *C. albicans*, clinically isolated drug-sensitive and drug-resistant *C. neoformans* fungi. The overall net cationic charge of the assemblies allowed sufficient electrostatic interactions with anionic fungal cell surfaces. The compounds **3a–3d** inhibited fungal growth at relatively low minimum inhibitory concentration (MIC) values, which were greater than their CMCs in the fungus culture medium (Table 1). In addition, MIC values remained unchanged when the fungal concentration varied from 10^2 to 10^5 CFU ml^{-1} (Supplementary Fig. S6). These findings indicated that the compounds were active as aggregate assemblies rather than discrete molecules. This is particularly important as the cell wall of *C. albicans* consists of multiple layers with low negative charges (zeta potential: -4 mV), which impairs the ability of cationic nanoparticles to

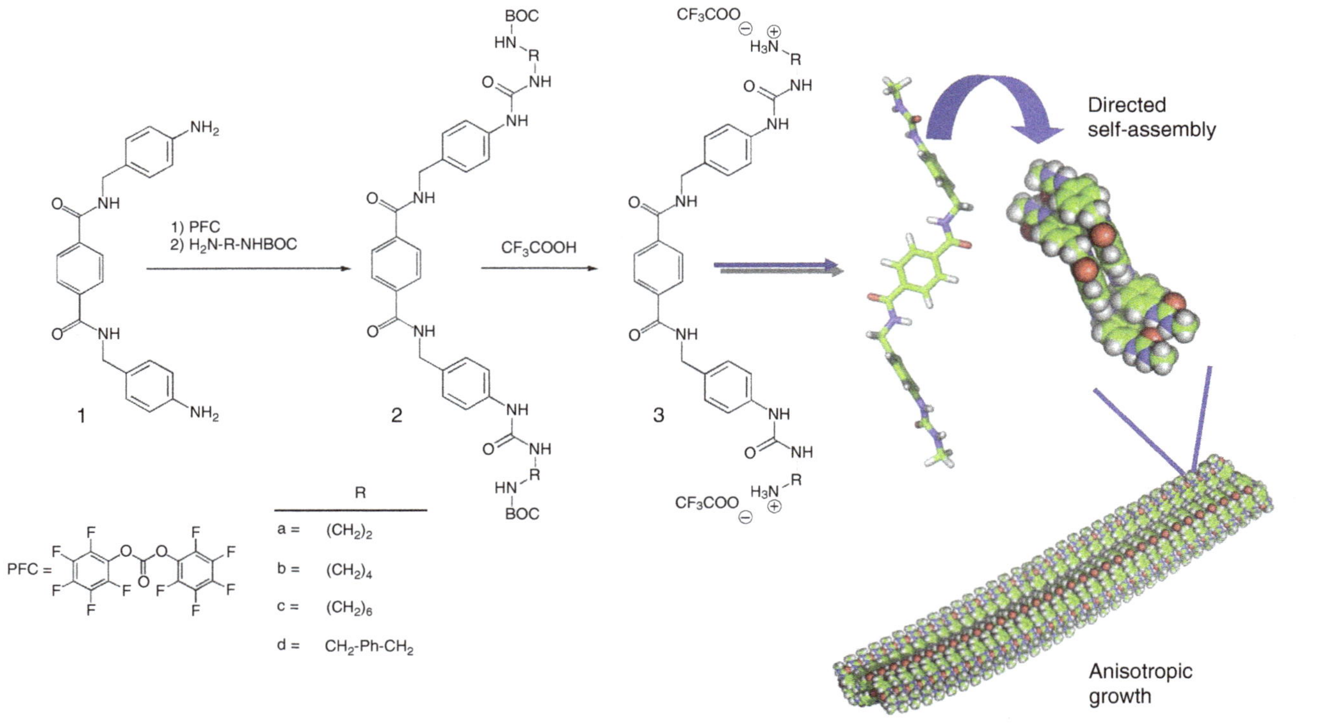

Figure 1 | Synthesis and characteristics of compounds 3a-d. Self-assembly motif with tunable functional groups. Molecular mechanics conformational analysis of the terephthalamide-bisurea structure revealed a zig-zag or bent structure with the distal benzyl urea groups perpendicular to the terephthalamide nanorod structure that is mechanically stable and is capable of generating high aspect structures.

adhere to the cell wall and cause membrane disruption and lysis. The antifungal activity might be attributed to the nanostructure formation (Fig. 2c), facilitating cell wall/membrane penetration. Additionally, increasing hydrophobicity of the terminal groups from $(CH_2)_2$ (**3a**) to $(CH_2)_4$ (**3b**) improved antifungal efficacy (Fig. 1). However, further increasing the hydrophobicity from $(CH_2)_4$ to $(CH_2)_6$ (**3c**) did not affect antifungal activity. The compound **3d** that can form rigid nanofibers had higher efficacy against *C. neoformans* as compared with **3a–3c**. In order to determine microbicidal properties, colony assays were performed. Fluconazole demonstrated fungistatic characteristic against *C. albicans* (MIC: $2\,mg\,l^{-1}$) (Fig. 3a) and *C. neoformans* (MIC: $8\,mg\,l^{-1}$) (Fig. 3b) even at $2 \times$ MIC. At these concentrations, the reduction in the viable colony counts of fungi after treatment with fluconazole was $<3\ \log_{10}$ as compared with the control without the treatment. This phenomenon was also reported by others[13]. However, *C. albicans* and *C. neoformans* treated with the assemblies for 24 h showed $>3\ \log_{10}$ reduction in the viable colony counts as compared with the control group (that is, >99.9% eradication) using concentrations at their MIC (Fig. 3a,b), and they were almost completely killed (~100%) at $2 \times$ MIC, indicating a fungicidal mechanism. The capability of cationic compounds for killing fungi was further investigated by analysing the viable colony counts of *C. albicans* upon treatment at MIC concentration utilizing various exposure times. Notably, >80% of *C. albicans* cells exposed to **3b** were killed at 30 min, and >99.9% eradication was found at 1 h (Supplementary Fig. S7).

The antifungal effect of **3a** and **3b** was further investigated against clinically isolated fluconazole-resistant *C. neoformans*. MIC of fluconazole against this strain of fungus increased from 2 (against drug-sensitive strain) to $62.5\,mg\,l^{-1}$, verifying that this strain of fungus was resistant to fluconazole[14]. The MICs of **3a** and **3b** were 125.0 and $62.5\,mg\,l^{-1}$, respectively, which were the same as those against drug-sensitive *C. neoformans*. At and above their MICs, both cationic assemblies removed almost 100% fluconazole-resistant *C. neoformans* cells, while fluconazole was fungistatic as expected (reduction in the viable colony counts of fungi after fluconazole treatment: $<3\ \log_{10}$ as compared with the control without the treatment) (Fig. 3c). These results indicated that **3a** and **3b** were effective against both drug-sensitive and drug-resistant fungi. Furthermore, multiple sub-lethal dose treatments of *C. albicans* with cationic assemblies did not induce resistance. In contrast, drug resistance was developed after six sub-lethal fluconazole exposures (Fig. 3d). In addition, the cationic assemblies were fungicidal at MIC with >99.9% killing efficiency of *C. albicans* at passages 1–11, while fluconazole was fungistatic towards *C. albicans* even at $62.5 \times$ MICs (Supplementary Fig. S8). These findings demonstrated great potential of the cationic assemblies against drug resistance.

Biofilm lysis. Medical implants beset by fungal biofilm formations, especially those that are resistant to clinical antifungal agents such as amphotericin B and fluconazole[15,16], are a major cause for device failures. To evaluate biofilm disruption ability, cationic assembly **3b** was utilized for the treatment of contact lenses having a *C. albicans* biofilm in order to mimic fungal keratitis *in vitro*[17]. The untreated biofilm consisted of both metabolically active oval and long tubular hyphae cell types (red region), where extracellular matrix (ECM) (green region) was bound in both of them (Fig. 4a,c). In contrast, **3b** treatment mediated a significant reduction in the metabolically active cells (Fig. 4d), and cell wall/membrane of *C. albicans* was broken and debris was observed after the treatment (Fig. 4b). XTT and Safranin assays further confirmed the drastic decrease in *C. albicans* survival and the biofilm disruption after **3b** treatment (Supplementary Fig. S9).

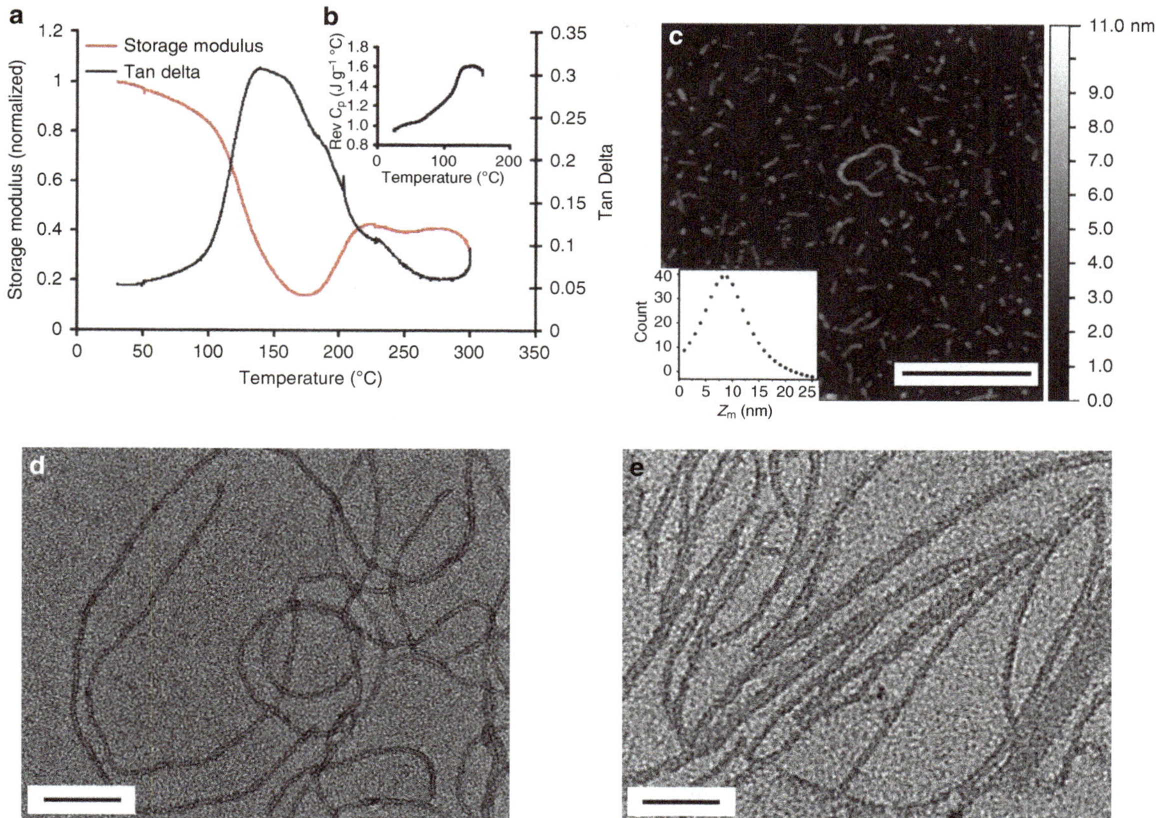

Figure 2 | Polymer-like properties. (**a**) DMA and (**b**) DSC thermograms of compound **3a**. (**c**) Topography micrograph of supramolecular assemblies of **3b** using AFM in fluid. Sample was prepared by direct dissolution of compound **3b** in water and imaged under water. The inset shows a distribution of statistical mean height (z_m) obtained through particle analysis. A Lorentzian fit to the distribution gives a z_m of ~8 nm in water. Scale bar: 500 nm. TEM micrographs of (**d**) compound **3b** and (**e**) compound **3d**. Scale bar: 100 nm.

Table 1 | Physicochemical and biological properties of the cationic compounds.

Compound	R	CMC* (mg l^{-1})	Zeta Potential (mV)	MIC (mg l^{-1})	
				C. A.	C. N.
3a	$(CH_2)_2$	100.0 (56.0)	32.2	62.5	125.0
3b	$(CH_2)_4$	20.0 (14.0)	36.7	31.2	62.5
3c	$(CH_2)_6$	15.0 (13.0)	35.3	31.2	62.5
3d	CH_2-Ph-CH_2	12.0 (6.0)	45.1	31.2	31.2

C. A., C. albicans; C. N., C. neoformans; MIC, minimum inhibitory concentration.
*Measured in DI water with 1,000 mg l^{-1}; the values in parenthesis were measured in yeast mould broth

Antifungal mechanism. The antifungal mechanism was studied by visualizing a typical cell structure (that is *C. neoformans* and *C. albicans*) before and after treatment via scanning electron microscopy (SEM) and TEM. Prior to treatment, all fungi showed smooth cellular exteriors and intact cell wall/membrane (Fig. 4e,g—control). After treatment with **3b**, cell wall and membrane damage was easily visible along with dead microbe remnants (Fig. 4f,h—treated). In particular, the membrane damage led to the release of cytoplast from *C. neoformans* cells (Fig. 4h). Fungal membrane damage was also evaluated by measuring the absorbance (260 nm) of cell culture media, which can be directly correlated with nucleic acid release post-treatment[18]. As shown in Supplementary Fig. S10, following treatment of *C. albicans* with **3b**, a significant amount of nucleic acids was observed in the culture media. Furthermore, nucleic acid release was found to be dose-dependent with elevated concentrations of **3b**, causing amplified membrane damage, thereby inducing more cytoplasmic leakage. We postulated that cationic nanorods exploited an associative mechanism (which required appropriately balanced hydrophobic and hydrophilic regions), whereby antifungal material became integrated within the cellular exterior causing membrane destabilization and lysis. This membrane-lytic antifungal mechanism might be the reason for preventing the development of drug resistance (Fig. 3d).

***In vitro* biocompatibility.** A major side effect caused by many cationic antimicrobial peptides and polymers is haemolysis. Haemolytic evaluations were conducted using rat red blood cells incubated with the compounds at various concentrations (Supplementary Fig. S11a). Negligible haemolytic activity was observed for all samples, even at concentrations well above the MIC (up to 1,000 mg l^{-1}), demonstrating excellent selectivity. To evaluate cytotoxicity towards mammalian cells, human dermal fibroblast viability was analysed via MTT assay after incubation with compounds at various concentrations (15.6–1,000 mg l^{-1}) for 24 h (Supplementary Fig. S11b). More than 83% of cells were viable at all concentrations tested, indicating excellent mammalian cell biocompatibility.

***In vivo* antifungal efficacy.** To evaluate the *in vivo* antifungal activity of cationic compounds, fungal keratitis was established in

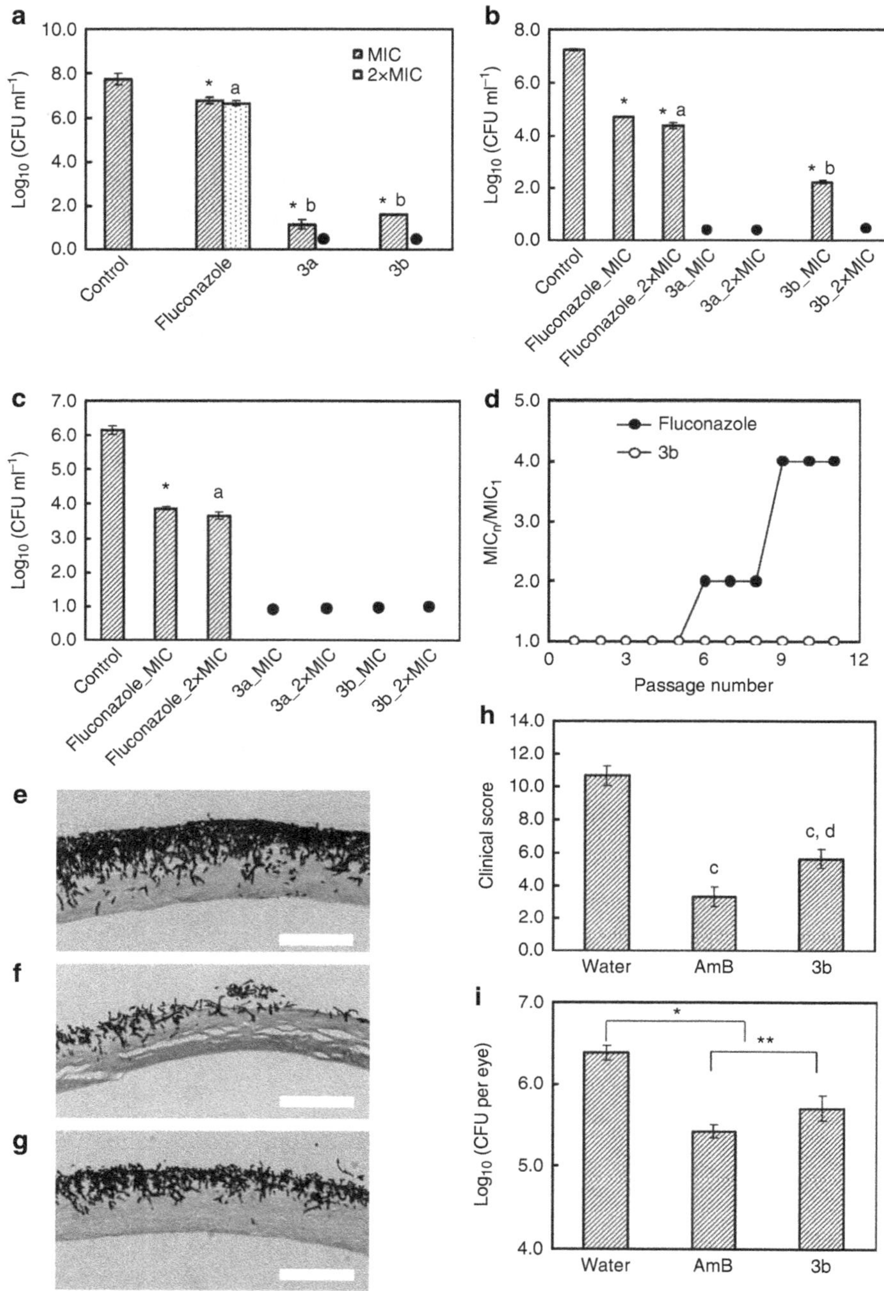

Figure 3 | *In vitro* and *in vivo* antifungal activity. Viable colony counts (Log_{10}) of (**a**) *C. albicans* and (**b**) *C. neoformans* after being treated with **3a**, **3b** and fluconazole at the specified concentrations for 24 h. (**c**) Viable colony counts (Log_{10}) of *C. neoformans* (clinically isolated fluconazole-resistant strain) after treatment with **3a** or **3b** at the specified concentrations for 24 h; fluconazole was used as the control. $^*P<0.01$, **3a**, **3b** and fluconazole at their respective MICs versus control; **a**: $P>0.05$, fluconazole at 2 × MIC versus fluconazole at MIC; **b**: $P<0.001$, **3a**, **3b** at MIC versus fluconazole at MIC. Filled black circles indicate that no colony was observed. (**d**) Changes in MICs of antifungal agents upon multiple sub-lethal exposures. (**e**-**g**) Representative histological sections of mouse cornea treated with water (**e**), AmB (**f**) and **3b** (**g**) (Grocott's methenamine silver stain, fungi in black). Scale bar: 100 μm. (**h**) Clinical scores for keratitis after treatment with the topical eye drop solutions. A total score of ≤5, 6-9 and >9 indicate mild, moderate and severe keratitis, respectively. **c**: $P<0.0005$, **3b** and AmB versus control; **d**: $P=0.008$, **3b** versus AmB. (**i**) CFU of *C. albicans* in mouse cornea treated with AmB and **3b**. The data are expressed as mean ± s.d. of 3-6 replicates. $^*P<0.01$, **3b** and AmB versus control. $^{**}P>0.05$, **3b** versus AmB.

mice by using contact lens-associated *C. albicans* biofilm infection[19,20]. The experimental protocol was approved by the Institutional Animal Care and Use Committee of Biological Research Centre, Agency for Science, Technology and Research (A*STAR), Singapore. This disease model was chosen because fungal keratitis is a severe eye infection and a major cause of ocular morbidity. An eye ulcer with dense opaque appearance was seen on the eyeballs of the mice with keratitis. The mice were randomly grouped and treated with three topical eye drop solutions: water solution (control), **3b** (2,000 mg l^{-1}) and amphotericin B (AmB) (1,500 mg l^{-1}). AmB was selected as positive control instead of fluconazole because AmB is a

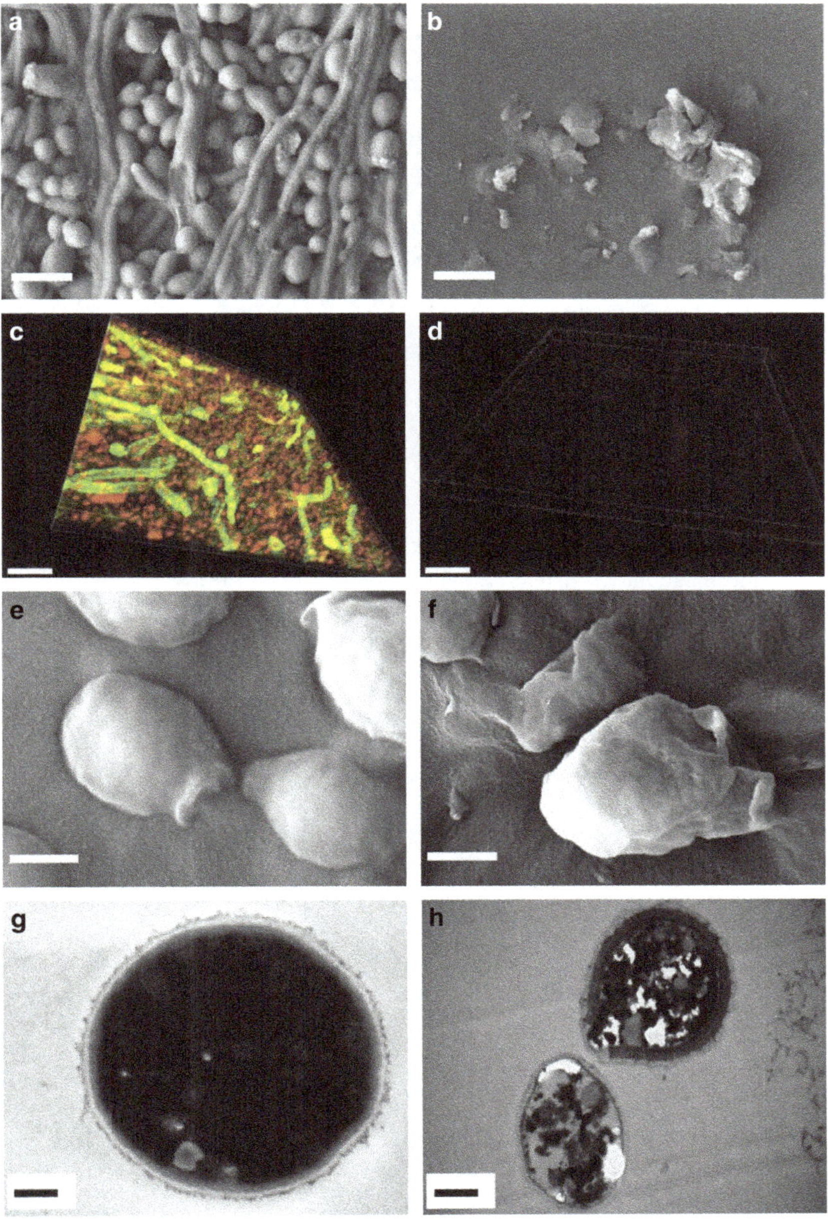

Figure 4 | Biofilm disruption and antifungal mechanism studies. SEM images of *C. albicans* biofilms (**a**) before and (**b**) after treatment with **3b** (scale bar: 5 μm). Confocal images of *C. albicans* biofilms (**c**) before and (**d**) after treatment with **3b** (scale bar: 20 μm). Areas of green fluorescence represents biofilm ECM stained with CON-A, and red fluorescence represents metabolically active cells stained with FUN-1. SEM images of *C. albicans* (**e**) before and (**f**) after treatment with **3b** (scale bar: 1 μm). TEM images of *C. neoformans* (**g**, scale bar: 0.5 μm) before and (**h**, scale bar: 1 μm) after treatment with **3b**.

clinically used strong antifungal agent, while fluconazole was unable to clear *C. albicans* biofilm *in vitro*. In control animals receiving water as eye drops, histological analysis showed extensive hyphal invasion into the corneal stroma (Fig. 3e). In contrast, treatments with **3b** and AmB resulted in significant reduction in the hyphal invasion (Fig. 3f,g and Supplementary Fig. S12), although AmB was relatively more potent. The maximal depth of fungal invasion in the cornea treated with AmB and **3b** was remarkably reduced as compared with that in the control group (18.0 ± 2.1 and 27.6 ± 1.5 μm versus 63.4 ± 5.6 μm) (Supplementary Fig. S12). Keratitis in the control, AmB- and **3b**-treated groups was further evaluated to provide clinical scores of 10.7 ± 0.6, 3.3 ± 0.6 and 5.7 ± 0.6, respectively (Fig. 3h and Supplementary Fig. S13), demonstrating that AmB and **3b** treatment significantly lessened the severity of keratitis ($P < 0.0005$). Importantly, **3b** treatment reduced the number of viable fungi remaining on the eyeballs (measured in colony-forming unit (CFU)) (5.79 $\log_{10}$ CFU per eye versus 6.38 $\log_{10}$ CFU per eye for control, 74.3% reduction, $P < 0.01$) as effectively as AmB (5.44 $\log_{10}$ CFU per eye, 88.7% reduction, $P > 0.05$ as compared with **3b** treatment) (Fig. 3i). Moreover, no significant erosion was observed in the epithelium of mouse cornea after topical administration of **3b** (Supplementary Fig. S14), indicating that **3b** was biocompatible to the corneal epithelium and underlying stroma. AmB has poor solubility in water and is unstable in aqueous, acidic or alkaline solution[21]. The water-soluble and stable antifungal compound **3b** is a better alternative to AmB.

Discussion

As fungi are metabolically similar to mammalian cells, limited fungi-specific targets are available for host differentiation. There is a pressing need to develop efficient and pathogen-specific antifungal agents to mitigate growing drug resistance problems. Our results show that a novel class of pathogen-specific, low-molecular weight antifungal agents have been successfully synthesized for self-assembly and therapeutic activity. These compounds have an exact molecular weight with a specific molecular recognition motif imparting polymer-like solid state properties—T_g and fibre-like assembly in water. The multivalent cationic charges of the self-assembled nanostructures facilitated lysis of fungal membranes with low MIC values and high selectivity. The cationic assemblies demonstrated efficient antifungal activity against clinically isolated drug-resistant strains, and effectively dispersed biofilms. In addition, they did not develop drug resistance after multiple sub-lethal treatments due to their membrane-lytic antifungal mechanism. Importantly, the nano-assemblies significantly decreased fungal counts, hindered hyphal corneal invasion and reduced the severity of keratitis in a fungal keratitis mouse model. They were also shown to have excellent *in vitro* and *in vivo* biocompatibility. Therefore, these small-molecule compounds hold great potential as antifungal agents for the prevention and treatment of topical fungus-induced infections where large and local doses can be administered.

Methods

PET degradation with 4-aminobenzylamine. PET flakes (9.61 g, 0.05 mol), 4-aminobenzylamine (28.2 g, 0.23 mol) and TBD (0.36 g, 2.5 mmol) were placed in a 250-ml flask, and then heated under nitrogen atmosphere at 120 °C for 3 h during which the reaction mixture solidified. The mixture was triturated and washed in isopropanol (200 ml). The residue was rinsed with THF and diethylether several times, and then dried in a vacuum oven at 80 °C, yielding a white powder as a product, bis(4-aminobenzyl)terephthalamide (4ABTA: 15.15 g, 81%). ^{1}H-NMR (400 MHz, dimethyl sulfoxide (DMSO)-d_6): δ 8.96 (*t*, *J* = 6 Hz, 2H, *NH*), 7.93 (*s*, 4H, Ar-*H*), 6.98 (*d*, *J* = 8 Hz, 4H, Ar-*H*), 6.51 (*d*, *J* = 8 Hz, Ar-*H*), 4.96 (*s*, 4H, NH_2), 4.30 (*d*, *J* = 6 Hz, 4H, CH_2). ^{13}C-NMR (100 MHz, DMSO-d_6): δ 165.4, 147.6, 136.7, 128.4, 127.3, 126.4, 113.8, 42.5. m.p. (DSC): 203 °C. The brief procedure for preparation of compound **3b** is given below as a typical example.

Synthesis of compound 3b. To a dry dimethylformamide (DMF) solution (16 ml) of pentafluorophenyl carbonate (PFC) (3.97 g, 10.1 mmol) was added a dry DMF solution (8 ml) of the diamine, N^1,N^4-bis(4-aminobenzyl)terephthalamide (4ABTA, **1**) (1.50 g, 4.0 mmol). The reaction mixture was stirred for 1 h at room temperature. Subsequently, *tert*-butyl (4-aminobutyl)carbamate (2.36 g, 12.6 mmol) was added, and the mixture was kept stirring overnight. To remove excess PFC and the amine reagent, the reaction mixture was precipitated in diethylether (250 ml). Thereafter, the product was filtered and dried in vacuum (60 °C) to yield **2b** (2.87 g, 90%). ^{1}H-NMR (400 MHz, DMSO-d_6): δ 9.08 (*t*, *J* = 5.8 Hz, 2H, Ar-CON*H*), 8.36 (*s*, 2H, Ar-N*H*), 7.95 (*s*, 4H, Ar-*H*), 7.32 (*d*, *J* = 8.4 Hz, 4H, Ar-*H*), 7.17 (*d*, *J* = 8.4 Hz, 4H, Ar-*H*), 6.82 (*t*, *J* = 5.6 Hz, 2H, N*H*COO), 6.07 (*t*, *J* = 5.6 Hz, 2H, N*H*CH_2), 4.39 (*d*, *J* = 5.6 Hz, 2H, Ar-CH_2), 3.09–3.00 (*m*, 4H, CH_2NHCOO), 2.95–2.86 (*m*, 4H, NHCH_2), 1.41–1.32 (*m*, 26H, CH_2 and CH_3). ^{13}C-NMR (100 MHz, DMSO-d_6): 165.3, 155.5, 155.1, 139.3, 136.6, 131.8, 127.7, 127.2, 117.4, 77.3, 42.2, 39.6, 38.7, 28.2, 27.2, 27.0.

The compound **2b** (2.50 g, 3.11 mmol) was added into trifluoroacetic acid (TFA, 10 ml) and the mixture was stirred overnight. As the deprotection proceeded, the reaction mixture became homogeneous. The reaction mixture was then precipitated in diethylether (200 ml), and the precipitate was filtered and washed with diethylether a few times, and dried in vacuum (60 °C) to yield **3b** (2.07 g, 80%). ^{1}H-NMR (400 MHz, DMSO-d_6): δ 9.09 (*t*, *J* = 5.8 Hz, 2H, Ar-CON*H*), 8.56 (*s*, 2H, Ar-N*H*), 7.95 (*s*, 4H, Ar-*H*), 7.72 (*b*, 6H, NH_3^+), 7.34 (*d*, *J* = 8.4 Hz, 4H, Ar-*H*), 7.17 (*d*, *J* = 8.4 Hz, 4H, Ar-*H*), 6.30 (*t*, *J* = 5.8 Hz, 2H, N*H*CH_2), 4.39 (*d*, *J* = 5.6 Hz, 2H, Ar-CH_2), 3.08 (*ddd*, *J* = 6.2, 6.2, 6.0 Hz, 4H, CH_2NH), 2.80 (*t*, *J* = 7.4 Hz, 4H, CH_3), 1.59–1.39 (*m*, 8H, CH_2). ^{13}C-NMR (100 MHz, DMSO-d_6): 165.3, 158.4, 155.3, 139.4, 136.6, 131.8, 127.7, 127.2, 117.5, 74.7(*t*), 42.2, 38.6, 38.3, 26.8, 24.4.

***In vitro* antifungal assays.** The MICs of the cationic compounds were measured using a broth microdilution method[22]. First, cationic compounds were dissolved in de-ionized (DI) water at 2,500 mg l^{-1}. The samples were further diluted to 31.25, 62.5, 125.0, 250.0, 500.0 and 1,000 mg l^{-1}. *C. albicans* and *C. neoformans* were grown in yeast mould broth (YMB) and Mueller Hinton broth (MHB), respectively, with vigorous shaking, and they were cultured at room temperature and 37 °C, respectively. The optical density ($OD_{600\,nm}$) of the fungus solution was adjusted to 0.1 by the addition of YMB or MHB. This fungus solution was further diluted to 10^5 CFU ml^{-1} using YMB or MHB. Cationic compound solution (100 μl) was transferred to each well of a 96-well plate (NUNC), followed by the addition of 100 μl of the fungus solution. YMB and MHB were used as the control. The optical density readings of fungus solutions were monitored by measuring $OD_{600\,nm}$ at predetermined times (0 h and 24 h) using a microplate reader (TECAN). The assay was performed in four replicates for each sample and the experiments were repeated at least three times.

Antifungal activities of cationic compounds were further tested through a spread plate method. Briefly, *C. albicans* and *C. neoformans* were treated at specific concentrations of cationic compounds. At predetermined time points, microbial suspensions (20 or 100 μl) were withdrawn and diluted sequentially and then plated on 1.5% LB agar plates. The plates were incubated for 48 h at room temperature. Microbial colonies were formed and counted. The results were expressed as mean log_{10} (CFU ml^{-1}). The experiments were performed in triplicates, and were repeated three times.

Drug resistance studies. *C. albicans* was used as a model microbe for drug resistance studies. Drug resistance was induced by treating the *C. albicans* repeatedly with antimicrobial agents[23]. The MIC of **3b** against *C. albicans* was tested for 11 passages of growth. MIC was determined using the broth microdilution method. *C. albicans* exposed to the sub-MIC concentration (1/8 of MIC at that particular passage) were re-grown to a logarithmic growth phrase, and re-used for the subsequent passage's MIC measurement for the same antimicrobial agent. Drug-resistant behaviour of *C. albicans* was evaluated by recording the changes in the MIC normalized to that of the first passage. Conventional antifungal agent fluconazole was used as the control.

Haemolysis assay. Fresh rat blood cells were diluted with PBS buffer to give a cell suspension (4% in volume). Cell suspension (100 μl) was introduced to each well of a 96-well plate, and 100 μl of cationic compound solution was then added to the well. PBS and Triton X-100 (0.2%) were used as the control. The plates were incubated for 1 h at 37 °C. The 96-well plates were centrifuged at 2,200 r.p.m. for 5 min. Aliquots (100 μl) of the supernatant were transferred to a new 96-well plate. Haemoglobin release was measured at 576 nm using a microplate reader (TECAN). The red blood cells in PBS were used as a negative control. Absorbance of wells with red blood cells lysed with 0.2% Triton X-100 was taken as 100% haemolysis. Percentage of haemolysis was calculated using the following formula: haemolysis (%) = [(OD_{576nm} in the sample − OD_{576nm} in PBS)/(OD_{576nm} in 0.2% Triton X-100 − OD_{576nm} in PBS)] × 100. The data were expressed as mean and s.d. of four replicates, and the tests were repeated three times.

MTT assay. The cytotoxicity tests of cationic compounds were performed in human dermal fibroblasts using MTT assay. The cells were cultured in Dulbecco's Modified Eagle Medium (DMEM) supplemented with 10% FBS, 5% penicillin, 2 mM L-glutamine (Sigma) and incubated at 37 °C in 5% CO_2. The cells were seeded onto 96-well plates at a density of 10,000 cells per well and incubated for 1 day. Cationic compounds were diluted with the growth medium to give final concentrations of 31.25, 62.50, 125.0, 250.0, 500.0 and 1,000 mg l^{-1}. The media were replaced with 100 μl of the pre-prepared samples. The plates were then returned to the incubator and maintained in 5% CO_2 at 37 °C for 24 h. Fresh growth media (100 μl) containing 10% MTT solution (5 mg ml^{-1}) were used to replace the mixture in each well after 24 h. The plates were then returned to the incubator, and maintained in 5% CO_2 at 37 °C for another 4 h. The growth medium and excess MTT in each well were then removed. DMSO (150 μl) was then added to each well to dissolve the internalized purple formazan crystals. An aliquot of 100 μl was taken from each well, and transferred to a new 96-well plate. Each sample was tested in eight replicates per plate. The plates were then assayed at 550 nm and 690 nm. The absorbance readings of the formazan crystals were taken to be that at 550 nm subtracted by that at 690 nm. The results were expressed as a percentage of the absorbance of the blank control.

SEM analysis. The *C. albicans* before and after incubation with cationic compound **3b** at MIC for 2 h were harvested by centrifugation at 4,000 r.p.m. for 5 min. They were washed by PBS three times, and then fixed in formalin solution containing 4% formaldehyde overnight. The cells were further washed with DI water, followed by dehydration using a series of ethanol solutions with different volume contents (35, 50, 75, 90, 95 and 100%). The sample was placed on a carbon tape, which was further coated with platinum. The morphologies of the *C. albicans* before and after the treatment were observed using a field emission scanning electron microscope (JEOL JSM-7400F) operated at an accelerating voltage of 10.0 kV and a working distance of 8.0 mm.

TEM analysis. The morphologies of the cationic compounds were analysed by TEM (FEI Tecnai G^2 F20 electron microscope). Samples were prepared by a membrane dialysis method. The cationic compounds (10 mg) were dissolved in

2 ml of DMF. The solution was then dialyzed against DI water at 20 °C for 24 h using a dialysis membrane with a molecular weight cutoff of 1,000 (Spectra/Por 7, Spectrum Laboratories Inc.). Cationic compounds solution (5 µl) was placed on a copper grid coated with carbon film and incubated for 1 min. Phosphotungstic acid (5 µl; 0.1 w/v%) was applied and incubated for another minute. The extra sample solution on the grid was absorbed by filter paper. The samples were air-dried at room temperature. The TEM studies were conducted with an electron kinetic energy of 200 keV.

The morphologies of the *C. neoformans* before and after treatment with cationic compound **3b** were observed under a JEM-1230 transmission electron microscope (JEOL, Japan) using an acceleration voltage of 80 keV. The *C. neoformans* (1.5 ml) were incubated with 0.5 ml of **3b** solution at 2 × MIC for 8 h. The solution was then centrifuged at 4,000 r.p.m. for 10 min, and the supernatants were removed. They were washed by PBS (pH 7.0) twice, and then fixed in formalin solution containing 2.5% glutaraldehyde overnight. The samples were then washed by PBS three times (15 min each), and post-fixed with 1% OsO_4 in the phosphate buffer (pH 7.0) for 1 h. The fixed samples were washed in the phosphate buffer three times (15 min each), followed by dehydration in a graded ethanol solution series. The samples were incubated with a mixture of acetone and Spurr resin (1:1 in volume) for 1 h at room temperature, and then transferred to a 1:3 mixture of acetone and Spurr resin for 3 h, and lastly to Spurr resin for overnight incubation. Ultrathin sections (70–90 nm) were obtained with a Reichert–Jung Ultracut E ultramicrotome, and post-stained with uranyl acetate and lead citrate for 15 min each prior to the TEM studies.

Membrane integrity test. To further elucidate that the fungal membrane was damaged after the treatment, the presence of 260 nm-absorbing molecules in the culture media was tested after 3 h of incubation with the nanostructures according to a previously reported protocol[18]. Briefly, overnight culture of *C. albicans* was first adjusted to contain 3×10^6 CFU ml^{-1} with sterile PBS. Antifungal solutions were prepared at different concentrations of **3b** by serial dilutions with sterile DI water. Equal volumes of fungal suspension and antifungal solution were then mixed to achieve the final **3b** concentrations ranging from MIC to 4 × MIC, and the mixture was incubated for 3 h. The microbial suspension was filtered with 0.22-mm filter to remove the fungal cells from the suspension, and the absorbance of the filtrate solution was measured at 260 nm using a ultraviolet-visible spectrophotometer (Nanodrop ND-1000, Biofrontiers Technology, Singapore). The experiment was performed in triplicate, and untreated fungal suspension was used as the negative control to normalize the absorbance reading of the experimental groups.

Biofilm formation. *C. albicans* biofilm was formed on contact lenses (Air optix, CIBA Vision). The contact lens was cut into pieces of 2 mm in diameter and transferred into a six-well plate. The samples were soaked in YMB overnight at 37 °C. Broth solution was withdrawn from the plates, followed by addition of 4 ml of *C. albicans* (10^7 CFU ml^{-1}) to each well. The plates were incubated at room temperature with shaking at 100 r.p.m. After 5 h of incubation, suspension was withdrawn and the lenses were washed by phosphate buffered saline (PBS) (pH 7.4) to remove any non-adherent cells, followed by the addition of 4 ml of fresh YMB. The plates containing the contact lenses with cells adhered were incubated at room temperature with shaking at 100 r.p.m. for 2 days to allow biofilm formation.

***In vitro* anti-biofilm assays.** Contact lenses containing biofilms were transferred to individual wells of a new 24-well plate. Biofilms were washed three times using PBS (pH 7.4) to remove non-adhered cells. Solution (500 µl) containing different concentrations of **3b** was added to each well containing biofilm, which was incubated for another day. Blank contact lenses were used as the control. After treatment, the solution was withdrawn from each well, and the biofilm was washed with PBS. The viability of cells in the biofilm was determined by XTT assay. This assay is based on the reduction of XTT tetrazolium salt to XTT formazan by mitochondrial dehydrogenases. Briefly, 200 µl of PBS containing 20 µl of XTT solution (1 mg ml^{-1}) and 4 µl of menadione solution (1 mM) were added to each well. Plates were then incubated at 37 °C for 3 h. The colorimetric change associated with cell viability was measured using the microplate reader at 490 nm. The results were expressed as a percentage of the absorbance of the untreated samples.

The ECM production was quantified by Safranin assay. Briefly, the biofilms were stained with 200 µl of aqueous solution containing 0.1% Safranin O for 15 min. The excess stain was removed by washing with PBS. The stained biofilm was solubilized with 200 µl of 70% ethanol for 15 min and the optical absorbance at 550 nm was recorded using the microplate reader. The assay was performed in four replicates for each sample, and the experiments were repeated at least three times. The readings were normalized to that of the untreated samples.

The biofilm samples before and after **3b** treatment (500 mg l^{-1}) for SEM images were prepared using a similar method as described earlier. The biofilms formed on contact lenses were also observed with confocal laser scanning fluorescence microscopy (CLSM). Briefly, contact lenses containing biofilms before and after **3b** treatment at 500 mg l^{-1} were washed three times using PBS, and transferred to individual wells of a new 24-well plate. The samples were stained with 1 ml of PBS solution containing 25 mg l^{-1} of green fluorescence CON-A (excitation wavelength: 488 nm; emission wavelength: 505 nm) and 10 µM of red fluorescence FUN-1 (excitation wavelength: 543 nm; emission wavelength: 560 nm) for 30 min at 37 °C, followed by rinsing with PBS solution. Samples were visualized by Carl Zeiss LSM 510 META confocal microscope (Germany). Three-dimensional (3D) reconstruction of images was obtained with Imaris software. All images were obtained under the same conditions.

***In vivo* toxicity evaluation.** C57BL/6 mice (8 weeks old, 18–22 g) were used for animal studies. The mice were randomly grouped. In each group, a total of three mice were used. The compound **3b** (2,000 mg l^{-1} in aqueous solution) was administered to the eyes every 5 min during the first hour and every 30 min during the next 7 h. All mice were killed after the administration of the last eye drop. The treated eyeballs were collected and fixed in 4% neutral buffered formalin. The fixed eyeballs were embedded in paraffin, sectioned and stained with hematoxylin (nucleus, blue) and eosin (cytoplasma, purple) by the standard protocol. The eyeballs treated with water were used as control.

Keratitis model. Keratitis model was established by a previously reported method[19,20]. The mice were immune suppressed via subcutaneously injecting cyclophosphamide (Sigma-Aldrich, 180 g per kg) at 5 days, 3 days and 1 day before inducing keratitis. The mice were anaesthetized by ketamine (150 mg per kg) and xylazine (10 mg ml^{-1}) by intraperitoneal injection. Additional corneal anaesthesia was also performed with 0.5% tetracaine hydrochloride eye drops (Bausch & Lomb, Tampa, Florida). A 2-mm filter paper disc moistened with 99% 1-heptanol (Sigma-Aldrich, Lausanne, Switzerland) was placed on the centre of the cornea for 40 s. The corneal epithelium was wiped off and the eyes were rinsed with PBS removing any remaining 1-heptanol. A 2 mm-diameter punch from the contact lens with *C. albicans* biofilm was then placed on the denuded cornea surface. The lids were closed with silk sutures to keep the contact lenses inside. Eye ulcer with a leathery, tough and raised surface was observed after *C. albicans* were introduced on the eyeball for 18 h. The eye lids were then opened and the lens was removed. The mice with keratitis were randomly grouped in groups of nine and treated with three topical eye drop solutions: water (control), 2,000 mg l^{-1} of **3b** and 1,500 mg l^{-1} of amphotericin B (AmB, Sigma-Aldrich, Lausanne, Switzerland). AmB was used as positive control. Eye drops (20 µl each) were administered to the mice every 5 min during the first hour and every 30 min during the next 7 h. The severity of keratitis was graded in clinical scores ranging from 1 to 12 based on the scoring system reported by Wu *et al.*[20] to evaluate treatment efficacy. A disease grading of 1–4 was assigned to the area of opacity, density of opacity and surface regularity (Supplementary Table S2). A total score of ≤ 5, 6–9 and >9 indicate mild, moderate and severe keratitis, respectively.

All mice were killed after the administration of the last eye drop. The treated eyeballs were collected immediately; three eyeballs from each group were collected for histology, and the remaining six eyeballs were homogenized (Pro200 tissue homogenizer) for quantitative analysis of fungal counts. Briefly, aliquots of serial dilutions were plated in triplicate on agar plates, and the plates were incubated for 48 h at room temperature before the colonies were counted. The number of CFUs recovered was expressed as mean $\log_{10}$ CFU per eye. The fixed eyeballs were embedded in paraffin, sectioned and stained with Grocott's methenamine silver or periodic acid-Schiff reagent by the standard protocol for histological analysis. To determine the extent of hyphal invasion into corneal stroma, each stained section obtained from cornea was imaged using a light microscope (Olympus, Japan). Three representative images per group with a total of 150 points (50 points for each image) were analysed for the absolute deepest depth of corneal penetration at each point using AutoCAD software.

Statistics analysis. The data were expressed as mean ± s.d. (s.d. is indicated by the error bars). Student's *t*-test was used to determine significance among groups. A value of $P < 0.05$ was considered to be significant.

References

1. Ostrosky-Zeichner, L., Casadevall, A., Galgiani, J. N., Odds, F. C. & Rex, J. H. An insight into the antifungal pipeline: selected new molecules and beyond. *Nat. Rev. Drug Discov.* **9**, 719–727 (2010).
2. Berman, J. & Sudbery, P. E. Candida albicans: a molecular revolution built on lessons from budding yeast. *Nat. Rev. Genet.* **3**, 918–930 (2002).
3. Wisplinghoff, H. *et al.* Nosocomial bloodstream infections in US hospitals: analysis of 24,179 cases from a prospective nationwide surveillance study. *Clin. Infect. Dis.* **39**, 309–317 (2004).
4. Anderson, J. B. Evolution of antifungal-drug resistance: Mechanisms and pathogen fitness. *Nat. Rev. Microbiol.* **3**, 547–556 (2005).
5. Cowen, L. E. The evolution of fungal drug resistance: modulating the trajectory from genotype to phenotype. *Nat. Rev. Microbiol.* **6**, 187–198 (2008).
6. Hartsel, S. & Bolard, J. Amphotericin B: new life for an old drug. *Trends Pharmacol. Sci.* **17**, 445–449 (1996).
7. Fanos, V. & Cataldi, L. Amphotericin B-induced nephrotoxicity: a review. *J. Chemother.* **12**, 463–470 (2000).

8. Brogden, K. A. Antimicrobial peptides: pore formers or metabolic inhibitors in bacteria? *Nat. Rev. Microbiol.* **3,** 238–250 (2005).
9. Nederberg, F. *et al.* Biodegradable nanostructures with selective lysis of microbial membranes. *Nat. Chem.* **3,** 409–414 (2011).
10. Liu, L. H. *et al.* Self-assembled cationic peptide nanoparticles as an efficient antimicrobial agent. *Nat. Nanotech.* **4,** 457–463 (2009).
11. Qiao, Y. *et al.* Highly dynamic biodegradable micelles capable of lysing Gram-positive and Gram-negative bacterial membrane. *Biomaterials* **33,** 1146–1153 (2011).
12. Silva, A. D. *et al.* A fundamental study on dissolution behavior of high-resolution molecular glass photoresists. *Chem. Mater.* **20,** 7292–7300 (2008).
13. Klepser, M. E., Ernst, E. J., Lewis, R. E., Ernst, M. E. & Pfaller, M. A. Influence of test conditions on antifungal time-kill curve results: proposal for standardized methods. *Antimicrob. Agents Chemother.* **42,** 1207–1212 (1998).
14. Rex, J. H. *et al.* Development of interpretive breakpoints for antifungal susceptibility testing: conceptual framework and analysis of *in vitro in vivo* correlation data for fluconazole, itraconazole, and Candida infections. *Clin. Infect. Dis.* **24,** 235–247 (1997).
15. Douglas, L. J. Candida biofilms and their role in infection. *Trends Microbiol.* **11,** 30–36 (2003).
16. Finkel, J. S. & Mitchell, A. P. Genetic control of *Candida albicans* biofilm development. *Nat. Rev. Microbiol.* **9,** 109–118 (2011).
17. Chandra, J., Mukherjee, P. K. & Ghannoum, M. A. *In vitro* growth and analysis of Candida biofilms. *Nat. Protoc.* **3,** 1909–1924 (2008).
18. Chen, C. Z. & Cooper, S. L. Interactions between dendrimer biocides and bacterial membranes. *Biomaterials* **23,** 3359–3368 (2002).
19. Goldblum, D., Frueh, B. E., Sarra, G. M., Katsoulis, K. & Zimmerli, S. Topical caspofungin for treatment of keratitis caused by *Candida albicans* in a rabbit model. *Antimicrob. Agents Chemother.* **49,** 1359–1363 (2005).
20. Wu, T. G., Wilhelmus, K. R. & Mitchell, B. M. Experimental keratomycosis in a mouse model. *Invest. Ophthalmol. Vis. Sci.* **44,** 210–216 (2003).
21. Keay, L. *et al.* Microbial keratitis: Predisposing factors and morbidity. *Ophthalmology* **113,** 109–116 (2006).
22. Wiegand, I., Hilpert, K. & Hancock, R. E. W. Agar and broth dilution methods to determine the minimal inhibitory concentration (MIC) of antimicrobial substances. *Nat. Protoc.* **3,** 163–175 (2008).
23. Dzidic, S., Suskovic, J. & Kos, B. Antibiotic resistance mechanisms in bacteria: biochemical and genetic aspects. *Food Technol. Biotechnol.* **46,** 11–21 (2008).

Acknowledgements

We would like to acknowledge the financial support from IBM Almaden Research Center, USA, and the Institute of Bioengineering and Nanotechnology (Biomedical Research Council, A*STAR, Singapore).

Author contributions

J.L.H. and Y.Y.Y. oversaw the project and project planning. J.L.H. and K.F. synthesized the compounds. S.L. performed compound characterization and biological studies. H.W. and S.L. conducted the animal study, which was supervised by J.Y.Y. A.C.E. and D.J.C. contributed to DSC analysis. H.M. conducted AFM analysis. J.P. contributed to the computational modelling. N.W. studied the release of C. albicans cytoplasmic contents. S.V. performed TEM analysis of the compounds. Y.H. and W.F. contributed to MIC and killing efficiency against *C. neoformans* and TEM of *C. neoformans*. All the authors contributed to the paper writing.

Additional information

Competing financial interests: The authors declare no competing financial interests.

11

A mitochondria-targeted inhibitor of cytochrome *c* peroxidase mitigates radiation-induced death

Jeffrey Atkinson[1,2], Alexandr A. Kapralov[1,3], Naveena Yanamala[1,4], Yulia Y. Tyurina[1,3], Andrew A. Amoscato[1,3], Linda Pearce[3], Jim Peterson[3], Zhentai Huang[1,3], Jianfei Jiang[1,3], Alejandro K. Samhan-Arias[1,3], Akihiro Maeda[1,3], Weihong Feng[1,3], Karla Wasserloos[3], Natalia A. Belikova[1,3], Vladimir A. Tyurin[1,3], Hong Wang[1,5], Jackie Fletcher[1,2], Yongsheng Wang[1,2], Irina I. Vlasova[1,3], Judith Klein-Seetharaman[4], Detcho A. Stoyanovsky[1,3], Hülya Bayîr[1,3,6], Bruce R. Pitt[3], Michael W. Epperly[1,7], Joel S. Greenberger[1,7] & Valerian E. Kagan[1,3]

The risk of radionuclide release in terrorist acts or exposure of healthy tissue during radiotherapy demand potent radioprotectants/radiomitigators. Ionizing radiation induces cell death by initiating the selective peroxidation of cardiolipin in mitochondria by the peroxidase activity of its complex with cytochrome *c* leading to release of haemoprotein into the cytosol and commitment to the apoptotic program. Here we design and synthesize mitochondria-targeted triphenylphosphonium-conjugated imidazole-substituted oleic and stearic acids that blocked peroxidase activity of cytochrome *c*/cardiolipin complex by specifically binding to its haem-iron. We show that both compounds inhibit pro-apoptotic oxidative events, suppress cyt *c* release, prevent cell death, and protect mice against lethal doses of irradiation. Significant radioprotective/radiomitigative effects of imidazole-substituted oleic acid are observed after pretreatment of mice from 1 h before through 24 h after the irradiation.

[1] Center for Free Radical and Antioxidant Health and Center for Medical Countermeasures against Radiation, University of Pittsburgh, Bridgeside Point, 100 Technology Drive, Suite 350, Pittsburgh, Pennsylvania 15219, USA. [2] Department of Chemistry & Centre for Biotechnology Brock University, St Catharines, Ontario, L2S 3A1 Canada. [3] Departments of Environmental and Occupational Health, University of Pittsburgh, 3501 Fifth Avenue, BST3 Rm. 2051, Pittsburgh, Pennsylvania 15219, USA. [4] Department of Structural Biology, University of Pittsburgh, Bridgeside Point, 100 Technology Drive, Suite 350, Pittsburgh, Pennsylvania 15261, USA. [5] Department of Biostatistics, Graduate School of Public Health, University of Pittsburgh, 201 North Craig Street, Suite 325 Sterling Plaza, Pittsburgh, Pennsylvania 15213, USA. [6] Department of Critical Care Medicine, School of Medicine, University of Pittsburgh, 3550 Terrace Street, Pittsburgh, Pennsylvania 15261, USA. [7] Department of Radiation Oncology, University of Pittsburgh Cancer Institute, 5150 Centre Avenue, Rm. 533, Pittsburgh, Pennsylvania 15232, USA. Correspondence and requests for materials should be addressed to V.E.K. (email: kagan@pitt.edu).

Despite having evolved from organisms adapted to massive irradiation during the early development of Earth's biosphere, the human body—with its abundance of water—is vulnerable to radiolysis by high-energy (ionizing) irradiation. Medical applications of irradiation critically consider this sensitivity of normal tissues, particularly in the use of total body exposure for bone marrow transplantation patients. However, in uncontrolled situations of exposure to radiation, such as during a terrorist attack, or the unavoidable radiation exposure of flight crews during extended space missions, the development of protective measures is lagging behind, and there is an immediate need for the stockpiling of safe and effective radioprotectors/radiomitigators.

Acute radiation syndrome is associated with damage to the haematopoietic system and gastrointestinal tract due to massive cell loss in radiosensitive tissues occurring largely via apoptosis[1–3]. Along with radicals generated by radiolysis of water, the execution of mitochondria-mediated apoptosis is universally associated with the production of reactive oxygen species[4,5]. Therefore, development of radiomitigators/radioprotectors for biodefense applications and radiotherapy has mostly focused on nonspecific thiol-based antioxidants that have shown clinically insignificant results[6–8]. Recently, reactive oxygen species production has been identified as a required step in selective peroxidation of a mitochondria-specific phospholipid, cardiolipin (CL), whose oxidation products are essential for the outer membrane permeabilization and release of pro-apoptotic factors[4,9]. The catalyst of the peroxidation reaction is cytochrome *c* (cyt *c*) that forms a high-affinity complex with CL exhibiting potent peroxidase activity towards polyunsaturated CLs[9]. In normal mitochondria, CL and cyt *c* are spatially separated: the former is confined almost exclusively to the inner mitochondrial membrane, whereas the latter is located in the intermembrane space[10]. Early in apoptosis, CL migrates from the inner to the outer mitochondrial membrane—a process likely facilitated by one of the four candidate mitochondrial proteins: scramblase-3, nucleoside diphosphate kinase, mitochondrial isoforms of creatine kinase and t-Bid[11–13]. Trans-membrane re-distribution of CL makes physical interaction of CL and cyt *c* possible resulting in the formation of cyt *c*/CL complexes[9]. Several previous studies have proposed that there are two types of interaction of cyt *c* with anionic phospholipids: an electrostatic interaction and a specific hydrophobic interaction. Whereas the electrostatic interaction is mainly driven by the charges between the protein and anionic lipids, the hydrophobic interaction involves the insertion of the lipid acyl chain in a hydrophobic channel present in the structure of cyt *c*. It has been shown that both interactions are essential for initiating the peroxidase activity of cyt *c*[9] leading to peroxidation of bound polyunsaturated molecular species of CL. Notably, accumulation of peroxidized CL is essential for the execution of the apoptotic program. Conversely, prevention of CL peroxidation leads to inhibition of apoptosis[14].

In the present study, we reason that the new 'pro-oxidant' enzymatic activity of cyt *c*/CL complexes represents a target for anti-apoptotic radioprotective drugs. Specifically, the peroxidase activity is due to CL-induced partial unfolding of the protein in the complex resulting in a 'loosened' liganding capacity of haem-iron by a distal Met_{80} (ref. 15). We hypothesize that 'locking' of the haem-iron coordination bond with a strong ligand delivered through the hydrophobic channel to the immediate proximity of the haem catalytic site would block the peroxidase activity, inhibit CL peroxidation and prevent the progression of apoptosis. Indeed, we demonstrate that mitochondria-targeted 3-hydroxypropyl-triphenylphosphonium (TPP)-conjugated imidazole-substituted oleic acid (**TPP-IOA**) and stearic acid (**TPP-ISA**) exert strong specific liganding of haem-iron in cyt *c*/CL complex, effectively suppressing its peroxidase activity and CL peroxidation, thus preventing cyt *c* release and cell death, and protecting mice against lethal doses of irradiation.

Results

Molecular modelling and docking studies. We have designed (Fig. 1) and synthesized (Supplementary Fig. S1) imidazole-substituted fatty acids and their esters—imidazole substituted oleic acid (**IOA**), stearic acid (**ISA**) (Fig. 1a,b), imidazole substituted methyl ester of oleic acid (**IEOA**, Fig. 1c) and imidazole substituted dodecanoic acid (**IDA**) (Fig. 1d)—assuming that these compounds will interact with cyt *c* by providing the imidazole group as a sixth ligand to the haem. A similar strategy was used to inhibit the terminal oxidation of fatty acids by CYP4A1 (ref. 16). Molecular modelling and docking studies of partially unfolded cyt *c* showed that 18-carbon-long **IOA** and **ISA** (Fig. 2a–c) as well as **IEOA** (Fig. 2d) with the imidazole moiety 7-carbon atoms away from the terminal methyl group indeed positioned the heterocycle close to haem such that the nitrogen atom of imidazole was within 2.4 Å (**IOA**), 2.5 Å (**IEOA**) and 2.7 Å (**ISA**) from the haem-iron. A hydrophobic channel formed by the displacement of the Met_{80}-containing loop in the partially unfolded cyt *c* structure stabilized the interaction (Fig. 2b, coloured in yellow). Notably, the truncated derivative **IDA**, with the imidazole-moiety attached to the terminal CH_2-group, this specific positioning was not achieved and the imidazole nitrogen was 6.9 Å away from the haem-iron (Fig. 2e).

Suppression of peroxidase activity of cyt *c* complexes. We next evaluated the effect of **ISA**, **IOA** and **IEOA** on the peroxidase activity of cyt *c* complexes with tetra-oleoyl-cardiolipin (TOCL) towards H_2O_2-driven oxidation of two prototypical phenolic substrates, Amplex Red (Fig. 3a) and etoposide (Fig. 3b). We found that **ISA**, **IOA** and **IEOA** acted as potent inhibitors of the peroxidase activity of cyt *c*/TOCL complexes with both substrates (Fig. 3). Computer modelling showed that **IOA** (Fig. 2a), **IEOA** (Fig. 2d) and **ISA** (Fig. 2c) bind to cyt *c* in a similar fashion. The truncated derivative **IDA**, did not exert any inhibitory effect (Fig. 3a), in line with our computer modelling data. Because catalytic reactive intermediates of cyt *c*/CL peroxidase complexes—protein-immobilized (tyrosyl) radicals (Tyr•)—can be detected by electron paramagnetic resonance (EPR) spectroscopy[17], we studied the effect of **IEOA** and **IOA** on H_2O_2-dependent formation of radicals (Fig. 3c). Both **IOA** and **IEOA** (but not **IDA**) effectively quenched generation of Tyr• radicals. Finally, we assessed the ability of **ISA** and **IEOA** to inhibit peroxidase activity using isolated mouse liver mitochondria.

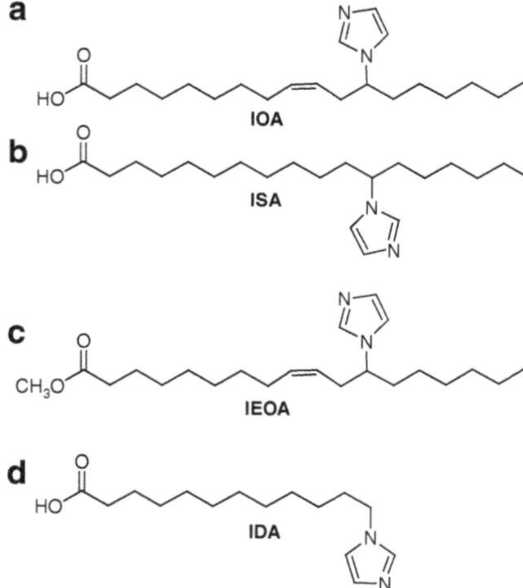

Figure 1 | Structural formulas of synthesized compounds. (**a**) 12-(1H-imidazol-1-yl)-(Z)-octadec-9-enoic acid (**IOA**); (**b**) 12-(1H-imidazol-1-yl) octadecanoic acid (**ISA**); (**c**) methyl 12-(imidazol-1-yl)-(Z)-octadec-9-enoate (**IEOA**); (**d**) 12-(imidazol-1yl)-dodecanoic acid (**IDA**). Synthetic and experimental details are provided in Supplementary Methods.

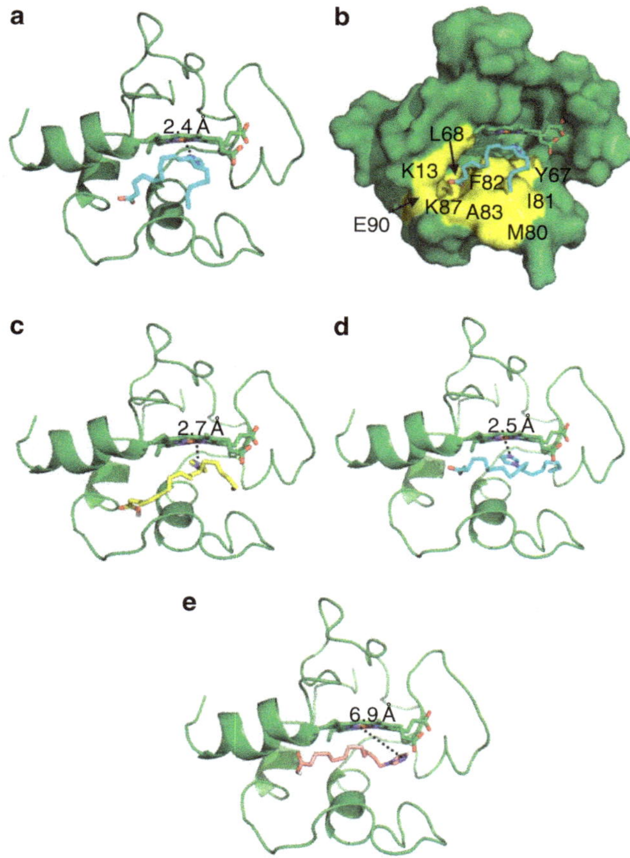

Figure 2 | Modelling of the binding of imidazole substituted fatty acids. (**a**,**b**) **IOA**, (**c**) **ISA**, (**d**) **IEOA**, and (**e**) **IDA**. Cyt *c* is coloured in green and represented as cartoon in (**a**,**c**,**d**,**e**) and as surface in (**b**). **IOA**, **IEOA**, **ISA**, **TPP-IOA**, **TPP-ISA**, **IDA** and haem are represented as sticks. **IOA** and **IEOA** are coloured in cyan; **ISA** is coloured in yellow and **IDA** is coloured in wheat. The hydrophobic surface corresponding to the predicted **IOA** binding site is coloured in yellow (**b**).

To avoid decomposition of H_2O_2 by catalase, we used *tert*-butyl hydroperoxide (tBOOH) as a source of oxidizing equivalents. Both **ISA** and **IEOA** suppressed peroxidase activity in a concentration-dependent manner (Supplementary Fig. S2).

Liganding of haem-iron in cyt *c*/TOCL complexes. To address whether **ISA** and **IEOA** act as strong ligands of haem-iron in cyt *c*/TOCL complexes, we used low-temperature EPR spectroscopy[18]. In the reduced form, cyt *c*/TOCL binds NO$^{\bullet}$ to produce haem-nitrosylated complexes with characteristic EPR spectra[9]. Indeed, at 77 K, typical spectra of penta-, and hexa-coordinated cyt *c* were detectable on incubation of cyt *c*/TOCL complexes in the presence of a source of nitroxyl (HNO), Angeli's salt (Fig. 3d). **ISA** and **IEOA** (Fig. 3d) caused a concentration-dependent decrease of the EPR signal. To provide evidence for coordination changes of the haem-iron in cyt *c*, we performed liquid-He EPR measurements. The X-band EPR spectrum of native ferri-cyt *c* at pH 7.4, recorded at 20 K, exhibited anisotropic, low-spin signals, with $g_z = 3.09$, $g_y = 2.24$ and $g_x \sim 1$ (usually unobserved) (Fig. 3e) indicative of His/Met axial coordination at the haem[19,20]. On the addition of **IOA**, there was no change in the EPR spectrum indicating retention of the native His/Met axial coordination (Fig. 3e). However, when **IOA** was added to the cyt *c*/TOCL complex, the EPR spectrum revealed the presence of another low-spin species ($g_z = 2.97$, $g_y = 2.27$, $g_x \sim 1.5$, Fig. 3e) with *g*-values entirely consistent with His/imidazole coordination[20,21].

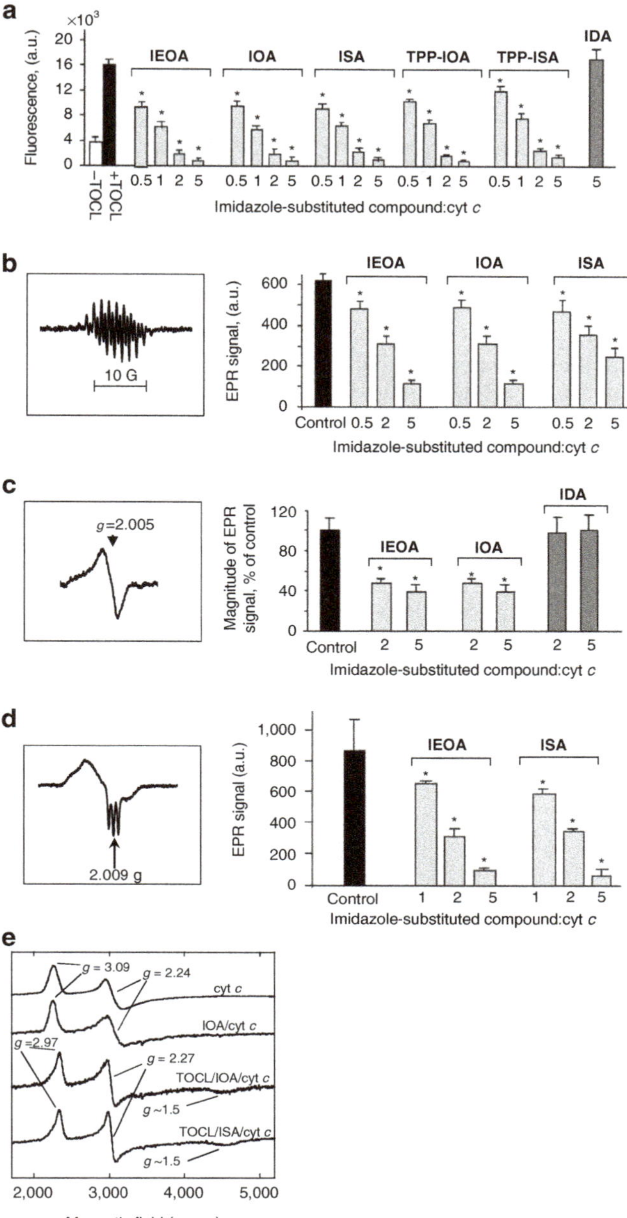

Figure 3 | Inhibition of peroxidase activity of cyt *c*/TOCL complexes. (**a**) Assessments of peroxidase activity of cyt *c*/TOCL by H_2O_2-induced oxidation of Amplex Red to resorufin. Data are means±s.d., $n = 4$, $*P < 0.01$ (Student's *t*-test) versus control (TOCL/cyt *c*/H_2O_2 with no **ISA** or **IOA** or **IEOA** or **TPP-IOA** or **TPP-ISA** added). (**b**) A typical EPR spectrum of etoposide phenoxyl radicals (left panel). Assessments of peroxidase activity of cyt *c*/TOCL by H_2O_2-induced oxidation of etoposide using EPR spectroscopy (right panel). (**c**) A typical low-temperature EPR spectrum of protein-immobilized (tyrosine) radicals (left panel). Assessments of protein-immobilized (tyrosine) radicals by low-temperature (77 K) EPR spectroscopy (right panel). (**d**) **ISA** and **IEOA** limit accessibility of haem to small molecules. A typical low-temperature (77 K) EPR spectrum of cyt *c*/TOCL complexes in the presence of Angeli's salt (left panel). Effects of **ISA** and **IEOA** on haem-nitrosylation of cyt *c*/TOCL induced by nitroxyl (HNO) generated from Angeli's salt (right panel). Data are means±s.d., $n = 3$, $*P < 0.05$ versus control (no **ISA** and **IEOA** added). (**e**) Liquid-He EPR evidence for ligation change in cyt *c* haem-iron. X-band liquid-He (20 K) EPR spectra of cyt *c*.

This signal was broadened on the low-field side, suggesting a combination of the native ferri-cyt *c* and a His/imidazole form. Spectral simulations (not shown) confirm an ~50:50 mixture of the native structure and the form in which Met_{80} has been replaced by the imidazole moiety of **IOA**. These were the only signals observed; in particular, there were none at *g* ~6, indicating the absence of any penta- or hexacoordinate high-spin species. Similarly, **ISA** was able to change haem-iron coordination in cyt *c*, whereby Met_{80} was substituted by the imidazole moiety (Fig. 3e). These results confirm experimentally that the imidazole moiety of imidazole fatty acids can indeed serve as a coordinating ligand for the haem substituting for Met_{80} ligation.

Inhibition of apoptosis by TPP-ISA and TPP-IOA. We then explored the ability of imidazole substituted fatty acids to inhibit apoptosis in cells. To target imidazole substituted fatty acids into mitochondria, we esterified them with TPP-derived propanol (Fig. 4a,b), an organic cationic alcohol with delocalized electron density—known to be effectively 'electrophoresed' because of the negative potential on the inside of the organelle's membrane[22]. By using computer modelling, we confirmed that conjugation of **ISA** and **IOA** with TPP did not significantly affect their positioning within the immediate proximity of the cyt *c*'s haem-iron, that is, the nitrogen atom of the imidazole of both **TPP-IOA** and **TPP-ISA** was within 2.9 Å from the haem-iron (Fig. 4c,d). Moreover, **TPP-ISA** and **TPP-IOA** were as effective as non-conjugated **ISA** and **IOA** in inhibiting peroxidase activity of cyt *c*/TOCL complexes (Fig. 3).

We further estimated the amounts of accumulated **TPP-IOA** in mitochondria of mouse embryonic cells using high-performance liquid chromatography (HPLC) and electrospray ionization mass spectrometry (ESI-MS) (Supplementary Fig. S3). We found that most of **TPP-IOA** was present in mitochondria (Supplementary Fig. S3). Assuming that the volume of mitochondria constitutes ~15–25% of the total volume of a cell, the mitochondrial enrichment factor becomes even greater such that the concentration of **TPP-IOA** in mitochondria may be as high as ~5 mM. It is likely that endogenous esterases can hydrolyse the ester-bond and release **IOA** and TPP-derived Propanol. To test this, we performed assessments of esterase activity of mitochondria and cytosolic fractions isolated from mouse embryonic cells based on HPLC measurements of **TPP-IOA** (Supplementary Fig. S3). We found that hydrolysis of **TPP-IOA** takes place in both mitochondria and the cytosol. The hydrolysis rate in mitochondria was comparable to that in the cytosolic fraction (Supplementary Fig. S3). Thus, both **TPP-IOA** and its de-esterifed form, **IOA**, could be present in mitochondria of mouse embryonic cells. Because TPP-conjugated imidazole-substituted fatty acids effectively partition into mitochondria, we examined whether they affected bioenergetic functions, particularly ATP production. Neither **TPP-IOA** nor **TPP-ISA** had any effect on ATP levels in mouse embryonic cells. Normally, mitochondria are the major source of superoxide radicals in mouse embryonic cells[23,24]. Assessments

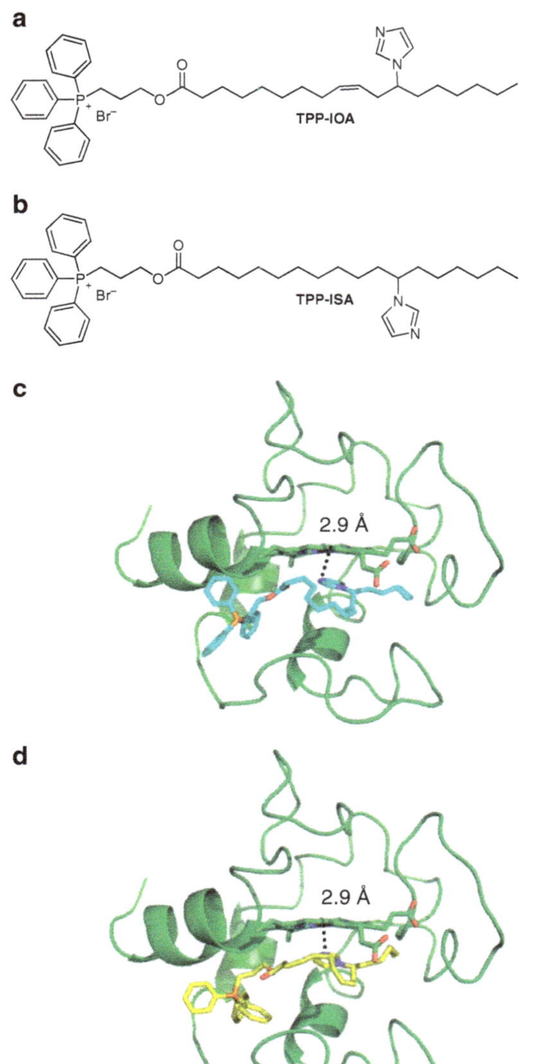

Figure 4 | Structures and molecular modelling of TPP-IOA and TPP-ISA. (**a**,**c**) 9-(Z)-(3-((12-imidazol-1-yl)octadeca-9-enoyloxy)propyl)triphenyl phosphonium bromide (**TPP-IOA**); (**b**,**d**) (3-(12-imidazol-1-yl)-octadecanoyl) propyl)triphenylphosphonium bromide (**TPP-ISA**); **TPP-IOA** is coloured in cyan, **TPP-ISA** is coloured in yellow.

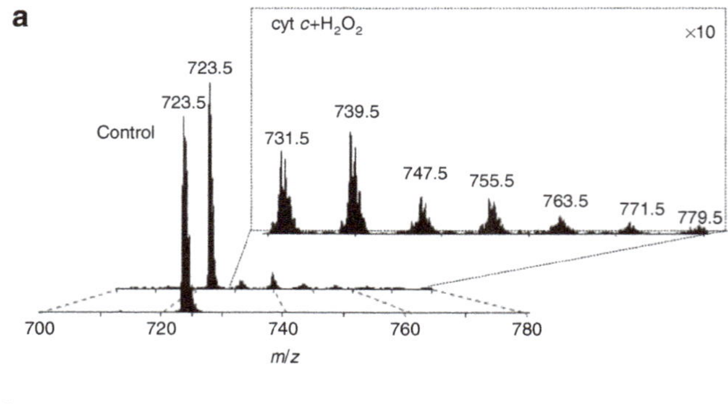

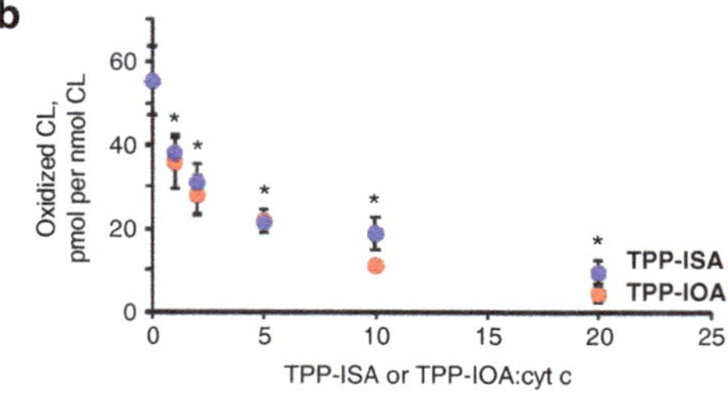

Figure 5 | Inhibition of H_2O_2-induced TLCL peroxidation. (**a**) Typical ESI mass spectra of doubly charged molecular ions of non-oxidized TLCL and TLCL oxidized by CL/cyt *c* and H_2O_2. Mass-to-charge (*m/z*; negative MS mode) values of 723.5 and 731.5, 739.5, 747.5, 755.5, 763.5, 771.5 and 779.5 were assigned to molecular clusters of non-oxidized TLCL and TLCL enriched with 1-7 oxygen atoms, respectively. (**b**) Quantitative assessment of TLCL and its oxidation products by ESI-MS. Data are means±s.d., $n=3$, $^{*}P<0.05$ (ANOVA) versus TLCL/cyt *c*/H_2O_2.

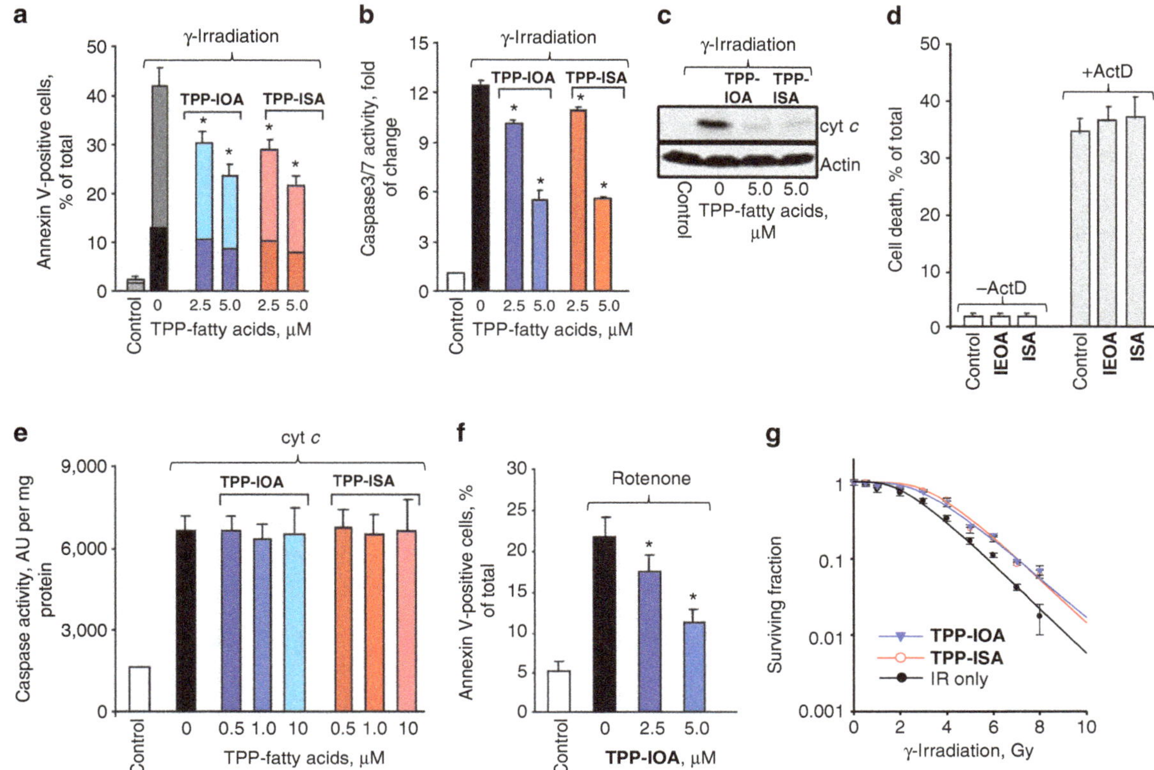

Figure 6 | Mitigative effects of TPP-ISA and TPP-IOA against apoptosis. Effect of **TPP-ISA** and **TPP-IOA** on γ-irradiation induced PS externalization (dark colour—Annexin V-positive, PI-positive cells; light colour—Annexin V-positive, PI negative cells) (**a**), caspase 3/7 activation (**b**), and cyt c release from mitochondria into the cytosol (anti-cyt c antibody, $0.2\,\mu g\,ml^{-1}$, 1:3,000, Pharmmingen) (**c**) in mouse embryonic cells. Cells were γ-irradiated to a dose of 10 Gy, and then incubated in the presence of different concentrations of **TPP-ISA** or **TPP-IOA** for 48 h. Data are means±s.d., $n=3$. *$P<0.01$ (Student's *t*-test) versus irradiated only cells. **TPP-ISA** or **TPP-IOA** was added to cells 30 min after γ-radiation. (**d**) Effect of **IEOA** and **ISA** on actinomycin D-induced cell death in mouse embryonic cells. **IEOA** or **ISA** were incubated in the presence of fatty acid-free bovine serum albumin (BSA) (Sigma) at a molar ratio of 5:1 at 37 °C for 30 min. Mouse embryonic cells were incubated with **IEOA**/BSA or **ISA**/BSA (100 μM) complexes for 30 min before the addition of $100\,ng\,ml^{-1}$ actinomycin D (ActD). After 18-h incubation with ActD, cell viability was analysed by flow cytometry using an Annexin V/PI kit. ActD-induced cell death in ~34.2% of cells. Treatment of cells with **ISA** or **IEOA** in concentrations ranging from 1 to 100 μM exerted no detectable protection against ActD-induced cell death. Representative data with 100 μM **IEOA**/BSA and **ISA**/BSA complexes are shown. Data are means±s.d., $n=3$. (**e**) Effect of **TPP-ISA** and **TPP-IOA** on caspase-3 activation in S-100 from mouse embryonic cells. Data are means±s.d., $n=3$. (**f**) Effect of **TPP-IOA** on mouse lung endothelial cells treated with rotenone (apoptosis was assessed by PS externalization). Data are means±s.d., $n=3$. *$P<0.05$ (Student's *t*-test) versus rotenone challenged cells. (**g**) Effect of **TPP-ISA** and **TPP-IOA** on clonogenic survival of mouse embryonic cells after γ-irradiation. The data were fitted to a single-hit multi-target model. Data are means±s.d., $n=3$. **TPP-IOA** or **TPP-ISA** was added to cells 30 min after γ-radiation.

of intracellular superoxide production using dihydroethidium showed that neither **TPP-IOA** nor **TPP-ISA** had any effect on superoxide production in cells with or without radiation treatment (Supplementary Fig. S4).

For the anti-apoptotic action, it is essential that proposed haem-iron ligation is effective in inhibiting peroxidation of polyunsaturated species of CL. Therefore, we used an oxidizable tetra-linoleoyl-cardiolipin (TLCL), and conducted experiments on its cyt c/H_2O_2-induced oxidation (Fig. 5). In the presence of H_2O_2, we detected accumulation of characteristic TLCL peroxidation products with multiple oxygenated linoleic acid residues detectable by ESI-MS (Fig. 5a). We found that both **TPP-IOA** and **TPP-ISA** inhibited cyt c/H_2O_2-induced oxidation of TLCL in a concentration-dependent manner. No difference in inhibition of TLCL oxidation between **TPP-IOA** and **TPP-ISA** was detected. The oxidation of TLCL was completely blocked at a ratio of cyt *c* to **TPP-IOA** or **TPP-ISA** of 1:20 (Fig. 5b).

We then employed a model of intrinsic apoptosis induced in mouse embryonic cells by γ-irradiation and assessed several biomarkers of apoptosis. We found that **TPP-IOA** and **TPP-ISA** had similar radiation mitigating effects on mouse embryonic cells as evidenced by phosphatidylserine (PS) externalization (Fig. 6a), caspase 3/7 activation (Fig. 6b) and cyt *c* release (Fig. 6c). In contrast, **IEOA** or **ISA**—devoid of a mitochondria-targeting TPP-moiety—exerted no protection against apoptosis in mouse embryonic cells (Fig. 6d). To verify that the protective effects were realized during mitochondrial stages of apoptosis, **TPP-ISA** were added to the *in vitro* 'caspase activation system' containing S100 fraction from mouse embryonic cells[25]. Caspase activation caused by exogenously added cyt *c* was completely insensitive to **TPP-ISA** and **TPP-IOA** (Fig. 6e) thus confirming that anti-apoptotic effects of **TPP-IOA** and **TPP-ISA** were realized in mitochondria. Furthermore, the anti-apoptotic activity was neither cell- nor stimulus-specific, as **TPP-IOA** effectively inhibited apoptosis, induced by a mitochondrial complex I inhibitor, rotenone, in cultured mouse lung endothelial cells (Fig. 6f).

Mitochondria are believed to be involved in orchestration of different cell death pathways[26,27]. We found that necrotic cells (propidium iodide (PI)-positive, Annexin V-positive) represented 12.9% while apoptotic cells (PI-negative, Annexin V-positive) were accountable for 28.9% of total PS-positive cells detectable after irradiation.

Treatment with **TPP-IOA** caused a twofold decrease in the number of apoptotic cells (to 14.8%) and 1.6-fold reduction in the number of necrotic cells (to 8.2%). Similarly, **TPP-ISA** protected via both anti-apoptotic and anti-necrotic mechanisms (to 13.9% of apoptotic and 7.8% necrotic cells, respectively). Overall, these results suggest that **PP-IOA** and **TPP-ISA** afforded the radiomitigation in mouse embryonic cells acting through both anti-apoptotic and anti-necrotic pathways. In addition to apoptosis, and necrosis, mitotic cell death can be also triggered in irradiated cells. Using clonogenic assay, that includes the mitotic cell death component, we demonstrated that post-irradiation treatment of mouse embryonic cells with **TPP-ISA** or **TPP-IOA** resulted in a significant protection. Using a single-hit multi-target model, we estimated that **TPP-ISA** or **TPP-IOA** increased D_0—the dose needed to reduce cell surviving fraction to 37% (1/*e*)—to 1.67±0.06 and 1.71±0.05, respectively, compared with 1.33±0.08 in untreated cells (Fig. 6g).

Radiomitigative effects of of TPP-IOA and TPP-ISA. Given the ability of **TPP-IOA** and **TPP-ISA** to act as radiomitigators *in vitro*, we assessed their potential to act as radioprotectors/radiomitigators *in vivo*. C57BL/6NTac female mice were exposed to 9.25 Gy total body irradiation at the dose rate of 80 cGy min^{-1} using the cesium irradiator. Three independent experiments (the total number of mice in each group was 31–35) yielded similar results: irradiation resulted in death of animals within 13–15 days (with survival of only 20% of animals by day 30). **TPP-IOA** or **TPP-ISA** (i.p. injection, 5 mg per kg body weight, 10 min after irradiation) showed a strong radiomitigative effect for both compounds (Fig. 7a). There was no statistically significant difference in radiomitigative potency of **TPP-IOA** and **TPP-ISA** (P=0.6389, a two-sided log-rank test). We also used a clinical linear accelerator to deliver the radiation dose. The mice (three groups with 22–23 animals in each) were irradiated to 9.25 Gy at the dose rate of 100 cGy min^{-1} using a Varian TrueBeam linear accelerator (Varian Medical Systems) and injected i.p. with 5 mg per kg body weight of either **TPP-ISA** or **TPP-IOA**, 10 min after irradiation. Similarly to the results with cesium irradiator, the survival curves over 52 days were statistically different for **TPP-IOA** (5 mg per kg body weight) and **TPP-ISA** (5 mg per kg body weight) versus irradiated controls (Table 1); however, there was no statistically significant difference between **TPP-IOA** and **TPP-ISA** (P=0.4567, a two-sided log-rank test). Thus, after multiple experiments, using two different irradiators, we demonstrated a high potency of both **TPP-IOA** and **TPP-ISA** in mitigating radiation damage without significant difference in radiomitigative activity between them. Therefore, all subsequent *in vivo* experiments were conducted with **TPP-IOA** and linear accelerator as the radiation source. We chose a dose of 5 mg per kg body weight of **TPP-IOA**, because a lower dose (2.5 mg per kg body weight) of drug was not effective in mitigating the mice against irradiation. When mice (10 per group) were irradiated and administered 2.5 mg per kg body weight (10 min after irradiation), there was a trend towards a greater survival that, however, did not reach the level of significance (P=0.0525, a two-sided log-rank test) (Table 1). We further tested whether **TPP-IOA** was protective if given at later time points (than 10 min) after irradiation (10 mice per group). Administration of **TPP-IOA** at 5 or 24 h after irradiation resulted in a significant increase in survival (Fig. 7b, Table 1). **TPP-IOA** was also protective if given 10 min or 1 h before irradiation (Fig. 7b; Table 1).

Given the high radioprotective/radiomitigative activity of **TPP-IOA**, we determined the extent to which it would be absorbed to reach radiosensitive tissues. This required the development of new LC-MS/MS protocols to quantitate **TPP-IOA** in tissue samples. These involved the establishment of a selective reaction monitoring protocol for **TPP-IOA** that provides high selectivity and sensitivity. Our direct assessments clearly demonstrated the presence of **TPP-IOA** in plasma (Supplementary Fig. S5) as well as in the two most important radiosensitive tissues, bone marrow and small intestine. **TPP-IOA** levels were highest in plasma (54.0 ng ml^{-1} of plasma), followed by small intestine (1.5 ng per g of tissue) and bone marrow (0.2 ng per g of tissue), at the 10 min time point after i.p. injection. The levels measured in plasma are consistent with those found for decyl-TPP, a closely related compound, as seen in the study by Porteous *et al.*[28] We showed that, after intravenous injection, the TPP-compounds are distributed rapidly to various tissues and less than 1% remains in plasma after 15 min. In addition, we assessed the hydrolysis of **TPP-IOA** in tissues (plasma, bone marrow and small intestine) yielding TPP and non-esterified **IOA** utilizing two different LC-MS/MS approaches: a selected reaction monitoring method to determine the levels of **IOA**, a likely hydrolysis product of **TPP-IOA**, in tissue samples, and multiple reaction monitoring

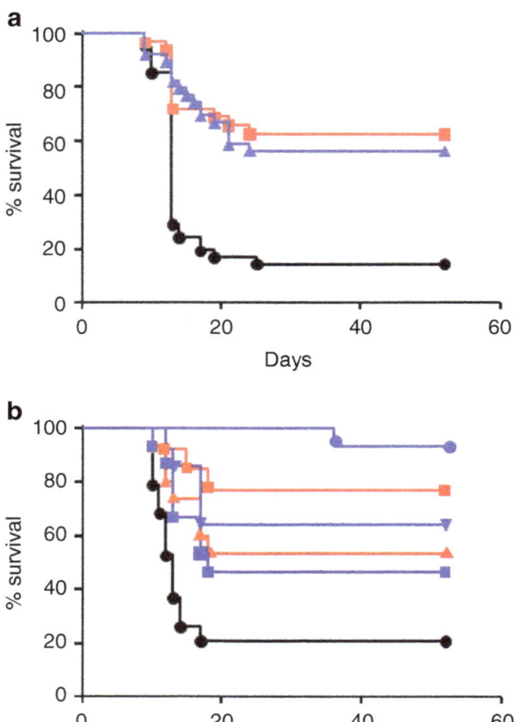

Figure 7 | Radiation protection and mitigation by TPP-IOA and TPP-ISA. C57BL/6NTac female mice were exposed to total body irradiation to a dose of 9.25 Gy using a cesium source (n=31–35 mice per group) (**a**) or a linear accelerator (n=10–23 mice per group) (**b**). (**a**) The mice were irradiated and injected i.p. with **TPP-IOA** or **TPP-ISA** (5 mg per kg body weight in 100 µl of water containing 25% ethanol) 10 min after irradiation. Mice exposed to: total body irradiation at the dose of 9.25 Gy only (black circles); to total body irradiation at the dose of 9.25 Gy and injected with **TPP-ISA** (5 mg per kg body weight) 10 min (blue triangles) or **TPP-IOA** (5 mg per kg body weight) 10 min (red squares) thereafter. P<0.0001 (a two-sided log-rank test)—**TPP-IOA** or **TPP-ISA** injected and exposed to total body irradiation mice versus mice exposed to total body irradiation only. (**b**) The mice were injected i.p. with **TPP-IOA** (5 mg per kg body weight in 100 µl of water containing 25% ethanol) at 1 h or 10 min before irradiation or 10 min, 5 or 24 h after irradiation. Mice exposed to: total body irradiation at the dose of 9.25 Gy only (black circles); to total body irradiation at the dose of 9.25 Gy and injected with **TPP-IOA** (5 mg per kg body weight) 10 min (blue circles), 5 h (blue triangles) and 24 h (blue squares) thereafter. Mice injected with **TPP-IOA** (5 mg per kg body weight) 10 min (red squares) and 1 h (red triangles) before total body irradiation (9.25 Gy). For assessments of significance see Table 1.

Table 1 | TPP-IOA and TPP-ISA increase survival of mice following irradiation.

Treatment group	Overall survival (52 days)		Survival over first 20 days		N
	Median survival (95% confidence interval)	P*	Median survival (95% confidence interval)	P*	
9.25 Gy	13 (11, 14)		13 (11, 14)		22
TPP-IOA 5 mg per kg body weight, 1 h before 9.25 Gy	— (12, —)	0.0230	— (12, —)	0.0230	10
TPP-IOA 5 mg per kg body weight, 10 min before 9.25 Gy	— (18, —)	0.0009	— (18, —)	0.0009	10
TPP-IOA 5 mg per kg body weight, 10 min after 9.25 Gy	— (—, —)	<0.00010.4567†	— (—, —)	<0.0001	23
TPP-IOA 5 mg per kg body weight, hr after 9.25 Gy	— (17, —)	0.0030	— (17, —)	0.0030	10
TPP-IOA 5 mg per kg body weight, 24 h after 9.25 Gy	18 (13, —)	0.0416	18 (13, —)	0.0416	10
TPP-IOA 2.5 mg per kg body weight, 10 min after 9.25 Gy	17 (14, —)	0.0525	17 (14, —)	0.0525	10
TPP-ISA 5.0 mg per kg body weight 10 min after 9.25 Gy	— (13, —)	0.0114	— (13, —)	0.0114	22

The two-sided log-rank test was used to examine the differences between irradiated mice with or without treatment with **TPP-ISA** or **TPP-IOA**.
Mice were irradiated to 9.25 Gy using a Varian TrueBeam linear accelerator (Varian Medical Systems) and injected i.p. with either **TPP-ISA** or **TPP-IOA** (2.5 or 5 mg per kg body weight in 100 µl of water containing 25% ethanol) at 1 h or 10 min before irradiation or 10 min, 5 or 24 h after irradiation.
***TPP-IOA** and **TPP-ISA** versus irradiated mice.
†**TPP-IOA** (5 mg per kg body weight 10 min after irradiation) versus **TPP-ISA** (5 mg per kg body weight 10 min after irradiation).

offering extremely high selectivity and sensitivity (Supplementary Fig. S6). Using these approaches, we determined that bone marrow had the least amount of hydrolysis, exhibiting a level of 0.6 ng per g tissue per min of the TPP-propyl hydrolysis product. This was followed by a level of 4.1 ng per g tissue per min and 19.0 ng per g tissue per min of the TPP hydrolysis product in plasma and small intestine, respectively. Simple calculations show that the total amounts of non-hydrolysed **TPP-IOA** plus hydrolysed (**IOA** + TPP) will be significantly (approximately two orders of magnitude) higher than those of the non-hydrolysed compound measured in the small intestine and bone marrow. The importance of this is underscored by our data that both **TPP-IOA** and **IOA** are effective inhibitors of peroxidase activity of cyt *c*/CL complexes (Fig. 3) and CL peroxidation (Fig. 5).

Discussion

In this work, we designed, synthesized and explored a new class of mechanism-based mitochondria-targeted inhibitors that act as strong ligands of iron in complexes of cyt *c* with CL. The compounds 'lock' the catalytic site of the enzymatic complex, inhibiting its ability to facilitate the development of pro-apoptotic oxidative events, and suppress release of cyt *c* from mitochondria into the cytosol thus inhibiting apoptotic cell death. We demonstrated that imidazole fatty acids specifically interact with partially unfolded cyt *c* and not with intact cyt *c*. Indeed, low-temperature (He) EPR experiments indicate that liganding of haem-iron in cyt *c* by **IOA** was dependent on the presence of CL. While it is possible that imidazole fatty acids may interact with other haemoproteins—for example, cytochromes P450 (ref. 16) their effects on the oxygenase/peroxidase activity of the haemoproteins might depend on several parameters such as redox potential, haem-coordination state, spin states. Notably, many haemoproteins with peroxidase function—cytochromes P450, myeloperoxidase, cyclooxygenase—do not require anionic (phospho)lipids for their activation.

Importantly, **TPP-ISA** and **TPP-IOA** exerted strong radoprotective/radiomitigative effects *in vivo* against lethal doses of irradiation of mice (from 1 h before through 24 h after the irradiation). One can envision two possible applications of our findings in clinical practice. One of them may be associated with the employment of the newly discovered radiomitigators for the treatment of victims of terrorist attacks with nuclear devices as well as individuals inadvertently exposed to irradiation resulting from catastrophic nuclear accidents. Intraperitoneal (i.p.) injections of **TPP-IOA** and **TPP-ISA** employed in this study is not the preferred route of drug administration in clinical practice, although it has been used for selected drugs in several disease states[29–31]. It is likely that pharmacologists would have to derive new formulations that could be given orally or as a skin patch. For radiation counterterrorism, a topical or trans-dermal delivery system would be preferred.

The second kind of applications may be relevant to organ-specific delivery of **TPP-IOA** and **TPP-ISA** to protect normal tissues from ionizing irradiation effects in clinical radiotherapy. Several highly effective chemotherapy drugs are known to interact with ionizing irradiation to promote tumour cell killing, but unfortunately, also exacerbate normal tissue toxicity. Local, tissue-specific delivery of **TPP-IOA** and **TPP-ISA** may be also important in amelioration of the toxicity of this combined modality cancer therapy. The design of a pharmacological formulation by which to facilitate delivery of **TPP-IOA** and **TPP-ISA** to the oral cavity or oropharynx during radiotherapy of head and neck cancer; to the oesophagus during radiotherapy of non-small cell lung cancer; to the bladder during brachytherapy or fractionated pelvic radiotherapy of endometrial or cervix cancer; and to the rectum, during fractionated radiotherapy of prostate cancer, could provide both normal tissue protection and decreased morbidity for conventional treatment protocols and potentially allow radiation dose-escalation to improve local control.

γ-Irradiation is a potent carcinogen by virtue of its ability to cause single- and double-strand DNA breaks[32]—the effect that is also associated with a massive p53-dependent cell death in radiosensitive targets (primary lymphoid organs and intestinal epithelium) leading to acute injury[33,34]. Although it is known that p53 acts as a potent and important tumour suppressor[35], it is believed that this tumour suppressor activity is not directly related to p53's acute pathological response to irradiation-induced systemic genotoxicity[34]. Indeed, there is substantial pharmacological[36] and genetic[34] evidence supporting the notion that temporary and reversible suppression of p53, resulting in massive rescue of cells in radiosensitive tissues, is not associated with an increase in carcinogenicity. Rather, the tumour suppressor activity of p53 is related to activities in cells several days after the irradiation-induced systemic genotoxicity. Thus, p53 inhibitors are expected to represent tissue protective drugs to be used under pathological conditions associated with massive apoptotic cell death[37]. Although p53 inhibitors hold therapeutic promise, their potential applications are limited by the tissue specificity of p53-dependent radiosensitivity. For example, despite the pronounced p53-dependent apoptosis that occurs among epithelial cells of the small intestine after irradiation, clinical gastrointestinal acute radiation syndrome develops independently of p53. Thus, radioprotection of the gastrointestinal tract should be based on p53-independent strategies[38], possibly other types of apoptosis inhibitors. The current work capitalizes on this principle by utilizing mitochondria-targeted inhibitors of cyt *c*/CL peroxidase activity—**TPP-IOA** and **TPP-ISA**—that demonstrated effectiveness in protecting against radiation-induced apoptosis as well as radioprotective and radiomitigative effects *in vivo*. The mechanism of radiation mitigation proposed herein will prevent acute radiation sickness while having no impact on p53-mediated tumour suppression. When treatment with the mitochondrial-targeted inhibitors of cyt *c* is withdrawn, those few cells that have acquired a radiation-induced oncogenic chromosome aberration will be eliminated by p53-mediated apoptosis. This acquired oncogenic stress will be present in these cells for many weeks before tumour onset allowing ample time for p53 to execute its function as a tumour suppressor.

This study was aimed at the discovery, rather than the development, of novel mitochondria-targeted radiomitigators and radioprotectors. However, further improvements of structural features and pharmacological characteristics of the proposed inhibitors may lead to an optimized series of radioprotectors and radiomitigators with a broad spectrum of biomedical applications in the biodefense area as well as in radiotherapy of cancer, by achieving increased resistance of normal tissues surrounding the tumour.

Methods

Animals. C57BL/6NTac female mice were anaesthetized with Nembutal (1 mg per 20 gm mouse), irradiated to a total body dose of 9.25 Gy using either a Shepherd Mark 1 Model 68 cesium irradiator at a dose rate of 80 cGy min^{-1} (31–35 mice per group) or a Varian TrueBeam linear accelerator (Varian Medical Systems) at 100 monitor units or 100 cGy min^{-1} using 6 MV photons with a 40 cm×40 cm field at 100 SSD (10–23 mice per group). Mice were injected intraperitoneally (i.p.) with 5 mg per kg body weight of **TPP-IOA** in a 100 µl volume of water containing 25% ethanol at 1 h before irradiation, 10 min before irradiation, 10 min after irradiation, 5 h after irradiation and 24 h after irradiation. Other groups were injected i.p. with 2.5 mg per kg body weight of **TPP-IOA** or 5 mg per kg body weight of **TPP-ISA** 10 min after irradiation. The mice were followed for the development of haematopoietic syndrome (at which time they were killed). The health of the non-irradiated mice was unexceptional and no adverse side effects were noticed over the period of study (52 days) after i.p. injection of either **TPP-IOA** or **TPP-ISA** (5 mg per kg body weight). The log-rank test was used for three analyses: the comparison of overall survival that is defined as the time from the date of radiation to the date of death for all mice under study; the comparison of short-term survival over the first 20 days, that is, the overall survival count at 20 days; and the comparison of conditional survival in mice surviving 20 or more days, that is, the time from the date of radiation to the date of death for all mice who survived 20 days or longer after radiation. All these comparisons were made between each of the treated groups and the radiation-only control group. All procedures were pre-approved and performed according to the protocols established by the Institutional Animal Care and Use Committee of the University of Pittsburgh.

Cells. Mouse embryonic cells (courtesy of Dr X. Wang, University of Texas, Dallas) were cultured in DMEM supplemented with 15% FBS, 25 mM Hepes, 50 mg per litre uridine, 110 mg per litre pyruvate, 2 mM glutamine, 1× nonessential amino acids, 50 µM β-mercaptoethanol, 0.5×10^6 U per litre mouse leukaemia inhibitory factor, 100 U per litre penicillin, and 100 mg per litre streptomycin in a humidified atmosphere of 5% CO_2, 95% air at 37 °C. Mouse lung endothelial cells were obtained as previously described[39]. Briefly, lungs were flushed with HBSS containing 10 U ml^{-1} heparin, then homogenized and digested in type I collagenase using a gentle MACs dissociator (Miltenyi). Pulmonary endothelial cells were isolated by magnetic beads coated with antibody (rat anti-mouse) to PECAM-1 (BD Pharmingen), and seeded for subculture (passage 1). At approximately passage 2, cells were incubated with fluorescently labelled diacetylated LDL followed by FACS sorting for further purification. The enriched PECAM and diacetylated LDL population was sub-cultured on a collagen/gelatin matrix in 2% O_2, 5% CO_2, 93% nitrogen in a Coy Hypoxic Glove Box/Chamber in Opti-MEM (Gibco), 10% FBS, 2 mM glutamine, 0.2% retinal-derived growth factor (Vec Technologies), 10 U ml^{-1} heparin, 0.1 mM non-essential amino acid supplement (Gibco) and 55 µM β-mercaptoethanol (Counted as passage 3). Cells at passage 4–6 were applied to do the experiments.

Phosphatidylserine externalization. Phosphatidylserine externalization was determined by Annexin V–FITC apoptosis detection kit (Biovision) according to the manufacturer's instruction.

Caspase 3/7 activity. Caspase-3/7 activity was measured using a luminescence Caspase-Glo 3/7 assay kit (Promega) according to the manufacturer's instruction.

Measurement of cyt *c* release by western blot analysis. Cells were collected after 48 h post-irradiation incubation and resuspended in lysis buffer containing 0.05% digitonin for 4 min on ice. Supernatants were collected after centrifugation for 10 min at 10,000*g*. Equal amounts of protein were subject to 15% SDS–PAGE, transferred onto a nitrocellulose membrane, and probed with antibodies against cyt *c* (clone 7H8.2C12, BD Pharmingen) or actin (Novus) (loading control) followed by horseradish peroxidase-coupled detection. The protein band profile was analysed by densitometry using Labworks image acquisition and analysis software (UVP).

Liquid-He EPR measurements of ISA and IEOA liganding. Conditions: native cyt *c* (300 µM), **IEOA**/cyt *c* (2:1), TOCL/ **IEOA**/cyt *c* (20:2:1), 20 mM HEPES buffer, pH 7.4. Samples (200 µl) were placed in 3 mm o.d. suprasil quartz EPR tubes and frozen in liquid nitrogen for subsequent spectroscopic measurements. X-band (9 GHz) EPR spectra were recorded on a Bruker ESP 300 spectrometer equipped with an Oxford Instruments ESR 910 flow cryostat for ultra-low-temperature measurements. Spectra were recorded at 9.8 G modulation amplitude and 200 µW microwave power. The microwave frequency was calibrated by a frequency counter and the magnetic field was calibrated with a gaussmeter. The temperature was calibrated with carbon–glass resistors (CGR-1-1000) from LakeShore. This instrument and the software (SpinCount) to analyse the EPR spectra were provided by Professor Mike Hendrich, Carnegie Mellon University.

Molecular docking. The structures of the ligands **ISA**, **IOA**, **IEOA**, **IDA**, **TPP-ISA** and **TPP-IOA** were docked to the partially unfolded structure of horse heart cyt *c* using the Lamarckian genetic algorithm provided by the Autodock 4.0 software[40,41]. The partially unfolded structure of cyt *c*, where the Met_{80} containing loop is displaced was obtained using the molecular dynamics simulation approach as described below. The X-ray crystal structure (Protein Database accession code: 1HRC) was used as the base structure for performing the MD simulations. The docking procedure used was similar to the studies performed earlier[42], except for the following changes. A cubic box positioned at *x*, *y*, and *z* 0.032, −0.399, and −0.36, respectively, as the centre was built around the protein with 70×52×54 points and a spacing of 0.375 Å between the grid points was used. A total of 25 genetic algorithm runs were considered in each case with an initial population of 300 and a maximum number of 5,000,000 energy evaluations. The top 25 resulting orientations that have less than or equal to 0.5 Å root mean square deviation were clustered together. The best ligand bound to the partially unfolded cyt *c* structure in each case was chosen based on lowest energy as well as the conformation where the imidazole group was closest to the haem iron.

Molecular dynamics simulation. Molecular dynamics simulations were performed using the MD software package NAMD[43] using the VEGA ZZ 2.3.2 (ref. 44) package as the user interface. The model structure of horse heart cyt *c* (PDB ID: 1HRC) was downloaded from the Protein Data Bank, and explicit hydrogens were added using the package VEGA ZZ 2.3.2 (ref. 44). A spherical solvent cluster with a radius of 48.5 Å positioned at geometric centre of the protein was built and Cl^- ions were added to neutralize the system. This system was energy minimized for 2,000 steps using conjugate gradient method. The energy-minimized structure was slowly heated from 0 to 310 K over a period of 100 ps. Following this, 2 ns molecular dynamics simulation was performed at 310 K to obtain the partially unfolded cyt *c* structure.

Statistics. For the *in vitro* experiments, the results are presented as means ± s.d. values from at least three experiments, and statistical analyses were performed by either paired/unpaired Student's *t*-test or one-way ANOVA. As an exploratory analysis, *P*-values were not adjusted for multiple comparisons. For the survival data, median survival and its 95% confidence interval were calculated for each group, and the two-sided log-rank test was used to examine the differences between irradiated mice and irradiated mice treated with **TPP-ISA** or **TPP-IOA**. In all these tests, a *P*-value of <0.05 was regarded as significant.

References

1. Paris, F. *et al.* Endothelial apoptosis as the primary lesion initiating intestinal radiation damage in mice. *Science* **293,** 293–297 (2001).
2. Merritt, A. J. *et al.* The role of p53 in spontaneous and radiation-induced apoptosis in the gastrointestinal tract of normal and p53-deficient mice. *Cancer Res.* **54,** 614–617 (1994).
3. Komarova, E. A. *et al.* Dual effect of p53 on radiation sensitivity *in vivo*: p53 promotes hematopoietic injury, but protects from gastro-intestinal syndrome in mice. *Oncogene* **23,** 3265–3271 (2004).
4. Ott, M., Gogvadze, V., Orrenius, S. & Zhivotovsky, B. Mitochondria, oxidative stress and cell death. *Apoptosis* **12,** 913–922 (2007).
5. Giorgio, M., Trinei, M., Migliaccio, E. & Pelicci, P. G. Hydrogen peroxide: a metabolic by-product or a common mediator of ageing signals? *Nat. Rev. Mol. Cell. Biol.* **8,** 722–728 (2007).
6. Weiss, J. F. & Landauer, M. R. Protection against ionizing radiation by antioxidant nutrients and phytochemicals. *Toxicology* **189,** 1–20 (2003).
7. Dziegielewski, J. *et al.* WR-1065, the active metabolite of amifostine, mitigates radiation-induced delayed genomic instability. *Free Radic. Biol. Med.* **45,** 1674–1681 (2008).
8. Dorr, R. T. Radioprotectants: pharmacology and clinical applications of amifostine. *Semin. Radiat. Oncol.* **8,** 10–13 (1998).
9. Belikova, N. A. *et al.* Peroxidase activity and structural transitions of cytochrome *c* bound to cardiolipin-containing membranes. *Biochemistry* **45,** 4998–5009 (2006).

10. Krebs, J. J., Hauser, H. & Carafoli, E. Asymmetric distribution of phospholipids in the inner membrane of beef heart mitochondria. *J. Biol. Chem.* **254,** 5308–5316 (1979).
11. Liu, J. *et al.* Phospholipid scramblase 3 controls mitochondrial structure, function, and apoptotic response. *Mol. Cancer Res.* **1,** 892–902 (2003).
12. Schlattner, U. *et al.* Mitochondrial kinases and their molecular interaction with cardiolipin. *Biochim. Biophys. Acta* **1788,** 2032–2047 (2009).
13. Sorice, M. *et al.* Cardiolipin and its metabolites move from mitochondria to other cellular membranes during death receptor-mediated apoptosis. *Cell. Death Differ.* **11,** 1133–1145 (2004).
14. Tyurina, Y. Y. *et al.* Oxidative lipidomics of hyperoxic acute lung injury: mass spectrometric characterization of cardiolipin and phosphatidylserine peroxidation. *Am. J. Physiol. Lung Cell. Mol. Physiol.* **299,** L73–L85 (2010).
15. Kagan, V. E. *et al.* Cytochrome *c* acts as a cardiolipin oxygenase required for release of proapoptotic factors. *Nat. Chem. Biol.* **1,** 223–232 (2005).
16. Lu, P., Alterman, M. A., Chaurasia, C. S., Bambal, R. B. & Hanzlik, R. P. Heme-coordinating analogs of lauric acid as inhibitors of fatty acid omega-hydroxylation. *Arch. Biochem. Biophys.* **337,** 1–7 (1997).
17. Qian, S. Y. *et al.* Identification of protein-derived tyrosyl radical in the reaction of cytochrome *c* and hydrogen peroxide: characterization by ESR spin-trapping, HPLC and MS. *Biochem. J.* **363,** 281–288 (2002).
18. Kon, H. Paramagnetic resonance study of Nitric Oxide hemoglobin. *J. Biol. Chem.* **243,** 4350–4357 (1968).
19. Gadsby, P. M., Peterson, J., Foote, N., Greenwood, C. & Thomson, A. J. Identification of the ligand-exchange process in the alkaline transition of horse heart cytochrome *c. Biochem. J.* **246,** 43–54 (1987).
20. Brautigan, D. L. *et al.* Multiple low spin forms of the cytochrome *c* ferrihemochrome. EPR spectra of various eukaryotic and prokaryotic cytochromes *c. J. Biol. Chem.* **252,** 574–582 (1977).
21. Carraway, A. D., Miller, G. T., Pearce, L. L. & Peterson, J. The Alkaline Transition of Bis(N-acetylated) Heme Undecapeptide. *Inorg. Chem.* **37,** 4654–4661 (1998).
22. Murphy, M. P. & Smith, R. A. Targeting antioxidants to mitochondria by conjugation to lipophilic cations. *Annu. Rev. Pharmacol. Toxicol.* **47,** 629–656 (2007).
23. Du, C. *et al.* Mitochondrial ROS and radiation induced transformation in mouse embryonic fibroblasts. *Cancer Biol. Ther.* **8,** 1962–1971 (2009).
24. Zhang, Y. *et al.* Loss of manganese superoxide dismutase leads to abnormal growth and signal transduction in mouse embryonic fibroblasts. *Free Radic. Biol. Med.* **49,** 1255–1262 (2010).
25. Liu, X., Kim, C. N., Yang, J., Jemmerson, R. & Wang, X. Induction of apoptotic program in cell-free extracts: requirement for dATP and cytochrome *c. Cell* **86,** 147–157 (1996).
26. Duprez, L., Wirawan, E., Vanden Berghe, T. & Vandenabeele, P. Major cell death pathways at a glance. *Microbes Infect.* **11,** 1050–1062 (2009).
27. Nagley, P., Higgins, G. C., Atkin, J. D. & Beart, P. M. Multifaceted deaths orchestrated by mitochondria in neurones. *Biochim. Biophys. Acta.* **1802,** 167–185 (2010).
28. Porteous, C. M. *et al.* Rapid uptake of lipophilic triphenylphosphonium cations by mitochondria *in vivo* following intravenous injection: implications for mitochondria-specific therapies and probes. *Biochim. Biophys. Acta.* **1800,** 1009–1017 (2010).
29. Logtenberg, S. J. *et al.* Health-related quality of life, treatment satisfaction, and costs associated with intraperitoneal versus subcutaneous insulin administration in type 1 diabetes: a randomized controlled trial. *Diabetes Care* **33,** 1169–1172 (2010).
30. Ishigami, H. *et al.* Phase II study of weekly intravenous and intraperitoneal paclitaxel combined with S-1 for advanced gastric cancer with peritoneal metastasis. *Ann. Oncol.* **21,** 67–70 (2010).
31. Kahokehr, A., Sammour, T., Srinivasa, S. & Hill, A. G. Systematic review and meta-analysis of intraperitoneal local anaesthetic for pain reduction after laparoscopic gastric procedures. *Br. J. Surg.* **98,** 29–36 (2011).
32. Ulsh, B. A. Checking the foundation: recent radiobiology and the linear no-threshold theory. *Health Phys.* **99,** 747–758 (2010).
33. Pawlik, T. M. & Keyomarsi, K. Role of cell cycle in mediating sensitivity to radiotherapy. *Int. J. Radiat. Oncol. Biol. Phys.* **59,** 928–942 (2004).
34. Christophorou, M. A., Ringshausen, I., Finch, A. J., Swigart, L. B. & Evan, G. I. The pathological response to DNA damage does not contribute to p53-mediated tumour suppression. *Nature* **443,** 214–217 (2006).
35. Lane, D. & Levine, A. p53 Research: the past thirty years and the next thirty years. *Cold Spring Harb. Perspect. Biol.* **2,** a000893 (2010).
36. Leonova, K. I. *et al.* A small molecule inhibitor of p53 stimulates amplification of hematopoietic stem cells but does not promote tumor development in mice. *Cell Cycle* **9,** 1434–1443 (2010).
37. Gudkov, A. V. & Komarova, E. A. Prospective therapeutic applications of p53 inhibitors. *Biochem. Biophys. Res. Commun.* **331,** 726–736 (2005).
38. Gudkov, A. V. & Komarova, E. A. Radioprotection: smart games with death. *J. Clin. Invest.* **120,** 2270–2273 (2010).
39. Tang, Z. L. *et al.* Roles for metallothionein and zinc in mediating the protective effects of nitric oxide on lipopolysaccharide-induced apoptosis. *Mol. Cell. Biochem.* **234/235,** 211–217 (2002).
40. Morris, G. M., Huey, R. & Olson, A. J. Using AutoDock for ligand-receptor docking. *Curr. Protoc. Bioinformatics*, Chapter 8: Unit 8. 14. (2008).
41. Goodsell, D. S., Morris, G. M. & Olson, A. J. Automated docking of flexible ligands: applications of AutoDock. *J. Mol. Recognit.* **9,** 1–5 (1996).
42. Yanamala, N., Tirupula, K. C. & Klein-Seetharaman, J. Preferential binding of allosteric modulators to active and inactive conformational states of metabotropic glutamate receptors. *BMC Bioinformatics* **9** (Suppl 1), S16 (2008).
43. Phillips, J. C. *et al.* Scalable molecular dynamics with NAMD. *J. Comput. Chem.* **26,** 1781–1802 (2005).
44. Pedretti, A., Villa, L. & Vistoli, G. VEGA—an open platform to develop chemo-bio-informatics applications, using plug-in architecture and script programming. *J. Comput. Aided Mol. Des.* **18,** 167–173 (2004).

Acknowledgements

This work was supported by NIH (U19AIO68021, HL70755, HL094488, CA119927), NIOSH (OH008282) and La Junta de Extremadura y el Fondo Social Europeo (2010063090).

Author contributions

J.A. designed and synthesized the compounds; J.F. and Y.W. contributed to synthesis of chemical compounds. A.A.K., A.M. and I.I.V. performed experiments on peroxidase activity of cytc/CL complexes. L.P. and J.P. performed liquid-He EPR experiments. N.Y. and J.K.S. performed computer modelling. Y.Y.T. and V.A.T. performed MS analysis of cardiolipin oxidation. A.A.A. and A.K.S. performed MS analysis of compounds in tissues. N.A.B. participated in HPLC analysis of compounds in cells. D.A.S. performed HPLC analysis of compounds in cells, and participated in the design of *in vivo* experiments on radioprotection. Z.H., J.J., W.F. and. K.W. perfomed cell experiments. H.B. and B.R.P. participated in design of experiments, discussion of results and writing the manuscript. M.W.E. and J.S.G. contributed to the design and performance of the *in vivo* experiment. H.W. performed statistical analysis of *in vivo* data. V.E.K. suggested the idea, designed the study and wrote the manuscript.

Additional information

Competing financial interests: The authors declare no competing financial interests.

12

Asymmetric synthesis of *N*-allylic indoles via regio- and enantioselective allylation of aryl hydrazines

Kun Xu[1,*], Thomas Gilles[1,*] & Bernhard Breit[1]

The asymmetric synthesis of *N*-allylic indoles is important for natural product synthesis and pharmaceutical research. The regio- and enantioselective *N*-allylation of indoles is a true challenge due to the favourable C3-allylation. We develop here a new strategy to the asymmetric synthesis of *N*-allylic indoles via rhodium-catalysed *N*-selective coupling of aryl hydrazines with allenes followed by Fischer indolization. The exclusive *N*-selectivities and good to excellent enantioselectivities are achieved applying a rhodium(I)/DTBM-Segphos or rhodium(I)/DTBM-Binap catalyst. This method permits the practical synthesis of valuable chiral *N*-allylated indoles, and avoids the *N*- or *C*-selectivity issue.

[1]Institut für Organische Chemie, Albert-Ludwigs-Universität Freiburg, Albertstrasse 21, Freiburg im Breisgau 79104, Germany. * These authors contributed equally to this work. Correspondence and requests for materials should be addressed to B.B. (email: bernhard.breit@chemie.uni-freiburg.de).

The asymmetric synthesis of indoles is of great interest because of their prevalence in bioactive molecules[1–6]. In particular, indoles bearing a α-chiral carbon centre on the *N* are important structural motifs in natural products and pharmaceutical drugs (Fig. 1a)[7–12]. For this reason, extensive efforts have been undertaken to explore the catalytic asymmetric allylation of indoles[13–24]. However, selective *N*-allylation of indoles is a true challenge due to the high nucleophilicity of C3 of the indole nucleus and the weak acidity of the N–H bond (Fig. 1b)[25,26]. As a consequence, efficient strategies for the synthesis of *N* α-chiral allylic indoles are still rare. Recent advances were achieved upon installation of an electron-withdrawing substituent at C2 or C3 positions, which tempers the nucleophilicity at C3 and increases the acidity of the N–H bond[22]. In addition, a two-step protocol by allylation/oxidation of indolines could avoid C3 selectivity issue (Fig. 1c)[24].

Potentially, chiral N^1-allylic aryl hydrazine could give access to various chiral *N*-allylic indoles by employing a well-established Fischer indole synthesis[27–30]. This method would allow flexible construction of complex chiral *N*-allylic indoles starting from commercially accessible materials (ketones and aldehydes). Challenge towards the synthesis of chiral N^1-allylic aryl hydrazines arises from the selectivity control: (1) N^1 and N^2 selectivity of aryl hydrazines[31–33]; (2) branched and linear selectivity of the allylic moiety; (3) enantioselectivity of the branched regioisomer. To address these issues, we envisioned that a transition metal-catalysed asymmetric N^1-selective coupling of aryl hydrazines with terminal allenes[34–40] could lead to the synthesis of chiral N^1-allylic aryl hydrazines. The N^1 and N^2 selectivities at the aryl hydrazine may differentiate in the oxidative addition step, in which the more acidic N–H bond at N^1 proceeds faster than the less acidic N–H bond at N^2. Furthermore, combination of a suitable transition metal catalyst and a chiral ligand may allow to control branched selectivity and enantioselectivity.

Herein we report a rhodium-catalysed regio- and enantioselective coupling of aryl hydrazines with terminal allenes, which lead to the asymmetric synthesis of *N*-allylic indoles by following a Fischer indolization (Fig. 1c).

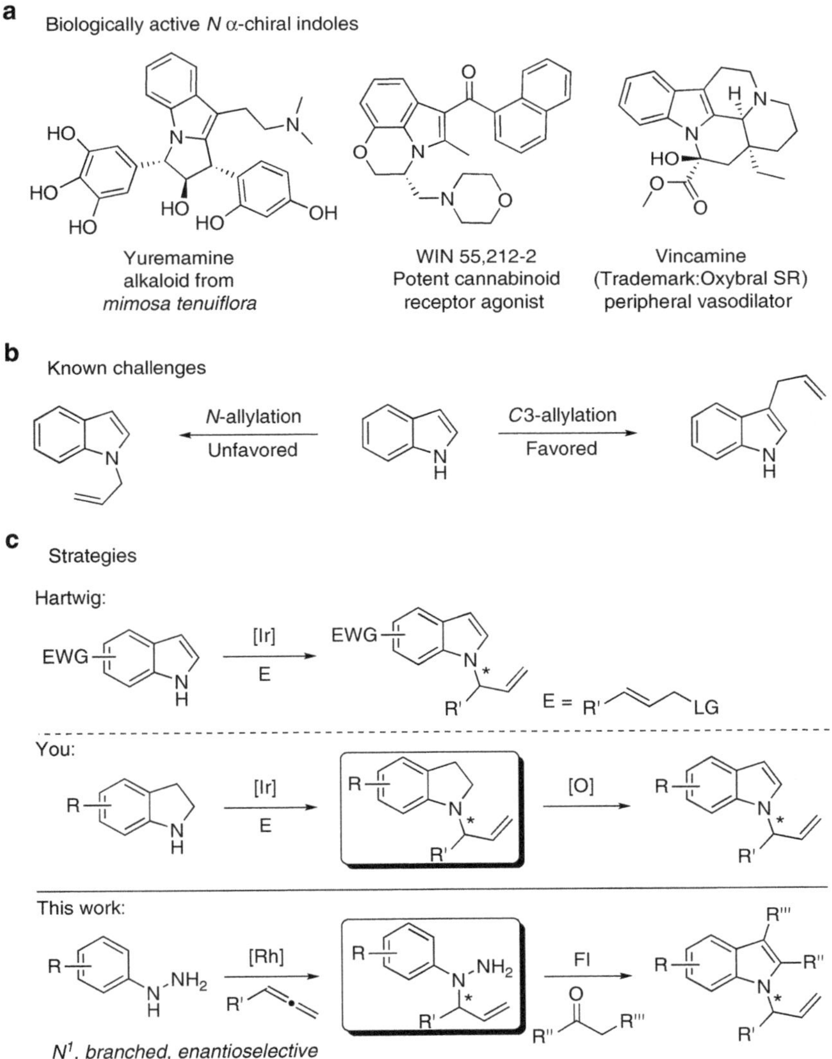

Figure 1 | Challenges for asymmetric synthesis of *N*-allylic indoles. (**a**) Selected examples of biologically active *N* α-chiral indoles. (**b**) Selectivity issue for allylation of indoles. (**c**) Strategies for transition metal-catalysed asymmetric synthesis of *N*-allylic indoles. LG, leaving group; EWG, electron-withdrawing group; FI, Fischer indolization.

Results

Reaction optimization of aryl hydrazine allylation. To evaluate our assumption, our studies began with the coupling reaction of phenyl hydrazine and cyclohexylallene in the presence of $[Rh(COD)Cl]_2$ (1.25 mmol%) and DPEphos (5.0 mmol%) in 1,2-dichloroethane at 80 °C. Surprisingly, the desired N^1-selective branched product was isolated with a promising 77% yield as a single regioisomer (Table 1, entry 1). Encouraged by the high N^1 and branched regioselectivities, we then tested a range of chiral bidentate phosphine ligands (Table 1, entries 2–10). The ligands Josiphos L and (*R*,*R*)-Diop led to low yield or poor enantioselectivity (Table 1, entries 2 and 3). After extensive screening (see Supplementary Table 1), we were pleased to observe that biaryl-type bisphosphine ligands led to high yield and promising enantiomeric excess (*ee*) (Table 1, entries 4–6). Increasing the steric effect of the Segphos-type ligand could significantly increase the enantioselectivity. The best *ee* was obtained with a bulky (*S*)-DTBM-Segphos ligand (Table 1, entries 6–8). Similarly, (*R*)-DTBM-Binap gave a comparable result (Table 1, entry 9). The enantiomeric purity could be enriched by a single recrystallization of the toluene sulfonic acid salt. Control experiments indicated that both rhodium catalyst and ligand are necessary for the coupling reaction of aryl hydrazine with allene to proceed (Table 1, entries 10 and 11).

Table 1 | Optimization of Rh-catalyzed coupling of phenyl hydrazine with cyclohexylallene.

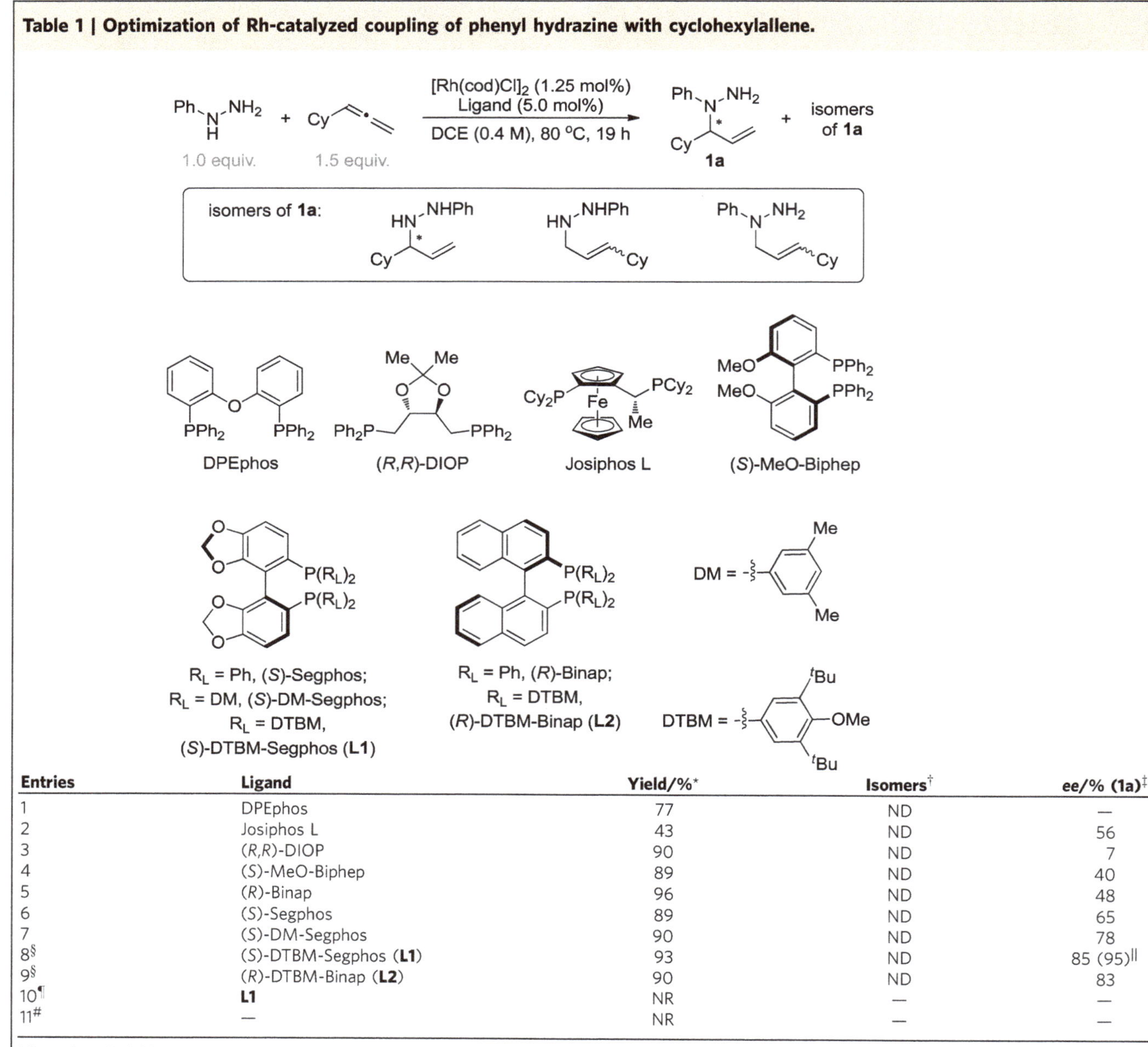

Entries	Ligand	Yield/%*	Isomers†	ee/% (1a)‡
1	DPEphos	77	ND	—
2	Josiphos L	43	ND	56
3	(*R*,*R*)-DIOP	90	ND	7
4	(*S*)-MeO-Biphep	89	ND	40
5	(*R*)-Binap	96	ND	48
6	(*S*)-Segphos	89	ND	65
7	(*S*)-DM-Segphos	90	ND	78
8§	(*S*)-DTBM-Segphos (**L1**)	93	ND	85 (95)‖
9§	(*R*)-DTBM-Binap (**L2**)	90	ND	83
10¶	**L1**	NR	—	—
11#	—	NR	—	—

ND, not determined; NR, no result.
*Isolated yield.
†Isomers of **1a** were determined by ^1H NMR of the crude reaction mixture.
‡Determined by chiral HPLC.
§$[Rh(cod)Cl]_2$ (1.0 mol%), **L1** (4.0 mol%).
‖*ee* after recrystallization from tosylic acid salt.
¶Without $[Rh(cod)Cl]_2$.
#Without ligand.

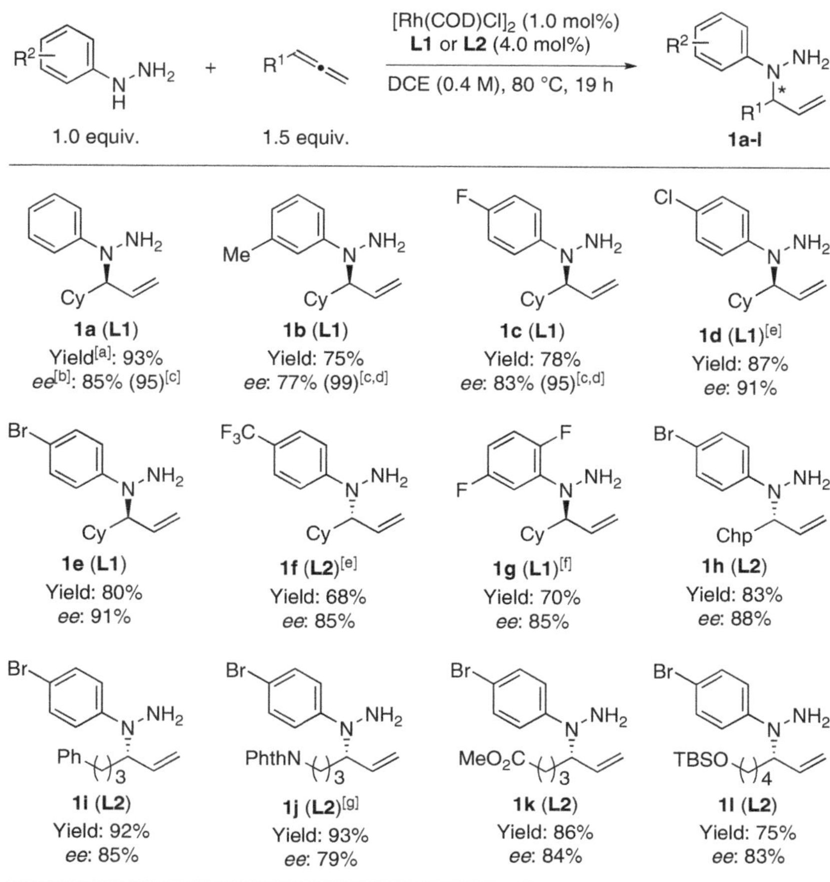

Figure 2 | Scope of Rh-catalysed coupling of aryl hydrazines with allene. [a]Isolated yield. [b]Determined by chiral HPLC. [c]*ee* after recrystallization from tosylic acid salt. [d]Reaction in 1.0 mmol scale. [e][Rh(cod)Cl]$_2$ (2 mol%), **L1** or **L2** (8.0 mol%). [f]Reaction at 100 °C. [g]The NMR spectrum of **1j** is not fully pure due to contamination of acetone (formation of hydrazone) during the purification. This problem can be avoided in the process of one-pot asymmetric synthesis of *N*-allylic indoles. Chp, cycloheptyl; HPLC, high-performance liquid chromatography; Phth, phaloyl; TBS, *tert*-butylsilyl.

Substrates scope of aryl hydrazine allylation. With the optimized conditions in hand, we then examined the scope of the addition of different aryl hydrazines with terminal allenes (Fig. 2). Various aryl hydrazines were coupled with cyclohexylallene in up to 93% isolated yield (**1a**) and up to 91% *ee* (**1d–e**). Practically, the *N*-allylated aryl hydrazines can be recrystallized from the corresponding tosylic acid salts to enrich the enantiomeric excess (**1a–c**). Several mono-substituted allenes were also tested (**1h–l**). Allenes bearing a phthaloyl-protected amine, an ester function and a silylether were suitable (**1g–l**).

One-pot asymmetric synthesis of *N*-allylic indoles. To investigate the compatibility of our strategy in the synthesis of *N*-allylic indoles via a one-pot process, the crude reaction mixture of the coupling step (**1a**) was subjected directly for the Fischer indolization with cyclohexanone in acetic acid at 70 °C. The desired *N*-allylic indole **2a** was obtained in 87% isolated yield over two steps with retention of the enantiomeric purity. Variation with other aryl hydrazines and allenes using this one-pot process led to the synthesis of the corresponding *N*-allylic indoles in up to 90% yield and up to 91% *ee* (**2b–f**). Furthermore, aldehydes, phenyl-substituted ketones as well as a dihydro-2*H*-thiopyran-4(3*H*)-one were well tolerated under standard conditions (Fig. 3).

To test the scalability and application for the synthesis of bioactive molecules, we applied the one-pot process for the late-stage indolization of (+)-testosterone acetate. To our delight, the desired indole product **3** was obtained in 59% yield and 17:1 diastereoselectivity in 1.06 gram scale, which indicates the practicality and usefulness of the method (Fig. 4).

Mechanistic investigations. To probe the possible reaction mechanism, a control experiment of 1-methyl-1-phenylhydrazine with cyclohexylallene was conducted under optimized conditions (Fig. 5a). The reaction was sluggish and gave only traces of the N^2-allylated product **4**, which is in accord with the lower reactivity of N^2 of the aryl hydrazine. Deuterium-labelling experiments with [D$_3$]phenylhydrazine under optimized conditions displayed that deuterium was only incorporated in the internal position of the double bond (Fig. 5b). Stoichiometric reaction of phenylhydrazine with [{Rh(COD)Cl}$_2$] and DPEphos in CDCl$_3$ was monitored by NMR spectroscopy. After 5 min at room temperature, the ^{1}H NMR spectrum (263 K) showed a major rhodium hydride species at $\delta = -15.4$ p.p.m. ($^1J_{Rh\text{-}H} = 14$ Hz), which is indicative of the oxidative addition of the N–H bond to rhodium (Fig. 5c).

On the basis of these observations, the following mechanism can be proposed (Fig. 5d). Oxidative addition of the phenyl hydrazine to Rh(I) generates Rh(III) complex (**A** or **A′**)[41]. The oxidative addition step favours the formation of intermediate **A** because of the higher acidity of N–H bond of N^1 than N^2. Hydrometalation of the less-substituted double bond could generate π-allyl-Rh (or δ-allyl-Rh) complex **B** (or **B′**)[42–45], which could generate the desired branched *N*-allylic aryl

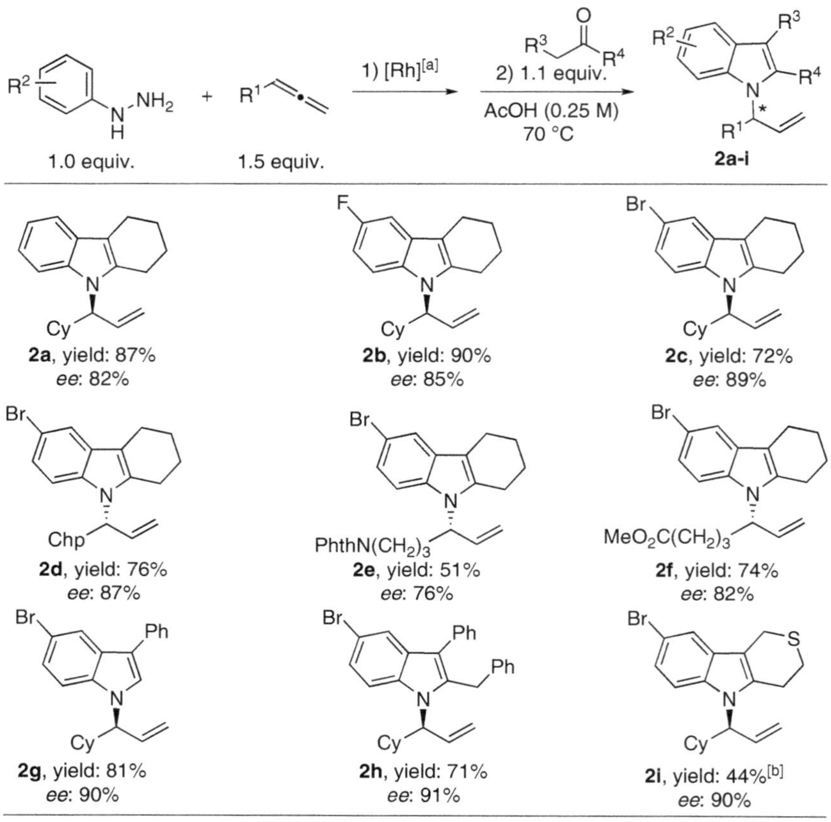

Figure 3 | Scope of one-pot asymmetric synthesis of *N*-allylic indoles. [a]Scope conditions of Fig. 2. [b]Reaction carried out at 100 °C.

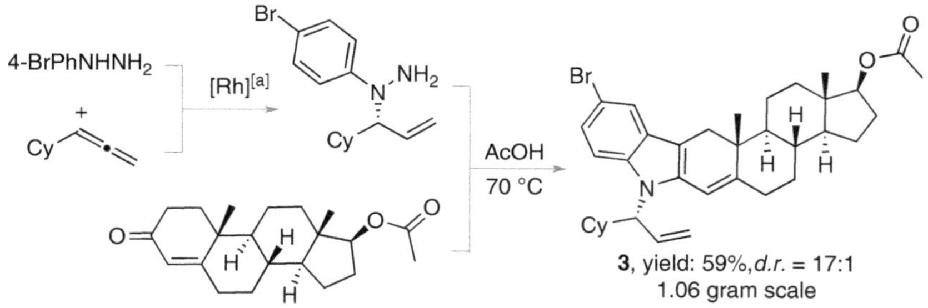

Figure 4 | One-pot late-stage indolization of (+)-testosterone acetate. [a][Rh(cod)Cl]$_2$ (1.0 mol%), **L2** (4.0 mol%), 1,2-dichloroethane (0.4 M), 80 °C, 19 h.

hydrazine **1a** via reductive elimination. The *N*-selectivity was determined within the oxidative addition step[46].

Discussion

We have developed the enantioselective *N*-selective coupling of aryl hydrazines with allenes via a rhodium(I)/DTBM-Segphos or rhodium(I)/DTBM-Binap catalyst system, which allowed the asymmetric synthesis of various valuable *N*-allylic indoles by following a one-pot Fischer indolization. *N*-selective allylation of aryl hydrazines using alkynes, target-oriented synthesis, and mechanistic investigations are currently underway in our laboratory and will be reported in due course.

Methods

Allylation of aryl hydrazines. To a screw-cap Schlenk tube was added [Rh(cod)Cl]$_2$ (0.005 mmol, 1 mol%), **L1** or **L2** (0.02 mmol, 4 mol%), aryl hydrazine (0.5 mmol, 1.0 equiv.), 1,2-dichloroethane (0.4 M) and allene (0.75 mmol, 1.5 equiv.). The Schlenk tube was sealed and the mixture was stirred for 19 h at 80 °C (or 100 °C). After cooling to room temperature, the solvent was removed by rotary evaporation. The crude product was purified by flash column chromatography to obtain the corresponding allylic hydrazine.

One-pot asymmetric synthesis of *N*-allylic indoles. To the reaction mixture of allylation of hydrazine was added ketone or aldehyde (0.55 mmol, 1.1 equiv.), and the mixture was stirred for half hour to form the corresponding hydrazine, then solvent was removed under reduced pressure. To the residue was added acetic acid (2.0 ml, 0.25 M), and the reaction mixture was stirred for 3–18 h at 70 °C (or 100 °C). The volatiles were removed by rotary evaporation and the crude reaction mixture was purified by flash column chromatography. The *ee* of each product was determined by HPLC analysis using chiral stationary phases. All new compounds were fully characterized. For NMR, high resolution mass spectrometry (HRMS) analysis and HPLC traces of the compounds in this article, see Supplementary Figs 1–53. General information, materials, synthesis and characterization of compounds in this article (**1a–l**, **2a–i**, **3**, **4** and **5**), and experimental part for mechanistic investigations see Supplementary Methods.

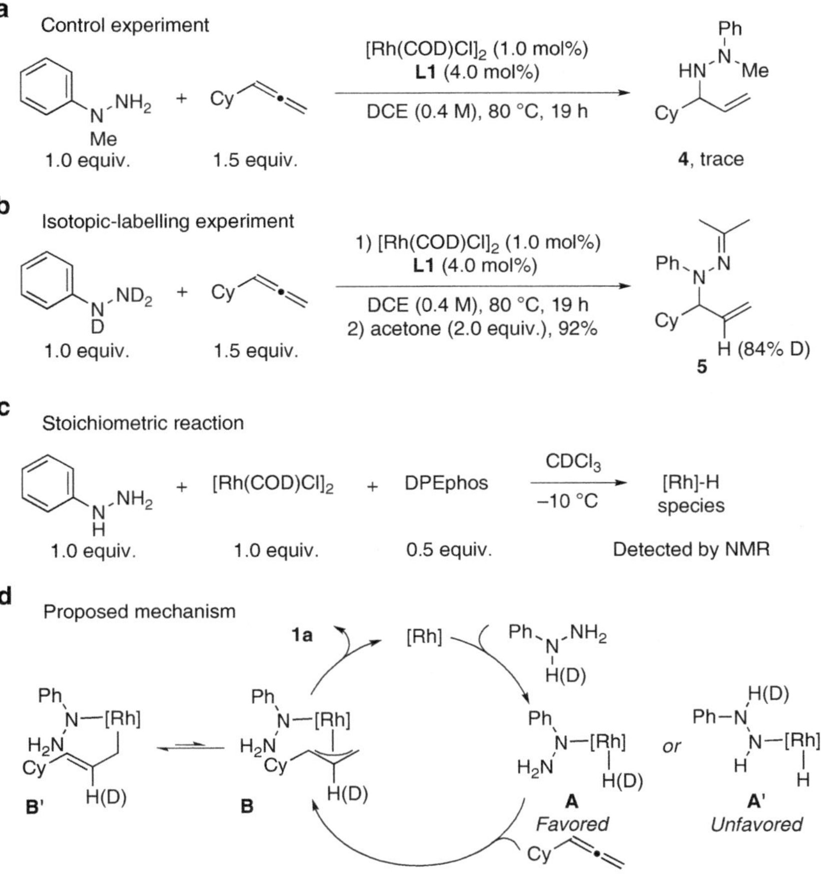

Figure 5 | Mechanistic investigations. (**a**) Control experiment with 1-methyl-1-phenylhydrazine. (**b**) Isotopic-labelling experiment with [D_3]phenylhydrazine. (**c**) Stoichiometric reaction of phenylhydrazine with catalysts. (**d**) Proposed mechanism.

References

1. Gul, W. & Hamann, M. T. Indole alkaloid marine natural products: an established source of cancer drug leads with considerable promise for the control of parasitic, neurological and other diseases. *Life Sci.* **78,** 442–453 (2005).
2. Pasquali, G., Porto, D. D. & Fett-Neto, A. G. Metabolic engineering of cell cultures versus whole plant complexity in production of bioactive monoterpene indole alkaloids: recent progress related to old dilemma. *J. Biosci. Bioeng.* **101,** 287–296 (2006).
3. Lewis, S. E. Recent advances in the chemistry of macroline, sarpagine and ajmaline-related indole alkaloids. *Tetrahedron* **62,** 8655–8681 (2006).
4. O'Connor, S. E. & Maresh, J. J. Chemistry and biology of monoterpene indole alkaloid biosynthesis. *Nat. Prod. Rep.* **23,** 532–547 (2006).
5. Higuichi, K. & Kawasaki, T. Simple indole alkaloids and those with a nonrearranged monoterpenoid unit. *Nat. Prod. Rep.* **24,** 843–868 (2007).
6. Kochanowska-Karamyan, A. J. & Hamann, M. T. Marine indole alkaloids: potential new drug leads for the control of depression and anxiety. *Chem. Rev.* **110,** 4489–4497 (2010).
7. Maincent, P., Verge, R. L., Sado, P., Couvreur, P. & Devissaguet, J. P. Disposition kinetics and oral bioavailability of vincamine-loaded polyalkyl cyanoacrylate nanoparticles. *J. Pharm. Sci.* **75,** 955–958 (1986).
8. Herzberg, U., Eliav, E., Bennett, G. J. & Kopin, I. J. The analgesic effects of *R*(+)-WIN 55,212-2 mesylate, a high affinity cannabinoid agonist, in a rat model of neuropathic pain. *Neurosci. Lett.* **221,** 157–160 (1997).
9. Rahbæk, L. & Christophersen, C. Marine alkaloids. 19. Three new alkaloids, securamines E-G, from the marine bryozoan *Securiflustra securifrons*. *J. Nat. Prod.* **60,** 175–177 (1997).
10. Vepsäläinen, J. J., Auriola, S., Tukiainen, M., Ropponen, N. & Callaway, J. C. Isolation and characterization of yuremamine, a new phytoindole. *Planta Med.* **71,** 1053–1057 (2005).
11. Fernandez, L. S., Buchanan, M. S., Carroll, A. R., Feng, Y. J. & Quinn, R. J. Flinderoles A-C: antimalarial bis-indole alkaloids from *Flindersia* species. *Org. Lett.* **11,** 329–332 (2009).
12. Vallakati, R., Smuts, J. P., Armstrong, D. W. & May, J. A. On the biosynthesis and optical activity of the flinderoles. *Tetrahedron Lett.* **54,** 5892–5894 (2013).
13. Kimura, M., Futamata, M., Mukai, R. & Tamaru, Y. Pd-catalyzed C3-selective allylation of indoles with allyl alcohols promoted by triethylborane. *J. Am. Chem. Soc.* **127,** 4592–4593 (2005).
14. Zaitsev, A. B. *et al.* Fast and highly regioselective allylation of indole and pyrrole compounds by allyl alcohols using Ru-sulfonate catalysts. *J. Am. Chem. Soc.* **130,** 11604–11605 (2008).
15. Liu, W., He, H., Dai, L. & You, S. Ir-catalyzed regio- and enantioselective friedel-crafts-type allylic alkylation of indoles. *Org. Lett.* **10,** 1815–1818 (2008).
16. Sundararaju, B. *et al.* Ruthenium (IV) complexes featuring P,O-chelationg ligands: regioselective substitution directly from allylic alcohols. *Angew. Chem. Int. Ed.* **49,** 2782–2785 (2010).
17. Jiao, L., Herdtweck, E. & Bach, T. Pd(II)-catalyzed regioselective 2- alkylation of indoles via a norbornene-mediated C-H activation: mechanism and applications. *J. Am. Chem. Soc.* **134,** 14563–14572 (2012).
18. Sevov, C. S. & Hartwig, J. F. Iridium-catalyzed intermolecular asymmetric hydroheteroarylation of bicycloalkenes. *J. Am. Chem. Soc.* **135,** 2116–2119 (2013).
19. Trost, B. M., Krische, M. J., Berl, V. & Grenzer, E. M. Chemo-, regio-, and enantioselective Pd-catalyzed allylic alkylation of indolocarbazole pro-aglycons. *Org. Lett.* **4,** 2005–2008 (2002).
20. Cui, H. *et al.* Chemoselective asymmetric N-allylic alkylation of indoles with Morita-Baylis-Hillman carbonates. *Angew. Chem. Int. Ed.* **48,** 5737–5740 (2009).
21. Luzung, M. R., Lewis, C. A. & Baran, P. S. Direct, chemoselective *N-tert*-prenylation of indoles by C-H functionalization. *Angew. Chem. Int. Ed.* **48,** 7025–7029 (2009).
22. Stanley, L. M. & Hartwig, J. F. Iridium-catalyzed regio- and enantioselective *N*-allylation of indoles. *Angew. Chem. Int. Ed.* **48,** 7841–7844 (2009).
23. Trost, B. M., Osipov, M. & Dong, G. Palladium-catalyzed dynamic kinetic asymmetric transformation of vinyl aziridines with nitrogen heterocycles: rapid access to biologically active pyrroles and indoles. *J. Am. Chem. Soc.* **132,** 15800–15807 (2010).
24. Liu, W., Zhang, X., Dai, L. & You, S. Asymmetric *N*-allylation of indoles through the iridium-catalyzed allylic alkylation/oxidation of indolines. *Angew. Chem. Int. Ed.* **51,** 5183–5187 (2012).
25. Lakhdar, S. *et al.* Nucleophilic reactivities of indoles. *J. Org. Chem.* **71,** 9088–9095 (2006).

26. Otero, N., Mandado, M. & Mosquera, R. A. Nucleophilicity of indole derivatives: activating and deactivating effects based on proton affinities and electron density properties. *J. Phys. Chem. A* **111,** 5557–5562 (2007).
27. Wagaw, S., Yang, B. H. & Buchwald, S. L. A palladium-catalyzed strategy for the preparation of indoles: a novel entry into the fisher indole synthesis. *J. Am. Chem. Soc.* **1998** 120 6621–6622 (2006).
28. Boal, B. W., Schammel, A. W. & Garg, N. K. An interrupted fischer indolization approach toward fused indoline-containing natural products. *Org. Lett.* **11,** 3458–3461 (2009).
29. Müller, S., Webber, M. J. & List, B. The catalytic asymmetric fischer indolization. *J. Am. Chem. Soc.* **133,** 18534–18537 (2011).
30. Gore, S., Baskaran, S. & König, B. Fischer indole synthesis in low melting mixtures. *Org. Lett.* **14,** 4568–4571 (2012).
31. Ragnarsson, U. *et al.* Acidity of di- and triprotected hydrazine derivatives in dimethyl sulfoxide and aspects of their alkylation. *J. Org. Chem.* **70,** 5916–5921 (2005).
32. Bredihhin, A., Groth, U. M. & Mäeorg, U. Efficient methodology for selective alkylation of hydrazine derivatives. *Org. Lett.* **9,** 1097–1099 (2007).
33. Johns, A. M., Liu, Z. & Hartwig, J. F. Primary *tert-* and *sec-* allylamines via palladium-catalyzed hydroamination and allylic substitution with hydrazine and hydroxylamine derivatives. *Angew. Chem. Int. Ed.* **46,** 7259–7261 (2007).
34. Zimmer, R., Dinesh, C., Nandanan, E. & Khan, F. A. Palladium-catalyzed reactions of allenes. *Chem. Rev.* **100,** 3067–3125 (2000).
35. Trost, B. M., Jäkel, C. & Plietker, B. Palladium-catalyzed asymmetric addition of pronucleophiles to allenes. *J. Am. Chem. Soc.* **125,** 4438–4439 (2003).
36. Nishina, N. & Yamamoto, Y. Gold-catalyzed intermolecular hydroamination of allenes with arylamines and resulting high chirality transfer. *Angew. Chem. Int. Ed.* **45,** 3314–3317 (2006).
37. Kim, I. S. & Krische, M. J. Iridium-catalyzed hydrocarboxylation of 1,1-dimethylallene: byproduct-free reverse prenylation of carboxylic acids. *Org. Lett.* **10,** 513–515 (2006).
38. Moran, J., Preetz, A., Mesch, R. A. & Krische, M. J. Iridium-catalyzed direct C-C coupling of methanol and allenes. *Nat. Chem.* **3,** 287–290 (2011).
39. Koschker, P., Lumbroso, A. & Breit, B. Enantioselective synthesis of branched allylic esters via rhodium-catalyzed coupling of allenes with carboxylic acids. *J. Am. Chem. Soc.* **133,** 20746–20749 (2011).
40. Xu, K., Thieme, N. & Breit, B. Unlocking the N^2 selectivity of benzotriazoles: regiodivergent and highly selective coupling of benzotriazoles with allene. *Angew. Chem. Int. Ed.* **53,** 7268–7271 (2014).
41. Ardizzoia, G. A. *et al.* Oxidative addition of N-H bonds to a metal center: synthesis, characterization, and crystal structure of new rhodium (III) hydrido-pyrazolate complexes. *Inorg. Chem.* **41,** 610–614 (2002).
42. Choi, J., Osakada, K. & Yamamoto, T. Single and multiple insertion of arylallene into the Rh-H bond to give (π-allyl)rhodium complexes. *Organometallics* **17,** 3044–3050 (1998).
43. Tran, N. & Cramer, N. Rhodium-catalyzed dynamic kinetic asymmetric transformations of racemic allens by the [3 + 2] annulation of aryl ketimines. *Angew. Chem. Int. Ed.* **52,** 10630–10634 (2013).
44. Evans, P. A. & Nelson, J. D. Conservation of absolute configuration in the acyclic rhodium-catalyzed allylic alkylation reaction: evidence for an enyl $(\delta + \pi)$ organorhodium intermediate. *J. Am. Chem. Soc.* **120,** 5581–5582 (1998).
45. Wucher, B., Moser, M., Schumacher, S. A., Rominger, F. & Kunz, D. First X-ray structure analyses of rhodium(III) η^1-allyl complexes and a mechanism for allylic isomerization reactions. *Angew. Chem. Int. Ed.* **48,** 4417–4421 (2009).
46. Gellrich, U. *et al.* Mechanistic investigations of the rhodium catalyzed propargylic CH activation. *J. Am. Chem. Soc.* **136,** 1097–1104 (2014).

Acknowledgements

This work was supported by the DFG, the International Research Training Group 'Catalysts and Catalytic Reactions for Organic Synthesis' (IRTG 1038), the Fonds der Chemischen Industrie and the Krupp Foundation. We thank Umicore, BASF and Wacker for generous gifts of chemicals. K.X. thanks Dr Y.Z. Xia and Dr C.K. Li for helpful discussions.

Author contributions

K.X. initiated the project, planned and carried out the initial optimization; K.X. and T.G. completed the experimental work and final characterizations; B.B. directed and coordinated the project; K.X wrote the manuscript with the assistance of the other authors.

Additional information

Competing financial interests: The authors declare no competing financial interests.

13

Spirocyclic hypervalent iodine(III)-mediated radiofluorination of non-activated and hindered aromatics

Benjamin H. Rotstein[1,*], Nickeisha A. Stephenson[1,*], Neil Vasdev[1] & Steven H. Liang[1]

Fluorine-18 ($t_{½} = 109.7$ min) is the most commonly used isotope to prepare radiopharmaceuticals for molecular imaging by positron emission tomography (PET). Nucleophilic aromatic substitution reactions of suitably activated (electron-deficient) aromatic substrates with no-carrier-added [^{18}F]fluoride ion are routinely carried out in the synthesis of radiotracers in high specific activities. Despite extensive efforts to develop a general ^{18}F-labelling technique for non-activated arenes there is an urgent and unmet need to achieve this goal. Here we describe an effective solution that relies on the chemistry of spirocyclic hypervalent iodine(III) complexes, which serve as precursors for rapid, one-step regioselective radiofluorination with [^{18}F]fluoride. This methodology proves to be efficient for radiolabelling a diverse range of non-activated functionalized arenes and heteroarenes, including arene substrates bearing electron-donating groups, bulky *ortho* functionalities, benzylic substituents and *meta*-substituted electron-withdrawing groups. Polyfunctional molecules and a range of previously elusive ^{18}F-labelled building blocks, compounds and radiopharmaceuticals are synthesized.

[1] Division of Nuclear Medicine and Molecular Imaging, Center for Advanced Medical Imaging Sciences, Massachusetts General Hospital & Department of Radiology, Harvard Medical School, 55 Fruit Street, Boston, MA 02114, USA. * These authors contributed equally to this work. Correspondence and requests for materials should be addressed to N.V. (email: vasdev.neil@mgh.harvard.edu) or to S.H.L. (email: liang.steven@mgh.harvard.edu).

Fluorine-18 (^{18}F; $t_{½} = 109.7$ min) labelled compounds and radiopharmaceuticals are the mainstay of functional molecular imaging by positron emission tomography (PET) for a broad range of applications including clinical diagnosis and drug discovery[1–5]. Consequently, there is a rapidly growing demand for new ^{18}F-labelled agents to probe biological processes and targets *in vivo*[6]. Fluorine-18 is most readily prepared in high specific activity as no-carrier-added [^{18}F]fluoride ion, by proton irradiation of [^{18}O]H_2O (^{18}O(p,n)^{18}F nuclear reaction) in medical cyclotrons. Most ^{18}F-labelling methodologies for nucleophilic aromatic substitution (S_NAr) reactions employ 'naked' [^{18}F]fluoride ion with appropriately activated (electron-deficient) aromatic/heteroaromatic substrates. However, radiofluorination of non-activated arenes represents a major challenge in the field and there is an urgent need for a general and practical methodology that can introduce ^{18}F into molecules that cannot be labelled using a conventional S_NAr reaction.

Reactions of non-activated arenes with [^{18}F]fluoride by Balz–Schiemann reactions with diazonium tetrafluoroborate salts[7] or Wallach reactions with triazene-based precursors[8] have proven to be inefficient and low yielding. Other efforts to achieve this goal include applications of triarylsulphonium salts[9], diarylsulphoxides[10] or the post-S_NAr conversion of activating, electron-withdrawing groups into electron-donating groups, for example, through Baeyer–Villiger oxidation[11], all of which are based on reactions towards electron-deficient arenes and have limited substrate scope. Alternatively, transition-metal-mediated fluorination reactions (Fig. 1a, **1**)[12,13] and oxidative fluorination of phenol derivatives[14] (Fig. 1a, **2**) have been investigated. Unfortunately, the latter two methods employ air-sensitive complexes of toxic metals (**1**) or have yet to demonstrate extensive substrate scope (**2**).

The introduction of [^{18}F]fluoride ion into electron-rich or -deficient arenes via diaryliodonium salt-based precursors (Fig. 1a, **3**)[15–17] has been recently reviewed[18,19]. This technology has been successfully used to prepare PET radiopharmaceuticals. However, ^{18}F-incorporation into the relatively electron-deficient (activated) arene is accompanied by production of undesired radioactive byproducts arising from the electron-rich aryl auxiliary.[17,20] Although diaryliodonium salts represent the most investigated class of hypervalent iodine(III) compounds in PET, there is scant patent literature[21] on how one might achieve the desired regiospecific radiofluorination based on the use of aryliodonium ylides ($ArI = CX_2$; X = electron-deficient substituent) as precursors with Meldrum's acid auxiliaries.

Here we report a spirocyclic hypervalent iodine(III)-mediated radiofluorination strategy, based on iodonium ylides (Fig. 1b, **4**), to afford ^{18}F-aryl fluorides in high radiochemical yields. The technique involves stable, easily purified precursors and is readily implemented with standard workup procedures. The conceptual advantages of excellent regioselectivity and viability of incorporation of ^{18}F into a wide array of non-activated (hetero)arenes make this methodology suitable for routine radiopharmaceutical production.

Results

Design of spirocyclic iodonium ylides for radiolabelling. The initial goal of the present work was to discover an optimally

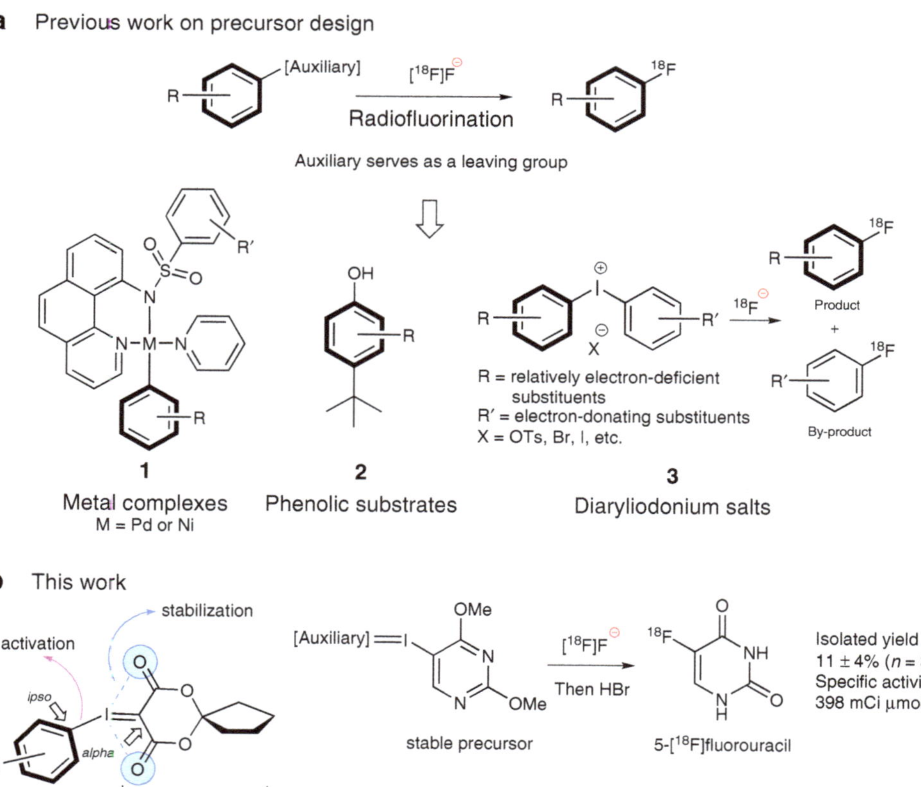

Figure 1 | Direct radiofluorination of non-activated arenes. (**a**) Previous work on precursor design. (**b**) This work.

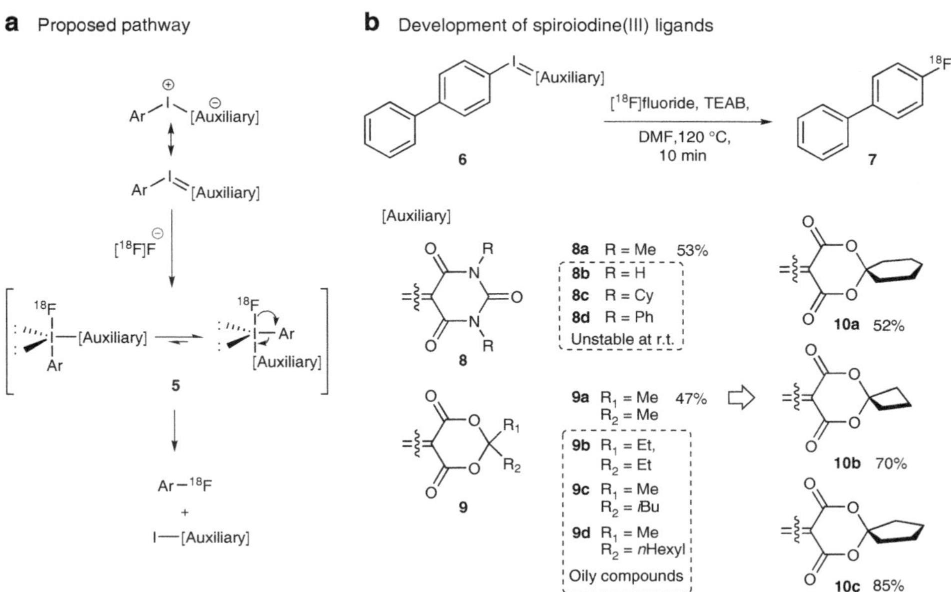

Figure 2 | Development of spirocyclic iodonium ylides for radiofluorination. (**a**) Proposed pathway. Radiofluorination of spiroiodonium ylides is proposed to occur through trigonal bipyramidal intermediate **5**. (**b**) Development and screening of spiroiodine(III) ligands. Conditions: biphenyl spiroiodine(III) precursor (2 mg), TEAB (7 mg), DMF (400 µl), 120 °C, 10 min. Incorporation yield and product identity were determined by radioTLC and radioHPLC, respectively ($n = 3$). TEAB, tetraethylammonium bicarbonate; DMF, *N,N*-dimethylformamide.

designed auxiliary (Fig. 1b, **4**) capable of stabilizing the I(III) centre of the iodonium ylide precursors, particularly if bound to non-activated arenes, thereby disfavouring notorious I(III) decomposition[22] and disproportionation[23] pathways. As shown in Fig. 2a, the extent of such stabilization should still enable the formation of ^{18}F-labelled products via the addition/reductive elimination mechanism[16,24] that has been invoked for diaryliodonium salts and other I(III) species[15–17,20,25,26]. Initial experiments (Fig. 2b) with derivatives of Meldrum's acid **9a** and barbituric acid **8a**, based on a challenging electron-neutral biphenyl substrate, provided radiochemical conversions of 47% and 53%, respectively. Analogues incorporating substituents on the nitrogen atoms of barbiturates **8b–d** or alkyl groups other than methyl on the quaternary carbon of diesters **9b–d** either exhibited poor stability at room temperature or were thick oils that were difficult to handle. These fruitless attempts led us to study a unique spirocyclic scaffold, which is rarely utilized in organic chemistry and has not been previously explored in radiochemistry. Gratifyingly, a spirocyclohexyl precursor, **10a**, was a stable crystalline solid that showed reactivity towards ^{18}F-fluoride ion similar to that of **9a** (52% incorporation yield). The well-tolerated initial reactions with **10a** inspired us to modulate smaller spirocycles and we discovered that cyclobutyl **10b** and cyclopentyl **10c** groups led to significantly increased conversions, 70% and 85%, respectively (Fig. 2b; Supplementary Fig. 1). The biphenyl precursor **10c** exhibited a significantly enhanced thermal stability over congeners incorporating alternative ligands under analogous radiolabelling conditions (DMF, 120 °C, 10 min).

The labelling precursors **13** (Fig. 3a) were easily synthesized from the corresponding aryl iodine(III) derivatives **12** or by a one-pot procedure from aryl iodide **11**. These reactions were typically carried out under 'open-flask' conditions (Supplementary Methods) and in all cases afforded crystalline products. Among many commonly-used radiolabelling conditions, a simple combination of dried $[^{18}F]$fluoride with tetraethylammonium bicarbonate (TEAB[27]) and spirocyclic iodine precursor in DMF was deemed to be optimal (Supplementary Table 1). The use of 2,2,6,6-tetramethyl-1-piperidinyloxy and butylated hydroxytoluene, as radical scavengers, offered no improvement of radiolabelling efficiency. As shown in Fig. 3b, hindered alkyl substituents without activating groups were successfully radiolabelled with ^{18}F in 45–56% incorporation yield (**15** and **16**, Supplementary Figs 2 and 3). Compound **15** represents a rare example of a highly sterically hindered ^{18}F-labelled benzene derivative bearing alkyl substituents. We next turned our attention to arenes with substituents at the benzyl position. Three substrates (**17–19**) underwent ^{18}F-incorporation in modest to good yields (Supplementary Figs 4–6). A protected form of 4-$[^{18}F]$fluorobenzyl amine (**18**)—an important building block—was prepared by the present method in 40% yield without the requirement of metal-mediated reduction from a nitrile precursor[28,29].

Radiolabelling of non-activated and/or hindered arenes. A range of other electron-rich arenes, the labelling of which constitutes an unmet need and a historical challenge, proved to be good substrates for the present ^{18}F-labelling strategy. This includes arenes incorporating alkoxy groups **20–23**, where **21–23** are concurrently challenged with hindered *ortho* substituents (Supplementary Figs 7–10). Bromo derivative **22** represents a new building block that could be further functionalized or linked to complex molecular motifs through cross-coupling reactions[30]. Notably, a radiosynthesis of *N*-acetyl 3-$[^{18}F]$fluoroaniline (**24**) revealed an advantage over previous methods by avoiding the undesired formation of $[^{18}F]$fluoromethane generated via the reaction of $[^{18}F]$fluoride with a *N,N,N*-trimethylammonium-3-nitrobenzene triflate precursor[31] (Supplementary Fig. 11). Indoline **25** and pyridine **26** were radiofluorinated in 34% and 65% incorporation yield, respectively, demonstrating the broad potential of our method for ^{18}F-labelling of nitrogen-containing heterocycles (Supplementary Figs 12 and 13).

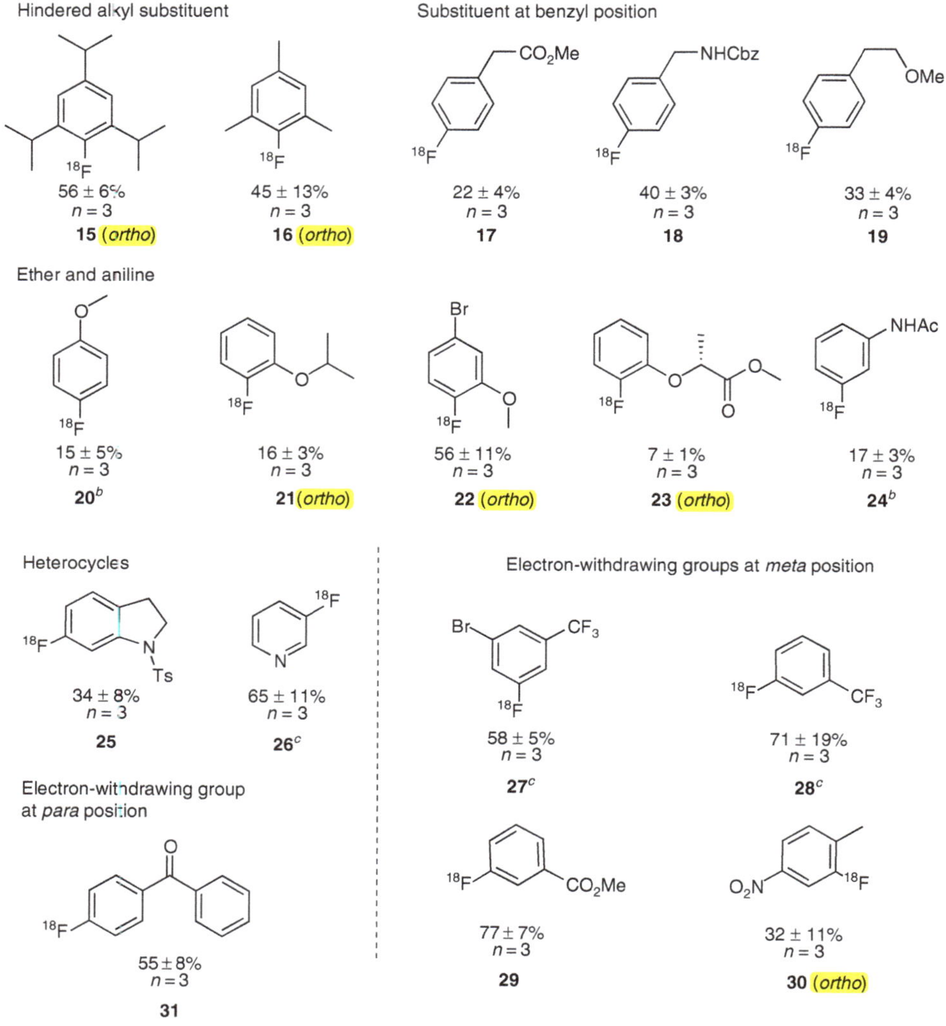

Figure 3 | Scope of spirocyclic hypervalent iodine(III)-mediated radiofluorination. (**a**) Preparation of spiroiodine(III) precursors and radiofluorination. (**b**) Fluorination of non-activated (hetero)arenes with [^{18}F]fluoride. [a]Radiolabelling conditions: precursor (2 mg), TEAB (7 mg), DMF (400 µl), [^{18}F]fluoride (1-3 mCi), 120 °C × 10 min. Incorporation yield was determined by radioTLC. The identity of labelled product was confirmed by radioHPLC. [b]Reaction temperature 150 °C. [c]Incorporation yield was determined by radioHPLC. Non-activated arenes with *ortho* functionalities are highlighted in yellow. TEAB, tetraethylammonium bicarbonate; *m*CPBA, *meta*-chloroperoxybenzoic acid.

Arenes displaying electron-withdrawing groups, including trifluoromethyl, halide, nitro and ester substituents at the *meta* (non-activated) positions (Fig. 3b, **27–30**), were also successfully radiofluorinated by the new protocol (Supplementary Figs 14–17). Two arene substrates with the CF_3 pharmacophore (**27** and **28**) were successfully radiolabelled with ^{18}F at the *meta*-position in excess of 45% conversion. Compound **27** demonstrates compatibility with aryl halides and could be further functionalized via coupling reactions[30]. Ester **29** was labelled in 77% conversion and may be directly converted to 3-[^{18}F]fluorobenzyl alcohol, which is a key fragment of [^{18}F]lapatinib[32]. In the example of fluorobenzophenone **31**, we demonstrated that our method

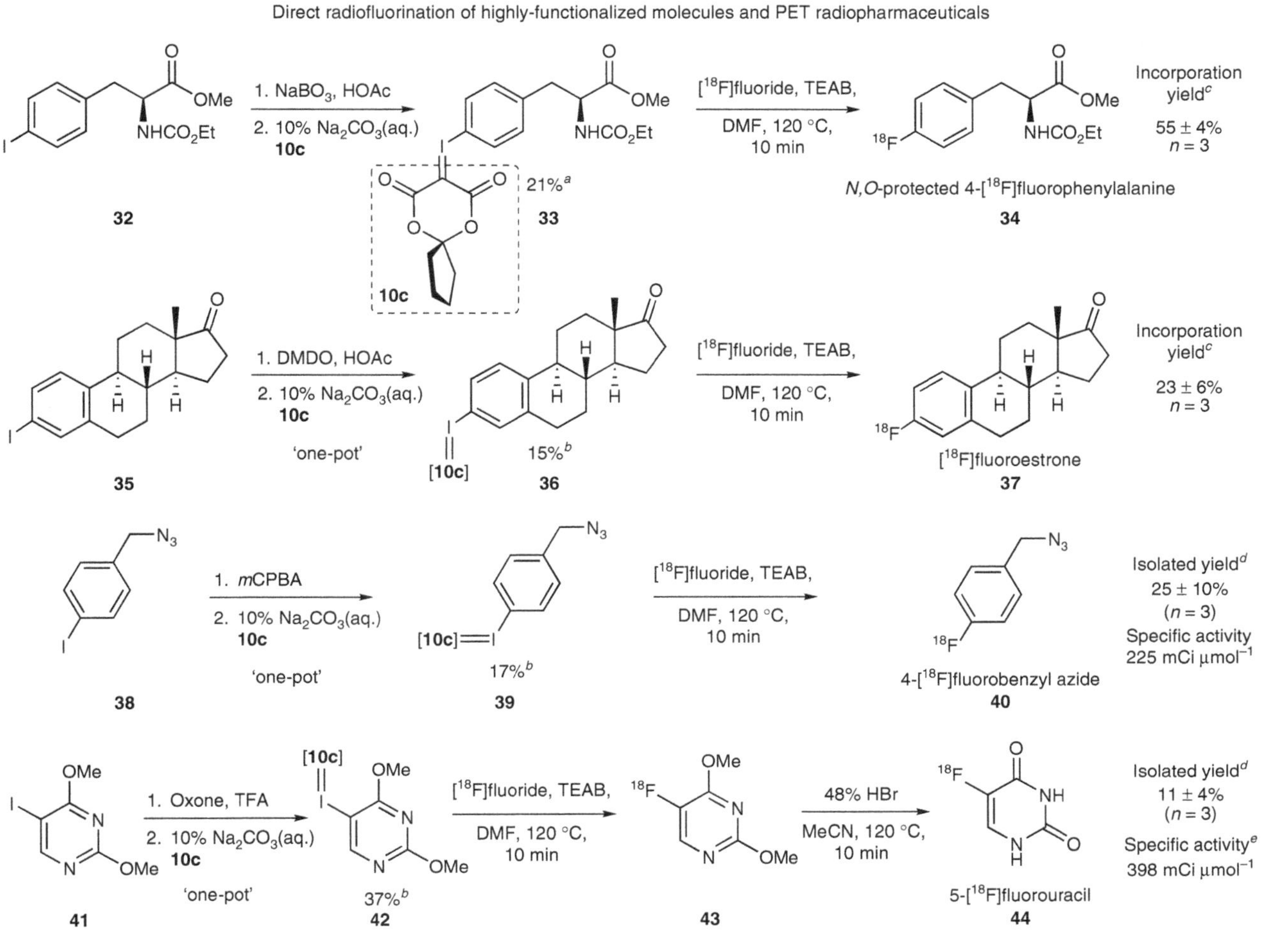

Figure 4 | Direct radiofluorination of highly functionalized molecules and PET radiopharmaceuticals. (**a**) Purified by recrystallization. (**b**) Purified by silica chromatography. (**c**) Incorporation yield and product identity were determined by radioTLC and radioHPLC, respectively ($n = 3$). (**d**) Reported as uncorrected radiochemical yield and isolated by solid-phase extraction technique ($n = 3$), radiochemical purity >95%. (**e**) Specific activity was determined based on intermediate **43**. DMDO, dimethyldioxirane; Oxone, potassium peroxysulphate; TFA, trifluoroacetic acid.

worked equally well for an activated arene with an electron-withdrawing group at the *para* position (Supplementary Fig. 18). Few exceptions for this methodology are expected, which includes precursors with unprotected hydroxy groups, amines and carboxylic acids. The above-mentioned examples demonstrate that this radiofluorination technology is widely applicable in six major classes of arenes and overcomes the challenges in previous methodologies as well as offers unique building blocks that were previously inaccessible.

Chromatographic analysis (radioTLC and radioHPLC) of crude reaction mixtures obtained in the course of this study showed that the sole radioactive products were the ^{18}F-radiolabelled arenes along with unreacted [^{18}F]fluoride. No other radioactive byproducts were detected. The unique selectivity can be, in part, explained by the substantial difference of electron densities between two carbon atoms attached to the I(III) center. A ^{13}C NMR study of our spirocyclic biphenyl based on **10c** revealed that the *ipso* carbon (Fig. 1, 4) resonates significantly downfield (114.3 p.p.m.) relative to the *alpha* carbon (57.2 p.p.m.) and is less shielded, indicating decreased electron density, and consequently greater propensity towards ^{18}F during reductive elimination. In contrast, diaryliodonium salts[22] do not exhibit a dramatic difference in ^{13}C chemical shifts, in accord with the reduced degree of regioselectivity in fluorination.

Translation to PET radiopharmaceuticals. To highlight the practical utility of spirocyclic hypervalent iodine(III)-based radiofluorination, we have demonstrated that established radiotracers that were previously accessible by [^{18}F]F_2 and known molecules with sensitive functionalities are well suited for labeling with [^{18}F]fluoride. As shown in Fig. 4, a *N,O*-protected [^{18}F]fluorophenylalanine, **34**, was successfully labelled via the corresponding spiroiodine(III) precursor in 55% incorporation yield (Supplementary Fig. 19). It is noteworthy that [^{18}F]fluorophenylalanine and its derivatives have only been synthesized via carrier-added [^{18}F]F_2[33–35] or through cumbersome multi-step reactions starting with [^{18}F]fluoride culminating with chiral HPLC separations[36]. [^{18}F]Fluoroestrone (**37**), previously prepared by transition-metal-mediated methods[12,13], was also synthesized, in 23% incorporation yield (Supplementary Fig. 20).

Fluorine-18-labelled azides have found widespread use in 'click' syntheses of ^{18}F-labelled peptides[37,38]. For example, 4-[^{18}F]fluorobenzyl azide (Fig. 4, **40**) is a common building block for such reactions that is synthesized by a lengthy four-step route[37] or via a diaryliodonium salt method using an esoteric flow device[39]. In the present work, we significantly improved and simplified the synthesis of **40** using a spiroiodine(III) precursor **39**, prepared from 4-iodobenzyl azide by a one-pot method, and directly radiolabelled and isolated **40** in 25%

uncorrected radiochemical yield within 40 min, relative to dried [^{18}F]fluoride (Supplementary Figs 21 and 22 and Supplementary Table 2). The methodology presented herein was also used to prepare a PET radiopharmaceutical, 5-[^{18}F]fluorouracil (**44**), which was difficult to achieve by S_NAr and was previously prepared by an electrophilic [^{18}F]F_2 method, that consequently results in low specific activity due to carrier F_2 (ref. 40). We converted 5-iodo-2,4-dimethoxypyrimidine to the corresponding spiroiodine(III) precursor **42**, which underwent a stepwise radiofluorination and deprotection by aqueous hydrobromic acid, to generate **44** in 11% isolated uncorrected radiochemical yield from dried [^{18}F]fluoride with a specific activity of 0.4 Ci μmol^{-1} (Supplementary Figs. 23 and 24 & Supplementary Table 3), representing the radiosynthesis of 5-[^{18}F]fluorouracil from nucleophilic [^{18}F]fluoride for the first time. This reaction was carried out using *ca.* 300 mCi of starting [^{18}F]fluoride for proof of concept. We are presently scaling up and automating this reaction for clinical radiopharmaceutical production.

Discussion

Spiroiodine(III)-based precursors are stable species that have proven to enable direct and regioselective ^{18}F-labelling of non-activated and sterically hindered arenes with remarkably broad functional group compatibility. A wide range of non-activated arenes with structurally diverse and/or *ortho* functional groups, including esters, carbamates, halides, amides, nitro groups, trifluoromethyl groups, ketones and heterocycles, were efficiently radiolabelled by the developed method. Several ^{18}F-PET tracers and building blocks were successfully synthesized from [^{18}F]fluoride ion for the first time and/or the corresponding radiosyntheses were significantly simplified and improved via one-step reactions. Radiotracers prepared by this methodology were shown to be easily isolated in high radiochemical yields and specific acitivies, suitable for clinical translation.

Methods

General methods for radioisotope production and preparation. A GE PETtrace 16.5 MeV cyclotron was used for [^{18}F]fluoride production by the ^{18}O(p,n)^{18}F nuclear reaction to irradiate ^{18}O-enriched water. [^{18}F]fluoride was delivered to a lead-shielded hot cell in ^{18}O-enriched water by nitrogen gas pressure. [^{18}F]fluoride was prepared for radiofluorination of aromatics by one of two methods: (A) A solution of base (for example, TEAB, 7 mg) in acetonitrile and water (1 ml, v/v 7:3) was added to an aliquot of target water ($\leq$1 ml) containing the appropriate amount of [^{18}F]fluoride in a V-shaped vial sealed with a teflon-lined septum. The vial was heated to 110 °C while nitrogen gas was passed through a P_2O_5-Drierite column followed by the vented vial. When no liquid was visible in the vial, it was removed from heat, anhydrous acetonitrile (1 ml) was added and the heating was resumed until dryness. This step was repeated an additional three times. The vial was then cooled at room temperature under nitrogen pressure. The contents were resolubilized in the desired solvent (for example, DMF). (B) An aliquot of target water containing the appropriate amount of [^{18}F]fluoride was slowly passed through an anion exchange cartridge (MP1, ORTG, TN, USA), preactivated by flushing with $NaHCO_{3(aq)}$ (8.4%, 1 ml) and water (2–3 ml, until neutral by a pH indicator). [^{18}F]fluoride was eluted using a solution of base (for example, TEAB, 7 mg) in acetonitrile and water (1 ml, v/v 7:3) into a V-shaped vial sealed with a teflon-lined septum. Drying and resolubilization were then performed as described above. For preparations involving crypt-222, drying was conducted at 95 °C.

General methods for analysis of radiofluorination reactions. Radioactivity was quantified using a Capintec Radioisotope Calibrator (CRC-712M) ion chamber. Radiochemical incorporation yields were determined by radioTLC. EMD TLC Silica gel 60 plates (10 × 2 cm^2) were spotted with an aliquot (1–5 μl) of crude reaction mixture ~1.5 cm from the bottom of the plate (baseline). Unless otherwise noted, TLC plates were developed in a chamber containing ethyl acetate until within 2 cm of the top of the plate (front). Analysis was performed using a Bioscan AR-2000 radio-TLC imaging scanner and WinScan software. Radiochemical identity and purity were determined by radioHPLC. A Phenomenex Luna C18, 250 × 4.6 mm, 5 μm HPLC column was used with a Waters 1515 Isocratic HPLC Pump equipped with a Waters 2487 Dual λ Absorbance Detector, a Bioscan Flow-Count equipped with a NaI crystal and Breeze software. Mobile phases and flowrates included 70% CH_3CN, 30% 0.1 M $NH_4 \cdot HCO_{2(aq)}$, 1 ml min^{-1}; 50% CH_3CN, 50% 0.1 M $NH_4 \cdot HCO_{2(aq)}$, 1 ml min^{-1}, and 5% EtOH, 95% 0.1% $AcOH_{(aq)}$, 1 ml min^{-1}.

In order to account for immobilized radioactivity (which would not be accounted for by radioTLC), reaction vessels were decanted after quenching, and residual and solution radioactivity were separately quantified. In all cases, $\geq$95% of radioactivity remained in solution.

General procedure for radiofluorination of arenes. Azeotropically dried [^{18}F]Et_4NF (typically 1–3 mCi, 37–110 MBq), resolubilized in DMF (400 μl), was added to a V-vial containing spiroiodine(III) precursor (**13**, 2 mg). The reaction was heated at 120 °C for 10 min, and quenched with HPLC buffer (for example, 60:40 CH_3CN:H_2O + 0.1 N ammonium formate, 1 ml). Fluorine incorporation and product identities were determined by radioTLC and radioHPLC ($n \geq 3$). For radioTLC and radioHPLC data, see Supplementary Figs 1–22.

Conditions were optimized for radiofluorination of **10c** to produce **[^{18}F]7**. Radiofluorination of all other substrates was performed under identical conditions and they remained unoptimized. For certain products that were detected in low yield (that is, **20**, **24**), a reaction temperature of 150 °C proved superior to the general procedure temperature of 120 °C.

Specific activity of isolated radioactive products. Specific activity was determined by measurement of the UV absorbance of a known amount of radioactivity under identical analytical HPLC conditions used to generate a calibration curve for the corresponding nonradioactive standard. See Supplementary Figs 22 and 24, and Supplementary Tables 2 and 3 for details.

General procedure for synthesis of iodonium ylides. To a solution of the auxiliary acid (**8–10**, 0.25 mmol) in 10% $Na_2CO_{3(aq)}$ (w/v, 0.75 ml, 0.33 M solution) was added ethanol (1 ml) followed quickly by diacetoxyiodoarene (**11**, 0.25 mmol). The reaction mixture was vigorously stirred at room temperature for 0.5–4 h, until full conversion of starting materials was determined by TLC. The reaction mixture was then diluted with water (~8 ml), and extracted with DCM (3 × 10 ml). The combined organic extracts were dried with anhydrous Na_2SO_4, filtered and concentrated. To the residue was added ethyl acetate and hexanes to induce precipitation (at room temperature or −25 °C). Solids were collected by filtration and purified by flash chromatography if necessary. For ^{1}H, ^{13}C and ^{19}F spectra of new compounds, see Supplementary Figs 25–118.

References

1. Fowler, J. S. & Wolf, A. P. Working against time: rapid radiotracer synthesis and imaging the human brain. *Acc. Chem. Res.* **30,** 181–188 (1997).
2. Phelps, M. E. Positron emission tomography provides molecular imaging of biological processes. *Proc. Natl Acad. Sci. USA* **97,** 9226–9223 (2000).
3. Ametamey, S. M., Honer, M. & Schubiger, P. A. Molecular imaging with PET. *Chem. Rev.* **108,** 1501–1516 (2008).
4. Cai, L., Lu, S. & Pike, V. W. Chemistry with [18F]fluoride ion. *Eur. J. Org. Chem.* **2008,** 2853–2873 (2008).
5. Miller, P. W., Long, N. J., Vilar, R. & Gee, A. D. Synthesis of 11C, 18F, 15O, and 13N radiolabels for positron emission tomography. *Angew. Chem. Int. Ed.* **47,** 8998–9033 (2008).
6. Holland, J. P. *et al.* Alternative approaches for PET radiotracer development in Alzheimer's disease: imaging beyond plaque.. *J. Labelled Compd. Radiopharm.* **57,** 323–331 (2014).
7. Balz, G. & Schiemann, G. Über aromatische Fluorverbindungen, I.: Ein neues Verfahren zu ihrer Darstellung. *Ber. dtsch. Chem. Ges. A/B* **60,** 1186–1190 (1927).
8. Wallach, O. Ueber das Verhalten einiger Diazo- und Diazoamidoverbindungen. *Justus Liebigs Ann. Chem.* **235,** 233–255 (1886).
9. Mu, L. *et al.* 18F-radiolabeling of aromatic compounds using triarylsulfonium salts. *Eur. J. Org. Chem.* **2012,** 889–892 (2012).
10. Chun, J.-H., Morse, C. L., Chin, F. T. & Pike, V. W. No-carrier-added [18F]fluoroarenes from the radiofluorination of diaryl sulfoxides. *Chem. Commun.* **49,** 2151–2153 (2013).
11. Wagner, F. M., Ermert, J. & Coenen, H. H. Three-step, "one-pot" radiosynthesis of 6-fluoro-3,4-dihydroxy-l-phenylalanine by isotopic exchange. *J. Nucl. Med.* **50,** 1724–1729 (2009).
12. Lee, E., Hooker, J. M. & Ritter, T. Nickel-mediated oxidative fluorination for PET with aqueous [18F] fluoride. *J. Am. Chem. Soc.* **134,** 17456–17458 (2012).
13. Lee, E. *et al.* A fluoride-derived electrophilic late-stage fluorination reagent for PET imaging. *Science* **334,** 639–642 (2011).
14. Gao, Z. *et al.* Metal-free oxidative fluorination of phenols with [18F]fluoride. *Angew. Chem. Int. Ed.* **51,** 6733–6737 (2012).
15. Pike, V. W. & Aigbirhio, F. I. Reactions of cyclotron-produced [18F]fluoride with diaryliodonium salts-a novel single-step route to no-carrier-added [18]fluoroarenes. *J. Chem. Soc. Chem. Commun.* 2215–2216 (1995).

16. Shah, A., Pike, V. W. & Widdowson, D. A. The synthesis of [18F]fluoroarenes from the reaction of cyclotron-produced [18F]fluoride ion with diaryliodonium salts. *J. Chem. Soc. Perkin Trans. 1* 2043–2046 (1998).
17. Ross, T. L., Ermert, J., Hocke, C. & Coenen, H. H. Nucleophilic 18F-fluorination of heteroaromatic iodonium salts with no-carrier-added [18F]fluoride. *J. Am. Chem. Soc.* **129,** 8018–8025 (2007).
18. Yusubov, M. S., Maskaev, A. V. & Zhdankin, V. V. Iodonium salts in organic synthesis. *ARKIVOC* **2011,** 370–409 (2011).
19. Yusubov, M. S., Svitich, D. Y., Larkina, M. S. & Zhdankin, V. V. Applications of iodonium salts and iodonium ylides as precursors for nucleophilic fluorination in positron emission tomography. *ARKIVOC* **2013,** 364–395 (2013).
20. Carroll, M. A., Jones, C. & Tang, S.-L. Fluoridation of 2-thienyliodonium salts. *J. Labelled Compd. Radiopharm.* **50,** 450–451 (2007).
21. Satyamurthy, N. & Barrio, J. R. No-carrier-added nucleophilic [F-18] fluorination of aromatic compounds. WO2010/117435 A2 (2010).
22. Moon, B. S. *et al.* Facile aromatic radiofluorination of [18F]flumazenil from diaryliodonium salts with evaluation of their stability and selectivity. *Org. Biomol. Chem.* **9,** 8346–8355 (2011).
23. Wang, B., Cerny, R. L., Uppaluri, S., Kempinger, J. J. & Dimagno, S. G. Fluoride-promoted ligand exchange in diaryliodonium salts. *J. Fluorine Chem.* **131,** 1113–1121 (2010).
24. Martin-Santamaria, S. *et al.* Fluoridation of heteroaromatic iodonium salts-experimental evidence supporting theoretical prediction of the selectivity of the process. *Chem. Commun.* 649–650 (2000).
25. Graskemper, J. W., Wang, B., Qin, L., Neumann, K. D. & DiMagno, S. G. Unprecedented directing group ability of cyclophanes in arene fluorinations with diaryliodonium salts. *Org. Lett.* **13,** 3158–3161 (2011).
26. Wang, B., Graskemper, J. W., Qin, L. & DiMagno, S. G. Regiospecific reductive elimination from diaryliodonium salts. *Angew. Chem. Int. Ed.* **49,** 4079–4083 (2010).
27. Reed, C. D., Launay, G. G. & Carroll, M. A. Evaluation of tetraethylammonium bicarbonate as a phase-transfer agent in the formation of [18F]fluoroarenes. *J. Fluorine Chem.* **143,** 231–237 (2012).
28. Turkman, N. *et al.* Synthesis and preliminary evaluation of [18F]-labeled 2-oxoquinoline derivatives for PET imaging of cannabinoid CB2 receptor. *Nucl. Med. Biol.* **39,** 593–600 (2012).
29. Koslowsky, I., Mercer, J. & Wuest, F. Synthesis and application of 4-[18F]fluorobenzylamine: a versatile building block for the preparation of PET radiotracers. *Org. Biomol. Chem.* **8,** 4730–4735 (2010).
30. Pretze, M., Große-Gehling, P. & Mamat, C. Cross-coupling reactions as valuable tool for the preparation of PET radiotracers. *Molecules* **16,** 1129–1165 (2011).
31. Vasdev, N. *et al.* Metabolic stability of 6,7-dialkoxy-4-(2-, 3- and 4-[18F]fluoroanilino)quinazolines, potential EGFR imaging probes. *Bioorg. Med. Chem.* **19,** 2959–2965 (2011).
32. Basuli, F. *et al.* A first synthesis of 18F-radiolabeled lapatinib: a potential tracer for positron emission tomographic imaging of ErbB1/ErbB2 tyrosine kinase activity. *J. Labelled Compd. Radiopharm.* **54,** 633–636 (2011).
33. Coenen, H. H., Franken, K., Kling, P. & Stöcklin, G. Direct electrophilic radiofluorination of phenylalanine, tyrosine and dopa. *Int. J. Radiat. Appl. Instrum.* **39,** 1243–1250 (1988).
34. Namavari, M., Satyamurthy, N., Phelps, M. E. & Barrio, J. R. Synthesis of 6-[18F] and 4-[18F]fluoro-l-m-tyrosines via regioselective radiofluorodestannylation. *Appl. Radiat. Isot.* **44,** 527–536 (1993).
35. VanBrocklin, H. F. *et al.* A new precursor for the preparation of 6-[18F]Fluoro-l-m-tyrosine ([18F]FMT): efficient synthesis and comparison of radiolabeling. *Appl. Radiat. Isot.* **61,** 1289–1294 (2004).
36. Lemaire, C., Guillaume, M., Christiaens, L., Palmer, A. J. & Cantineau, R. A new route for the synthesis of [18F]fluoroaromatic substituted amino acids: no carrier added L-p-[18F]fluorophenylalanine. *Appl. Radiat. Isot.* **38,** 1033–1038 (1987).
37. Thonon, D., Kech, C., Paris, J., Lemaire, C. & Luxen, A. New strategy for the preparation of clickable peptides and labeling with 1-(azidomethyl)-4-[18F]-fluorobenzene for PET. *Bioconjugate Chem.* **20,** 817–823 (2009).
38. Campbell-Verduyn, L. S. *et al.* Strain-promoted copper-free "click" chemistry for 18F radiolabeling of Bombesin. *Angew. Chem. Int. Ed.* **50,** 11117–11120 (2011).
39. Chun, J.-H. & Pike, V. W. Single-step radiosynthesis of "18F-labeled click synthons" from azide-functionalized diaryliodonium salts. *Eur. J. Org. Chem.* **2012,** 4541–4547 (2012).
40. Fowler, J. S., Finn, R. D., Lambrecht, R. M. & Wolf, A. P. The synthesis of 18F-5-fluorouracil. VII. *J. Nucl. Med.* **14,** 63–64 (1973).

Acknowledgements

B.H.R. is a Natural Sciences and Engineering Research Council of Canada (NSERC) Postdoctoral Fellow. We thank Dr Thomas Lee Collier, Dr Jason P. Holland, Professor Thomas J. Brady and Professor Marco A. Ciufolini for helpful discussions. We also thank Jon Patteson, Rebecca Lewis and Alina Kassenbrock for technical support, and Dr Ronald Moore and David F. Lee, Jr., for isotope production.

Author contributions

B.H.R. and N.A.S. contributed equally to the work and performed the synthesis and radiofluorination experiments. All authors contributed to the design and development of the method and application. N.V. and S.H.L. prepared the manuscript, guided and supervised the project. All the authors discussed the experimental results and commented on the manuscript.

Additional information

Competing financial interests: The authors declare no competing financial interests.

14

Influenza neuraminidase operates via a nucleophilic mechanism and can be targeted by covalent inhibitors

Christopher J. Vavricka[1,2,*], Yue Liu[2,*], Hiromasa Kiyota[3], Nongluk Sriwilaijaroen[4,5], Jianxun Qi[2], Kosuke Tanaka[3], Yan Wu[2], Qing Li[2,6], Yan Li[2], Jinghua Yan[2], Yasuo Suzuki[5] & George F. Gao[1,2,6,7]

Development of novel influenza neuraminidase inhibitors is critical for preparedness against influenza outbreaks. Knowledge of the neuraminidase enzymatic mechanism and transition-state analogue, 2-deoxy-2,3-didehydro-*N*-acetylneuraminic acid, contributed to the development of the first generation anti-neuraminidase drugs, zanamivir and oseltamivir. However, lack of evidence regarding influenza neuraminidase key catalytic residues has limited strategies for novel neuraminidase inhibitor design. Here, we confirm that influenza neuraminidase conserved Tyr406 is the key catalytic residue that may function as a nucleophile; thus, mechanism-based covalent inhibition of influenza neuraminidase was conceived. Crystallographic studies reveal that 2α,3ax-difluoro-*N*-acetylneuraminic acid forms a covalent bond with influenza neuraminidase Tyr406 and the compound was found to possess potent anti-influenza activity against both influenza A and B viruses. Our results address many unanswered questions about the influenza neuraminidase catalytic mechanism and demonstrate that covalent inhibition of influenza neuraminidase is a promising and novel strategy for the development of next-generation influenza drugs.

[1] Research Network of Immunity and Health (RNIH), Beijing Institutes of Life Science (BIOLS), Beijing 100101, China. [2] CAS Key Laboratory of Pathogenic Microbiology and Immunology, Institute of Microbiology, Chinese Academy of Sciences, Beijing 100101, China. [3] Graduate School of Agricultural Science, Tohoku University, Aoba-ku Sendai 981-8555, Japan. [4] Faculty of Medicine, Thammasat University, Pathumthani 12120, Thailand. [5] College of Life and Health Sciences, Chubu University, Aichi 487-8501, Japan. [6] School of Life Sciences, University of Science and Technology of China, Hefei, Anhui Province 230027, China. [7] Chinese Center for Disease Control and Prevention (China CDC), Beijing 102206, China. *These authors contributed equally to this work. Correspondence and requests for materials should be addressed to G.F.G. (email: gaof@im.ac.cn).

It has recently been demonstrated that highly pathogenic H5N1 avian influenza can easily adapt to become airborne-transmissible in mammals[1,2], reminding the world about the pandemic potential of avian influenza viruses[3,4]. Moreover, only two drugs, zanamivir and oseltamivir, that function as influenza neuraminidase (NA) inhibitors are currently recommended for use worldwide. Therefore, the development of novel influenza drugs is critical for preparedness against possible future influenza epidemics and pandemics.

The influenza A virus genome comprises 8 negative strand RNA segments encoding 13 proteins[5]. Two major glycoproteins, hemagglutinin (HA) and NA, as well as the M2 ion channel, are on the surface of the virions and are therefore highly accessible targets for drug development[6,7]. Of these three transmembrane proteins, only NA is known to function as an enzyme and is therefore an ideal target for the design of competitive inhibitors that can mimic catalytic transition-state intermediates[8]. Accordingly, influenza NA is currently the most successful drug-target against influenza virus.

Besides NA inhibitors, only M2 ion channel inhibitors have been fully developed; however, the influenza M2 inhibitors amantadine and rimantadine are no longer in use due to serious problems with drug resistance[8]. The design of influenza NA inhibitors is regarded a classical example of rational structure-based drug design, but there are currently only two NA inhibitors, oseltamivir and zanamivir, that are approved for use worldwide[8]. Furthermore, oseltamivir resistance was reported to be highly prevalent in seasonal H1N1 isolates from September 2008 to January 2009[9], whereas zanamivir is not orally active and has a short duration of action. Two more recently developed NA inhibitors, laninamivir and peramivir, are approved for use in Japan and still under phase III clinical trials in the United States. All of these current NA inhibitors were designed based upon the structure of 2-deoxy-2,3-didehydro-*N*-acetylneuraminic acid (Neu5Ac2en), a putative NA transition-state analogue[8,10–12]. Insight into the NA catalytic mechanism and the proposed oxocarbenium ion transition-state intermediate were crucial for the design of Neu5Ac2en analogues with potent NA inhibitory activity[13,14]. However, evidence regarding the key influenza NA catalytic residues has remained elusive and the successful design of highly effective next-generation influenza NA inhibitors has proven to be a difficult task.

Influenza NA is a retaining glycosidase that cleaves the α-ketosidic bond of terminally linked sialic acid, notably *N*-acetylneuraminic acid (Neu5Ac), the predominant sialic acid in humans[8]. A majority of known retaining glycosidases utilize a pair of conserved active-site carboxylate residues with one functioning as a catalytic nucleophile in a double-displacement mechanism[15,16]. Retaining NA mechanisms, on the other hand, appear to be quite distinct. Biochemical analysis of NA from various microorganisms has revealed that a conserved active-site tyrosine can function as a nucleophile and may be the most important catalytic residue[17–19].

Although influenza NAs share very little sequence identity with NAs from other microorganisms, their active sites are highly conserved, which suggests that they all may function in a similar manner[8]. Leaving group effect and kinetic isotope effect experiments with influenza NA carried out by Guo *et al.*[16] and Chou *et al.*[20] are compatible with the classical mechanism that includes a covalent enzyme-sialosyl intermediate. Studies by Burmeister *et al.*[21] and Ghate *et al.*[22] also suggest that Tyr406 has an important role in the influenza NA mechanism. However, numerous studies still indicate that the influenza NA may possibly function in a unique manner. For example, 4-guanidino-Neu5Ac2en (zanamivir), 4-amino-Neu5Ac2en and even Neu5Ac2en all exhibit selectivity for influenza NA over NA from other species[10]; a computational study by Thomas *et al.* [23]concluded that a direct hydroxylation mechanism with no covalent influenza NA-sialosyl intermediate is actually the energetically preferred pathway; moreover, some bacterial NAs that possess the same canonical protein fold and conserved active-site tyrosine still produce completely different products[16,24]. Taken together, the above studies clearly illustrate that the influenza virus NA catalytic mechanism may be quite unique. Therefore, experimental evidence is necessary to determine whether the influenza NA conserved active-site tyrosine is really a key catalytic residue and whether covalent inhibition of influenza NA is even possible.

In this study, we first confirmed the catalytic role of the conserved active-site tyrosine (Tyr406, N2 numbering is used throughout the text) of influenza NA in order to explore the possibility of developing covalent influenza NA inhibitors. Influenza N2 was used as a classical example in this study, as N2-containing viruses are among the most common seasonal strains. Furthermore, the pathogenic agents of the 1957 H2N2 pandemic (Asian flu) and 1968 H3N2 pandemic (Hong Kong flu) are both N2-containing influenza A viruses. NMR and crystal soaking experiments clearly demonstrated that substitution of N2 Tyr406 with aspartic acid results in a switch of the influenza NA catalytic mechanism from a retaining glycosidase mechanism to an inverting mechanism. This further indicated that Tyr406 likely functions as a catalytic nucleophile; therefore, 2α,3ax-difluoro-Neu5Ac was synthesized and explored as a potential covalent influenza virus NA inhibitor. Soaking of N2 crystals with 2α,3ax-difluoro-Neu5Ac produced the first influenza virus NA covalent complex structure, proving that influenza NA Tyr406 functions as a catalytic nucleophile and that covalent NA inhibition is indeed possible. Most importantly, the covalent inhibitor 2α,3ax-difluoro-Neu5Ac achieved potent inhibition against both influenza A and B viruses as well as oseltamivir-resistant His274Tyr-NA.

Results

Tyr406 is the key catalytic residue of influenza NA. Although Ghate *et al.*[22] were successful with the analysis of Tyr406Phe NA from influenza B[22], a previous report by Lentz *et al.*[25] demonstrated that the phenylalanine 406 substitution actually results in an aberrantly processed influenza A N2 with loss of NA activity. Therefore, we chose a different approach by using a baculovirus expression system to produce recombinant N2 (rN2) from pandemic A/RI/5+/1957(H2N2) with a Tyr406Asp substitution. Substitution of Tyr406 with aspartic acid yielded a stable protein (rN2-Tyr406Asp) that was purified to homogeneity. rN2-Tyr406Asp had 100-fold reduced K_{cat} and two-fold reduced K_m as shown using kinetic analysis with a standard 4-methylumbelliferyl-Neu5Ac-based fluorescent assay (Table 1). This confirms that Tyr406 is a critical factor for the catalytic activity of influenza NA. The enzymatic reaction of rN2 and rN2-Tyr406Asp was further monitored with ^{1}H NMR using the avian influenza receptor analogue 3′-sialyllactose. According to previous studies confirming that influenza NA is a retaining

Table 1 | Fluorescence-based kinetic analysis of wild-type influenza rN2 compared with rN2-Tyr406Asp.

Enzyme	K_m (μM) (95% CI)	Relative K_{cat}*
rN2	46.5 (40.1-53.0)	100 ± 2
rN2-Tyr406Asp	103.2 (87.0-119.4)	1.11 ± 0.02

*The absolute K_{cat} value for WT is 21.3 ± 0.4 s^{-1}.

glycosidase[13], wild-type rN2 initially produced α-Neu5Ac, which mutarotates to form the more stable β-Neu5Ac over time. Interestingly, the β-anomer of Neu5Ac was detected as the initial product of 3′-sialyllactose after incubation with rN2-Tyr406Asp, which demonstrates that rN2-Tyr406Asp has switched from a retaining to inverting glycosidase mechanism (Fig. 1a and b).

A novel β-Neu5Ac-influenza NA complex structure. rN2-Tyr406Asp was then crystallized and crystal soaking experiments were performed using 3′-sialyllactose. Despite its impaired catalytic activity, rN2-Tyr406Asp still hydrolysed the avian receptor analogue during soaking, resulting in the first influenza NA-β-Neu5Ac complex structure, at a resolution of 1.50 Å (Fig. 2b). Crystallographic data and refinement statistics are shown in Table 2. Free sialic acids are much more stable in their β-anomeric configuration in solution; nevertheless, Neu5Ac always binds to wild-type NA as the α-anomer in a boat conformation[8] (Fig. 2b). The additional space created by substitution of Tyr406 with a smaller aspartic acid residue allows for the Neu5Ac to adopt a β-conformation where the C-2 hydroxy group in the N2-Tyr406Asp-β-Neu5Ac complex occupies the same region as the Tyr406 hydroxyl group of the wild-type complex. Furthermore, substitution of Tyr406 with Asp406 creates space for additional two water molecules between the C-2 hydroxyl group and Asp406 side-chain (Fig. 2b). Taken together, these results reveal that Tyr406 is indeed the key influenza NA catalytic residue and suggest that Tyr406 likely functions as a nucleophile that can be targeted by covalent inhibitors.

Targeting influenza NA Tyr406 with a covalent inhibitor. Based on our biochemical and structural analysis regarding the conserved Tyr406, we hypothesized that there was a high probability of targeting influenza virus NA with covalent inhibitors. In order for Tyr406 to undergo nucleophilic attack of the Neu5Ac anomeric carbon, a good leaving group should replace the C-2 hydroxyl group[26]. Another electronegative group at the C-3 position should also be present to destabilize any oxocarbenium ion transition-state intermediate, thereby stabilizing the potential Tyr406-inhibitor covalent bond[26]. Fluorinated compounds have been investigated for their anti-NA activity for quite some time and are excellent choices for covalent influenza NA inhibitors[26–30]. Although 2β,3eq-difluoro-Neu5Ac, which has been explored as an inhibitor of parainfluenza virus, was readily available from our previous studies[30], structural analysis clearly demonstrates that the compound should be in the α-anomeric configuration so that the

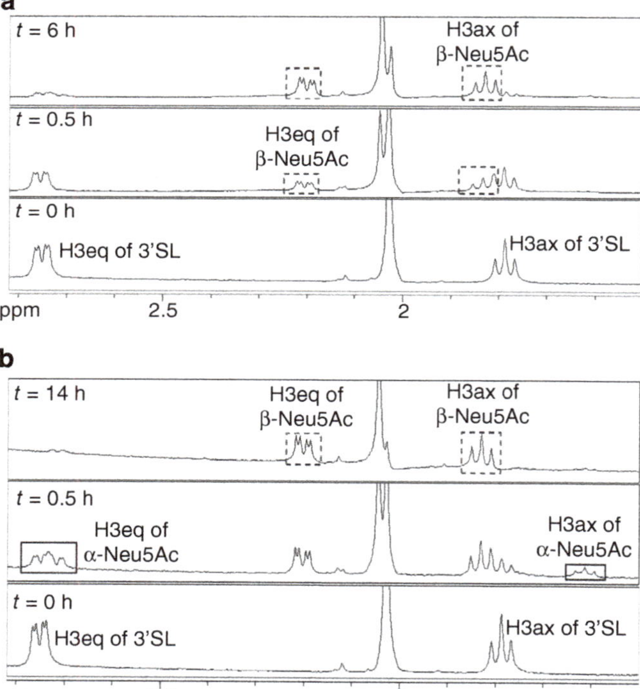

Figure 1 | Conserved Tyr406 is the key catalytic residue of influenza neuraminidase. (**a**) ^{1}H NMR analysis shows the initial and continuous production of β-Neu5Ac after incubation of rN2-Tyr406Asp with avian influenza receptor analogue 3′-sialyllactose, demonstrating that rN2-Tyr406Asp has shifted to an inverting glycosidase mechanism. (**b**) Wild-type influenza NA, in this case rN2, follows a retaining mechanism and therefore initially produces α-Neu5Ac from 3′-sialyllactose; the α-Neu5Ac undergoes mutarotation to form the more stable anomer, β-Neu5Ac, over time.

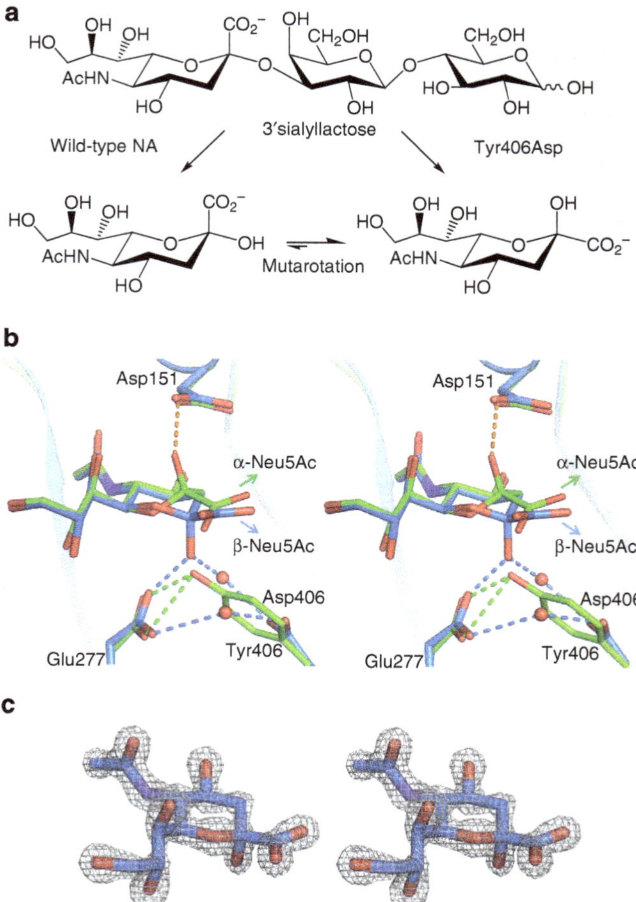

Figure 2 | N2-Tyr406Asp operates via an inverting sialidase mechanism. (**a**) Scheme outlining the initial formation of α-Neu5Ac by wild-type influenza NA and initial formation of β-Neu5Ac by influenza NA with a Tyr406Asp substitution. (**b**) Stereo illustration of the novel N2-Tyr406Asp-β-Neu5Ac complex (marine) in comparison to wild-type A/Tokyo/3/1967(H2N2) N2 complexed with α-Neu5Ac (green) (PDB ID: 2BAT). Two additional water molecules present in the N2-Tyr406Asp-β-Neu5Ac active site are coloured cyan. (**c**) Stereo illustration of β-Neu5Ac when bound to the N2-Tyr406Asp active site with the 2|Fo|-|Fc|map contoured at 2.0σ.

leaving group can face toward the outside of the NA active site cavity and depart easily (Fig. 3a). Therefore, 2α,3ax-difluoro-Neu5Ac was our primary target for a potential influenza virus NA covalent inhibitor.

2α,3ax-difluoro-Neu5Ac is a potent influenza virus inhibitor. 2α,3ax-difluoro-Neu5Ac indeed displayed potent *in vitro* NA inhibition, using both rN2 and live A/Jiangxi/262/2005(H3N2) virus, with IC_{50} values of 201 and 286 nM, respectively (Table 3). Inhibition of viral replication of seasonal A/Aichi/102/2008(H3N2) and A/Aichi/75/2008(H3N2) by 2α,3ax-difluoro-Neu5Ac in an AX4 cell-based assay was even more potent, both with IC_{50} values of 16.1 nM (Table 3). 2α,3ax-difluoro-Neu5Ac was also a highly potent low nanomolar level inhibitor of B/Lee/40 influenza B virus (Table 3, Fig. 4). Although no dramatic time dependent effects on influenza A virus NA inhibition were observed when using submicromolar concentrations of 2α,3ax-difluoro-Neu5Ac, inhibition of NA from B/Lee/40 resulted in more pronounced time-dependent effects, even at concentrations of 10–100 nM (Fig. 4).

In a previous mass spectrometric based analysis, binding of zanamivir and Neu5Ac2en to an 09N1 peptide containing Tyr406 was successfully detected[31]. Furthermore, covalent modification of the conserved active-site tyrosine was also detected in *Trypanosoma rangeli* sialidase using mass spectrometric methods[26]. Despite our attempts, we were unable to detect the covalent intermediate using similar methods; however, the observation of time-dependent inhibition indicates that the covalent intermediate is being formed in solution with influenza NA.

One major concern for the use of fluorinated covalent inhibitors is toxicity; however, we observed no cytotoxicity to MDCK cells when using up to 1 mM 2α,3ax-difluoro-Neu5Ac as determined by an MTT assay. Interestingly, 2β,3eq-difluoro-Neu5Ac was a better inhibitor of rN2-Tyr406Asp than wild-type

Table 2 | Crystallographic data collection and refinement statistics.

	N2-covalent	N2-Tyr406Asp-β-Neu5Ac
Data collection		
Space group	C2221	P21
Cell dimensions		
a, b, c (Å)	114.70, 139.70, 140.07	83.22, 114.83, 84.26
α, β, γ (°)	90, 90, 90	90, 99.7, 90
Resolution (Å)	50-1.80 (1.86-1.80)	50-1.50 (1.55-1.50)
R_{merge}	0.101 (0.385)	0.098 (0.367)
$I/\sigma I$	19.6 (4.9)	15.9 (3.7)
Completeness (%)	100.0 (100.0)	99.9 (99.8)
Redundancy	7.4 (7.5)	4.6 (4.6)
Refinement		
Resolution (Å)	38.82-1.80	39.05-1.50
No. reflections	103136	248190
R_{work}/R_{free}	0.1513/0.1749	0.1400/0.1613
No. atoms		
Protein	6235	12485
Ligand/ion	44	162
Water	927	2189
B-factors		
Protein	17.5	10.4
Ligand/ion	15.6	14.7
Water	33.2	23.7
R.M.S. deviations		
Bond lengths (Å)	0.007	0.007
Bond angles (°)	1.199	1.366

*Values in parentheses are for the highest-resolution shell.

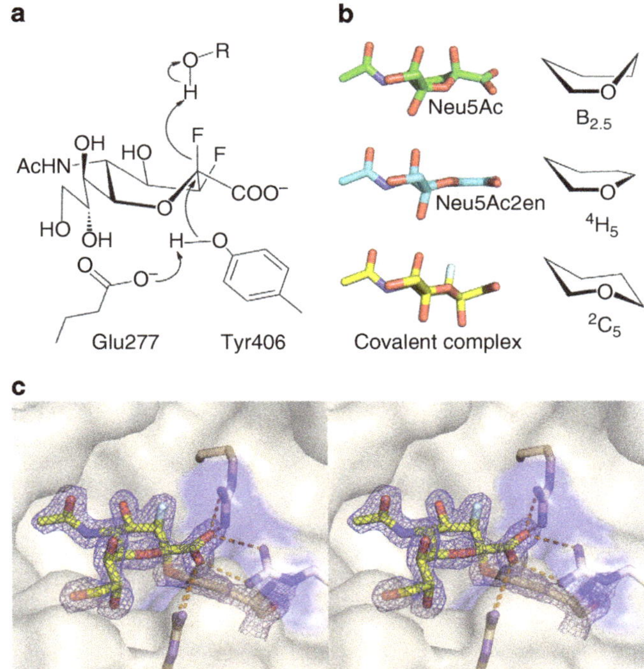

Figure 3 | Structure-based design and analysis of the first influenza NA covalent inhibitor. (**a**) Scheme for the mechanism-based design of covalent inhibition targeting influenza NA using 2α,3ax-difluoro-Neu5Ac. (**b**) Neu5Ac (green) adopts a boat conformation after binding to NA active site (PDB ID: 2BAT). Neu5Ac2en (cyan), a putative oxocarbenium ion transition state analogue, adopts a half-chair conformation(PDB ID: 1F8B). The covalently bound 3ax-fluoro-Neu5Ac moiety (yellow) adopts a chair conformation where C-2 moves toward Tyr406. This illustrates that in order to arrive at a covalently-linked intermediate, the reaction trajectory must still involve a planar intermediate. (**c**) Stereo illustration of the first influenza NA covalent complex, formed between rN2 Tyr406 (wheat) and a 3ax-fluoro-Neu5Ac moiety (yellow). The 2|Fo|-|Fc|map for the 3ax-fluoro-Neu5Ac moiety and Tyr406 is shown contoured at 2.0σ.

Table 3 | 2α,3ax-difluoro-Neu5Ac is a potent inhibitor of influenza virus NA and influenza virus replication.

	IC_{50} (nM)	95% CI (nM)
rN2-Tyr406Asp*	$>20 \times 10^6$	—
rN2*	201	179-226
A/Jiangxi/262/2005(H3N2)*	286	271-303
A/Aichi/102/2008†	16.1	10.5-24.6
A/Aichi/75/2008†	16.1	7.67-33.7
r09N1*	226	196-261
r09N1-His274Tyr*	247	233-261
B/Lee/40*	56.8	50.9-63.4
B/Lee/40§	9.85	4.30-22.6

Inhibition of NA activity from rN2, rN2-Tyr406Asp, A/Jiangxi/262/2005(H3N2), r09N1, r09N1-His274Tyr and B/Lee/40 by 2α,3ax-difluoro-Neu5Ac. Inhibition of A/Aichi/102/2008(H3N2) and A/Aichi/75/2008(H3N2) viral replication in AX4 cells by 2α,3ax-difluoro-Neu5Ac. MDCK cell-based inhibition of B/Lee/40 viral replication by 2α,3ax-difluoro-Neu5Ac in a plaque-reduction assay.
*Inhibition of NA enzymatic activity.
†Inhibition of viral replication in an AX4 cell-based assay. §Inhibition of viral replication in a MDCK cell-based plaque-reduction assay.

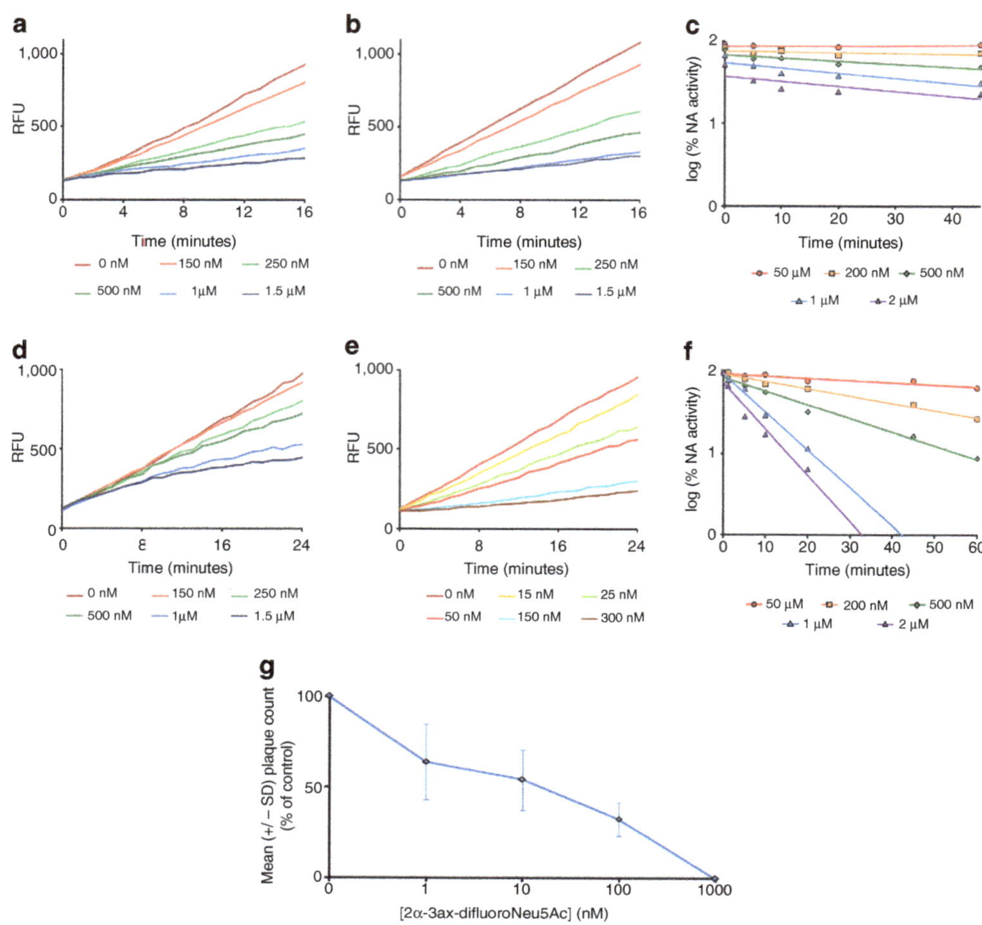

Figure 4 | Inhibition of A/Jiangxi/262/2005(H3N2) and B/Lee/40 influenza viruses. (**a**) Inhibition of A/Jiangxi/262/2005(H3N2) NA activity using no preincubation of virus with 0-1.5 µM 2α,3ax-difluoro-Neu5Ac (final concentration). (**b**) Inhibition of A/Jiangxi/262/2005(H3N2) NA activity using 30 min preincubation of virus with 0-1.5 µM 2α,3ax-difluoro-Neu5Ac (final concentration). (**c**) Plot of log[% H3N2 NA activity] versus incubation time for different preincubation concentrations of 2α,3ax-difluoro-Neu5Ac. (**d**) Inhibition of B/Lee/40 NA activity using no preincubation of virus with 0-1.5 µM 2α,3ax-difluoro-Neu5Ac (final concentration). (**e**) Inhibition of B/Lee/40 NA activity using 20 min preincubation of virus with 0-300 nM 2α,3ax-difluoro-Neu5Ac (final concentration). (**f**) Plot of log[% B/Lee/40 NA activity] versus incubation time for different preincubation concentrations of 2α,3ax-difluoro-Neu5Ac. (**g**) Inhibition of B/Lee/40 plaque formation by 1 nM, 10 nM, 100 nM and 1 µM 2α,3ax-difluoro-Neu5Ac. Each point with error bars represents the mean % plaque count (based upon 4 values for 1 nM and 6 values for 0 nM, 10 nM, 100 nM and µM) ± s.d.

rN2 (2 mM 2β,3eq-difluoro-Neu5Ac produced 54% inhibition of rN2-Tyr406Asp and only 25% inhibition of wild-type rN2). This can be explained by the rN2-Tyr406Asp-β-Neu5Ac complex structure, where the additional space resulting from the substitution of tyrosine with aspartic acid can better accommodate 2β,3eq-difluoro-Neu5Ac. The poor inhibition of rN2-Tyr406Asp by 2α,3ax-difluoro-Neu5Ac (>20 mM, Table 3) further indicated that it targets Tyr406 as a covalent inhibitor in solution.

Probing the influenza virus NA covalent intermediate. To determine if a covalent complex is really formed between influenza virus NA and 2α,3ax-difluoro-Neu5Ac, quality rN2 protein crystals were soaked with inhibitor and the complex crystal structure was solved at 1.80 Å. A N2-covalent complex structure was successfully obtained, with clear electron density revealing a 1.46 Å covalent bond between the Tyr406 terminal oxygen and the C-2 of a 3ax-fluoro-Neu5Ac moiety (Fig. 3c). The 3ax-fluoro-Neu5Ac moiety carboxylate is shifted closer toward Arg118 and away from Arg292 relative to N2 complexed with Neu5Ac. As expected, the C-2 fluoride leaving group is not present, confirming that it has departed during the formation of the molecular bond with Tyr406. Although no method is readily available to directly detect a naturally occurring covalent NA intermediate, the ability to obtain the influenza NA covalent complex using 2α,3ax-difluoro-Neu5Ac still suggests that a covalently bound intermediate is a critical step during hydrolysis of natural NA substrates. Therefore, we propose that influenza NA follows a double-displacement mechanism similar to the classical retaining glycosidase mechanism[16].

The covalently linked 3ax-fluoro-Neu5Ac moiety adopts a chair conformation, whereas α-Neu5Ac and Neu5Ac2en adopt boat and half-chair conformations[10], respectively, when bound to influenza NA (Fig.3b). In our N2-covalent complex, the unique C-3 fluorine of the 3ax-fluoro-Neu5Ac moiety is 3.51–3.55 Å away from the closest neighbouring residue Arg118. Aside from the differences regarding C-2 due to a novel covalent bond and chair conformation, the remaining interactions between the 3ax-fluoro-Neu5Ac moiety and influenza NA highly resemble those of α-Neu5Ac and Neu5Ac2en.

Effective covalent inhibition of oseltamivir-resistant NA. The similarity of the 3ax-fluoro-Neu5Ac moiety binding mode to the natural NA ligand Neu5Ac is a strong indication that the covalent inhibitor 2α,3ax-difluoro-Neu5Ac should be effective against drug-resistant NA. This is also illustrated by the high similarity between the binding modes of the covalent inhibitor and zanamivir, which remain effective against oseltamivir-resistant His274Tyr NA[32] (Fig. 5). Therefore, we also tested inhibition against oseltamivir-resistant rN1-His274Tyr from the 2009 H1N1 pandemic in comparison to wild-type rN1. Although His274Tyr N1 has been reported to exhibit more than 200-times lower inhibition by oseltamivir than by wild-type N1[32], the covalent inhibitor 2α,3ax-difluoro-Neu5Ac inhibited recombinant 2009 pandemic N1 (r09N1-His274Tyr) at the same level as wild-type recombinant 2009 pandemic N1 (r09N1) (Table 3). This demonstrates that 2α,3ax-difluoro-Neu5Ac is an effective inhibitor against the most common oseltamivir-resistant NA.

Discussion

In this study, we confirm that the conserved active site Tyr406 has an integral role in the catalytic mechanism of influenza virus NA and that Tyr406 can be successfully targeted for the design of covalent inhibitors. Furthermore, due to its importance in the catalytic cycle, drug-resistant mutations leading to substitution of Tyr406 are extremely unfavourable for the influenza virus. This is further illustrated by the fact that Tyr406 is almost 100% conserved among all influenza virus NA proteins. Therefore, the targeting of Tyr406 with covalent inhibitors is a next-generation strategy for influenza inhibitor development, which is highly advantageous in terms of drug resistance.

However, the first generation of influenza NA competitive inhibitors are still highly vulnerable to drug resistance. Long before the widespread circulation of natural oseltamivir-resistant influenza virus strains, it had been proposed that inhibitors that more closely resemble natural NA ligands are less likely to develop drug resistance[33]. Oseltamivir contains a hydrophobic pentyl ether group in place of the glycerol moiety of the natural NA ligand Neu5Ac and therefore oseltamivir resistance is easily developed. Upon binding of natural NA ligands, Glu276 hydrogen bonds with the ligand glycerol moiety. However, in order to accommodate oseltamivir, Glu276 must rotate to form a salt bridge with Arg224. The most common oseltamivir-resistant mutations, like His274Tyr, interfere with the rotation of Glu276, which is necessary to accommodate oseltamivir[32].

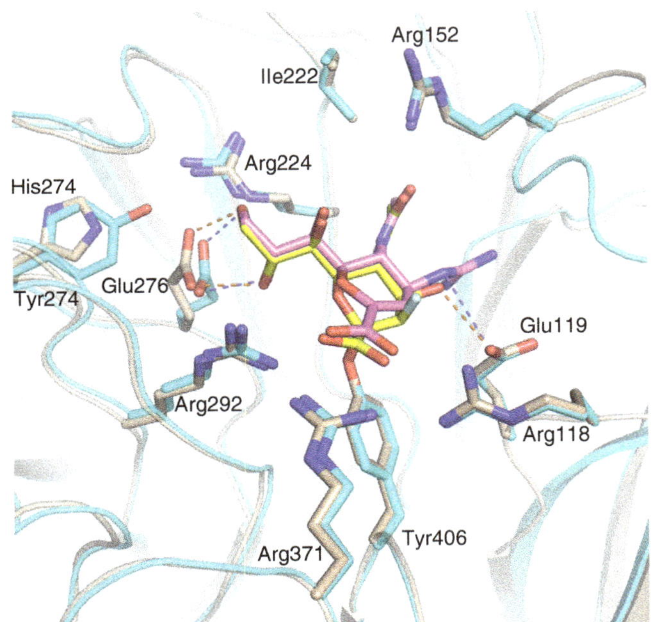

Figure 5 | Structural comparison of the N2-covalent complex with the oseltamivir-resistant N1-His274Tyr zanamivir complex. The binding mode of the 3ax-fluoro-Neu5Ac moiety (yellow) in N2 (wheat) and zanamivir (violet) in N1-His274Tyr (cyan) (PDB ID: 3CKZ) is highly similar, indicating that 2α,3ax-difluoro-Neu5Ac should remain effective against common oseltamivir-resistant influenza viruses.

Although zanamivir resistance is not as common as oseltamivir resistance due to a higher similarity with Neu5Ac, amino-acid substitutions, like Glu136Lys, can still arise that interfere with the binding of the zanamivir C-4 guanidino group. Aside from the similarity with the natural NA ligand, Neu5Ac, zanamivir is also not as commonly used as oseltamivir, which contributes to the lower frequency of zanamivir-resistant viruses. Nevertheless, the oseltamivir hydrophobic pentyl ether and the zanamivir C-4 guanidino that contribute to drug resistance are the key modifications that contribute to their potency. Therefore, 2α,3ax-difluoro-Neu5Ac, which more closely resembles the natural NA ligand, can still exhibit highly potent inhibition due to its action as a covalent inhibitor, and thus possesses significant advantages.

Still, rational modification of 2α,3ax-difluoro-Neu5Ac should be vigorously pursued to produce more potent next-generation covalent influenza virus NA inhibitors. As we observe stronger time-dependent inhibition (Fig. 4) in combination with a significant increase in potency (Table 3) for influenza B NA, the increased time dependence must be a result of an increased lifetime of a reversible covalent intermediate rather than an effect of slow inhibitor binding[34]. Therefore, this illustrates that further stabilization of the covalent intermediate is a promising strategy to improve the effectiveness of next-generation covalent influenza virus NA inhibitors.

Two major strategies can be taken for the stabilization of the influenza NA Tyr406-inhibitor covalent bond: modification of the covalent inhibitor to disrupt steric effects imposed by the NA active site that destabilize the favored chair conformation of the covalent intermediate, and modification of the covalent inhibitor to further destabilize build-up of positive charge around C-2, thereby stabilizing the covalent intermediate.

In regards to the first strategy, it is difficult to predict from our complex structure, what specific modifications will stabilize the chair conformation of the covalent intermediate. In regards to the second strategy, a stronger C-3 electron-withdrawing group might increase the lifetime of the covalent intermediate. As observed in the N2-covalent complex structure, there is no significant interaction between the 3-ax-fluoro-Neu5Ac moiety 3-ax-fluorine with influenza N2, indicating that the C-3 fluorine contributes to the inhibition potency by stabilization of the covalent intermediate. The lack of interactions between the 3-ax-fluorine and the NA active site should also allow for sufficient room to accommodate a bulkier, stronger C-3 electron-withdrawing group that may further stabilize the NA covalent intermediate. Although the closed conformation of the 150-loop in group 2 NA structures as well as the 2009 pandemic N1[40] could potentially hinder the binding of a bulkier C-3 group, recent studies have demonstrated that the 150-loop is inherently flexible[35] and, therefore, is able to accommodate bulkier electron-withdrawing groups.

In conclusion, this study contributes the first proof-of-concept for the use of covalent influenza NA inhibitors as a true next-generation strategy for influenza drug development. The first-generation influenza NA inhibitors, zanamivir and oseltamivir, are regarded as a classical example of structure-based competitive inhibitor design; however, novel strategies for NA inhibition has remained limited. The first covalent influenza NA-complex offered here provides a framework for the rational and structure-based development of highly potent next-generation influenza virus inhibitors of the future.

Methods

Cells and viruses. AX4 cells, MDCK cells with increased levels of sialyl-α2,6-galactose moieties, were grown and maintained following previous protocols[36,37]. The seasonal influenza virus isolates A/Aichi/102/2008(H3N2), A/Aichi/75/2008(H3N2) (Aichi Pref. Inst. Public Health, Japan), A/Jiangxi/262/2005(H3N2) (China CDC) and recombinant B/Lee/40 were amplified in MDCK cells. Viral culture supernatants were harvested, concentrated and stored at − 80 °C.

Expression and purification of influenza NAs. Recombinant NAs were purified to homogeneity after being expressed in a baculovirus expression system, based on the original method by Xu *et al.*[38–41] with modifications. For rN2-Tyr406Asp and 2009 pandemic rN1-His274Tyr, point mutations were introduced by site-directed mutagenesis based upon the corresponding wild-type NAs (Generay, China).

Enzymatic kinetics. The activity of rN2 and rN2-Tyr406Asp was monitored using a fluorometric assay based on methods from Potier *et al.*[42] NA activity was monitored using 0–500 μM 4-methylumbelliferyl-Neu5Ac (J&K Scientific) with 33 mM MES and 4 mM $CaCl_2$ (pH 6.0). The final concentration of enzymes used for wild-type rN2 and rN2-Tyr406Asp were 1 and 167 nM, respectively. Reactions were performed in a total volume of 50 μl at 37 °C, and monitored every 30 s over the course of 30 min on a SpectraMax M5 (Molecular Devices) at excitation and emission wavelengths of 355 and 460 nm, respectively. All assays were performed in no less than triplicates and the final data were fitted to the Michaelis–Menten equation using GraphPad Prism to determine the Michaelis–Menten constant (K_m) and maximum velocity of substrate conversion (V_{max}).

***In vitro* NA inhibition assay**. A 4-methylumbelliferyl-Neu5Ac-based fluorometric NA assay was also used to test competitive NA inhibition[42]. Recombinant NA or live influenza virus was diluted until NA activity was in the appropriate range for fluorescence detection of liberated 4-methylumbelliferone on a SpectraMax M5 (Molecular Devices), using excitation and emission wavelengths of 355 and 460 nm, respectively. 4-methylumbelliferyl-Neu5Ac was used at a final concentration of 100 μM. Five concentrations of 0–5 μM 2α,3ax-difluoro-Neu5Ac and a positive control with an equivalent volume of PBS were used for each replicate. For quantification of the B/Lee/40 half maximal inhibitory concentration (IC_{50}), 2α,3ax-difluoro-Neu5Ac was preincubated with live B/Lee/40 virus for 20 min before starting the reaction. For influenza A NA, all components were mixed simultaneously at the start of the reaction. Each assay was done in no less than triplicates. IC_{50} values were determined by plotting log[inhibitor] versus per cent inhibition using the sigmoidal dose response (variable slope) function in GraphPad Prism.

^{1}H NMR NA activity assay. ^{1}H NMR spectroscopy (600 MHz Bruker DXM-600, Bruker, CAS Institute of Biophysics) was employed to monitor the hydrolysis of 3′-sialyllactose (Carbosynth) catalysed by NA until the reactions reached equilibrium. For each reaction, a total volume of 500 μl with the ratio of D_2O to H_2O of 1:9 was used, containing enzyme, 2 mM substrate, 20 mM phosphate, 100 mM NaCl and 1 mM $CaCl_2$ (pH 6.0). The final concentrations for wild-type rN2 and rN2-Tyr406Asp were 32 nM and 13 μM, respectively. Spectral data were collected at 37 °C with 64 scans and a relaxation delay of 2 s. An initial spectrum containing only substrate and buffer (without NA) was acquired and referred to as time zero. The same reactions were also performed at 25 °C for monitoring and no obvious difference was seen.

Crystallization, soaking and data collection. The baculovirus expression system allows for the production of high quantities of soluble NA for crystallization experiments; however, despite our recent success with the structural characterization of 09N1 (ref. 40), we were unable to obtain enough quality N1 crystals for the soaking experiments carried out in this study. Instead, quality rN2 crystals were obtained as previously described[41], and rN2-Tyr406Asp crystals were grown by vapour diffusion in hanging drops that consist of 1 μl concentrated protein (6 mg ml^{-1}) and 1 μl reservoir solution (0.1 M MES monohydrate pH 6.0, 14% w/v polyethylene glycol 4000). rN2 and rN2-Tyr406Asp crystals were soaked in the corresponding mother liquor containing 10 mM of 2α,3ax-difluoro-Neu5Ac2 at 4 °C for 45 min and 10 mM 3′-sialyllactose at 18 °C for 180 min, respectively. After flash-cooling at 100 K with cryoprotection, diffraction data were collected at SSRF beamline BL17U and KEK beamline BL17A for the N2-Tyr406Asp-β-Neu5Ac complex and N2-covalent complex, respectively.

Data processing and structure solution. Diffraction data were processed and scaled using HKL2000 (ref. 43) and the statistics are outlined in Table 2. The structure of N2-Tyr406Asp complexed with β-Neu5Ac and the wild-type N2-covalent complex were both determined by molecular replacement using Phaser[44] from the CCP4 suite[45] with the structure of A/Tokyo/3/1967(H2N2)N2 (PDB ID: 1IVG) as the search model. REFMAC5 (ref. 46) and COOT[47] were employed for initial restrained rigid-body refinement and model building, respectively. Further cycles of refinement were carried out with phenix.refine implemented in the Phenix package[48]. The stereochemical quality of the obtained model was finally assessed using Procheck[49].

Cytotoxicity assay. Cytotoxicity was assessed in MDCK cells following a standard MTT assay protocol[50].

AX4 cell-based virus inhibition assay. Inhibition of influenza virus propagation was measured using AX4 cells in the presence of serial dilutions of 2α,3ax-difluoro-Neu5Ac (0.1–100 μM)[37,51]. Influenza virus at a multiplicity of infection of 0.03 was preincubated with a medium containing 2 μg ml^{-1} acetylated trypsin in the absence or presence of serially diluted inhibitor for 1 h at 4 °C. Then, the inhibitor–virus mixture was added onto the AX4 cell monolayers, which were incubated for 18–20 h at 37 °C. Infected cells were fixed and permealized with methanol followed by staining with antiviral NP mouse antibody and β-galactosidase-conjugated anti-mouse IgG. A substrate solution containing 4-methylumbelliferyl-β-D-galactoside and $MgCl_2$ was added to initiate the galactosidase reaction. 4-methylumbelliferyl was detected with an excitation wavelength of 355 nm and an emission wavelength of 460 nm on a Mithras LB940 microplate reader (Berthold Technologies, Pforzheim, Germany) to determine the virus titre in the infected cells.

The infectious foci were also observed using a peroxidase-based chromogenic assay. The cells were treated with HRP-conjugated goat anti-mouse IgG antibody and influenza virus was stained blue by incubation with H_2O_2, *N,N*-diethyl-*p*-phenylenediamine dihydrochloride and 4-chloro-1-naphthol. EC_{50} values were calculated graphically with GraphPad Prism using the fluorescent assay data. Eleven replicates were used for A/Aichi/102/2008 H3N2 and six replicates were used for A/Aichi/75/2008 H3N2.

Plaque-reduction assay. The effectiveness of 2α,3ax-difluoro-*N*-acetylneuraminic acid against influenza plaque reduction was assessed with recombinant B/Lee/40 influenza virus based on a previously reported method[52]. MDCK cell monolayers were inoculated with virus (~40 PFU per well) and the plates were incubated for 1 h at 37 °C. The inoculum was then removed and an agarose overlay containing appropriate inhibitor dilution was added. After 2 days of incubation at 37 °C, the results of plaques reduction were recorded, and the EC_{50} values were calculated graphically using GraphPad Prism. Six replicates were used for the plaque-reduction assay.

References

1. Imai, M. *et al.* Experimental adaptation of an influenza H5 HA confers respiratory droplet transmission to a reassortant H5 HA/H1N1 virus in ferrets. *Nature* **486,** 420–428 (2012).
2. Herfst, S. *et al.* Airborne transmission of influenza A/H5N1 virus between ferrets. *Science* **336,** 1534–1541 (2012).
3. Guan, Y. *et al.* The emergence of pandemic influenza viruses. *Protein Cell* **1,** 9–13 (2010).
4. Gao, G. F. & Sun, Y. It is not just AIV: from avian to swine-origin influenza virus. *Sci. China Life Sci.* **53,** 151–153 (2010).
5. Jagger, B. W. *et al.* An overlapping protein-coding region in influenza A virus segment 3 modulates the host response. *Science* **337,** 199–204 (2012).
6. Vavricka, C. J. *et al.* Special features of the 2009 pandemic swine-origin influenza A H1N1 hemagglutinin and neuraminidase. *Chin. Sci. Bull.* **56,** 1747–1752 (2011).
7. Sun, Y. *et al.* *In silico* characterization of the functional and structural modules of the hemagglutinin protein from the swine-origin influenza virus A (H1N1)-2009. *Sci. China Life Sci.* **53,** 633–642 (2010).
8. von Itzstein, M. *Influenza Virus Sialidase—A Drug Discovery Target* (Springer, Basel, 2012).
9. Centers for Disease Control and Prevention. Influenza activity-United States and worldwide, 2007–08 season. *Morb. Mortal. Wkly. Rep.* **58,** 115–119 (2009).
10. von Itzstein, M. *et al.* Rational design of potent sialidase-based inhibitors of influenza virus replication. *Nature* **363,** 418–423 (1993).
11. Kim, C. U. *et al.* Influenza neuraminidase inhibitors possessing a novel hydrophobic interaction in the enzyme active site: design, synthesis, and structural analysis of carbocyclic sialic acid analogues with potent anti-influenza activity. *J. Am. Chem. Soc.* **119,** 681–690 (1997).
12. Yamashita, M. *et al.* CS-8958, a prodrug of the new neuraminidase inhibitor R-125489, shows long-acting anti-influenza virus activity. *Antimicrob. Agents Chemother.* **53,** 186–192 (2009).

13. Chong, A. K., Pegg, M. S., Taylor, N. R. & von Itzstein, M. Evidence for a sialosyl cation transition-state complex in the reaction of sialidase from influenza virus. *Eur. J. Biochem.* **207,** 335–343 (1992).
14. Taylor, N. R. & von Itzstein, M. Molecular modeling studies on ligand binding to sialidase from influenza virus and the mechanism of catalysis. *J. Med. Chem.* **37,** 616–624 (1994).
15. Rye, C. S. & Withers, S. G. Glycosidase mechanisms. *Curr. Opin. Chem. Biol.* **4,** 573–580 (2000).
16. Guo, X., Laver, W. G., Vimir, E. & Sinnott, M. L. Catalysis by two sialidases with the same protein fold but different stereochemical courses: a mechanistic comparison of the enzymes from influenza A virus and *Salmonella typhimurium*. *J. Am. Chem. Soc* **116,** 5572–5578 (1994).
17. Watson, J. N., Dookhun, V., Borgford, T. J. & Bennet, A. J. Mutagenesis of the conserved active-site tyrosine changes a retaining sialidase into an inverting sialidase. *Biochemistry* **42,** 12682–12690 (2003).
18. Watts, A. G., Oppezzo, P., Withers, S. G., Alzari, P. M. & Buschiazzo, A. Structural and kinetic analysis of two covalent sialosyl-enzyme intermediates on *Trypanosoma rangeli* sialidase. *J. Biol. Chem.* **281,** 4149–4155 (2006).
19. Chan, J. *et al.* Bacterial and viral sialidases: contribution of the conserved active site glutamate to catalysis. *Biochemistry* **51,** 433–441 (2012).
20. Chou, D. T. H., Watson, J. N., Scholte, A. A., Borgford, T. J. & Bennet, A. J. Effect of neutral pyridine leaving groups on the mechanisms of influenza type A viral sialidase-catalyzed and spontaneous hydrolysis reactions of α-D-*N*-acetylneuraminides. *J. Am. Chem. Soc.* **122,** 8357–8364 (2000).
21. Burmeister, W. P., Henrissat, B., Bosso, C., Cusack, S. & Ruigrok, R. W. H. Influenza B virus neuraminidase can synthesize its own inhibitor. *Structure* **1,** 19–26 (1993).
22. Ghate, A. A. & Air, G. M. Site-directed mutagenesis of catalytic residues of influenza virus neuraminidase as an aid to drug design. *Europ. J. Biochem.* **258,** 320–331 (1998).
23. Thomas, A., Jourand, D., Bret, C., Amara, P. & Field, M. J. Is there a covalent intermediate in the viral neuraminidase reaction? A hybrid potential free-energy study. *J. Am. Chem. Soc.* **121,** 9693–9702 (1999).
24. Xu, G. G. *et al.* Three Streptococcus pneumoniae sialidases: three different products. *J. Am. Chem. Soc.* **133,** 1718–1721 (2011).
25. Lentz, M. R., Webster, R. G. & Air, G. M. Site-directed mutation of the active-site of influenza neuraminidase and implications for the catalytic mechanism. *Biochemistry* **26,** 5351–5358 (1987).
26. Watts, A. G. & Withers, S. G. The synthesis of some mechanistic probes for sialic acid processing enzymes and the labeling of a sialidase from Trypanosoma rangeli. *Can. J. Chem.* **82,** 1581–1588 (2004).
27. Nakajima, T., Hori, H., Ohrui, H., Meguro, H. & Ido, T. Synthesis of *N*-acetyl-3-fluoro-neuraminic acids. *Agr. Biol. Chem. Tokyo* **52,** 1209–1215 (1988).
28. Tsuchiya, T. Chemistry and developments of fluorinated carbohydrates. *Adv. Carbohydr. Chem. Biochem.* **48,** 91–277 (1990).
29. Hagiwara, T., Kijimasuda, I., Ido, T., Ohrui, H. & Tomita, K. Inhibition of bacterial and viral sialidases by 3-fluoro-*N*-acetylneuraminic acid. *Carbohydr. Res.* **263,** 167–172 (1994).
30. Ikeda, K. *et al.* 2β,3β-difluorosialic acid derivatives structurally modified at the C-4 position: synthesis and biological evaluation as inhibitors of human parainfluenza virus type 1. *Carbohydr. Res.* **339,** 1367–1372 (2004).
31. Swaminathan, K. & Downard, K. M. Anti-viral binding to influenza neuraminidase by MALDI mass spectrometry. *Anal. Chem.* **84,** 3725–3730 (2012).
32. Collins, P. J. *et al.* Crystal structures of oseltamivir-resistant influenza virus neuraminidase mutants. *Nature* **453,** 1258–1261 (2008).
33. Varghese, J. N. *et al.* Drug design against a shifting target: a structural basis for resistance to inhibitors in a variant of influenza virus neuraminidase. *Structure* **6,** 735–746 (1998).
34. Singh, J., Petter, R. C., Baillie, T. A. & Whitty, A. The resurgence of covalent drugs. *Nat. Chem. Biol.* **10,** 307–317 (2011).
35. Amaro, R. E., Cheng, X., Ivanov, I., Xu, D. & McCammon, J. A. Characterizing loop dynamics and ligand recognition in human- and avian-type influenza neuraminidases via generalized born molecular dynamics and end-point free energy calculations. *J. Am. Chem. Soc.* **131,** 4702–4709 (2009).
36. Hatakeyama, S. *et al.* Enhanced expression of an α2,6-linked sialic acid on MDCK cells improves isolation of human influenza viruses and evaluation of their sensitivity to a neuraminidase inhibitor. *J. Clin. Microbiol.* **43,** 4139–4146 (2005).
37. Sriwilaijaroen, N. *et al.* Mechanisms of the action of povidone-iodine against human and avian influenza A viruses: its effects on hemagglutination and sialidase activities. *Virol. J.* **6,** 124 (2009).
38. Xu, X., Zhu, X., Dwek, R. A., Stevens, J. & Wilson, I. A. Structural characterization of the 1918 influenza virus H1N1 neuraminidase. *J. Virol.* **82,** 10493–10501 (2008).
39. Zhang, W. *et al.* Crystal structure of the swine-origin A (H1N1) - 2009 influenza A virus hemagglutinin (HA) reveals similar antigenicity to that of the 1918 pandemic virus. *Protein Cell* **1,** 459–467 (2010).
40. Li, Q. *et al.* The 2009 pandemic H1N1 neuraminidase N1 lacks the 150-cavity in its active site. *Nat. Struct. Mol. Biol.* **17,** 1266–1268 (2010).
41. Vavricka, C. J. *et al.* Structural and functional analysis of laninamivir and its octanoate prodrug reveals group specific mechanisms for influenza NA inhibition. *PLoS Pathog.* **7,** e1002249 (2011).
42. Potier, M., Mameli, L., Belisle, M., Dallaire, L. & Melancon, S. B. Fluorometric assay of neuraminidase with a sodium (4-methylumbelliferyl-α-D-*N*-acetylneuraminate) substrate. *Anal. Biochem.* **94,** 287–296 (1979).
43. Otwinowski, Z. & Minor, W. Processing of X-ray diffraction data collected in oscillation mode. *Method. Enzymol.* **276,** 307–326 (1997).
44. Read, R. J. Pushing the boundaries of molecular replacement with maximum likelihood. *Acta Crystallogr. D Biol. Crystallogr.* **57,** 1373–1382 (2001).
45. Collaborative Computational Project, Number 4. The CCP4 suite: programs for protein crystallography. *Acta Crystallogr. D Biol. Crystallogr.* **50,** 760–763 (1994).
46. Murshudov, G. N., Vagin, A. A. & Dodson, E. J. Refinement of macromolecular structures by the maximum-likelihood method. *Acta Crystallogr. D Biol. Crystallogr.* **53,** 240–255 (1997).
47. Emsley, P. & Cowtan, K. Coot: model-building tools for molecular graphics. *Acta Crystallogr. D Biol. Crystallogr.* **60,** 2126–2132 (2004).
48. Adams, P. D. *et al.* PHENIX: a comprehensive python-based system for macromolecular structure solution. *Acta Crystallogr. D Biol. Crystallogr.* **66,** 213–221 (2010).
49. Laskowski, R. A., Macarthur, M. W., Moss, D. S. & Thornton, J. M. Procheck – a program to check the stereochemical quality of protein structures. *J. Appl. Crystallogr.* **26,** 283–291 (1993).
50. Mosmann, T. Rapid colorimetric assay for cellular growth and survival: application to proliferation and cytotoxicity assays. *J. Immunol. Methods* **65,** 55–63 (1983).
51. Sriwilaijaroen, N. *et al.* Antiviral effects of *Psidium guajava* Linn. (guava) tea on the growth of clinical isolated H1N1 viruses: Its role in viral hemagglutination and neuraminidase inhibition. *Antivir. Res.* **94,** 139–146 (2012).
52. Hayden, F. G., Cote, K. M. & Douglas, Jr. R. G. Plaque inhibition assay for drug susceptibility testing of influenza viruses. *Antimicrob. Agents Chemother.* **17,** 865–870 (1980).

Acknowledgements

Research in G.F.G.'s lab is supported by the National 973 project (Grant No. 2011CB504703) and the National Natural Science Foundation of China (NSFC, Grant No. 81021003). G.F.G. is a leading principal investigator of the NSFC Innovative Research Group. C.J.V. is supported by the Chinese Academy of Sciences Fellowship for Young International Scientists (Grant No. 2011Y2SA01) and the NSFC Research Fund for Young International Scientists (Grant No. 31250110214). H.K. is supported by a grant-in-aid from Japan Society for the Promotion of Science (Grant No. 17580092 and 19580120). Y.S. is supported by a grant from the MEXT COE project for private universities. We acknowledge Hongna Huang and Yanfang Zhang for help with protein production, and Shuhua Zhou (NMR facility at Institute of Biophysics, CAS) for help with NMR experiments. We thank Professor Yoshihiro Kawaoka for providing the plasmids used to rescue B/Lee/40 influenza B virus and the AX4 cells used in this study. Finally, we are grateful to Hiroshi Ohrui (Yokohama College of Pharmacy, Yokohama, Japan) and Yoshitomo Suhara (Shibaura Institute of Technology, Tokyo, Japan) for their synthetic research of fluorinated sialic acid derivatives which contributed to this work.

Author contributions

C.J.V., Y.L., H.K., Y.S. and G.F.G. designed the research; C.J.V., Y.L., H.K., N.S., J.Q., K.T., Y.W., Q.L. and Y.L. performed the research; all authors analysed the data; and C.J.V., Y. L., and G.F.G. wrote the paper.

Additional information

Accession Code: Atomic coordinates and structure factors for the N2-Tyr406Asp-β-Neu5Ac and N2-covalent complexes have been deposited in the Protein Data Bank under the accession codes 4H53 and 4H52, respectively.

Competing financial interests: The authors declare no competing financial interests.

15

Late-stage C–H functionalization of complex alkaloids and drug molecules via intermolecular rhodium-carbenoid insertion

Jing He[1], Lawrence G. Hamann[1], Huw M.L. Davies[2] & Rohan E.J. Beckwith[1]

Alkaloids constitute a large family of natural products possessing diverse biological properties. Their unique and complex structures have inspired numerous innovations in synthetic chemistry. In the realm of late-stage C–H functionalization, alkaloids remain a significant challenge due to the presence of the basic amine and a variety of other functional groups. Herein we report the first examples of dirhodium(II)-catalysed intermolecular C–H insertion into complex natural products containing nucleophilic tertiary amines to generate a C–C bond. The application to a diverse range of alkaloids and drug molecules demonstrates remarkable chemoselectivity and predictable regioselectivity. The capacity for late-stage diversification is highlighted in the catalyst-controlled selective functionalizations of the alkaloid brucine. The remarkable selectivity observed, particularly for site-specific C–H insertion at *N*-methyl functionalities, offers utility in a range of applications where efficient installation of synthetic handles on complex alkaloids is desired.

[1] Department of Global Discovery Chemistry, Novartis Institutes for BioMedical Research, 250 Massachusetts Avenue, Cambridge, Massachusetts 02139, USA. [2] Department of Chemistry, Emory University, 1515 Dickey Drive, Atlanta, Georgia 30322, USA. Correspondence and requests for materials should be addressed to H.M.L.D. (email: hmdavie@emory.edu) or to R.E.J.B. (email: rohan.beckwith@novartis.com).

The decline in the number of new drug approvals in recent years despite high levels of R&D investment has spurred a number of alternative approaches towards drug discovery within the pharmaceutical industry[1]. This includes a resurgence in phenotypic screens, and along with that a renewed interest in exploiting the unique structural diversity of natural products to modulate disease-relevant processes[2–5]. Drug-discovery efforts around natural product optimization have been underexplored, owing in part to the synthetic challenge of effecting useful modifications in the face of structural complexity and diverse functionality. Advances in synthetic methodology are therefore essential to enable progression of natural product hits of compelling phenotype into suitable probes for elucidating mechanism of action and towards the development of new therapeutics[6,7].

C–H functionalization is one such approach that has the potential to revolutionize how complex organic molecules, such as natural products, are made through the ability to selectively and efficiently transform C–H bonds in a predictable manner under mild conditions. Over the last two decades, the field of C–H functionalization has experienced explosive growth, and a number of highly effective transformations have been developed. Many compelling examples have been reported on the utilization of C–H functionalization as key strategic reactions in total synthesis, illustrating novel retrosynthetic analysis and step-economical synthesis[8–13]. In recent years, considerable efforts have been expended on the late-stage C–H functionalization of biologically compelling natural products and drug-like molecules[14–22]. This has been challenging, because although the pace of advances in C–H functionalization has been impressive, in many instances the new methodology is limited to a narrow range of substrates and functional groups. Many of the most effective C–H functionalization processes rely on the use of directing groups, which need to be introduced and then removed[23]. Consequently, the late-stage C–H functionalization examples demonstrated to date often use rather specialized substrates and are of limited generality.

Our aim is to select structurally complex molecules of compelling biological activity and then attempt to devise approaches to execute site-selective modification of C–H bonds in such compounds bearing multiple functional groups. The overarching goal is to establish a toolkit of reactions and reagents amenable to effecting functionalizations on a variety of complex molecules in a relatively predictive and selective manner for broad application. Alkaloids represent an extremely challenging class of natural products for direct C–H functionalization, because they typically contain a basic amine and a variety of other reactive functionality. In particular, a basic amine can impede many C–H-activation methodologies, as the nitrogen functionality may coordinate to and poison the catalyst[24–26] or generate undesirable side reactions[27,28]. Only a few examples of selective oxidation[29,30] or C–H amination of alkaloid derivatives have been reported, although in the case of the latter aza-ylide products are also formed and in many cases are the exclusive product[27]. One of the most effective methods for site-selective C–H functionalization, without resorting to the use of directing groups, has been the C–H insertion chemistry of rhodium-bound donor/acceptor carbenes[31]. Herein we demonstrate for the first time that such highly reactive intermediates are indeed capable of undergoing site-selective C–H functionalization of a range of complex alkaloids and drug molecules possessing a tertiary amine. We show that our effective strategy enables C–H functionalization at methyl, methylene or methine sites proximal to the basic amine, with little to no aza-ylide formation. This study constitutes a proof of concept that we envision can be readily extended to a wide range of applications, where efficient installation of synthetic handles on complex alkaloids may find utility. For instance, such a paradigm would be expected to greatly facilitate the ability to derivatize payloads for attachment to monoclonal antibodies for antibody–drug conjugate systems[32], and in probe design for target identification or mechanism of action studies in a chemical genetics context[27,33].

Results

Rhodium-carbenoid-mediated C–H functionalization of brucine. Brucine (**1**) is a readily available complex natural product, which contains 22 C–H bonds in different chemical environments. The presence of two doubly activated allylic sites, a complex multi-ring architecture, a lactam functionality, an electron-rich phenyl ring, methyl ethers, as well as a basic tertiary amine offered a challenging target on which to commence these studies. A metal-free carbene approach to derivatize brucine was recently reported, which yielded a ring-expanded product through formation of an aza-ylide species followed by a [1,2]-Stevens rearrangement[34]. Indeed, the use of metallocarbenoids to access an aza-ylide intermediate followed by ring expansion has been widely described[35–37]. Interested in effecting C–H insertions via a carbenoid approach, we were intrigued as to whether the presence of a suitable rhodium catalyst and appropriate temperature might influence the nature of the reaction with brucine, allowing for C–H insertion over aza-ylide formation or catalyst poisoning, despite the presence of the nucleophilic amine. To the best of our knowledge, the ability to effect such chemistry on substrates possessing a tertiary amine, especially in structurally complex alkaloids, has not been previously reported[31,38].

As illustrated in Fig. 1a, we first compared the influence of a dirhodium catalyst in contrast to a metal-free system. Brucine was treated with excess methyl-*p*-bromophenyl diazoacetate (**2**) in the presence or absence of the well-established carbenoid C–H insertion catalyst Rh_2(*S*-DOSP)$_4$ (ref. 31) in trifluorotoluene at 83 °C (oil bath temperature). We observed that the Rh_2(*S*-DOSP)$_4$-catalysed reaction provided C–H insertion product **3** in 20% yield as a single diastereomer, in addition to the expected Stevens rearrangement product **4** in 58% yield with 1.2:1 diastereomeric ratio (dr). When the same reaction was carried out in the absence of Rh_2(*S*-DOSP)$_4$, formation of **3** and **4** was not observed, strongly suggesting that effective functionalization of brucine was mediated via the dirhodium catalyst. Attempting the Rh_2(*S*-DOSP)$_4$-catalysed reaction at ambient temperature in either dichloromethane or trifluorotoluene failed to afford compound **3** or **4**. The differential outcome observed when conducting the reaction at room temperature as opposed to 83 °C led us to rationalize that a higher temperature enables a more rapid kinetic dissociation of the amine from the dirhodium catalyst. No longer incapacitated, the catalyst is free to effect diazo decomposition and carbenoid formation.

Control experiment. Having isolated aza-ylide **5**, we postulated whether formation of C–H insertion product **3** actually proceeded through a non-rhodium-bound ylide intermediate (as proposed in the formation of **4**)[34] aided by thermal activation. Accordingly, a control experiment was conducted as presented in Fig. 1b. Aza-ylide **5** was alternatively prepared *in situ* through deprotonation of the corresponding trifluoroacetate salt **6** at 0 °C. The reaction was heated to 83 °C in a pressure vessel for 30 min, yielding exclusively [1,2]-Stevens rearrangement product **4** in 1:1 dr. Since C–H insertion product **3** was not observed, it suggests that ylide formation and carbenoid C–H insertion proceed through different reaction pathways. Indeed, we speculate that product **3** is formed via direct C–H insertion

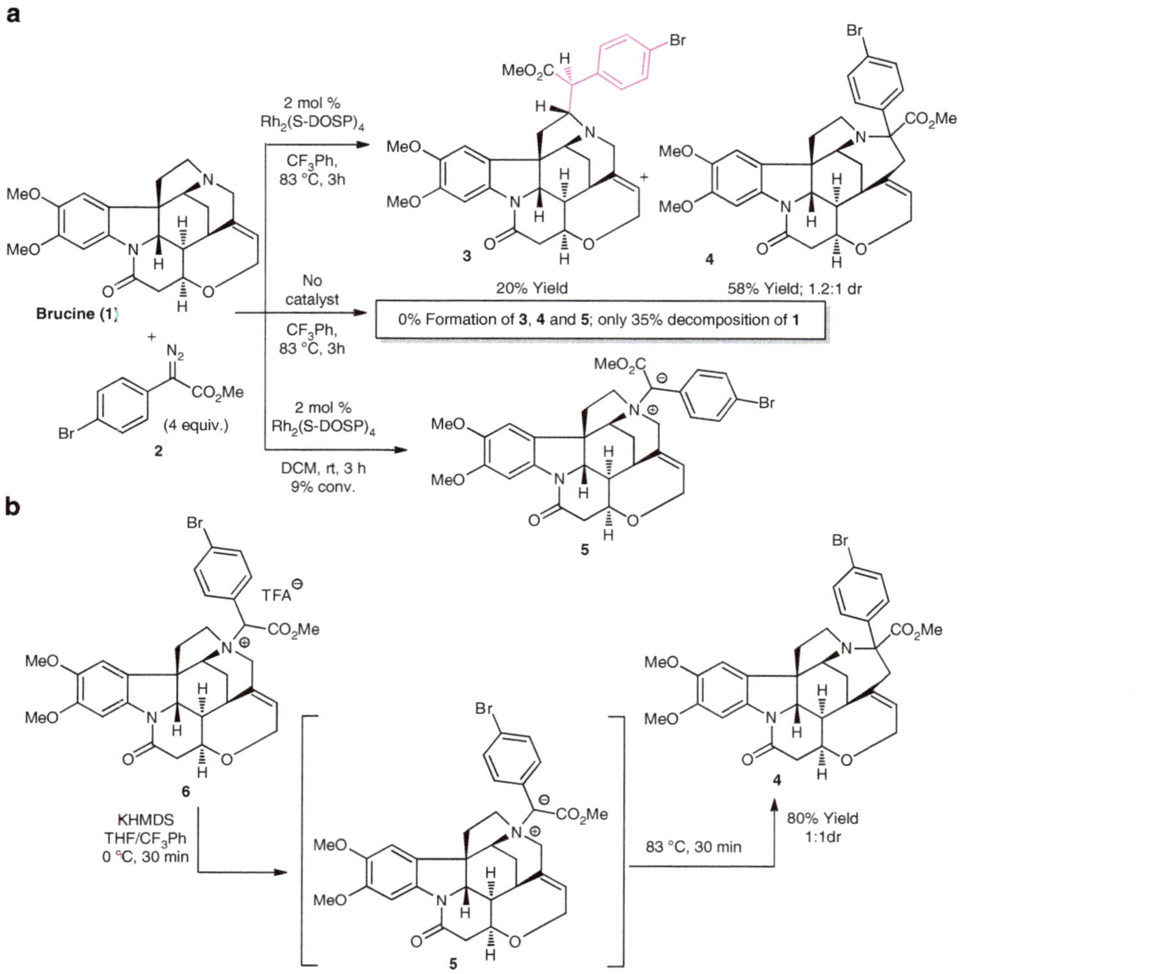

Figure 1 | Donor/acceptor rhodium-carbenoid-mediated functionalization of brucine (1). (**a**) Investigations into the role of the catalyst and temperature. (**b**) Control experiment provided mechanistic insights for the formation of C-H insertion product **3**. Conversion, yield and dr were determined by ^{1}H NMR with addition of 4-dimethylaminopyridine (DMAP) after work-up as an internal standard. rt, room temperature.

induced by the metal carbene[39,40]. This being the case, it is remarkable that **3** is the sole C–H insertion product observed from a molecule that has numerous potential sites for C–H functionalization. The subtle balance between electronic, steric and stereoelectronic effects can often result in exquisite regiocontrol in the C–H functionalization reactions of donor/acceptor rhodium carbenes[31], but such control has not been previously demonstrated with such a complex substrate.

Influence of dirhodium catalysts. The electrophilicity and steric environment of the metallocarbenoids can be affected by the nature of the catalyst[31]. Hence, we were eager to explore what influence various dirhodium catalysts would have on the site selectivity of the reaction (Table 1). The bulky dirhodium catalyst $Rh_2(TPA)_4$ promoted formation of the C–H insertion product, giving **3** in 50% yield as a single diastereomer. Subsequent investigations into other achiral rhodium catalysts (Table 1, entries 2–5) revealed that $Rh_2(TPA)_4$ is the most effective catalyst for carbenoid-mediated C–H insertion. In addition, the formation of Stevens rearrangement product **4** is a competing pathway for which the chemoselectivity between the formation of compounds **3** and **4** is catalyst dependent. Furthermore, the two enantiomers of chiral catalysts afforded different results. For example, only the use of the *S*-enantiomer of the DOSP ligand allowed for C–H insertion (Table 1, entries 7 and 8). A most unexpected result was obtained with the very bulky chiral catalyst $Rh_2(BTPCP)_4$ refs 41,42. Under the standard reaction conditions, the $Rh_2(BTPCP)_4$-catalysed reactions suffered very poor conversion, irrespective of whether the *R*- or *S*-enantiomer of the catalyst was used (Table 1, entries 11 and 12). Careful ^{1}H nuclear magnetic resonance (NMR) analysis of the crude reaction mixture revealed an alternative C–H insertion product (**7**) had been generated in low yield with $Rh_2(S\text{-}BTPCP)_4$. Increasing the catalyst loading of $Rh_2(S\text{-}BTPCP)_4$ to 20 mol% afforded compound **7** in 39% yield as a single diastereomer, albeit with moderate conversion (Fig. 2a). Extensive one- and two-dimensional NMR experiments confirmed that this new compound **7** was generated through C–H insertion into the tertiary C–H bond adjacent to the amine. The ability for $Rh_2(S\text{-}BTPCP)_4$ to enable selective C–H insertion at the methine position is unexpected, because a bulky catalyst should generally favour functionalization of a less-sterically encumbered C–H bond[42]. The catalyst screen reveals that one can manipulate the favoured site for functionalization in a catalyst-controlled manner, allowing one to rapidly probe three alternative sites on a complex molecule (Fig. 2a).

Table 1 | Influence of dirhodium catalyst on C-H carbene insertion of brucine (1).

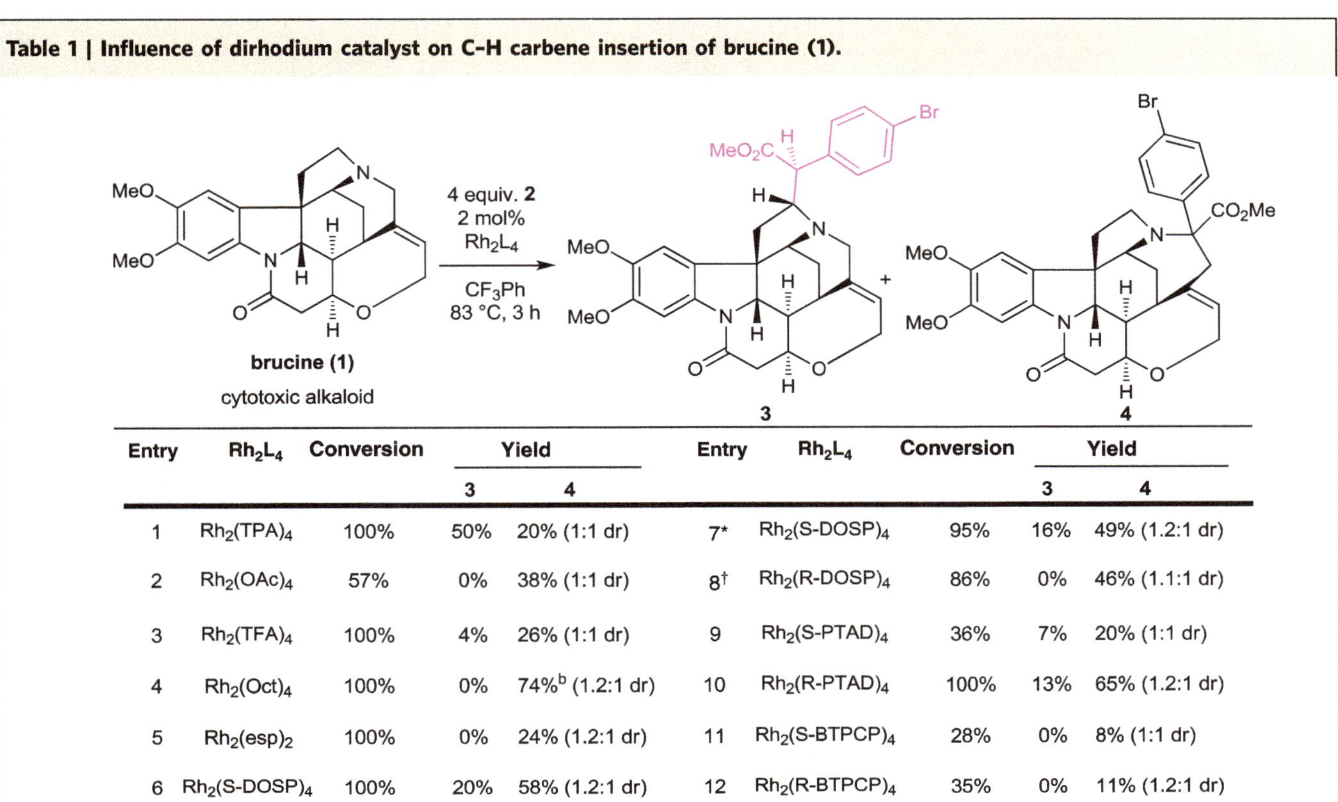

Entry	Rh_2L_4	Conversion	Yield 3	Yield 4	Entry	Rh_2L_4	Conversion	Yield 3	Yield 4
1	$Rh_2(TPA)_4$	100%	50%	20% (1:1 dr)	7*	$Rh_2(S\text{-}DOSP)_4$	95%	16%	49% (1.2:1 dr)
2	$Rh_2(OAc)_4$	57%	0%	38% (1:1 dr)	8†	$Rh_2(R\text{-}DOSP)_4$	86%	0%	46% (1.1:1 dr)
3	$Rh_2(TFA)_4$	100%	4%	26% (1:1 dr)	9	$Rh_2(S\text{-}PTAD)_4$	36%	7%	20% (1:1 dr)
4	$Rh_2(Oct)_4$	100%	0%	74%[b] (1.2:1 dr)	10	$Rh_2(R\text{-}PTAD)_4$	100%	13%	65% (1.2:1 dr)
5	$Rh_2(esp)_2$	100%	0%	24% (1.2:1 dr)	11	$Rh_2(S\text{-}BTPCP)_4$	28%	0%	8% (1:1 dr)
6	$Rh_2(S\text{-}DOSP)_4$	100%	20%	58% (1.2:1 dr)	12	$Rh_2(R\text{-}BTPCP)_4$	35%	0%	11% (1.2:1 dr)

Conversion, yield and dr were determined by ^{1}H NMR analysis with addition of DMAP during work-up as an internal standard, unless otherwise specified.
*1,2-Dichloroethane was used as solvent.
†Isolated yield.

Diazo scope. Studies with a small set of aryldiazoacetates of distinct electronic properties indicate that the nature of the carbenoid also plays a role in the chemoselectivity of the rhodium-carbenoid insertion (Table 2, entries 1-3). Donor/acceptor carbenoids bearing electron-deficient aryl substituents favoured C–H insertion product **9** over aza-ylide formation (Table 2, entries 1 and 3), whereas an electron-donating substituent provides a less-electrophilic rhodium-carbenoid for which exclusive formation of ring-expanded product **10** was observed (Table 2, entry 2). Reaction with methyl diazomalonate (**8c**) or ethyl diazoacetate (**8d**) failed to generate any C–H insertion or Stevens rearrangement product (Table 2, entries 4 and 5), suggesting the importance of the donor group in the efficiency of intermolecular C–H insertion reactions under these conditions.

C–H functionalization of securinine. To explore reaction generality, we applied the $Rh_2(TPA)_4$-mediated approach to other structurally complex alkaloids and tertiary amine-containing drug molecules (Figs 3 and 4). The $GABA_A$ antagonist securinine (**12**) is a tricyclic alkaloid possessing two olefins in conjugation with a lactone functionality, in addition to the tertiary amine (Fig. 3a). Treatment of **12** with methyl-*p*-bromophenyl diazoacetate (**2**) and $Rh_2(TPA)_4$ in trifluorotoluene at 83 °C selectively gave C–H insertion product **13** (44% yield, 2.2:1 dr), with no competing cyclopropanation at either olefin[43]. Furthermore, although securinine contains four C–H bonds adjacent to the amine (two methine and two diastereotopic methylene in nature), only a single methylene C–H bond undergoes carbene insertion. Unlike the case of brucine in which substrate control afforded a highly diastereoselective C–H insertion product, with securinine the diastereoselectivity was rather moderate, and was influenced by the dirhodium catalyst itself (Fig. 3a).

C–H functionalization of apovincamine. Further application of this method to apovincamine (**14a**) led to bis-cyclopropanation of the electron-rich indole ring **16,** with only minimal formation of the C–H insertion product (Fig. 3b)[44]. Attempts with other dirhodium catalysts provided similar reaction outcomes. It is well established that aromatic rings are sterically protected from reaction with rhodium donor/acceptor carbenoids when they are at least 1,4-disubstituted[45]. Accordingly, the iodinated apovincamine analogue **14b** was prepared and evaluated in the reaction, and in this instance the C–H insertion product **15b** was obtained in improved yield (47% yield) as a single diastereomer. Although **14b** contains one methine and four methylene C–H bonds adjacent to the amine, the C–H insertion occurred selectively at the benzylic methylene site rather than alpha to the amine. Previously, it has been reported that benzylic C–H bonds are also favourable sites for C–H insertion, due to the capacity of π-systems to stabilize the neighbouring buildup of positive charge in the transition state[46].

Selective *N*-methyl C–H insertion. C–H functionalization induced by dirhodium-bound donor/acceptor carbenoids has been shown to be initiated by a hydride transfer event, and sites that are capable of stabilizing positive charge buildup at carbon are electronically favoured[40]. However, the general order of reactivity of C–H bonds in competition reactions is typically methine $\sim$ methylene $>$ methyl, because although tertiary sites are

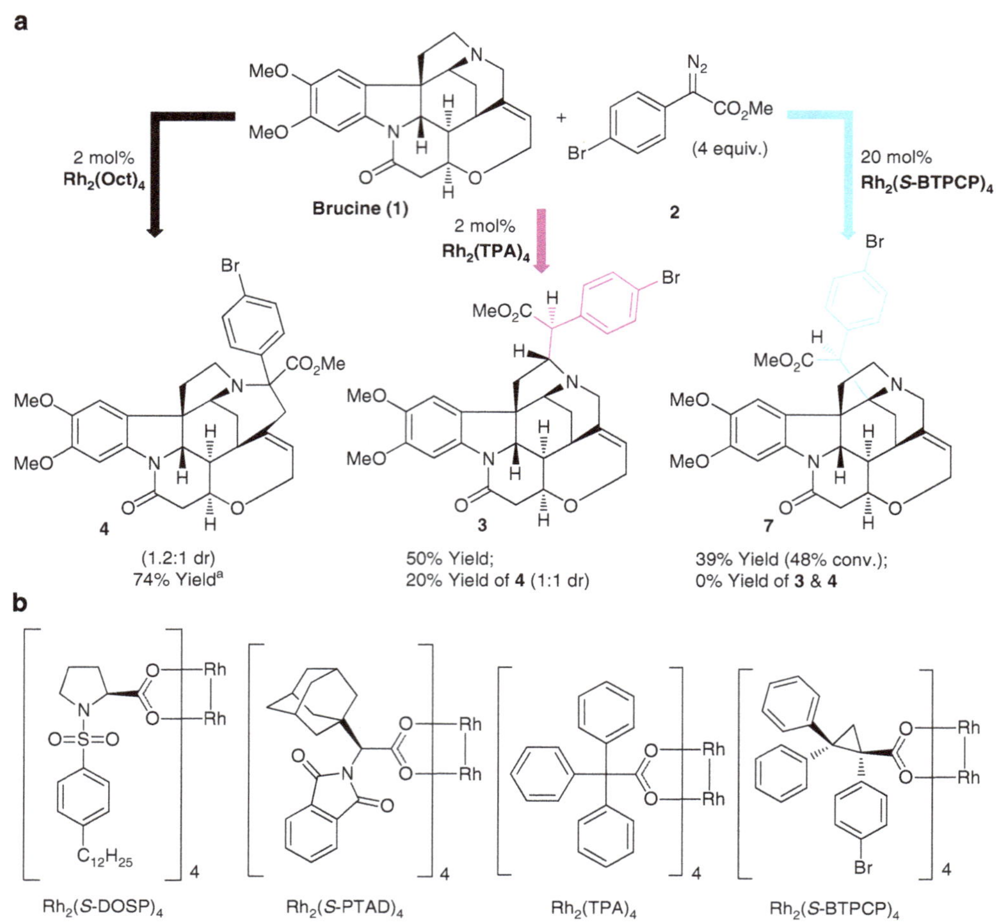

Figure 2 | Optimization of rhodium-catalysed C-H carbene insertion of brucine (1). (**a**) Catalyst influence on site-selective C-H functionalization of brucine (**1**). (**b**) Structures of dirhodium catalysts. Conversion, yield and dr were determined by ^1H NMR analysis with addition of 4-dimethylaminopyridine after work-up as an internal standard, unless otherwise specified. [a]Isolated yield.

electronically most activated, donor/acceptor carbenoids are sterically very demanding[31]. In the alkaloids studied so far the reactions have been remarkably site selective, suggesting that the majority of electronically activated methine and methylene sites in these alkaloids are sterically inaccessible. Therefore, we chose to explore the reactions of alkaloids containing *N*-methyl groups. Functionalization of electronically activated methyl C–H bonds has been observed, but only a few examples of C–H insertion into methyl C–H bonds in the presence of activated methylene and/or methine C–H bonds have been reported[42,47–49], and none of those feature a basic amine. We found for alkaloids possessing an *N*-Me functionality, the most favoured product in each case arose from C–H insertion into the said *N*-methyl group (Fig. 4). With dextromethorphan (**17**), for example, carbene insertion at the *N*-methyl C–H bond was the most favoured product despite methylene sites adjacent to the nitrogen atom and the phenyl ring. It is worth noting that no insertion was observed at the accessible methyl ether site. Indeed, C–H insertion at the *N*-methyl site was such a favoured pathway that we were able to effect the reaction at room temperature affording 87% yield of C–H insertion product (1:1 dr), with complete conversion of **17**. The structurally related yet more elaborate thebaine (**18**) smoothly underwent C–H insertion at the *N*-methyl site (52%, 1.4:1 dr), without any competing reactivity despite the electron-rich aryl group and the 1,3-diene functionality. It appears that regardless of conformation or neighbouring functionalities, in all systems explored the donor/acceptor carbenoid derived from **2** selectively inserts into the primary C–H bond adjacent to nitrogen. In addition, the apparent ease of insertion into the *N*-methyl group enables some reactions to be conducted at room temperature, with diazo **2** used as the limiting reagent, as was the case with noscapine (**19**), although the structurally related bicuculline (**20**) required more forcing conditions. Generally, the diastereoselectivity of the $Rh_2(TPA)_4$-mediated *N*-methyl insertion reactions afforded diastereomeric ratios in the 1:1-2:1 range, and the application of chiral dirhodium catalysts failed to improve on this (Table 3). Sercloremine (**21**) represents an interesting substrate in that its relatively simple structure suggests little potential for steric differentiation between the methylene sites and the terminal methyl site adjacent to the amine, however, the *N*-methyl C–H insertion product is again exclusively formed in 62% yield. It should be noted that Stevens-type rearrangement products were not observed in any of the *N*-methyl-containing systems explored in this study and presumably is no longer a competing pathway. It is likely that the ease of accessibility the primary C–H bond offers has a significant impact on the site-selectivity of this reaction.

We have successfully devised and implemented an effective strategy for non-directed C–H functionalization of nucleophilic tertiary amine-containing complex natural products and drug molecules. We demonstrate that these traditionally challenging substrates are capable of undergoing rhodium-

Table 2 | Influence of diazo reagents on rhodium-catalysed carbene insertion of brucine (1).

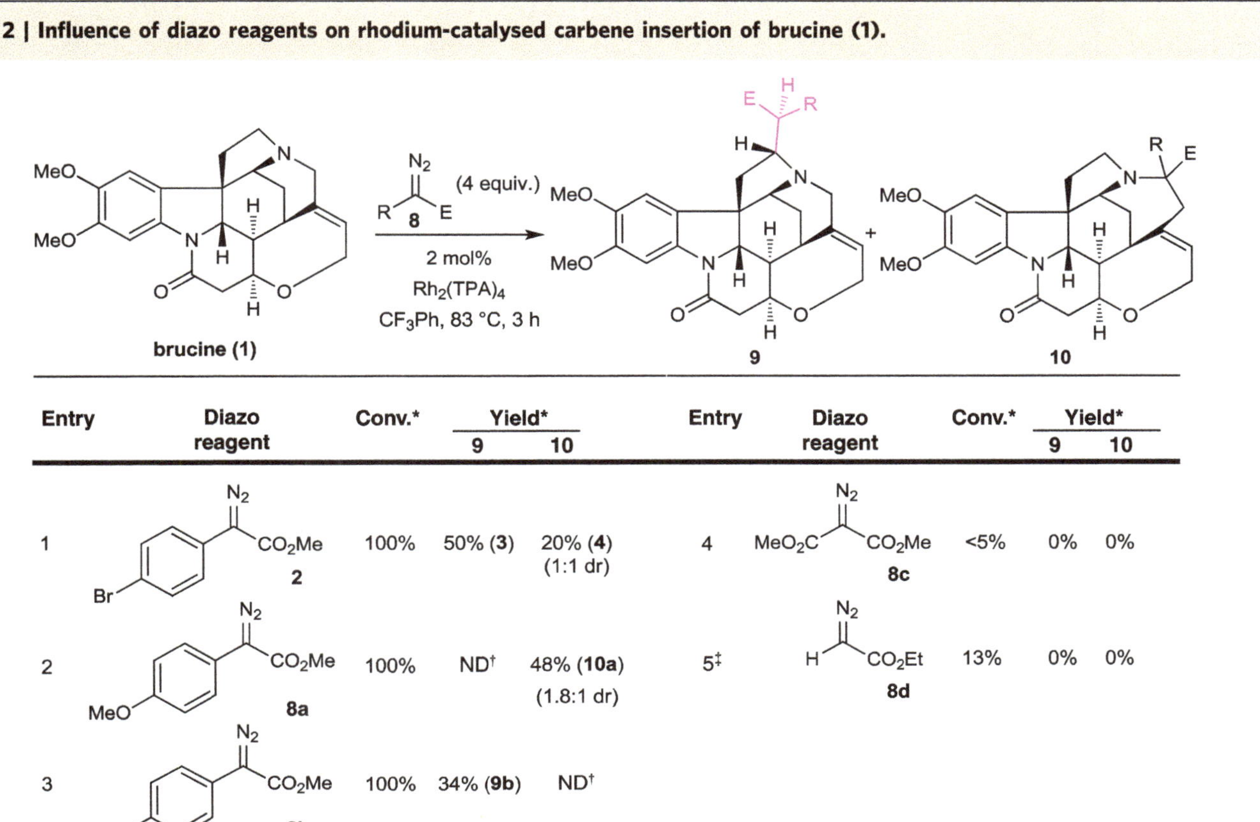

Entry	Diazo reagent	Conv.*	Yield* 9	Yield* 10
1	2	100%	50% (**3**)	20% (**4**) (1:1 dr)
2	8a	100%	ND†	48% (**10a**) (1.8:1 dr)
3	8b	100%	34% (**9b**)	ND†
4	8c	<5%	0%	0%
5‡	8d	13%	0%	0%

DMAP, 4-dimethylaminopyridine; NMR, nuclear magnetic resonance.
*Conversion, yield and dr were determined by ^{1}H NMR analysis with addition of DMAP during work-up as an internal standard, and where formed, the corresponding product is given in bold font in parentheses next to the yield.
†Not determined, but cannot be excluded owing to the presence of a small amount of material isolated as an intractable mixture of products.
‡The corresponding aza-ylide **11** was obtained as trifluoroacetate salt in 4% isolated yield.

Figure 3 | Rhodium-catalysed C-H insertion of alkaloids securinine and apovincamine. (**a**) Diastereoselective C-H carbene insertion is achieved by using chiral rhodium catalysts. (**b**) Introduction of steric hindrance could protect electron-rich aromatic rings from cyclopropanation and enable desired C-H insertion. Yield and dr were determined by ^{1}H NMR analysis with addition of 4-dimethylaminopyridine after work-up as an internal standard, unless otherwise specified.

Figure 4 | C-H insertion in *N*-methyl-containing natural products and drug molecules. [a]Yield and dr were determined by ^{1}H NMR with 4-dimethylaminopyridine as an internal standard. [b]Reaction was carried out in dichloromethane under room temperature. [c]Reaction was carried out with 0.5 equiv. of **2** in dichloromethane at room temperature (54% recovered SM). [d]Reaction was carried out with 0.5 equiv. of **2** (52% recovered SM). [e]Isolated yield.

Table 3 | Chiral dirhodium catalysts screen using bicuculline (20) as a substrate.

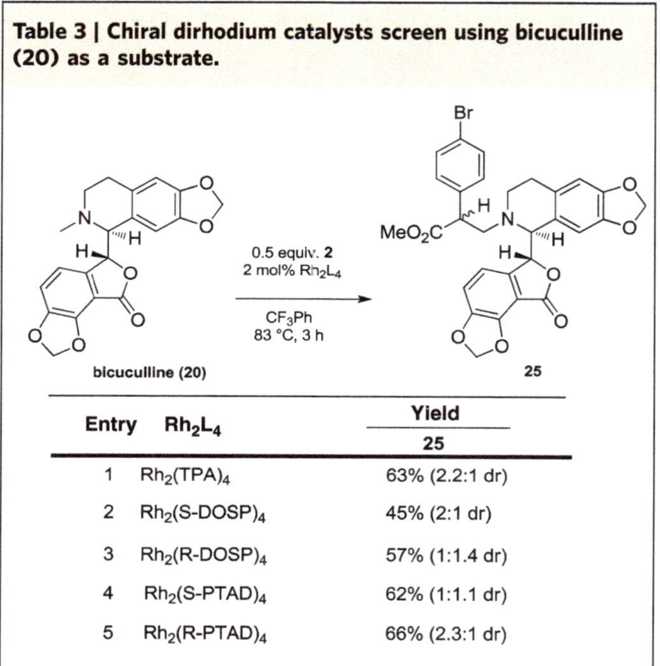

Entry	Rh_2L_4	Yield 25
1	$Rh_2(TPA)_4$	63% (2.2:1 dr)
2	$Rh_2(S\text{-}DOSP)_4$	45% (2:1 dr)
3	$Rh_2(R\text{-}DOSP)_4$	57% (1:1.4 dr)
4	$Rh_2(S\text{-}PTAD)_4$	62% (1:1.1 dr)
5	$Rh_2(R\text{-}PTAD)_4$	66% (2.3:1 dr)

DMAP, 4-dimethylaminopyridine; NMR, nuclear magnetic resonance.
Yield and dr were determined by ^{1}H NMR analysis with addition of DMAP during work-up as an internal standard.

catalysed C–H insertion reactions to selectively install a new C–C bond. The methods we describe are effectively implemented on a diverse set of alkaloids possessing a wide variety of architectures, functionalities and potentially reactive sites. The use of donor/acceptor carbenoids is the key to our ability to achieve such remarkable chemoselectivity and predictable regioselectivity. In addition, our approach obviates the challenging issue of undesired aza-ylide formation commonly observed with carbenoids in the presence of basic nitrogen-containing substrates, and in doing so the work significantly expands and enables the scope of this field[27]. The highly efficient generation of three distinct brucine derivatives in a catalyst-controlled fashion (Fig. 2a), showcases the potential of this approach to offer late-stage diversification of complex molecules. It is worth noting that the site of C–H insertion is routinely in proximity to the amine moiety. We look upon this consistency, in particular the remarkable selectivity for C–H insertion into *N*-methyl-containing alkaloids, as a robust and highly predictable approach for site-specific functionalization of complex molecules, which could be applied late on in a synthetic route for direct derivatization adjacent to an amine, or for the introduction of a synthetic handle for use in bioconjugation strategies for chemical biology studies.

Methods

Materials. Materials were obtained from commercial suppliers and used as received, or prepared according to standard procedures, unless otherwise noted. Sercloremine (**21**) and apovincamine (**14a**) were obtained from the Novartis compound archive. Methyl-*p*-bromophenyl diazoacetate (**2**) as well as its analogues **8a** and **8b** were synthesized according to a previously reported procedure[43]. All reactions were conducted under an inert atmosphere of dry nitrogen. Analytical thin-layer chromatography was performed on Kieselgel 60 F254 (250 μm silica gel) glass plates and compounds were visualized with ultraviolet light 254 nm). Flash column chromatography was performed using Kieselgel 60 (230–400 mesh) silica gel with ethyl acetate/hexanes as eluent, unless indicated otherwise.

General spectroscopic methods. ^{1}H NMR spectra were measured at 400 MHz on a Bruker Avance instrument and reported in parts per million (δ, p.p.m.). Coupling constants (*J*-values) were reported in Hertz (Hz), with multiplicity reported following usual convention: s = singlet, d = doublet, t = triplet, q = quartet, dd = doublet of doublets, m = multiplet and br = broad. The proton signal of the residual, non-deuterated solvent (δ 7.26 for $CHCl_3$) was used as an internal reference for ^{1}H NMR spectra. ^{13}C NMR spectra were completely hetero-decoupled and measured at 100 MHz. Residual chloroform (δ 77.23) was used as an internal reference. Preparative high-performance liquid chromatography was performed using Waters Autopurification system with a photodiode array detector. Preparative supercritical fluid chromatography was performed using a Thar (Waters) SFC 80 preparative system with a Waters 2489 UV/visible detector. All tested compounds were found to be >95% pure (unless stated otherwise) as determined by liquid chromatography-UV (LC-UV)/electrospray ionization (ESI)-mass spectrometry (MS), recorded using an Acquity G2 Xevo OTof mass spectrometer (accuracy <5 p.p.m.) with an electrospray ionization source and Acquity ultra performance liquid chromatograph (conditions: Acquity UPLC BEH C18 1.7 μm 2.1 × 50 mm column, solvent A: water + 0.1% formic acid, solvent B: acetonitrile + 0.1% formic acid, gradient: from 2 to 98% B in 4.4 min, 1.0 ml min^{-1} flow rate and 50 °C). Ammonium salts, which were generated in preparative high-performance liquid chromatography with trifluoroacetic acid or formic acid as a modifier, were converted to the corresponding free amine with 4 equiv. MP-carbonate (Biotage) in 0.1 M dichloromethane for 1 h at room temperature. ^{1}H NMR, ^{13}C NMR and high-resolution mass spectra (HRMS) are provided for all compounds. For NMR spectra and detailed analysis of NMR assignments, see

Supplementary Figs 1–28; Supplementary Notes 1–5, respectively. For supercritical fluid chromatography analysis and ion chromatography analysis of **6** see Supplementary Notes 6,7. See Supplementary Methods for the characterization data of compounds not listed in this section.

Synthesis of 3. An oven-dried 10 ml two-necked round-bottom flask fitted with a condenser was charged with brucine (**1**) (133.2 mg, 0.338 mmol) and $Rh_2(TPA)_4$ (9.7 mg, 6.8 μmol) in degassed trifluorotoluene (3.0 ml) under a nitrogen atmosphere. A solution of methyl-*p*-bromophenyl diazoacetate (**2**) (345 mg, 1.35 mmol) in degassed trifluorotoluene (3.8 ml) was slowly added via a syringe pump over 1 h under nitrogen atmosphere at 83 °C (oil bath temperature). The mixture was stirred at this temperature for 2 h and then concentrated *in vacuo*. ^{1}H NMR analysis with addition of 5.0 mg 4-dimethylaminopyridine as an internal standard indicated **3** was obtained in 50% yield as a single diastereomer and **4** in 20% yield (1:1 dr). The resulting crude was then purified through flash column chromatography (0–50% EtOAc/heptane) twice to afford **3** as a white solid (92.9 mg, 44% isolated yield, Rf = 0.04 in 50% EtOAc/heptane). To aid analysis, **3** was isolated as the corresponding TFA salt. ^{1}H NMR (400 MHz, chloroform-*d*) δ 7.76 (s, 1H), 7.59 (d, J = 8.0 Hz, 2H), 7.44 (d, J = 8.0 Hz, 2H), 6.91 (s, 1H), 6.01 (t, J = 4.0 Hz, 1H), 4.77 (br, 1H), 4.36 (d, J = 8.0 Hz, 1H), 4.35 (m, 1H), 4.24 (dd, J = 16.0, 8.0 Hz, 1H), 4.06 (d, J = 12.0 Hz, 1H), 3.96–4.06 (m, 2H), 3.91 (s, 3H), 3.90 (s, 3H), 3.86 (d, J = 16.0 Hz, 1H), 3.63 (s, 3H), 3.26 (br, 1H), 3.20 (dd, J = 16.0, 8.0 Hz, 1H), 2.73 (dd, J = 16.0, 4.0 Hz, 1H), 2.42–2.51 (m, 2H), 2.29 (t, J = 16.0 Hz, 1H), 2.17 (d, J = 16.0 Hz, 1H), 1.67 (d, J = 16.0 Hz, 1H), 1.39 (dt, J = 8.0, 4.0 Hz, 1H). ^{13}C NMR (100 MHz, chloroform-*d*) δ 170.9, 169.2, 161.7 (CF_3), 150.7, 147.5, 135.9, 135.5, 133.2, 132.9, 132.7, 130.3, 124.1, 118.8, 105.1, 101.3, 76.9, 66.7, 64.2, 63.5, 59.7, 56.5, 53.2, 52.5, 52.0, 51.4, 47.1, 46.1, 42.1, 30.5, 25.6. HRMS (ESI-time of flight (TOF)) $[M+H]^+$ calculated for $C_{32}H_{34}BrN_2O_6$: 621.1600; found: 621.1575. LC-UV/ESI-MS retention time: 1.70 min. Purification of the crude reaction mixture also afforded **4** contaminated with small amount of impurity. A subsequent purification through flash column chromatography (0–50% EtOAc/heptane) provided the two diastereomers of **4** as separate compounds (24.2 mg, 11% isolated yield, Rf = 0.30 in 50% EtOAc/heptane; 17.2 mg, 8% isolated yield, Rf = 0.25 in 50% EtOAc/heptane). **4a**, diastereomer 1: ^{1}H NMR (400 MHz, chloroform-*d*) δ 7.82 (s, 1H), 7.54 (d, J = 8.6 Hz, 2H), 7.40 (d, J = 8.6 Hz, 2H), 6.72 (s, 1H), 5.86 (q, J = 3.8 Hz, 1H), 4.38 (dd, J = 16.4, 5.0 Hz, 1H), 4.27 (m 1H), 4.10 (dm, J = 16.4 Hz, 1H), 3.98 (d, J = 11.1 Hz, 1H), 3.94 (s, 1H), 3.90 (s, 3H), 3.89–3.85 (m, 4H), 3.63 (s, 3H), 3.33–3.22 (m, 1H), 3.03 (d, J = 16.0 Hz, 1H), 2.97 (t, J = 7.5 Hz, 1H), 2.93 (m, 2H), 2.83 (s, 1H), 2.00 (dt, J = 16.0, 4.0 Hz, 1H), 1.96–1.81 (m, 2H), 1.60 (dt, J = 8.0, 4.0 Hz, 1H), 1.41 (d, J = 15.5 Hz, 1H). ^{13}C NMR (100 MHz, chloroform-*d*) δ 173.3, 170.0, 149.4, 146.3, 142.8, 138.3, 135.9, 131.7, 128.8, 128.4, 123.8, 121.5, 105.9, 101.1, 75.8, 68.7, 65.2, 62.9, 59.6, 56.8, 56.4, 53.2, 53.1, 49.4, 48.3, 47.0, 42.4, 39.5, 35.3, 31.7. HRMS (ESI-TOF) $[M+H]^+$ calculated for $C_{32}H_{34}BrN_2O_6$: 621.1600; found: 621.1594. LC-UV/ESI-MS retention time: 2.88 min. **4b**, diastereomer 2: ^{1}H NMR (400 MHz, chloroform-*d*) δ 7.81 (s, 1H), 7.48 (d, J = 8.2 Hz, 2H), 7.26 (br, 2H), 6.67 (s, 1H), 5.52 (s, 1H), 4.28–4.13 (m, 2H), 4.09 (d, J = 10.4 Hz, 1H), 4.00 (dm, J = 14.8 Hz, 1H), 3.94 (s, 3H), 3.90 (s, 3H), 3.89 (s, 3H), 3.68 (d, J = 15.2 Hz, 1H), 3.46 (d, J = 4.2 Hz, 1H), 3.10 (dd, J = 16.2, 8.3 Hz, 1H), 2.96 (s, 1H), 2.88–2.59 (m, 3H), 2.50–2.29 (m, 2H), 2.07–1.95 (m, 1H), 1.75–1.61 (m, 2H), 1.43 (dt, J = 10.5, 4.5 Hz, 1H). ^{13}C NMR (100 MHz, chloroform-*d*) δ 173.9, 170.5, 149.1, 146.5, 142.9, 142.1, 136.6, 131.5, 128.3, 128.1 (br), 124.1, 121.6, 105.7, 101.2, 79.3, 68.5, 67.0, 64.5, 60.4, 56.8, 56.4, 53.0, 52.1, 49.1, 47.9, 45.8, 42.2, 40.8, 35.2, 29.3. HRMS (ESI-TOF) $[M+H]^+$ calculated for $C_{32}H_{34}BrN_2O_6$: 621.1600; found: 621.1600. LC-UV/ESI-MS retention time: 3.03 min.

References

1. Bunnage, M. E. Getting pharmaceutical R&D back on target. *Nat. Chem. Biol.* **7**, 335–339 (2011).
2. Romo, R. & Robles, O. Chemo- and site-selective derivatizations of natural products enabling biological studies. *Nat. Prod. Rep.* **31**, 318–334 (2014).
3. Carlson, E. E. Natural products as chemical probes. *ACS Chem. Biol.* **5**, 639–653 (2010).
4. Metz, J. T. & Hajduk, P. J. Rational approaches to targeted polypharmacology: creating and navigating protein–ligand interaction networks. *Curr. Opin. Chem. Biol.* **14**, 498–504 (2010).
5. Fishman, M. C. & Porter, J. A. Pharmaceuticals: a new grammar for drug discovery. *Nature* **437**, 491–493 (2005).
6. Kesavan, S. & Marcaurelle, L. A. Translational synthetic chemistry. *Nat. Chem. Biol.* **9**, 210–213 (2013).
7. Bauer, A. & Brönstrup, M. Industrial natural product chemistry for drug discovery and development. *Nat. Prod. Rep.* **31**, 35–60 (2014).
8. Godula, K. & Sames, D. C-H bond functionalization in complex organic synthesis. *Science* **312**, 67–72 (2006).
9. Yamaguchi, J., Yamaguchi, A. D. & Itami, K. C-H bond functionalization: emerging synthetic tools for natural products and pharmaceuticals. *Angew. Chem. Int. Ed.* **51**, 8960–9009 (2012).
10. McMurray, L., O'Hara, F. & Gaunt, M. J. Recent developments in natural product synthesis using metal-catalyzed C–H bond functionalisation. *Chem. Soc. Rev.* **40**, 1885–1898 (2011).
11. Wencel-Delord, J. & Glorius, F. C–H bond activation enables the rapid construction and late-stage diversification of functional molecules. *Nat. Chem.* **5**, 369–375 (2013).
12. Davies, H. M. L. & Denton, J. R. Application of donor/acceptor-carbenoids to the synthesis of natural products. *Chem. Soc. Rev.* **38**, 3061–3071 (2009).
13. Gutekunst, W. R. & Baran, P. S. C–H functionalization logic in total synthesis. *Chem. Soc. Rev.* **40**, 1976–1991 (2011).
14. Wender, P. A., Hilinski, M. K. & Mayweg, A. V. W. Late-Stage intermolecular CH activation for lead diversification: a highly chemoselective oxyfunctionalization of the C-9 position of potent bryostatin analogues. *Org. Lett.* **7**, 79–82 (2005).
15. Lapointe, D., Markiewicz, T., Whipp, C. J., Toderian, A. & Fagnou, K. Predictable and site-selective functionalization of poly(hetero)arene compounds by palladium catalysis. *J. Org. Chem.* **76**, 749–759 (2011).
16. Dai, H.-X., Stepan, A. F., Plummer, M. S., Zhang, Y.-H. & Yu, J.-Q. Divergent C–H functionalizations directed by sulfonamide pharmacophores: late-stage diversification as a tool for drug discovery. *J. Am. Chem. Soc.* **133**, 7222–7228 (2011).
17. O'Hara, F., Blackmond, D. G. & Baran, P. S. Radical-based regioselective C–H functionalization of electron-deficient heteroarenes: scope, tunability, and predictability. *J. Am. Chem. Soc.* **135**, 12122–12134 (2013).
18. Sawayama, A. M. *et al.* A panel of cytochrome P450 BM3 variants to produce drug metabolites and diversify lead compounds. *Chem.Eur. J.* **15**, 11723–11729 (2009).
19. Gormisky, P. E. & White, M. C. Catalyst-controlled aliphatic C–H oxidations with a predictive model for site-selectivity. *J. Am. Chem. Soc.* **135**, 14052–14055 (2013).
20. Zhang, K., Shafer, B. M., Demars, II M. D., Stern, H. A. & Fasan, R. Controlled oxidation of remote sp^3 C–H bonds in artemisinin *via* P450 catalysts with fine-tuned regio- and stereoselectivity. *J. Am. Chem. Soc.* **134**, 18695–18704 (2012).
21. Lee, J. S., Cao, H. & Fuchs, P. L. Ruthenium-catalyzed mild C–H oxyfunctionalization of cyclic steroidal ethers. *J. Org. Chem.* **72**, 5820–5823 (2007).
22. Larsen, M. A. & Hartwig, J. F. Iridium-catalyzed C–H borylation of heteroarenes: scope, regioselectivity, application to late-stage functionalization, and mechanism. *J. Am. Chem. Soc.* **136**, 4287–4299 (2014).
23. Rousseau, G. & Breit, B. Removable directing groups in organic synthesis and catalysis. *Angew. Chem. Int. Ed.* **50**, 2450–2494 (2011).
24. Malik, H. A. *et al.* Non directed allylic C–H acetoxylation in the presence of Lewis basic heterocycles. *Chem. Sci.* **5**, 2352–2361 (2014).
25. Davies, H. M. L. & Townsend, R. J. Catalytic asymmetric cyclopropanation of heteroaryldiazoacetates. *J. Org. Chem.* **66**, 6595–6603 (2001).
26. Aller, E. *et al.* N-H insertion reactions of rhodium carbenoids. Part 1. Preparation of α-amino acid and α-aminophosphonic acid derivatives. *J. Chem. Soc. Perkin Trans.* **1**, 2879–2884 (1996).
27. Li, J. *et al.* Simultaneous structure–activity studies and arming of natural products by C–H amination reveal cellular targets of eupalmerin acetate. *Nat. Chem.* **5**, 510–517 (2013).
28. Padwa, A. & Hornbuckle, S. F. Ylide formation from the reaction of carbenes and carbenoids with heteroatoms lone pairs. *Chem. Rev.* **91**, 263–309 (1991).
29. Kim, J., Ashenhurst, J. A. & Movassaghi, M. Total synthesis of (+)-11,11′-dideoxyverticillin A. *Science* **324**, 238–241 (2009).
30. Su, S., Seiple, I. B., Young, I. S. & Baran, P. S. Total syntheses of (±)-massadine and massadine chloride. *J. Am. Chem. Soc.* **130**, 16490–16491 (2008).
31. Davies, H. M. L. & Beckwith, R. E. J. Catalytic enantioselective C–H activation by means of metal-carbenoid-induced C–H insertion. *Chem. Rev.* **103**, 2861–2903 (2003).
32. Zhou, Q. *et al.* Bioconjugation by native chemical tagging of C-H bonds. *J. Am. Chem. Soc.* **135**, 12994–12997 (2013).
33. Ziegler, S., Pries, V., Hedberg, C. & Waldmann, H. Target identification for small bioactive molecules: finding the needle in the haystack. *Angew. Chem. Int. Ed.* **52**, 2744–2792 (2013).
34. Hansen, S. R., Spangler, J. E., Hansen, J. H. & Davies, H. M. L. Metal-free N-H insertions of donor/acceptor carbenes. *Org. Lett.* **14**, 4626–4629 (2012).
35. Vanecko, J. A., Wan, H. & West, F. G. Recent advances in the Stevens rearrangement of ammonium ylides. Application to the synthesis of alkaloid natural products. *Tetrahedron* **62**, 1043–1062 (2006).
36. Sharma, A., Guénée, L., Naubron, J.-V. & Lacour, J. One-step catalytic asymmetric synthesis of configurationally stable Tröger bases. *Angew. Chem. Int. Ed.* **50**, 3677–3680 (2011).
37. Osipov, S. N., Sewald, N., Kolomiets, A. F., Fokin, A. V. & Burger, K. Synthesis of α-trifluoromethyl substituted α-amino acid derivatives from methyl 3,3,3-trifluoro-2-diazopropionate. *Tetrahedron Lett.* **37**, 615–618 (1996).
38. Davies, H. M. L. & Morton, D. Guiding principles for site selective and stereoselective intermolecular C–H functionalization by donor/acceptor rhodium carbenes. *Chem. Soc. Rev.* **40**, 1857–1869 (2011).

39. Nakamura, E., Yoshikai, N. & Yamanaka, M. Mechanism of C–H bond activation/ C-C bond formation reaction between diazo compound and alkane catalyzed by dirhodium tetracarboxylate. *J. Am. Chem. Soc.* **124,** 7181–7192 (2002).
40. Hansen, J., Autschbach, J. & Davies, H. M. L. Computational study on the selectivity of donor/acceptor-substituted rhodium carbenoids. *J. Org. Chem.* **74,** 6555–6563 (2009).
41. Qin, C. *et al.* D_2-Symmetric dirhodium catalyst derived from a 1,2,2-triarylcyclopropanecarboxylate ligand: design, synthesis and application. *J. Am. Chem. Soc.* **133,** 19198–19204 (2011).
42. Qin, C. & Davies, H. M. L. Role of sterically demanding chiral dirhodium catalysts in site-selective C–H functionalization of activated primary C–H bonds. *J. Am. Chem. Soc.* **136,** 9792–9796 (2014).
43. Wang, H., Guptill, D. M., Varela-Alvarez, A., Musaev, D. G. & Davies, H. M. L. Rhodium-catalyzed enantioselective cyclopropanation of electron-deficient alkenes. *Chem. Sci.* **4,** 2844–2850 (2013).
44. Hedley, S. J., Ventura, D. L., Dominiak, P. M., Nygren, C. L. & Davies, H. M. L. Investigation into factors influencing stereoselectivity in the reactions of heterocycles with donor-acceptor-substituted rhodium carbenoids. *J. Org. Chem.* **71,** 5349–5356 (2006).
45. Davies, H. M. L., Jin, Q., Ren, P. & Kovalevsky, A. Y. Catalytic asymmetric benzylic C–H activation by means of carbenoid-induced C–H insertions. *J. Org. Chem.* **67,** 4165–4169 (2002).
46. Davies, H. M. L., Hansen, J. H. & Churchill, M. R. Catalytic asymmetric C–H activation of alkanes and tetrahydrofuran. *J. Am. Chem. Soc.* **122,** 3063–3070 (2000).
47. Davies, H. M. L. & Venkataramani, C. Catalytic enantioselective synthesis of β^2-amino acids. *Angew. Chem. Int. Ed.* **41,** 2197–2199 (2002).
48. Davies, H. M. L. & Yang, J. Influence of a β-alkoxy substituent on the C–H activation chemistry of alkyl ethers. *Adv. Synth. Catal.* **345,** 1133–1138 (2003).
49. Davies, H. M. L. & Jin, Q. Double C–H activation strategy for the asymmetric synthesis of C_2-symmetric anilines. *Org. Lett.* **6,** 1769–1772 (2004).

Acknowledgements

We acknowledge support from Novartis Institutes for BioMedical Research and the NSF under the CCI Center for Selective C–H Functionalization, CHE-1205646. We thank Professor Djamaladdin G. Musaev (Emory University), Dr Andrew Patterson and Dr Hasnain Malik for insightful discussion. J.H. gratefully acknowledges the Education Office of the Novartis Institutes for BioMedical Research Inc. for receipt of a Presidential Postdoctoral Fellowship. We thank Changming Qin (Emory University) for providing $Rh_2(BTPCP)_4$ catalyst. We thank Jinhai Gao and Melissa Grondine for providing NMR and preparative SFC separation support, respectively.

Author contributions

R.E.J.B. and H.M.L.D. conceived and supervised this study. J.H., L.G.H., H.M.L.D. and R.E.J.B. were involved with experimental design and results discussion. J.H. conducted the experiments and analysed the data. J.H., H.M.L.D. and R.E.J.B. wrote the manuscript. All authors edited the manuscript.

Additional information

Competing financial interests: The authors declare no competing financial interests.

16

An influenza virus-inspired polymer system for the timed release of siRNA

Nghia P. Truong[1,*], Wenyi Gu[1,2,*], Indira Prasadam[2], Zhongfan Jia[1], Ross Crawford[2], Yin Xiao[2] & Michael J. Monteiro[1]

Small interfering RNA silences specific genes by interfering with mRNA translation, and acts to modulate or inhibit specific biological pathways; a therapy that holds great promise in the cure of many diseases. However, the naked small interfering RNA is susceptible to degradation by plasma and tissue nucleases and due to its negative charge unable to cross the cell membrane. Here we report a new polymer carrier designed to mimic the influenza virus escape mechanism from the endosome, followed by a timed release of the small interfering RNA in the cytosol through a self-catalyzed polymer degradation process. Our polymer changes to a negatively charged and non-toxic polymer after the release of small interfering RNA, presenting potential for multiple repeat doses and long-term treatment of diseases.

[1] Australian Institute for Bioengineering and Nanotechnology, The University of Queensland, Brisbane Queensland 4072, Australia. [2] Institute of Health and Biomedical Innovation, Queensland University of Technology, Kelvin Grove Campus, Brisbane Queensland 4059, Australia. *These authors are joint first author. Correspondence and requests for materials should be addressed to M.J.M. (email: m.monteiro@uq.edu.au).

Small interfering RNA (siRNA) silences specific genes by interfering with mRNA translation, and therefore acts to modulate or inhibit specific biological pathways[1–3]. The siRNA-based therapy holds great promise in the cure of cancers and many other diseases. However, the naked siRNA is susceptible to degradation by plasma and tissue nucleases and is unable to cross the cell membrane due to its negative charge. This has necessitated the design of delivery vehicles to overcome the inherent siRNA cell transport barriers. Amongst many investigated approaches, the initial work with viral delivery carriers showed great promise for delivering DNA and other biomolecules[4,5]. Viruses have evolved with exquisite strategies to deliver their payload efficiently within a cell; for example, the enveloped influenza virus easily appropriates the cellular machinery to replicate itself[6]. This virus first becomes endocytosed, and utilizes this transportation process to reach the inner parts of the cell. Before reaching the lysosome, the acidic pH triggers a rapid geometric conformational change of the haemagglutinin (HA) protein, releasing the HA2 membrane fusion peptide that binds and facilitates fusion of the virus with the endosome membrane. The virus escapes into the cytosol where it then proceeds to replicate its genome[7]. However, despite the above advantages, viral delivery devices have associated safety concerns due to non-specific interruption of genes and induction of an immune response[4,5].

Development of non-viral siRNA delivery systems incorporating the strategies of the virus could provide a safer, cheaper and effective treatment for various diseases[8,9]. Among synthetic delivery vehicles, cationic polymers and lyposomes are widely known as nanocarriers for siRNA; they bind via electrostatic interactions to form complexes with the siRNA that are rapidly taken up by cells[10,11]. The polymer carriers usually incorporate a pH buffering molecule that acts as a 'proton sponge' or binds to the endosome membrane to facilitate their escape[12,13]. Although such systems have demonstrated utility in nonhuman primate studies for liver-related diseases due to the natural accumulation of the carrier in the liver[14–17], the permanent cationic charge of the nanocarriers[18,19] makes release of the siRNA difficult[20–22]. The accumulation of cationic species could result in unwanted toxicity especially when administered in multiple doses. To overcome the release problem of siRNA, polymers have been designed to incorporate side chain molecules that trigger a release when stimulated using temperature[23], pH[24], redox potential[25,26], light[27], electrical pulse[28,29] and enzymatic degradation[30,31]. Such release mechanisms rely on either external (remote) or environmental stimuli. The complication arises in that many tissues and organs are not remotely accessible, and environmentally triggered stimuli can vary between cell lines and even within the same tissue or organ. Furthermore, after degradation, the polymers should form biologically benign particles avoiding toxic buildup in the tissues[32,33].

In the work reported here, we overcame these delivery challenges by designing our polymer carrier to deliver siRNA using some of the strategies inspired by viruses. The polymer carrier consists of a diblock copolymer with a first block of poly(2-dimethylaminoethyl acrylate) (PDMAEA, p*Ka* ~ 7.1). The PDMAEA block is cationic at physiological pH and degrades into the negatively charged and non-toxic poly(acrylic acid) (PAA) (Fig. 1a) in water through a self-catalyzed hydrolysis mechanism[32]. The degradation time to form PAA is independent of pH (as tested between pH 5.5 and 10.1) and the molecular weight of PDMAEA. This block segment can therefore bind strongly to siRNA and release it at a defined time (that is, 'timed release') independent of the physiological pH, allowing the delivery of siRNA into tissues not accessible through external or environmental triggers. The resulting negatively charged polymer should be relatively benign after release even after multiple doses. A second block consisting of P(*N*-(3-(1*H*-imidazol-1-yl)propyl) acrylamide (PImPAA) and poly(butyl acrylate) (PBA)[18] was designed to induce fusion with the endosome membrane (and act in a similar way to the fusion peptide HA2) that results in escape of the polymer/siRNA complex to the cytosol where release of the siRNA can occur after degradation to PAA (see Fig. 1a). In this work, we designed a range of block copolymers (Fig. 1b) to examine the mode of delivery and release using an osteosarcoma cell line as a proven siRNA model system, and determine cell death through siRNA knockdown of the polo-like kinase 1 (PLK1) pathway. The best polymer carrier from this study was then trialed *in vitro* to silence the MAPK–ERK1/2 pathway in primary chondrocytes.

Results

Synthesis and physiochemical properties of polymers. Single electron transfer-living radical polymerization (SET-LRP)[34,35] of DMAEA produced PDMAEA (polymer A in Supplementary Methods and Supplementary Table S1 in Supporting Information) with a number-average molecular weight (M_n) of 4,200 and a polydispersity index (PDI) of 1.29 determined by size exclusion chromatography based on polystyrene standards and neglecting differences in polymer hydrodynamic volume (see Supplementary Figs S1–S3). A more accurate value of 9,430 determined by ^{1}H NMR showed that the polymer consisted of 65 DMAEA units. This polymer was previously tested as a delivery vehicle for siRNA, showing $>90\%$ cell uptake after 4 h and low cytotoxicity[32,33], and thus was used as the first block in this work. $PDMAEA_{65}$ was extended with blocks containing units of ImPAA, BA and/or dimethylacrylamide (DMA) comonomers as shown in Fig. 1b using the SET-LRP technique. Conversion of monomer to polymer was kept low ($<40\%$) to avoid high levels of radical–radical termination and further maintain a high -Cl chain-end functionality to produce block copolymers (A–B1 to A–D3) with PDIs below 1.3 (Supplementary Table S1). The number of repeating units for all comonomers was given in Fig. 1b and Supplementary Table S1 based on ^{1}H NMR analysis (see Supplementary Figs S4–S7).

Complexation of an oligo DNA (23 bp) with the A–B polymer series in water showed an increase in size (i.e. diameter, D_h) from ~ 5 to 200 nm with an increase in the N/P ratio (i.e. nitrogen to phosphorus ratio) from 0 to 10 (see Supplementary Table S2). A similar trend was found for the A–C and A–D series, but here the initial D_h (at N/P = 0) showed that the incorporation of the hydrophobic monomers, BA and ImPAA, in the second block gave small polymeric micelles of ~ 15 to 20 nm (A–C1 to A–C3). The A–C3 polymer candidate showed that at an N/P ratio of 10 at pH 7.6, these small 20 nm nanoparticles aggregated with the oligo DNA to result into a narrow particle size distribution close to 200 nm in size as shown in Fig. 1c. Leaving the complex of A–C3/oligo DNA in water at pH 7.6 resulted in its degradation after 17 h, whereby the size decreased from 200 to 20 nm and the oligo DNA was fully released (see the Agarose gel in Fig. 1c). A similar profile was found when the complex was kept at pH 5.5, with full release of the oligo DNA after 25 h and a size decrease to 5 nm (Fig. 1c) corresponding to the size of an individual polymer coil (i.e. unimer) in solution. This result suggests that the siRNA (with a similar size to the oligo DNA) can still be complexed with the polymer in the low pH environment of the endosome, and if escape from the endosome is faster than the release time of ~ 17 h, the siRNA has a great chance of being released within the cytosol. The similar degradation profiles of A–C3 in pH 5.5 and 7.6 further supported a non-triggered and timed-release mechanism of the siRNA from the polymer carrier. In addition,

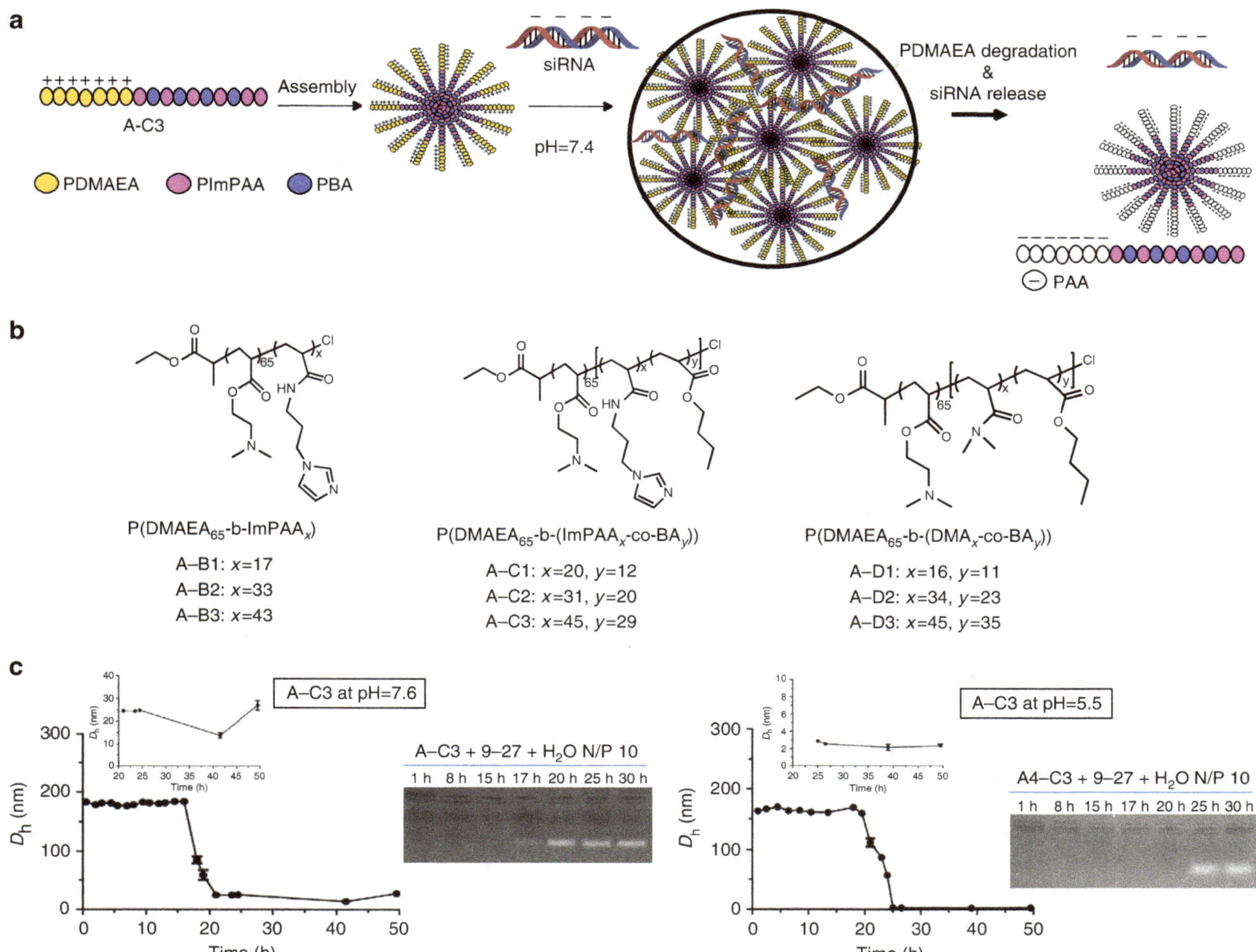

Figure 1 | Polymer structure and assembly. (**a**) Mechanism for polymer assembly, binding with siRNA and release of siRNA through a self-catalyzed degradation of PDMAEA, (**b**) chemical structures of the nine block copolymers, and (**c**) degradation profile of polymer A-C3 at pH 7.6 and 5.5 when complexes with oligo DNA as measured by DLS, and the time for release of the oligo DNA from the polymer carrier.

the degradation profiles for A-B3 and A-D3 at pH 7.6 and 5.5 were all similar to A-C3, suggesting that only the degradation of PDMAEA to PAA plays the dominant role for release of oligo DNA (see Supplementary Figs S9–S14).

***In vitro* RNAi-mediated knockdown of PLK1 in osteosarcoma.** Osteosarcoma is a bone cancer prevalent in young people, with poor survival rates. Polo-like kinase 1 (PLK1) has an important role in maintaining tumorgenic phenotype of osteosarcoma cells[36]. Its knockdown using siRNA delivery should induce selective growth arrest and cell death. In this work, we used the U-2OS cell line as an *in vitro* model system to test our polymers (from Fig. 1b) for knockdown using a previously screened siRNA[36]. We evaluated the knockdown of U-2OS cells using our polymer-loaded siRNA complexes via a cell viability assay. Four siRNAs were used: (i) siRNA targeting PLK1, (ii) universal negative control (Mission siRNA, Sigma-Aldrich), (iii) scrambled siRNA for PLK, and (iv) a negative control S10 siRNA that targets another pathway[37]. The polymer-loaded siRNA complexes were also compared with oligofectamine/siRNA complexes, in which oligofectamine is regarded as the gold standard for siRNA delivery. Solutions of the polymer and siRNA in PBS buffer at various N/P ratios (that is, 0 to 10) were mixed and incubated for 30 min at room temperature. The complex was then added to the cells in complete DMEM media at 37 °C, and after 4 h, the cells were washed to remove any complex not taken up by the cells and incubated for another 48 h. The concentration of siRNA used in this assay was 50 nM.

It can be seen that polymer A loaded with siRNA by itself (that is, $PDMAEA_{65}$) showed little toxicity and little or no knockdown compared with oligofectamine-loaded siRNA targeting PLK1 (see Supplementary Fig S15A). Incorporating an ImPAA second block (A–B series) to act as either a proton sponge or fusogenic polymer also showed little toxicity and little or no cell death irrespective of the molecular weight of the second block when loaded with PLK1 siRNA(Fig. 2a and Supplementary Fig. S15B–D). The results suggest that even with the inclusion of ImPAA (similar functional group to histidine), the polymer carrier could not escape the endosome. Polymer series A–C incorporating not only ImPAA but hydropobic BA was synthesized to further assist in endosome escape. The cell viability data (Fig. 2b and Supplementary Fig. S16) using A–C2 and A–C3 loaded with PLK1 siRNA showed little or no cell death at N/P ratios below 10. At an N/P ratio of 10, both polymers loaded with PLK1 siRNA complexes showed excellent knockdown (>80%) and little toxicity. This amount of cell viability loss specific to targeting the PLK1 pathway was substantially better than

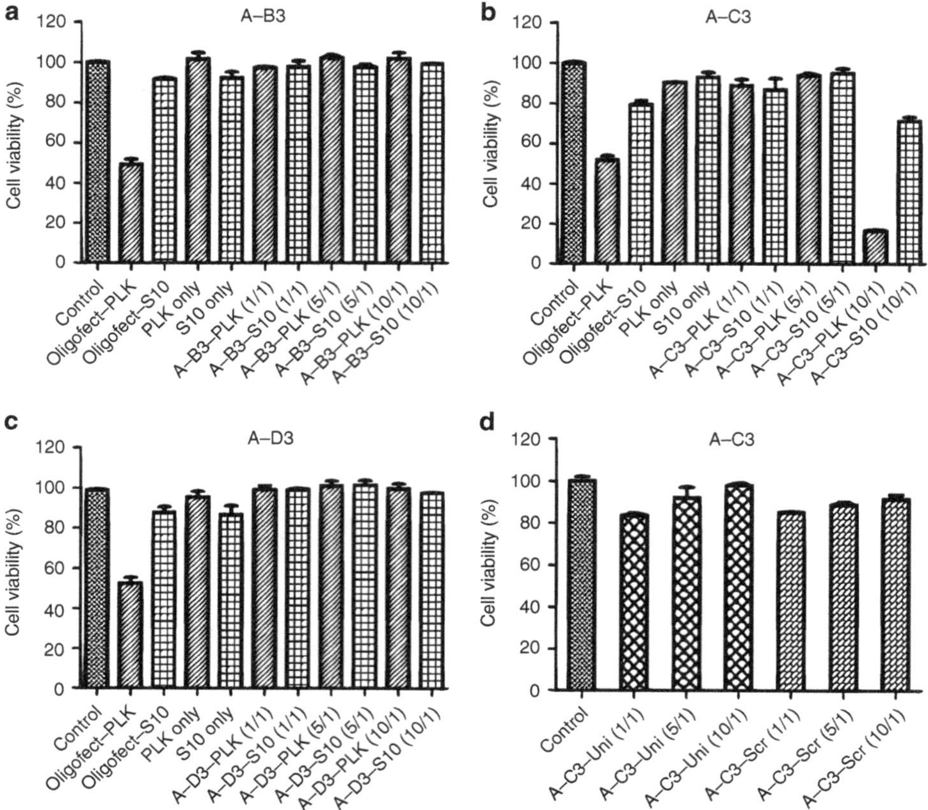

Figure 2 | *In vitro* knockdown efficiencies. U-2OS cell *in vitro* knockdown efficiency of (**a**) P(DMAEA$_{65}$-b-ImPAA$_{43}$) (A-B3), (**b**) P(DMAEA$_{65}$-b-(ImPAA$_{45}$-co-BA$_{29}$)) (A-C3), and (**c**) P(DMAEA$_{65}$-b-(DMA$_{45}$-co-BA$_{35}$)) (A-D3) complexes with siRNA targeting PLK and negative siRNA control S10 at N/P ratios of 1, 5 and 10 after 30 min complexation in water. The polymers were added to the cells and left to transfect for 4 h, and further incubated for 48 h. Controls used were untreated (Control), PLK/Oligofectamine complex (Oligofect-PLK), S10/Oligofectamine (Oligofect-S10) complexes, PLK siRNA only (PLK only) and S10 siRNA only (S10 only). Concentrations of PLK and S10 used was 50 nM. The data are reported as the mean ± s.e.m. of three replicates. (**d**) U-2OS cell viability of P(DMAEA)$_{65}$-P(ImPAA$_{45}$-co-BA$_{29}$) (A-C3) complexes with universal siRNA (Uni) and scrambled siRNA (Scr) at N/P ratio 1, 5 and 10 after 30 min complexation in water, 4 h transfection and 48 h incubation. Controls used are untreated (Control). Concentration of universal siRNA and scrambled siRNA used is 50 nM. The data are reported as the mean ± standard error of the mean of two replicates. Values in parenthesis are N/P ratios.

oligofectamine/siRNA. To test whether cell death was due to the combination of ImPAA and BA in the second block or as a result of only BA, we synthesized the A–D polymer series consisting of BA and DMA in the second block. The results for A–D3 (Fig. 2c) and A–D1 and A–D2 (Supplementary Fig. S17) showed that without ImPAA there was no observed cell death. The combination of ImPAA and BA in the second block demonstrates that both comonomers act synergistically to allow escape of the polymer/siRNA complex from the endosome into the cytosol, most probably due to the combined ionic and hydrophobic interactions with the endosome membrane. To confirm that cell death was primarily due to siRNA targeting PLK, we tested two different control siRNAs (universal negative control (denoted as Uni) and a scrambled siRNA (denoted as Scr)) delivered with polymer A–C3, and the data given in Fig. 2d shows that there is no knockdown with either of these siRNAs. Further, the cell viability of polymer A–C3 alone before (Supplementary Fig. S19A) and after (Supplementary Fig. S19B) degradation (that is, self-catalyze to poly(acrylic acid)) of the PDMAEA block in A–C3 showed little or no cell toxicity even at an NP ratio of 20. These results collectively demonstrate the excellent knockdown potential of A–C3 with little or no cytotoxicity.

Escape from the endosome is thus a key feature of our polymer carrier that allows effective delivery of the siRNA to the cytosol. Two mechanisms have been proposed for pH-responsive polymers (for example, with imidazole groups) to facilitate escape[12,13]: (i) an osmotic gradient caused by a flux of counter ions to maintain the ionic strength in the endosome and thus induce endosome lysis, or (ii) interaction of the imidazole groups with the endosome membrane. Our results showed that the siRNA targeting PLK gave ~80% knockdown with little or no toxicity from the polymer A–C3. The requirement for the combination of ImPAA and BA in the second block (A–C series) demonstrates the capability of these monomer units to fuse with the endosome membrane and facilitate escape. The ImPAA (that is, imidazole) side groups become highly protonated when the pH drops below its p*K*a of ~6, which should enable these positive charges to interact with the negatively charged endosome membrane and induce a bilayer phase separation. The BA monomer units should further interact with the membrane through hydrophobic interactions and facilitate fusion with the membrane leading to escape. As described earlier, the fusogenic second block in A–C2 and A–C3 is located in the core of the micelle with a size of ~20 nm (Supplementary Table S2), and must therefore be exposed to the surface of the micelles when the pH drops in the endosome to interact with the endosome membrane, mimicking structural reorganization found for the influenza virus. When the polymer without siRNA was

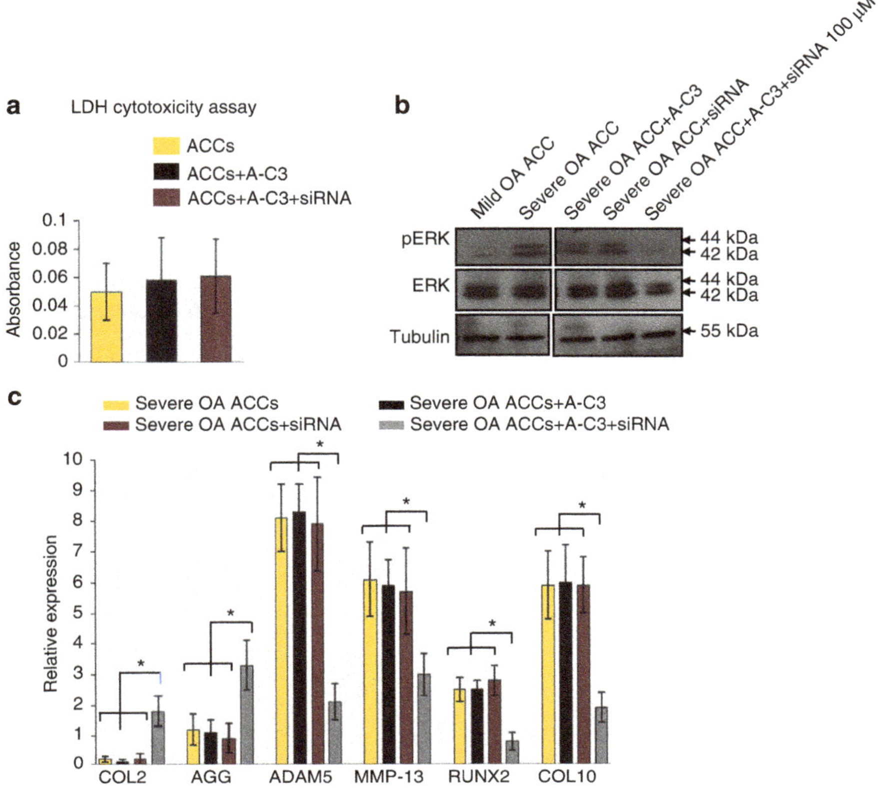

Figure 3 | *In vitro* effects of ERK siRNA delivery on OA ACCs. (**a**) Cell cytotoxicity of ACCs treated with polymer and polymer + ERK siRNA after 48 h of transfection. Compared with control, there is no significant difference in cell cytotoxicity in either polymer or polymer + ERK siRNA group ($P > 0.05$; $n = 5$ in all instances). (**b**) Western blotting image showing the substantial downregulation of ERK in polymer + siRNA-treated severe OA ACCs. A representative bands obtained from three patients with similar results was shown. (**c**) qRT-PCR showed that chondrogenic markers such as *COL2* and *AGG* were upregulated and degradative and hypertrophic markers such as ADAMTS5, MMP-13 and *COL10* were downregulated in severe OA ACCs treated with Polymer + ERK siRNA. mRNA levels were normalized against 18 S rRNA and the relative fold change gene expression is presented. Results are shown as mean ± s.d. *$P < 0.05$. Values are representative of five patients with similar results.

self-assembled in water at pH 7.6, small micelles formed with a size of ~20 nm (Supplementary Table S3). When the pH was decreased to 5.5, the polymer was fully water soluble and the polymer chains dissociated from the micelle forming unimers of ~5 nm. Increasing the pH back to 7.6 resulted in reconstitution (self-assembly) of the unimers back to small ~20 nm particles. The polymer (A–C3)/oligo DNA complex showed no change in particle size when the pH was decreased from 7.6 to 5.5 (Fig. 1). These results suggested that the 20 nm polymer particles when complex with the siRNA formed a large 200 nm aggregate, and when in the endosome, the size of the aggregate did not change due to the strong ionic binding between the siRNA and polymer chains even though the ImPAA groups were now cationic and hydrophilic. Our observations are consistent with the fully water soluble ImPAA and BA second block reorganizing in the endosome to be exposed to the exterior of the aggregate, allowing fusion and escape from the endosome membrane. Once in the cytosol, release of the siRNA occurs after 17 h, which acts to interfere with the specific mRNA.

***In vitro* RNAi-mediated knockdown of ERK in osteoarthritis chrondrocytes.** The MAPK–ERK (mitogen activated protein kinase-extracellular signal-regulated kinase) cell signaling pathway has been identified as one of the central regulatory factors in osteoarthritis (OA) progression, especially in the altered communication between the osteoarthritic cartilage and the subchondral bone[38]. We evaluated the efficiency of the polymer A–C3 loaded with siRNA targeting ERK in OA chondrocytes. Articular cartilage cells (ACCs) were isolated from OA cartilage, and the early passage cells (P1-2) were used in the *in vitro* experiments. The polymer/siRNA concentrations used in this study showed no significant cytotoxic effects in siRNA treatment groups using the standard LDH (lactate dehydrogenase) assay (Fig. 3a). The A-C3 polymer loaded with ERK siRNA diminished ERK1/2 (ERK1/2) levels in severe OA ACCs measured using the western blot analysis after 48 h (Fig. 3b). This *in vitro* knockdown of ERK enhanced chondrocyte differentiation and impaired pathological phenotytic changes in severe OA ACCs (Fig. 3c). The polymer A–C3 alone was not toxic to the OA ACCs even at an NP ratio of 20 before (Supplementary Fig. S20A) and after (Supplementary Fig. S20B) degradation of the PDMAEA part of the polymer. Knockdown by siRNA specific to the ERK pathway was further demonstrated using a universal negative siRNA control and a scrambled siRNA, both of which showed no knockdown capability (Supplementary Fig. S21). ACCs from severe OA knee cartilage (Mankin score ≥6) showed a poor capacity for chondrogenic differentiation with higher levels of hypertrophic and degenerative markers. When A–C3-loaded ERK siRNA was delivered to the severe OA ACCs, the degradative enzymes of ADAMTS5 (disintegrin and metalloproteinase with thrombospondin motifs 5), MMP-13 (matrix metalloproteinases 13) and pathological hypertrophic markers of type 10 collagen (COL10) and Runt-related transcription factor-2 (RUNX2) were significantly decreased. In contrast, we observed increased levels of chondrogenic markers COL2 and AGAN (Fig. 3c). These findings collectively indicated that ERK siRNA loaded into our polymer (A–C3) improved the chondrogenic differentiation and inhibited the pathological degradative and hypertrophic changes in OA ACCs.

Discussion

We demonstrate the use of a sophisticated polymer delivery carrier for the delivery of siRNA to silence distinct pathways. Our polymer was designed where one block binds electrostatically with siRNA and then degrades to a negatively charged side groups that repels and releases the siRNA. It takes 17 h in pH 7.6 to release the siRNA. This is more than sufficient time for the polymer carrier/siRNA to escape the endosome and release the siRNA in the cytosol. The second block consisting of ImPAA and BA resulted in a polymer carrier mimicking the escape mechanism of the influenza virus from the endosome into the cytosol. A distinct advantage of our polymer is that it forms a non-toxic negatively charged polymer, allowing the potential for multiple doses and effective treatment of the disease. Our polymer carrier was effective in siRNA knockdown with >80% of cell death when targeting the PLK1 pathway for osteosarcoma cancer cells, and when targeting the ERK1/2 pathway shown to be the key regulatory pathway in OA. These results demonstrate great promise for the application of our A–C3 polymer as an effective and safe siRNA delivery carrier for further applications in many diseases.

Methods

Synthesis and characterization of polymers. Details of the syntheses including materials used, and complete polymer characterization by size exclusion chromatography, ^{1}H nuclear magnetic resonance and dynamic light scattering and provided in the Supplementary Methods section, along with details of the agarose gel assays for binding and release studies.

Osteocarcoma model assays. Details of the osteocarcoma model assays, including *in-vitro* studies of knockdown of osteosarcoma U-2OS cells and examination of cell viability of osteosarcoma U-2OS cells using Cell Titer-Glo assay are provided in the Supplementary Methods section.

Osteoarthritis model assays. Details of the osteoarthritis model assays, including *in-vitro* cytotoxicity studies and examination of cell viability of osteosarcoma OA ACCs cells using Cell Titer-Glo assay are provided in the Supplementary Methods section.

References

1. Fire, A. *et al.* Potent and specific genetic interference by double-stranded RNA in *Caenorhabditis elegans*. *Nature* **391,** 806–811 (1998).
2. Turchinovich, A., Zoidl, G. & Dermietzel, R. Non-viral siRNA delivery into the mouse retina in vivo. *BMC Ophthalmol.* **10,** 25 (2010).
3. Leung, R. K. M. & Whittaker, P. A. RNA interference: from gene silencing to gene-specific therapeutics. *Pharmacol. Therapeut.* **107,** 222–239 (2005).
4. Lammers, T., Hennink, W. E. & Storm, G. Tumour-targeted nanomedicines: principles and practice. *Br. J. Cancer* **99,** 392–397 (2008).
5. Dincer, S., Turk, M. & Piskin, E. Intelligent polymers as nonviral vectors. *Gene Therapy* **12,** S139–S145 (2005).
6. Cho, Y. W., Kim, J. D. & Park, K. Follycation gene delivery systems: escape from endosomes to cytosol. *J. Pharm. Pharmacol.* **55,** 721–734 (2003).
7. Le Blanc, I. *et al.* Endosome-to-cytosol transport of viral nucleocapsids. *Nat. Cell Biol.* **7,** 653–U625 (2005).
8. Zhang, S. B., Zhao, B., Jiang, H. M., Wang, B. & Ma, B. C. Cationic lipids and polymers mediated vectors for delivery of siRNA. *J. Control Release* **123,** 1–10 (2007).
9. Davis, M. E., Chen, Z. & Shin, D. M. Nanoparticle therapeutics: an emerging treatment modality for cancer. *Nat. Rev. Drug Discov.* **7,** 771–782 (2008).
10. Pack, D. W., Hoffman, A. S., Pun, S. & Stayton, P. S. Design and development of polymers for gene delivery. *Nat. Rev. Drug Discov.* **4,** 581–593 (2005).
11. Whitehead, K. A., Langer, R. & Anderson, D. G. Knocking down barriers: advances in siRNA delivery. *Nat. Rev. Drug Discov.* **8,** 129–138 (2009).
12. Midoux, P., Kichler, A., Boutin, V., Maurizot, J. C. & Monsigny, M. Membrane permeabilization and efficient gene transfer by a peptide containing several histidines. *Bioconjug. Chem.* **9,** 260–267 (1998).
13. Pichon, C., Roufai, M. B., Monsigny, M. & Midoux, P. Histidylated oligolysines increase the transmembrane passage and the biological activity of antisense oligonucleotides. *Nucleic Acids Res.* **28,** 504–512 (2000).
14. Ozpolat, B., Sood, A. K. & Lopez-Berestein, G. Nanomedicine based approaches for the delivery of siRNA in cancer. *J. Intern. Med.* **267,** 44–53 (2010).
15. Soutschek, J. *et al.* Therapeutic silencing of an endogenous gene by systemic administration of modified siRNAs. *Nature* **432,** 173–178 (2004).
16. Zimmermann, T. S. *et al.* RNAi-mediated gene silencing in non-human primates. *Nature* **441,** 111–114 (2006).
17. Judge, A. D. *et al.* Confirming the RNAi-mediated mechanism of action of siRNA-based cancer therapeutics in mice. *J. Clin. Invest.* **119,** 661–673 (2009).
18. Convertine, A. J. *et al.* pH-responsive polymeric micelle carriers for siRNA drugs. *Biomacromolecules* **11,** 2904–2911 (2010).
19. Smith, D., Holley, A. C. & McCormick, C. L. RAFT-synthesized copolymers and conjugates designed for therapeutic delivery of iRNA. *Polym. Chem.* **2,** 1428–1441 (2011).
20. Miyata, K. *et al.* Block catiomer polyplexes with regulated densities of charge and disulfide cross-linking directed to enhance gene expression. *J. Am. Chem. Soc.* **126,** 2355–2361 (2004).
21. Schaffer, D. V., Fidelman, N. A., Dan, N. & Lauffenburger, D. A. Vector unpacking as a potential barrier for receptor-mediated polyplex gene delivery. *Biotechnol. Bioeng.* **67,** 598–606 (2000).
22. Plank, C., Tang, M. X., Wolfe, A. R. & Szoka, F. C. Branched cationic peptides for gene delivery: Role of type and number of cationic residues in formation and *in vitro* activity of DNA polyplexes. *Hum. Gene. Ther.* **10,** 319–322 (1999).
23. Kurisawa, M., Yokoyama, M. & Okano, T. Gene expression control by temperature with thermo-responsive polymeric gene carriers. *J. Control Release* **69,** 127–137 (2000).
24. Mehrotra, S., Lee, I. & Chan, C. Multilayer mediated forward and patterned siRNA transfection using linear-PEI at extended N/P ratios. *Acta Biomater.* **5,** 1474–1488 (2009).
25. McKenzie, D. L., Smiley, E., Kwok, K. Y. & Rice, K. G. Low molecular weight disulfide cross-linking peptides as nonviral gene delivery carriers. *Bioconjug. Chem.* **11,** 901–909 (2000).
26. Pichon, C. *et al.* Poly[Lys-(AEDTP)]: a cationic polymer that allows dissociation of pDNA/cationic polymer complexes in a reductive medium and enhances polyfection. *Bioconjug. Chem.* **13,** 76–82 (2002).
27. Handwerger, R. G. & Diamond, S. L. Biotinylated photocleavable polyethylenimine: Capture and triggered release of nucleic acids from solid supports. *Bioconjug. Chem.* **18,** 717–723 (2007).
28. Dieguez, L., Darwish, N., Graf, N., Voros, J. & Zambelli, T. Electrochemical tuning of the stability of PLL/DNA multilayers. *Soft Matter* **5,** 2415–2421 (2009).
29. Yamauchi, F., Kato, K. & Iwata, H. Layer-by-layer assembly of poly(ethyleneimine) and plasmid DNA onto transparent indium-tin oxide electrodes for temporally and spatially specific gene transfer. *Langmuir* **21,** 8360–8367 (2005).
30. Ren, K. F., Ji, J. & Shen, J. C. Tunable DNA release from cross-linked ultrathin DNA/PLL multilayered films. *Bioconjug. Chem.* **17,** 77–83 (2006).
31. Saurer, E. M., Jewell, C. M., Kuchenreuther, J. M. & Lynn, D. M. Assembly of erodible, DNA-containing thin films on the surfaces of polymer microparticles: toward a layer-by-layer approach to the delivery of DNA to antigen-presenting cells. *Acta Biomater.* **5,** 913–924 (2009).
32. Truong, N. P., Jia, Z. F., Burges, M., McMillan, N. A. J. & Monteiro, M. J. Self-catalyzed degradation of linear cationic poly(2-dimethylaminoethyl acrlyate) in water. *Biomacromolecules* **12,** 1876–1882 (2011).
33. Truong, N. P. *et al.* Self-catalyzed degradable cationic polymer for release of DNA. *Biomacromolecules* **12,** 3540–3548 (2011).
34. Percec, V. *et al.* Ultrafast synthesis of ultrahigh molar mass polymers by metal-catalyzed living radical polymerization of acrylates, methacrylates, and vinyl chloride mediated by SET at 25 degrees C. *J. Am. Chem. Soc.* **128,** 14156–14165 (2006).
35. Rosen, B. M. & Percec, V. Single-electron transfer and single-electron transfer degenerative chain transfer living radical polymerization. *Chem. Rev.* **109,** 5069–5119 (2009).
36. Duan, Z. F. *et al.* Lentiviral shRNA screen of human kinases identifies PLK1 as a potential therapeutic target for osteosarcoma. *Cancer Lett.* **293,** 220–229 (2010).
37. Wu, S. *et al.* Systemic delivery of E6/7 siRNA using novel lipidic particles and its application with cisplatin in cervical cancer mouse models. *Gene Therapy* **18,** 14–22 (2011).
38. Prasadam, I. *et al.* Osteoarthritic cartilage chondrocytes alter subchondral bone osteoblast differentiation via MAPK signalling pathway involving ERK1/2. *Bone* **46,** 226–235 (2010).

Acknowledgements

M.J.M. acknowledges the support of the Australian Research Council under the Discovery Grant.

Author contributions

M.J.M., W.G. and Y.X. proposed the concept of this work. Z.J. and N.P.T. designed, synthesized and characterized the polymers. I.P. and W.G. conducted the *in vitro* cell work. M.J.M. and Y.X. supervised the research. M.J.M., Y.X., W.G., Z.J., N.P.T., I.P. and R.C. wrote the manuscript.

Additional information

Competing financial interests: The authors declare no competing financial interests.

17

The key role of the scaffold on the efficiency of dendrimer nanodrugs

Anne-Marie Caminade[1,2], Séverine Fruchon[3,4], Cédric-Olivier Turrin[1,2], Mary Poupot[5,6], Armelle Ouali[1,2], Alexandrine Maraval[1,2], Matteo Garzoni[7], Marek Maly[8], Victor Furer[9], Valeri Kovalenko[10], Jean-Pierre Majoral[1,2], Giovanni M. Pavan[7] & Rémy Poupot[3,4]

Dendrimers are well-defined macromolecules whose highly branched structure is reminiscent of many natural structures, such as trees, dendritic cells, neurons or the networks of kidneys and lungs. Nature has privileged such branched structures for increasing the efficiency of exchanges with the external medium; thus, the whole structure is of pivotal importance for these natural networks. On the contrary, it is generally believed that the properties of dendrimers are essentially related to their terminal groups, and that the internal structure plays the minor role of an 'innocent' scaffold. Here we show that such an assertion is misleading, using convergent information from biological data (human monocytes activation) and all-atom molecular dynamics simulations on seven families of dendrimers (13 compounds) that we have synthesized, possessing identical terminal groups, but different internal structures. This work demonstrates that the scaffold of nanodrugs strongly influences their properties, somewhat reminiscent of the backbone of proteins.

[1] Laboratoire de Chimie de Coordination du CNRS, UPR 8241, 205 route de Narbonne, BP 44099, 31077 Toulouse Cedex 4, France. [2] Université de Toulouse, UPS, INP, LCC, F-31077 Toulouse, France. [3] Centre de Physiopathologie de Toulouse Purpan, F-31300 Toulouse, France. [4] INSERM, U1043; CNRS, U5282; Université de Toulouse, UPS, Toulouse, France. [5] Centre de Recherche en Cancérologie de Toulouse, F-31300 Toulouse, France. [6] INSERM, U1037; CNRS, U5294; Université de Toulouse, UPS, Toulouse, France. [7] Department of Innovative Technologies, University of Applied Sciences and Arts of Southern Switzerland, Galleria 2, 6928 Manno, Switzerland. [8] Faculty of Science, J.E. Purkinje University, Ceske mladeze 8, 400 96 Ústí nad Labem, Czech Republic. [9] Kazan State Architect and Civil Engineering University, Zelenaya 1, Kazan 420043, Russia. [10] A.E. Arbuzov Institute of Organic and Physical Chemistry of Kazan Scientific Center of Russian Academy of Science, Arbuzov Str., 8, Kazan 420088, Russia. Correspondence and requests for materials should be addressed to A.-M.C. (email: anne-marie.caminade@lcc-toulouse.fr) or to G.M.P. (email: giovanni.pavan@supsi.ch) or to R.P. (email: remy.poupot@inserm.fr).

The large number of potential applications of dendrimers[1] generates each year a tremendous amount of work, often connected to their biological properties. Emphasis is generally put on the modification of the terminal groups and of their number (related to the generation, that is, the number of layers), in connection with the multivalency effect that is the most important property recognized for dendrimers[2–5]. The possibility to design molecules with controlled multivalency is particularly important for biological applications[6], polyvalent interactions being ubiquitous in many biological systems[7]. Only very few publications have experimentally reported so far the influence of the internal structure of dendrimers on their properties, even if among the five critical nanoscale design parameters recently proposed by Tomalia[8] (size, shape, surface chemistry, flexibility and architecture), at least three of them are related to the internal structure. Comparison between PAMAM (polyamidoamine)[9] and PPI (polypropyleneimine)[10] dendrimers has emphasized the difference of the length of branches as the most important characteristics for their use as sensor[11], and for obtaining nanoparticles[12]. Comparison of the physical properties have shown important differences between PAMAM and poly(L-lysine) dendrimers[13], whereas rigid branches of dendrimers with azobenzene core induce significant differences for the isomerization, compared with less rigid branches[14]. In biology, a few examples have compared the efficiency of specific dendrimers with that of PAMAM dendrimers, with particular emphasis on transfection experiments[15]. However, there is no example to date of a study assessing the influence of a large number of dendritic scaffolds on the biological properties *per se*, and getting insights on the reasons for the differences.

Immunogenicity of dendrimers has been investigated for years, and these studies show absence or only weak immunogenicity of these molecules[16]. On the other hand, it is known that phagocytes of the immune system (that is, monocytes and macrophages that are immune white cells playing multiple roles in the immune system[17]) engulf nanoparticles, which in some cases leads to their activation[18]. Moreover, due to their involvement in many different diseases, monocytes are relevant targets to promote curative immunomodulation[19,20]. Some of us have already shown that a first-generation poly(phosphorhydrazone) dendrimer ended by azabis(phosphonic acid) groups has unprecedented biological properties. This compound is able to modulate *in vitro* the response of the human immune system, in particular, by inducing the multiplication of natural killer cells[21,22], activating monocytes[23] through an anti-inflammatory pathway[24]. The efficacy of this molecule has been proven *in vivo* in a mouse model of experimental arthritis relevant to human rheumatoid arthritis[25]. In this model, there is a constitutive inflammatory activation of monocytes/macrophages that is responsible for the onset and the development of the pathology. We have shown that this particular azabis(phosphonic acid)-ended dendrimer targets monocytes/macrophages and inhibits the main physiopathological features of the disease—systemic inflammation, cartilage degradation and bone resorption. The potential of this nanodrug candidate against rheumatoid arthritis has been highlighted[26,27]. This preliminary work has demonstrated that the $N(CH_2P(O)(OH)(ONa))_2$ pincer is the most active part within the structure. Variation on the structure of the pincer strongly decreases the biological activity[21], whereas the replacement of phosphonic acids by carboxylic acids or sulfonic acids precludes any activity[28]. Furthermore, the azabisphosphonic pincer has to be linked to the first-generation poly(phosphorhydrazone) dendrimer (12 terminal groups) through the nitrogen atom. These poly(phosphorhydrazone) dendrimers are still very active with a lower number of such terminal functions (8 or 10), but become poorly active with 6, 4 or 2 terminal functions, and the monomer is non-active at all[29], emphasizing the fact that these dendrimers are not drug carriers[30], but drugs by themselves. An increased number of terminal functions (16, 24 (generation 2)[21] or 30) has also a detrimental influence on the efficiency[29].

Such types of terminal groups appear appealing for studying and rationalizing the influence of the nature of the scaffold on the properties of dendritic nanodrugs. Therefore, we describe the grafting of azabisphosphonic acids as terminal groups (4 to 12 functions) to a series of dendrimers having different internal structures. Seven different families of dendrimers (13 compounds) having identical terminal groups (azabisphosphonic derivatives), but different internal structures (PAMAM, PPI, poly(carbosilane)[31], poly(L-Lysine)[32] and three different types of phosphorus-containing dendrimers) are synthesized. Their efficiency for the activation of human monocytes is described. To identify the reasons of the original and surprising biological results obtained, the modelling of the structures of the dendrimers in aqueous solution by means of all-atom molecular dynamics (MD) simulations is carried out for obtaining high-resolution (atomistic) details of the configuration they assume in the real environment (solvated state).

Results

Syntheses of the dendrimers. The seven different families of dendrimers (13 compounds) ended by azabisphosphonic groups that we have synthesized and tested are shown in Figs 1 and 2. Owing to the different terminal groups of the dendrimers before their functionalization by the azabis(phosphonic acid) groups, we have used two different linkers and developed different synthetic strategies.

The first linker is tyramine, which affords $OC_6H_4CH_2CH_2N(CH_2P(O)(OH)(ONa))_2$ terminal groups. In addition to the first-generation poly(phosphorhydrazone) dendrimer **1-G₁** (12 terminal functions) already synthesized[21], this linker has been used for another type of poly (phosphorhydrazone) dendrimer having internal branches extended by an arylether linkage, **2-G₁** (12 terminal functions), as well as for poly(thiophosphate)[33] dendrimers **3-G₁** (6 terminal functions) and **3-G₂** (12 terminal functions) and for a poly(carbosilane) dendrimer **4-G₁** (8 terminal functions; Fig. 1).

The second type of linker is obtained from the NH_2 terminal groups of the initial dendrimers via an amide linkage ($NHC(O)(CH_2)_xN(CH_2P(O)(OH)(ONa))_2$ with $x = 1$ or 3; Fig. 2). These terminal groups have been grafted also to the surface of the first-generation poly(phosphorhydrazone) dendrimer[34] via the tyramine function, to afford dendrimers **5a-G₁** ($x = 1$) and **5b-G₁** ($x = 3$) (12 terminal functions for both). The other types of dendrimers that we have synthesized with this second type of linker are different generations of PPI dendrimers, **6a-G₁** ($x = 1$) and **6b-G₁** ($x = 3$; 4 terminal functions for both) and **6b-G₂** ($x = 3$; 8 terminal functions); different generations of PAMAM dendrimers, **7a-G₁** ($x = 1$; 4 terminal functions) and **7b-G₂** ($x = 3$; 8 terminal functions); and the poly(L-lysine) dendrimer, **8a-G₂** ($x = 1$; 8 terminal functions). In all cases, the azabisphosphonic terminal groups are grafted to the dendrimers in the form of the corresponding methyl ester phosphonates, to carry out the reaction in organic solvents in which both reagents are soluble.

As shown in Fig. 3, we have used different strategies for grafting the azabisphosphonates to the various types of dendrimers. The first step of the synthesis of dendrimer **2-G₁** is the nucleophilic substitution on the $P(S)Cl_2$ terminal groups by the phenol moieties of the functionalized tyramine **9** in basic conditions; this method is identical to that used for the synthesis

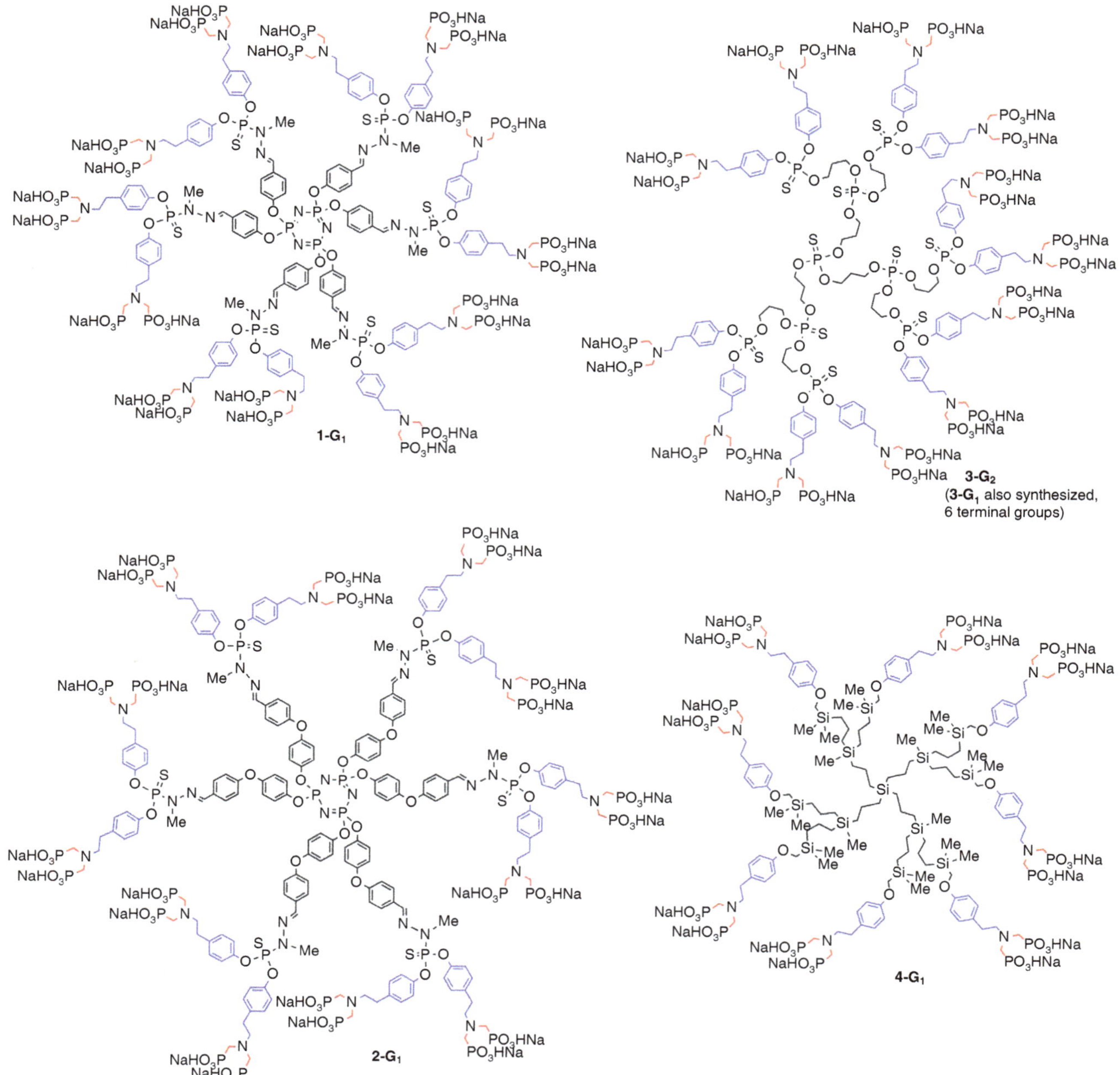

Figure 1 | Chemical structure of dendrimers 1-G$_1$–4-G$_1$. The azabisphosphonic salts are in red, the linkers in blue and variable internal structures in black.

of **1-G$_1$** (ref. 21). The same phenol **9** was used for the nucleophilic substitution on the CH_2I terminal groups of the carbosilane dendrimer, to finally afford **4-G$_1$**. The phosphane bisphosphonate **10** was used for phosphitylation of the alcohol end groups of the thiophosphate dendrimers, followed by oxidation of P^{III} with sulphur, finally affording **3-G$_1$** or **3-G$_2$**, depending on the generation of the starting dendrimer. The other types of tyramine derivatives **11a,b** (**a**: CH_2 spacer, **b**: $CH_2CH_2CH_2$ spacer) were also used for nucleophilic substitutions on $P(S)Cl_2$ terminal groups, to obtain dendrimers **5a-G$_1$** and **5b-G$_1$**. Compounds **11a** and **11b** were obtained by reaction of the carboxylic acids **12a** and **12b** with the NH_2 function of tyramine via peptide coupling. In the case of dendrimers ended by NH_2 groups (PPI, PAMAM, polylysine), this peptide coupling was carried out directly on the dendrimers with the derivatives **12a** and **12b**, affording finally the series of dendrimers **6a-G$_1$**, **6b-G$_1$**, **6b-G$_2$** (PPI-type), **7a-G$_1$**, **7b-G$_2$** (PAMAM-type) and **8a-G$_2$** (Poly-L-lysine type).

The terminal methyl ester phosphonate groups were converted to phosphonic acid salts by reaction with bromotrimethylsilane, MeOH and then NaOH in water. Remarkably, this process induced the cleavage of the terminal phosphonic ester groups, without destroying the internal structure of the dendrimers, even in the case of dendrimers **3-G$_1$** and **3-G$_2$**, which have other types of alkyl phosphonates in their internal structure.

Monocyte activation by dendrimers. On stimulation, monocytes/macrophages undergo morphological changes, that is, increase of their size and granularity[35], indicative of an activated

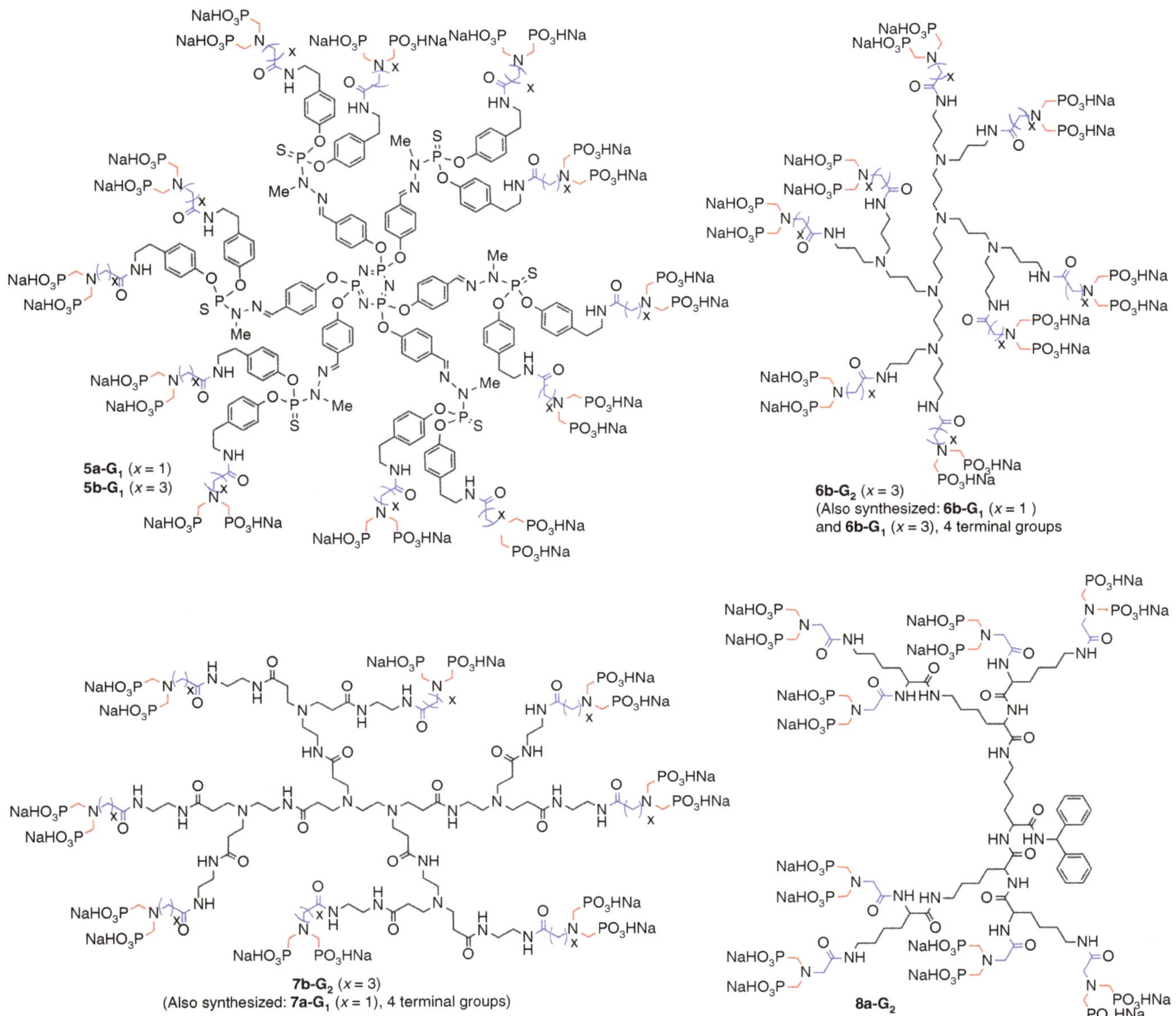

Figure 2 | Chemical structure of dendrimers 5a,b-G_1–8a-G_1. The azabisphosphonic salts are in red, the linkers in blue and variable internal structures in black.

status. In particular, we have shown that phosphorus-containing anti-inflammatory dendrimers induce these morphological changes of monocytes[23]. Therefore, we have screened the biological properties of the series of dendrimers synthesized for this study by measuring the morphological features of human monocytes (Figs 4 and 5; the negative control, without any dendrimer, is given first in Fig. 5). These changes appear within a few days in *in vitro* cultures of monocytes, and can be quantified by flow cytometry. These tests were conducted at three different concentrations of dendrimer (20, 2 and 0.2 μM). The more monocytes are activated by the dendrimers, the more their size and granularity are increased. So far, dendrimer **1-G_1** appears as the most active among all the dendrimers we have tested[23,25,29]. Thus, this molecule is the standard indicator of the activation of human monocytes in this study. As the dendrimers are dissolved in pure water, the negative control of the tests consists in treating the monocytes with the accurate volume of water. The qualitative results of monocyte activation are shown in Fig. 4 for the active dendrimers and in Fig. 5 for the non-active dendrimers, with indication of the efficiency score, from + + + for the most active to 0 for the least active (non-active) dendrimers. Dendrimer **1-G_1** is the only one displaying strong activity at 2 μM, and which is still active at 0.2 μM. It appears also that dendrimers **2-G_1**, **3-G_n**, **4-G_1** and **5a,b-G_1** display good activity (average for **3-G_1**) (Fig. 4), whereas dendrimers **6a,b-G_n**, **7a,b-G_n** ($n = 1$, 2) and **8a-G_2** are not active at all (Fig. 5). Dendrimers **5a-G_1** and **5b-G_1** only differ by the length of the linker between the azabisphosphonate terminations and the proximal branching points ($x = 1$ versus $x = 3$, Fig. 2). The bioactivity of these molecules appears to be equivalent. The same observation is made with dendrimers **6a-G_1** and **6b-G_1**, which are both inactive.

All-atom MD simulations of the dendrimers in explicit solvent. Molecular modelling was used to understand the striking differences observed in the biological properties. To gain molecular-level information about the dendrimers in the biological conditions, all-atom MD simulations of the 13

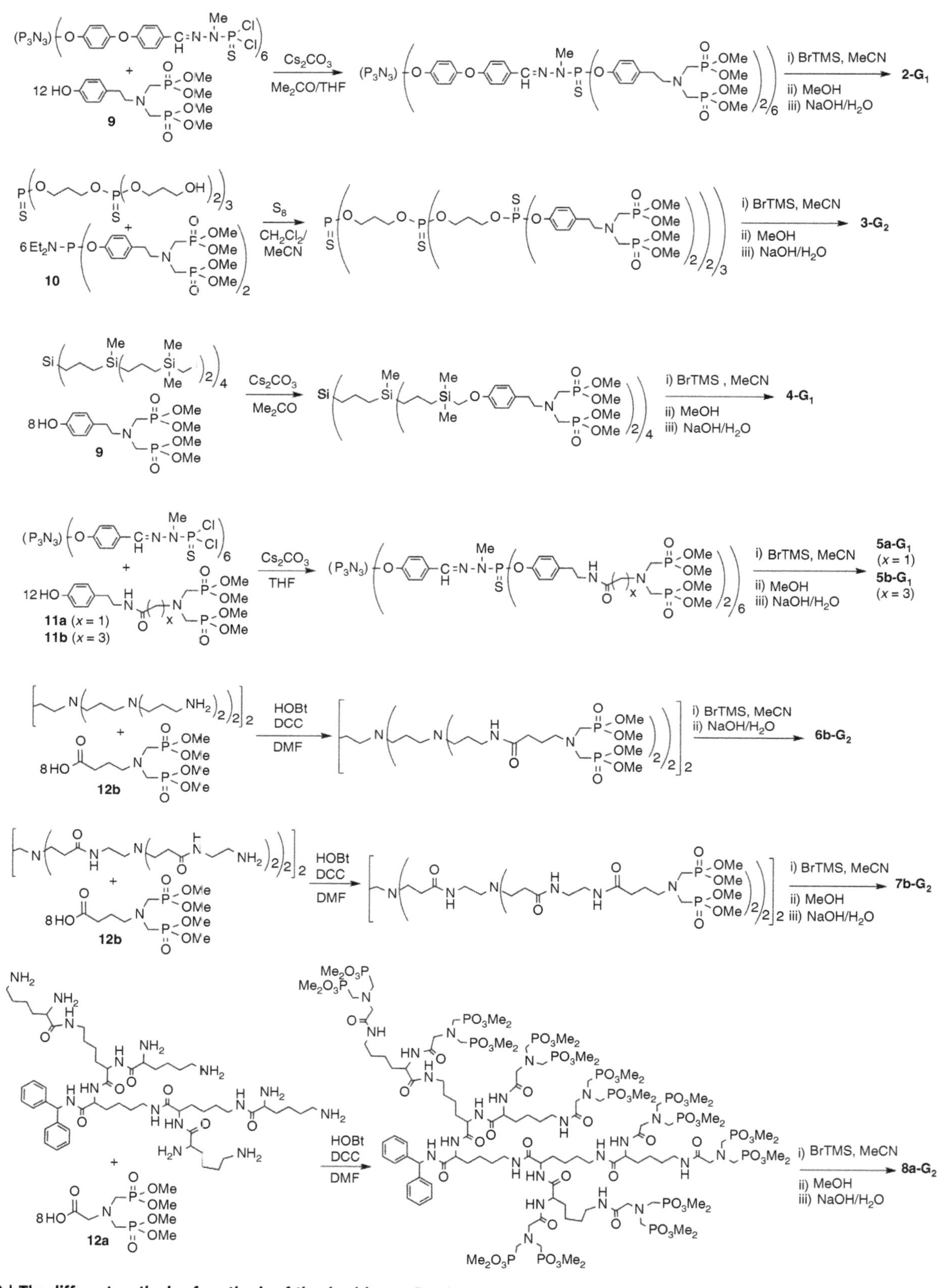

Figure 3 | The different methods of synthesis of the dendrimers. Dendrimer **3-G$_1$** is synthesized as **3-G$_2$**; dendrimers **6a-G$_1$** and **6b-G$_1$** as **6b-G$_2$**; and dendrimers **7a-G$_1$** as **7b-G$_2$** (HOBt: hydroxybenzotriazole, DCC: *N,N'*-dicyclohexylcarbodiimide, BrTMS: bromotrimethylsilane).

dendrimers in solution were carried out at 37 °C in presence of explicit water molecules and NaCl (150 mM). Each molecular system was equilibrated during 200 ns of MD simulation (Supplementary Fig. 1). Different data were extracted from the equilibrated phase MD trajectories. Figure 6a reports the equilibrated size data (that is, the radius of gyration, R_g) for the

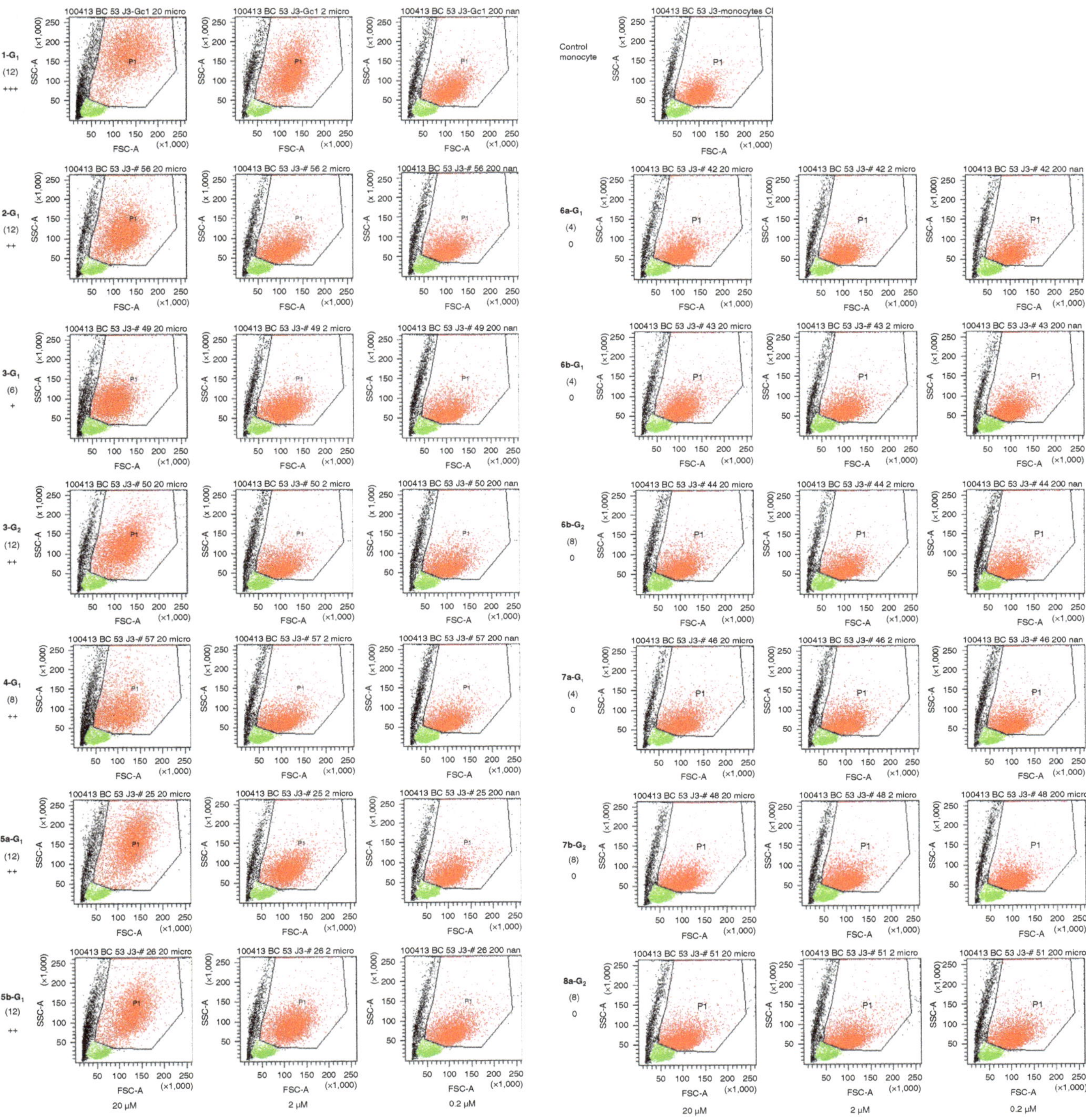

Figure 4 | Activation of human monocytes by the series of dendrimers 1-G$_1$, 2-G$_2$, 3-G$_1$, 3-G$_2$, 4-G$_1$, 5a-G$_1$ and 5b-G$_1$. The bioactivity of the dendrimers is analysed by flow cytometry. Each dot in the plots is indicative of morphological change (size—the Forward Scatter (FSC) parameter on the *x* axis—and granularity—the Side Scatter (SSC) parameter on the *y* axis) undergone by purified monocytes in the presence of the different dendrimers at 20, 2, and 0.2 μM (left, middle, and right graphs respectively). Red points are monocytes (gated in the polygon), green points are remaining lymphocytes after purification, black points are died or dying cells. For each dendrimer, the number of terminal functions is indicated in parentheses. The score attributed to each dendrimer appears in red on the left, from 0 (no activation) to + + + (the highest activity, attributed to **1-G$_1$**). Data are from one representative experiment out of six.

Figure 5 | Activation of human monocytes by the series of dendrimers 6a-G$_1$, 6b-G$_1$, 6b-G$_2$, 7a-G$_1$, 7b-G$_2$ and 8a-G$_2$. The bioactivity of the dendrimers is analysed by flow cytometry. Each dot in the plots is indicative of morphological change (size—the forward scatter (FSC) parameter on the *x* axis—and granularity—the side scatter (SSC) parameter on the *y* axis) undergone by purified monocytes in the presence of the different dendrimers at 20, 2, and 0.2 μM (left, middle and right graphs, respectively). Red points are monocytes (gated in the polygon), green points are remaining lymphocytes after purification, black points are died or dying cells. For each dendrimer, the number of terminal functions is indicated in parentheses. The score attributed to each dendrimer appears in red on the left, 0 means no activation. The negative control, without any dendrimer, is given first. Data are from one representative experiment out of six.

dendrimers in solution. Comparison of the R_g data with the number of terminal groups indicates that neither the size (generation) of the dendrimers (we used generations 1 and 2), nor the number of terminal functions are exclusively important criteria for the biological activity of each molecule. For instance, the activity of dendrimer **4-G$_1$** (8 terminal functions) is marked + +, as that of dendrimers **2-G$_1$**, **3-G$_1$** and **5b-G$_1$** (12 terminal functions); nevertheless, dendrimers **6b-G$_2$**, **7b-G$_2$** and **8a-G$_2$** also have 8 terminal functions, but no activation properties towards monocytes.

The equilibrated snapshots taken from the MD simulations reported in Fig. 6b clearly show that the three-dimensional (3D)-geometrical arrangements of these dendrimers in the solvent are very different. Several information can be extracted from the MD simulations. Analysis of the principal moments of inertia (I_x, I_y and I_z), of the aspect ratio and of anisotropy of the equilibrated dendrimers highlight that some of them assume spherical-like rather than elongated shape in the real environment (see Supplementary Fig. 2). However, comparison of these data with the biological activity (Figs 4, 5 and 6a) demonstrates that even the overall shape of the dendrimers is not a unique discriminant parameter for their activity. The same is true for the dendrimers solvent-accessible surface area (see Supplementary Fig. 2).

However, deeper structural analysis reveals other important differences related to the location of the active surface groups in the dendrimers structure. Interestingly, as emphasized by the circle drawn around the equilibrated dendrimers in Fig. 6b, dendrimers **3-G$_1$**, **6a,b-G$_1$**, **6b-G$_2$**, **7a-G$_1$**, **7b-G$_2$** and **8a-G$_2$** are much more symmetrical than the other ones. The azabisphosphonic terminal functions are spread all over the molecular surface (sphere) for these non-active dendrimers, while, at the equilibrium, the biologically active dendrimers **1-G$_1$**, **2-G$_1$**, **3-G$_2$**, **4-G$_1$** and **5a,b-G$_1$** appear as directional molecules, as in these cases the azabisphosphonic groups are gathered in half-sphere (see also Supplementary Movies 1 and 2: 1 MD 3D structure of **1-G$_1$**, and 2 MD 3D structure of **7b-G$_2$**). Thus, the solvated state of the different dendrimers—namely, the conformation assumed in the 'real' environment in terms of localization and density of azabisphosphonic functions on the dendrimers surface—is morphologically very different between active and non-active dendrimers. Since the surface functionalization is identical among all dendrimers, this effect is intimately related to the different internal structure.

Further analysis on the terminal groups' location quantified these structural differences. Plots in Fig. 7a display the radial distribution functions—*g(r)*—of the azabisphosphonate terminal groups (END) calculated with respect to the core unit (CEN) of the dendrimers (Fig. 7a: END to CEN) and respect to each other (END to END: Fig. 7c). The *g(r)* curves provide indication on the relative probability to find the terminal functions at a certain distance from the centre of the dendrimer or from each other (data are averaged over the last 50 ns of the equilibrated MD trajectories). The positions of the *g(r)* maximum peaks are particularly interesting. Figure 7b,d shows the normalized peaks of the *g(r)* curves—only the topmost 10%—revealing the average (most probable) distance for the azabisphosphonic terminal groups (END) respect to the dendrimers central unit (CEN) or respect to each other. Plots in Fig. 7a,b show that, in general, the surface groups are displayed at a larger distance from the dendrimer centre for the active compounds than in the case of the inactive ones ($\sim 1.5\,R_g$ versus $\sim R_g$). Moreover, *g(r)* maximum peaks related to the distance between the different surface groups (Fig. 7d) show that the azabisphosphonate terminal functions are more densely packed in the active dendrimers (the distance between the terminal branching points (N atom) is $\sim 0.5\,R_g$) than in the case of the inactive dendrimers ($\sim R_g$). These data provide a picture where active dendrimers look like directional molecules with all surface functions gathered together into 'clusters', far from the dendrimers core unit (CEN), while non-active dendrimers assume a more symmetric configuration in salt water.

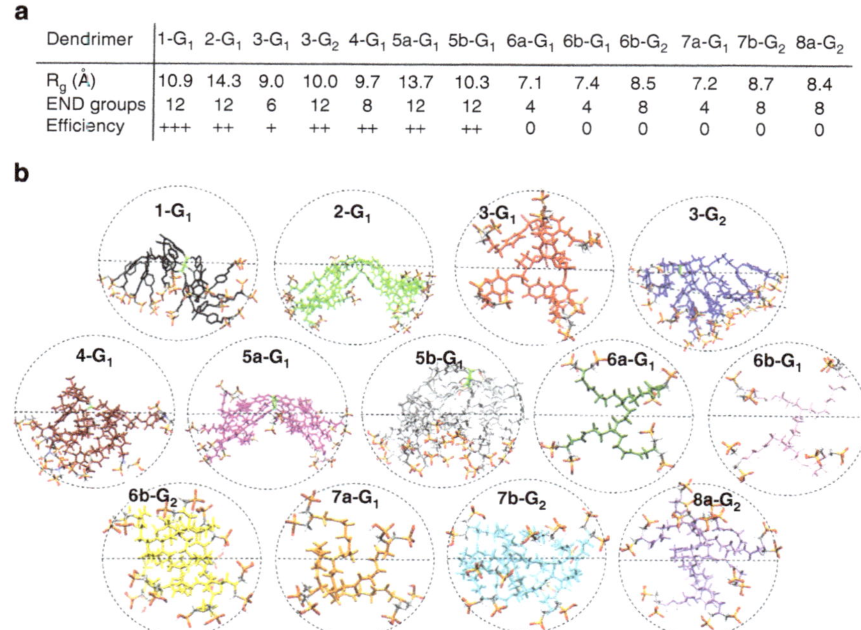

a

Dendrimer	1-G$_1$	2-G$_1$	3-G$_1$	3-G$_2$	4-G$_1$	5a-G$_1$	5b-G$_1$	6a-G$_1$	6b-G$_1$	6b-G$_2$	7a-G$_1$	7b-G$_2$	8a-G$_2$
R_g (Å)	10.9	14.3	9.0	10.0	9.7	13.7	10.3	7.1	7.4	8.5	7.2	8.7	8.4
END groups	12	12	6	12	8	12	12	4	4	8	4	8	8
Efficiency	+++	++	+	++	++	++	++	0	0	0	0	0	0

b

Figure 6 | Equilibrated configurations of the 13 dendrimers and their size, obtained from the MD simulations. (**a**) Radius of gyration (R_g) of the different dendrimers extracted from the equilibrated phase of the MD simulations in solution, number of azabisphosphonic surface groups (END) and biological efficiency score. Shape analysis: (**b**) MD equilibrated snapshots of the thirteen dendrimers displaying their shape. Dotted circles are added around the dendrimers to emphasize differences in the displacement of the azabisphosphonic functions around the dendrimers surface (symmetrical or directional molecules).

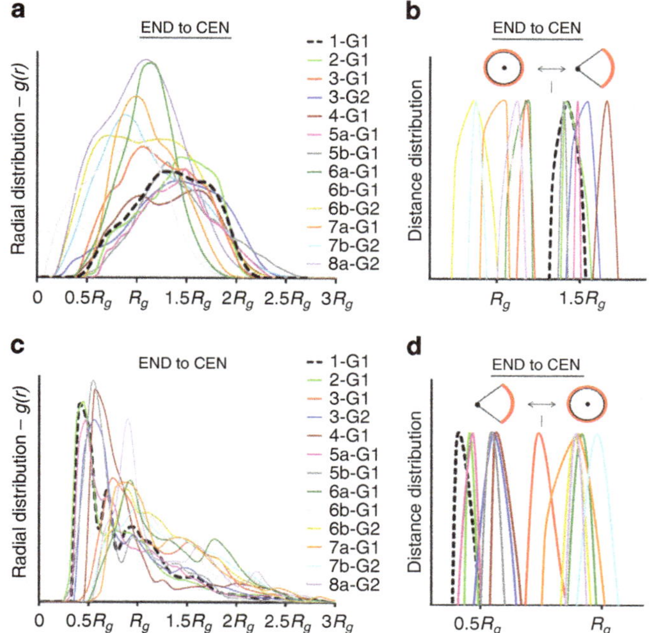

Figure 7 | Radial distribution functions of the dendrimer terminal groups. (**a**) Radial distribution functions—*g(r)*—of the terminal groups (END) with respect to the dendrimer core unit (CEN); (**b**) normalized peaks of the *g(r)* curves (only the topmost 10%) revealing the average (most probable) END to CEN distances in the dendrimers; (**c**) radial distribution functions, *g(r)*, of the terminal groups with respect to each other; (**d**) normalized peaks of the *g(r)* curves of **c** (only the topmost 10%) revealing the average (most probable) END to END distances. In all graphs, the distance (*x* axis) is expressed in R_g units to allow comparison between different size dendrimers, and the data corresponding to dendrimer **1-G₁** is given in dotted black lines.

To further characterize the solvated state of the dendrimers, the solvation energy (G_{sol})—namely, the solute-solvent interaction energy, or the energy necessary to drag the dendrimers out from water—was also extracted from the equilibrated phase MD simulations (the last 100 ns) and used as a descriptor of molecular hydrophilicity[36]. In general, the higher (the more negative) the G_{sol}, the more favourable the interactions of the dendrimer with water, which is a signal of overall hydrophilicity[36]. The G_{sol} data were further normalized for the MW of each dendrimer for comparison between different size, generation and structure of dendrimers (Fig. 8c)[36]. Additional information on the hydration of the dendrimers' interior (water penetration into the scaffold) was also extracted from the MD simulations (the last 100 ns) corroborating this analysis (see Supplementary Fig. 3).

Discussion

As evidenced from Figs 4 and 5, the various dendrimers induced very different results for the activation of monocytes (measured by the increase of size and granularity), despite their identical terminal groups. It is also clear from Fig. 6a that the number of terminal functions is not exclusively an important criterion. As the striking differences in the properties of all these dendrimers do not seem related to the terminal groups, we hypothesized that they could be related to the internal structure. At first glance, from the chemical structure point of view, the dendrimers could be divided into two families—those having aromatic groups in their structure and those essentially constituted of alkyl linkages. All dendrimers having aromatics in their structure (**1-G$_1$**, **2-G$_1$**, **5b-G$_1$**) are indeed active, but several dendrimers composed of alkyl linkages (**3-G$_1$**, **3-G$_2$**, **4-G$_1$**) are also active.

In view of these puzzling biological results, theoretical calculations have been carried out to try to rationalize them. We have employed all-atom MD simulations for the 13 different dendrimers immerged in a solvation box containing explicit water molecules and salt ions to gain a molecular-level detailed description of these macromolecules in the real environment.

The radii of gyration (R_g) of the equilibrated dendrimers (Fig. 6a) demonstrate that, similar to the number of terminal groups, size is not a discriminant factor controlling molecular activity. One reasonable hypothesis was that dendrimers' activity is somehow related to the shape or configuration assumed by the dendrimers in solution. However, the aspect ratio and the anisotropy parameters for the equilibrated dendrimers extracted from the MD simulations show that even the overall molecular shape is not a key parameter controlling activity (see Supplementary Fig. 2). Nevertheless, the equilibrated conformations assumed by the dendrimers in solution present other interesting differences. In particular, the structure of the active dendrimers is segregated in salt water, with all the hydrophilic terminal functions compacted on one side and the hydrophobic scaffold exposed to the external media (Fig. 6b). On the contrary, the non-active dendrimers have a more symmetrical structure with terminal groups displayed all around the dendrimer surface. Thus, our MD simulations divide the dendrimers into two categories identified by either a directional or a spherical configuration. The radial distribution functions *g(r)* data of the azabisphosphonic terminal groups (END) provide quantification for this observation (Fig. 7). In particular, the high *g(r)* peaks at short END–END distance (Fig. 7d) show that the terminal functions are more densely packed in the biologically active dendrimers, in particular for the most active **1-G$_1$**. In general, if the azabisphosphonic terminal groups packing density (position of the END–END *g(r)* peak) is taken as a score of molecular directionality, Fig. 7c,d show that the latter is in remarkable trend with biological activity.

To better quantify the structure–activity relationships, we have assessed the biological property of the set of dendrimers towards the activation of human monocytes, as there are major players in many different diseases[19,20,25] The biological activity of the molecules has been quantified by flow cytometry. Data shown in Figs 4 and 5 indicate that the different length of the linker ($x=1$ or $x=3$) has negligible effect within the same series of dendrimers (**5a-G$_1$/5b-G$_1$** and **6a-G$_1$/6b-G$_1$**). A similar comment can be done also on the results from MD, both in terms of 3D geometrical arrangement of the molecules and of quantification of the structural differences (Figs 6 and 7). Therefore, we discarded the three molecules **5a-G$_1$**, **6a-G$_1$** and **7a-G$_1$** from the initial set of 13. Figure 8a displays the biological activity of the 10 remaining dendrimers, as a function of the number of terminal groups. As taken alone the cell size parameter is poorly discriminating between the dendrimers, we have quantified and used the relative granularity of monocytes (at the highest concentration of dendrimers, that is, 20 µM; Fig. 8b): the more granulous the monocytes, the more active the dendrimer.

For better understanding the key parameters of the dendrimers structure for the biological activity, several other information have been extracted from the MD data. The G_{sol} energies extracted from the equilibrated phase (the last 100 ns) MD simulations of the dendrimers in solution are representative of the level of hydrophilicity/hydrophobicity of their solvated state. Figure 8c shows that also G_{sol} data are in good trend with the molecular activity of the dendrimers (Fig. 8a), which suggests that both hydrophilicity/hydrophobicity (Fig. 8c), and molecular directionality (Fig. 8d) are key discriminant parameters for

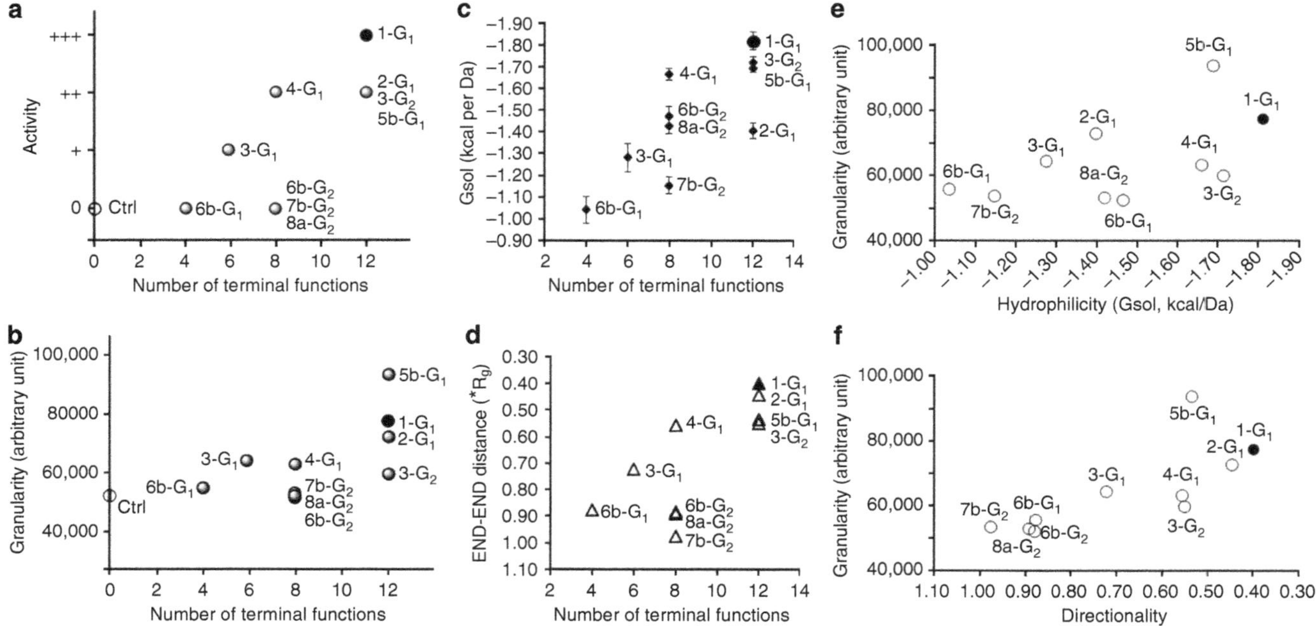

Figure 8 | Comparison of biological activity and data from MD simulations for 10 dendrimers. (**a**) The number of terminal groups of dendrimers versus the biological efficiency. (**b**) Quantification of relative granularity (arbitrary units, means from three donors) of the monocytes treated with the dendrimers and of negative control monocytes. (**c**) G_{sol} values from MD (relative hydrophilicity). (**d**) Calculated distance between terminal groups (in R_g units), as an indication of molecular directionality. (**e**,**f**) Comparison between biological data and MD data: granularity versus hydrophilicity (**e**) and granularity versus directionality (**f**). The black dots correspond in all cases to the lead compound **1-G$_1$**.

biological activity (Fig. 8a). In fact, the most active dendrimers, with particular emphasis on dendrimer **1-G$_1$**, possess the most favourable solvation energy (G_{sol}) and the highest directionality scores (the smaller the END–END distance, the higher molecular directionality), which also points towards a direct correlation between dendrimers multivalency and activity. In fact, at the molecular level, a higher density of active functions can impact biological efficiency because it intuitively amplifies cooperativity and favours multivalent interactions. As last, we put in direct correlation biological activity (granularity) with hydrophilicity (G_{sol}) and molecular directionality. The results are shown in Fig. 8e,f, respectively, showing remarkable trends. Indeed, looking at these dendrimers in solution, these analyses suggest that the dense concentration of active functions in regions of the dendrimers surface and the level of hydrophilicity/hydrophobicity of the structure are crucial to molecular activity. This is the case also of biological molecules like proteins, where the features of the surface, presence of charged or active patches, and overall and local hydrophobicity and hydrophilicity levels produce remarkable effects through a delicate network of multiscale interactions and molecular recognition.

In conclusion, this work carried out on seven different families of dendrimers clearly demonstrates that the internal structure of dendrimers cannot be anymore regarded as an 'innocent' support for active functions, but plays a crucial role, especially when considering biological properties. Indeed, the geometry of the dendrimers with identical terminal groups may be very different intrinsically, and the differences can be amplified in a real environment such as a water solution or biological materials (like blood, biological barriers and cell membranes), depending on the nature of the scaffold. Structural differences induce changes in shape and in the distribution of the terminal active functions of the dendrimers, which are responsible for the biological activity. Regarding monocyte activation, the most active dendrimers are those in which the surface functions are gathered on one side (directional molecules), a suitable orientation to maximize multivalent interactions with cells. Definitely, this work shows how changing one single parameter, even in the internal moieties, may totally modify the properties of dendrimers. Therefore, the implementation of extensive MD simulation studies of dendrimers appears as a pivotal asset when designing new bio-oriented dendritic devices or to optimize existing dendritic systems. Such finding exceeds the field of dendrimers and embraces those more general of macromolecules and nanostructures. The direct relationships traced here between hydrophobicity/hydrophilicity and activity, and between activity and surface characteristics (that is, directionality in the localization of functional groups) recall the main features of biological macromolecules such as proteins. Our results are reminiscent to what is known about the interplay between natural networks and their surroundings.

Methods

General information about the synthesis of dendrimers. All manipulations are performed under argon using standard Schlenk techniques. Commercial samples were used as received from Aldrich (PAMAM dendrimers, DAB dendrimers, Lysine dendrimer and all other chemicals). The following compounds have been prepared according to published procedures: tyramine azabisphosphonate **9** (ref. 21) and dendrimer **1-G$_1$** (ref. 21), Salamonczyk's thiophosphite dendrimers[33], chlorine-ended carbosilane dendrimers[37] and phosphorhydrazone dendrimers ended by 12 chlorine atoms[38]. All solvents were dried and distilled according to routine procedure before use. Thin-layer chromatography was carried out on Merck Kieselgel 60F254 precoated silicagel plates. Preparative chromatography was performed on Merck Kieselgel. ^{1}H, ^{13}C, ^{31}P NMR, HMQC and HMBC measurements were performed on Bruker AC200, AM250 and AV300 and AMX400. All dendrimers have been characterized by ^{1}H, $^{13}C\{^{1}H\}$ and $^{31}P\{^{1}H\}$ NMR, and two-dimensional NMR spectra when necessary. All details of the synthesis and the NMR data for all compounds are given in the Supplementary Information. The experimental information for the synthesis of all dendrimers is also given in the Supplementary Methods for chemistry. The synthesis of dendrimer **5a-G$_1$** is given below as a typical example.

Typical example for the synthesis of dendrimers. Synthesis of **5a-G$_1$**, *first step*: 0.017 mmol of generation 1 phosphorus-containing dendrimer (12 Cl terminations)[38] are placed in solution in 3 ml of dry tetrahydrofuran. Cs_2CO_3

(5.04 mmol), then 0.23 mmol of the tyramine azabisphosphonate **11a** ($x = 1$) in solution in 3 ml of dry tetrahydrofuran are successively added to this solution. The mixture is stirred overnight at room temperature and then filtered on celite. The reaction medium is evaporated under reduced pressure then the dry residue is dissolved in a minimum volume of dichloromethane. The product is then precipitated in a large volume of ether. This operation is repeated three times to eliminate the slight excess of starting tyramine derivative. The dendrimer with methylphosphonate terminations is obtained as an off-white powder (88% yield). *Second step*: 0.015 mmol of dendrimer with methylphosphonate terminations are placed in solution under an inert atmosphere in 3 ml of distilled acetonitrile. The solution is taken to 0 °C then 48 equivalents of BrTMS (0.73 mmol) are added dropwise under argon. The mixture is stirred for 30 min at 0 °C, then overnight at room temperature and finally evaporated to dryness under reduced pressure. The residue thus obtained is treated with methanol (2×15 ml), then evaporated to dryness and washed with dry ether (20 ml) to afford the dendrimer with phosphonic acid terminations (63% yield). *Third step*: the sodium salt is obtained by reaction of 24 equivalents of NaOH solution at 0.1955 N on one equivalent of dendrimer with phosphonic acid terminations, to produce, after stirring 1 h at room temperature and freeze drying, the expected dendrimer **5a-G$_1$** (70% yield).

Purification and activation of human monocytes. Preparation of PBMC (peripheral blood mononuclear cells) from healthy volunteers and subsequent purification of monocytes are performed as already described[24]. Purity of the monocytes (>95%) is assessed by flow cytometry on a LSR-II device (BD Biosciences, San Diego, CA, USA).

For activation cultures, purified monocytes are cultured in multi-well plates for 72 h at 10^6 cells ml^{-1} of complete RPMI 1640 medium (Roswell Park Memorial Institute medium), that is, supplemented with 10% of heat-inactivated fetal calf serum, 1 mM sodium pyruvate, 2 mM L-glutamine (all from Invitrogen Corporation, Paisley, UK), penicillin and streptomycin, both at 100 U ml^{-1} (Cambrex Bio Science). Dendrimers are added at the beginning of the cultures at 20, 2 and 0.2 μM.

Flow cytometry analyses. At the end of the culture, monocytes are washed with PBS with 5% fetal calf serum and their morphology (size and granularity) is analysed by flow cytometry (LSR-II device from BD Biosciences) and quantified using FACSDiva software (BD Biosciences). The most activated monocytes are the most granular, and biggest they appear. A score (from 0 to + + +) is attributed to each dendrimer on these morphological criteria. A score of 0 is given to dendrimers that do not induce morphological changes (monocytes with the same morphology than control, non-activated, monocytes). A score of + + + is given to dendrimer **1-G$_1$**, the most active one which induces dramatic morphological changes at 20 and 2 μM, still detectable at 0.2 μM. A score of + + is given to dendrimers whose effect is comparable to the one of dendrimer **1-G$_1$** at 20 μM but with no or weak detectable effect at 2 μM. A score of + is given to dendrimers which has a detectable effect, although weak, at 20 μM.

All-atom MD simulations. The MD simulation work is conducted by using the AMBER 12 software[39]. The molecular models for all dendrimers are created and parametrized according to a validated procedure for the simulation of dendrimers in aqueous solution (see Supplementary Table 1 for details)[36,40,41]. The force field parameters for the **4-G$_1$** carbosilane dendrimer are obtained as previously reported[42]. All the dendrimer models are immerged in a periodic box containing explicit TIP3P water molecules[43] and 150 mM of NaCl to reproduce the experimental conditions. All systems are simulated for 200 ns in NPT conditions at 37 °C. Analyses of the structural features and of the solvation energies (G_{sol}) of the dendrimers are performed on the equilibrated phase MD trajectories (Supplementary Fig. 1). Details on the computational procedures are given in the Supplementary Methods and Supplementary Movies 1 and 2 obtained from the MD simulations showing the 3D structures of **1-G$_1$** (MD 3-D structure of **1-G$_1$**) and **7b-G$_2$** (MD 3D structure of **7b-G$_2$**) as representative cases of directional and symmetrical molecules.

References

1. Caminade, A. M., Turrin, C. O., Laurent, R., Ouali, A. & Delavaux-Nicot, B. *Dendrimers: Towards Catalytic, Material and Biomedical Uses* (John Wiley & Sons, 2011).
2. Page, D., Zanini, D. & Roy, R. Macromolecular recognition: Effect of multivalency in the inhibition of binding of yeast mannan to concanavalin A and pea lectins by mannosylated dendrimers. *Bioorg. Med. Chem.* **4,** 1949–1961 (1996).
3. Pavan, G. M., Danani, A., Pricl, S. & Smith, D. K. Modeling the multivalent recognition between dendritic molecules and DNA: understanding how ligand 'sacrifice' and screening can enhance binding. *J. Am. Chem. Soc.* **131,** 9686–9694 (2009).
4. Pavan, G. M. Modeling the interaction between dendrimers and nucleic acids—a molecular perspective through hierarchical scales. *ChemMedChem* **9,** 2623–2631 (2014).
5. Darbre, T. & Reymond, J. L. Peptide dendrimers as artificial enzymes, receptors, and drug-delivery agents. *Acc. Chem. Res.* **39,** 925–934 (2006).
6. Lee, C. C., MacKay, J. A., Fréchet, J. M. J. & Szoka, F. C. Designing dendrimers for biological applications. *Nat. Biotechnol.* **23,** 1517–1526 (2005).
7. Mammen, M., Choi, S. K. & Whitesides, G. M. Polyvalent interactions in biological systems: implications for design and use of multivalent ligands and inhibitors. *Angew. Chem. Int. Ed.* **37,** 2754–2794 (1998).
8. Tomalia, D. A. Dendrons/dendrimers: quantisized, nano-element like building blocks for soft-soft and soft-hard nano-compound synthesis. *Soft Matter* **6,** 456–472 (2010).
9. Tomalia, D. A. *et al.* A new class of polymers—Starburst dendritic macromolecules. *Polym. J.* **17,** 117–132 (1985).
10. De Brabander-van den Berg, E. M. M. & Meijer, E. W. Poly(Propylene Imine) dendrimers—large-scale synthesis by heterogeneously catalyzed hydrogenations. *Angew. Chem. Int. Ed.* **32,** 1308–1311 (1993).
11. Mynar, J. L., Lowery, T. J., Wemmer, D. E., Pines, A. & Fréchet, J. M. J. Xenon biosensor amplification via dendrimer-cage supramolecular constructs. *J. Am. Chem. Soc.* **128,** 6334–6335 (2006).
12. Juttukonda, V. *et al.* Facile synthesis of tin oxide nanoparticles stabilized by dendritic polymers. *J. Am. Chem. Soc.* **128,** 420–421 (2006).
13. Tomalia, D. A., Hall, M. & Hedstrand, D. M. Starburst dendrimers.3. The importance of branch junction symmetry in the development of topological shell molecules. *J. Am. Chem. Soc.* **109,** 1601–1603 (1987).
14. Liao, X. L., Stellacci, F. & McGrath, D. V. Photoswitchable flexible and shape-persistent dendrimers: comparison of the interplay between a photochromic azobenzene core and dendrimer structure. *J. Am. Chem. Soc.* **126,** 2181–2185 (2004).
15. Merkel, O. M. *et al.* Triazine dendrimers as nonviral gene delivery systems: effects of molecular structure on biological activity. *Bioconjugate Chem.* **20,** 1799–1806 (2009).
16. Jain, K., Kesharwani, P., Gupta, U. & Jain, N. K. Dendrimer toxicity: let's meet the challenge. *Int. J. Pharm.* **394,** 122–142 (2010).
17. Ginhoux, F. & Jung, S. Monocytes and macrophages: developmental pathways and tissue homeostasis. *Nat. Rev. Immunol.* **14,** 392–404 (2014).
18. Zolnik, B. S., Gonzalez-Fernandez, A., Sadrieh, N. & Dobrovolskaia, M. A. Minireview: nanoparticles and immune system. *Endocrinology* **151,** 458–465 (2010).
19. Murray, P. J. & Wynn, T. A. Protective and pathogenic functions of macrophage subsets. *Nat. Rev. Immunol.* **11,** 723–737 (2011).
20. Sica, A. & Mantovani, A. Macrophage plasticity and polarization: *in vivo* veritas. *J. Clin. Invest.* **122,** 787–795 (2012).
21. Griffe, L. *et al.* Multiplication of human natural killer cells by nanosized phosphonate-capped dendrimers. *Angew. Chem. Int. Ed.* **46,** 2523–2526 (2007).
22. Portevin, D. *et al.* Regulatory activity of azabisphosphonate-capped dendrimers on human CD4$^+$ T cell proliferation for ex-vivo expansion of NK cells from PBMCs and immunotherapy. *J. Transl. Med.* **7,** 82 (2009).
23. Poupot, M. *et al.* Design of phosphorylated dendritic architectures to promote human monocyte activation. *FASEB J.* **20,** 2339–2351 (2006).
24. Fruchon, S. *et al.* Anti-inflammatory and immuno-suppressive activation of human monocytes by a bio-active dendrimer. *J. Leukocyte Biol.* **85,** 553–562 (2009).
25. Hayder, M. *et al.* Phosphorus-based dendrimer as nanotherapeutics targeting both inflammation and osteoclastogenesis in experimental arthritis. *Sci. Transl. Med.* **3,** 81ra35 (2011).
26. Leah, E. Experimental arthritis: dendrimer drug mends monocytes. *Nat. Rev. Rheumatol.* **7,** 376 (2011).
27. Lou, K.-J. Dendrimer throws a blanket on RA. *SciBX* **4,** doi:10.1038/scibx.2011.561 (2011).
28. Rolland, O. *et al.* Efficient synthesis of phosphorus-containing dendrimers capped with isosteric functions of amino-bis(methylene) phosphonic acids. *Tetrahedron Lett.* **50,** 2078–2082 (2009).
29. Rolland, O. *et al.* Tailored control and optimisation of the number of phosphonic acid termini on phosphorus-containing dendrimers for the *ex-vivo* activation of human monocytes. *Chem. Eur. J.* **14,** 4836–4850 (2008).
30. Wang, Y., Guo, R., Cao, X., Shen, M. & Shi, X. Encapsulation of 2-methoxyestradiol within multifunctional poly(amidoamine) dendrimers for targeted cancer therapy. *Biomaterials* **32,** 3322–3329 (2011).
31. Garber, S. B., Kingsbury, J. S., Gray, B. L. & Hoveyda, A. H. Efficient and recyclable monomeric and dendritic Ru-based metathesis catalysts. *J. Am. Chem. Soc.* **122,** 8168–8179 (2000).
32. Denkewalter, R. G., Kolc, J. & Lukasavage, W. J. Macromolecular highly branched homogeneous compound based on lysine units. US patent 4,289,872 (1981).
33. Salamonczyk, G. M., Kuznikowski, M. & Skowronska, A. A divergent synthesis of thiophosphate-based dendrimers. *Tetrahedron Lett.* **41,** 1643–1645 (2000).
34. Launay, N., Caminade, A. M., Lahana, R. & Majoral, J. P. A general synthetic strategy for neutral phosphorus-containing dendrimers. *Angew. Chem. Int. Ed.* **33,** 1589–1592 (1994).
35. Shafer, L. L., McNulty, J. A. & Young, M. R. Brain activation of monocyte lineage cells: brain-derived soluble factors differentially regulate BV2 microglia and peripheral macrophage immune functions. *Neuroimmunomodulation* **10,** 283–294 (2002).

36. Pavan, G. M., Barducci, A., Albertazzi, L. & Parrinello, M. Combining metadynamics simulation and experiments to characterize dendrimers in solution. *Soft Matter* **9,** 2593–2597 (2013).
37. de Groot, D., Reek, J. N. H., Kamer, P. C. J. & van Leeuwen, P. W. N. M. Palladium complexes of phosphane-functionalised carbosilane dendrimers as catalysts in a continuous-flow membrane reactor. *Eur. J. Org. Chem.* **2002,** 1085–1095 (2002).
38. Launay, N., Caminade, A. M. & Majoral, J. P. Synthesis of bowl-shaped dendrimers from generation 1 to generation 8. *J. Organomet. Chem.* **529,** 51–58 (1997).
39. Case, D. A. *et al. AMBER 12* (University of California, 2012).
40. Garzoni, M., Okuro, K., Ishii, N., Aida, T. & Pavan, G. M. Structure and shape effects of molecular glue on supramolecular tubulin assemblies. *ACS Nano* **8,** 904–914 (2014).
41. Simanek, E. E., Enciso, A. E. & Pavan, G. M. Computational design principles for the discovery of bioactive dendrimers: [s]-triazines and other examples. *Exp. Opin. Drug Disc.* **8,** 1057–1069 (2013).
42. Fuentes-Paniagua, E. *et al.* Carbosilane cationic dendrimers synthesized by thiol–ene click chemistry and their use as antibacterial agents. *RSC Adv.* **4,** 1256–1265 (2014).
43. Jorgensen, W. L., Chandrasekhar, J., Madura, J. D., Impey, R. W. & Klein, M. L. Comparison of simple potential functions for simulating liquid water. *J. Chem. Phys.* **79,** 926–935 (1983).

Acknowledgements

This work was financially supported by Rhodia (grant to S.F. and A.O.), CNRS (Centre National de la Recherche Scientifique), INSERM (Institut National de la Santé et de la Recherche Médicale), UPS (Université Paul Sabatier) and FRM (Fondation pour la Recherche Médicale, grant DCM20111223039).

Author contributions

A.-M.C. conceived the idea of the comparison between different types of dendrimers, supervised all the chemical work and wrote most of this paper. C.-O.T. was the day-to-day supervisor of the chemical work. S.F. performed most of the biological experiments under the direct guidance of M.P. A.O. synthesized dendrimers **2-G$_1$**, **3-Gn** ($n = 1, 2$) and **4-G$_1$**. A.M. synthesized dendrimers **5a,b-G$_1$**, **6a,b-G$_n$** ($n = 1, 2$), **7a-G$_1$**, **7b-G$_2$** and **8a-G$_2$** from commercial sources. G.M.P. is responsible for the modelling part, which has been performed with the help of M.G., M.M., V.F. and V.K., and wrote the simulation part of this paper. J.-P.M. was helpful in discussing the chemical part and obtained the grant for A.O. R.P. supervised all the biological work and wrote the biological part of this paper.

Additional information

Competing financial interests: The authors declare no competing financial interests.

Design of a bioactive small molecule that targets r(AUUCU) repeats in spinocerebellar ataxia 10

Wang-Yong Yang[1], Rui Gao[2], Mark Southern[3], Partha S. Sarkar[2] & Matthew D. Disney[1]

RNA is an important target for chemical probes of function and lead therapeutics; however, it is difficult to target with small molecules. One approach to tackle this problem is to identify compounds that target RNA structures and utilize them to multivalently target RNA. Here we show that small molecules can be identified to selectively bind RNA base pairs by probing a library of RNA-focused small molecules. A small molecule that selectively binds AU base pairs informed design of a dimeric compound (**2AU-2**) that targets the pathogenic RNA, expanded r(AUUCU) repeats, that causes spinocerebellar ataxia type 10 (SCA10) in patient-derived cells. Indeed, **2AU-2** (50 nM) ameliorates various aspects of SCA10 pathology including improvement of mitochondrial dysfunction, reduced activation of caspase 3, and reduction of nuclear foci. These studies provide a first-in-class chemical probe to study SCA10 RNA toxicity and potentially define broadly applicable compounds targeting RNA AU base pairs in cells.

[1] Departments of Chemistry and Neuroscience, The Scripps Research Institute, Scripps Florida, Jupiter, Florida 33458, USA. [2] Mitchell Center for Neurodegenerative Disorders, Department of Neurology, Neuroscience and Cell Biology, University of Texas Medical Branch, Galveston, Texas 77555, USA. [3] Informatics Core, The Scripps Research Institute, Scripps Florida, Jupiter, Florida 33458, USA. Correspondence and requests for materials should be addressed to M.D.D. (email: Disney@scripps.edu).

RNA has diverse cellular functions. For example, messenger RNAs (mRNAs) encode protein, microRNAs regulate the lifetime of mRNAs, and the ribosome translates mRNAs into proteins[1,2]. In bacteria, riboswitches control the production of proteins by binding to small molecule metabolites[3,4]. In fact, many non-coding RNAs have been found to play significant roles in cellular biology, and these discoveries expand even further the known functions of RNA[5].

Because of the important cellular functions of RNA under normal conditions, it is not surprising that mutations in RNA can cause disease. Single-nucleotide polymorphisms can give rise to cryptic alternative pre-mRNA splicing sites, leading to production of aberrant, defective proteins, as is the case with β-thalassaemia[6,7]. Expanded RNA repeats can also contribute to disease and can be present in 5′ and 3′ untranslated regions (UTRs; fragile X-associated tremor ataxia syndrome (FXTAS)[8] and myotonic dystrophy type 1 (DM1)[9]), introns (spinocerebellar ataxia type 10 (SCA10)[10] and myotonic dystrophy type 2 (DM2)[11]) or coding regions (Huntington's disease (HD)[12]). Small molecules that target these RNA and inhibit its dysfunction are thus highly desirable.

The bacterial ribosome is the most widely exploited RNA target[13,14]. Ribosomes and ribosomal RNA (rRNA) are privileged targets as (i) ribosomes play essential roles in cellular homeostasis and modulation of ribosome activity can have drastic cellular consequences, and (ii) rRNA comprises about 80–90% of the total RNA content of a cell[15]. Riboswitches are also emerging and established targets of RNA-directed small molecules. Compounds identified to bind to and modulate riboswitches generally mimic the structure of the RNA's natural metabolite[3,16], akin to substrate mimicry to design enzyme inhibitors[17]. Most RNA targets to which a small molecule binder is desired, however, are of low abundance and have no natural metabolite to inform drug design.

To aid RNA-targeting endeavours, our group has developed two-dimensional combinatorial screening (2DCS) to identify optimal (high affinity and selective) RNA motif–small molecule interactions. These interactions are deposited into a database and can be used to design small molecules to target RNAs by comparing motifs in the desired target to the database. This approach has been used to design small molecules targeting the RNAs that cause DM[18–20], FXTAS[21] and HD[22]. All of the interactions that are presently in the RNA motif–small molecule database are between small molecules and RNA loops such as hairpins, bulges and internal loops. Herein, we report small molecules that bind selectively to RNA base pairs. Among a variety of compounds tested, small molecules with benzamidine moieties were identified to bind selectively to AU base pairs. These data were leveraged to design the first bioactive small molecule to target the expanded r(AUUCU) repeat that causes SCA10, an incurable neuromuscular disorder. The compound targets the central AU base pairs in r(AUUCU)^{exp} and its dimeric compound (**2AU-2**) displaces sequestered proteins and improves defects in patient-derived cells. The observation that base pair-binding modules can provide bioactive compounds suggests that many other RNAs can be exploited as targets of small molecules.

Results and Discussion

Binding of RNA-focused small molecules to RNA base pairs. By using chemical similarity searching, small molecules with features that should pre-dispose them for binding RNA[23,24] were collected from both the National Cancer Institute's and The Scripps Research Institute's chemical libraries, including benzimidazole, benzamidine, aniline moieties. Compounds were further restrained to be fluorescent to allow for easy screening of binding events, affording 104 small molecules (Fig. 1a and Supplementary Table 1).

Compounds were screened for binding to different base pairs using four model constructs with stretches of AU and GC base pairs embedded in the stem of a common hairpin loop (Fig. 1b). The four RNAs display AU or GC pairs with different nearest neighbours. AUAU and AAUU RNAs have 5′AU/3′UA or 5′AAUU/3′UUAA stretches, respectively, while GCGC and GGCC have 5′GC/3′CG or 5′GGCC/3′CCGG stretches, respectively. Due to significant differences in the thermodynamic stability of the hairpins, RNAs with AU pairs had 12 base pairs in the stem while RNAs with GC pairs had 8 (ref. 25). The $\Delta G°_{37}$ for AUAU and AAUU is -8.5 and $-6.7\,\text{kcal mol}^{-1}$, respectively, while for GCGC and GGCC it is -17.5 and $-19.1\,\text{kcal mol}^{-1}$, respectively. If only eight AU base pairs were present, then the free energy drops considerably to -3.7 and $-2.5\,\text{kcal mol}^{-1}$, respectively.

In initial compound screens, each small molecule was incubated with the four RNAs and the change in emission was measured (Fig. 1c). Changes in emission were not only analysed for statistical significance for binding to these RNAs in general, but also for binding to the different RNA structures. For this compound collection, 29% of the compounds exhibited a

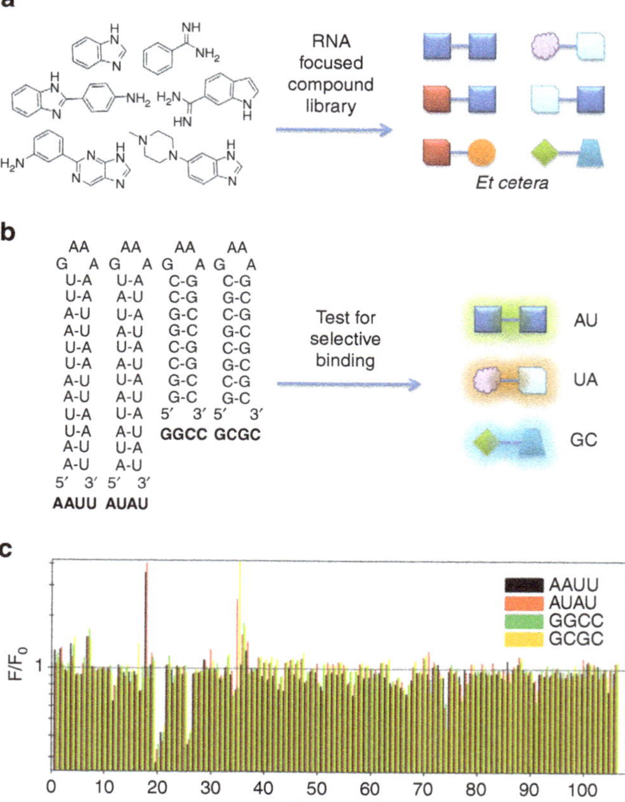

Figure 1 | Overall scheme to identify small molecules that bind to RNA base pairs. (**a**) A small molecule library was collected in which the small molecules have chemotypes present in compounds known to bind RNA. (**b**) The RNA-focused small molecule library was tested for binding to four different RNAs that have different orientations and identities of RNA base pairs. (**c**) Compounds were tested in a fluorescence emission assay for selectively binding to RNAs with different paired elements. Compounds that were selective were further analysed.

change in emission upon binding to any of the RNAs used in this study, and 18% of the compounds showed preferential binding to AU or GC pair-containing duplexes (Supplementary Table 2).

On the basis of the substructures within compounds that bind, a Venn diagram was constructed to correlate chemotypes and binding to AU and GC base pairs (Fig. 2). For example, various functionalized purines bound to RNAs with GC base pairs. Previously, other compounds that bind RNA base pairs have been identified. For example, the Beal group has used threading intercalators with acridine or other aromatic functionalities to target RNA bulges with nearby GC pairs[26]. Thus, it appears that acridine, and related compounds, can provide a GC base-pair-binding module. The group of Tor has shown that ethidium bromide is a 20-fold selective binder to poly r(A)-poly r(U) over poly r(G)–poly r(C)[27].

Each small molecule from the initial screen was tested for saturable binding when incubated with serially diluted RNA. The benzamidine compounds **1** and **2** provided the most robust and saturable change in emission and were found to bind selectively to AU base pairs (Supplementary Figs 1, 2 and 3). Due to the binding of these compounds to AU base pairs and their saturable emission properties, these compounds were selected for further study. This assay, by nature of using emission to study binding, could generate false negatives; however, it allowed us to further characterize positive hits and produce a first-in-class bioactive ligand that targets r(AUUCU), *vide infra*.

Compounds 1 and 2 bind selectively to AU base pairs. The selectivities of compounds **1** and **2** were further assessed by measuring EC_{50}s for all four RNAs. The EC_{50}s for **1** for binding to AAUU, AUAU, GGCC and GCGC are 170, 45, 390 and 240 nM, respectively, while the EC_{50}'s for **2** are 170, 190, 8,550 and 6,950 nM, respectively (Table 1). On the basis of these data, **2** is much more selective for AU base pairs than **1**, with an AU pair selectivity of ~40-fold (Fig. 3). Measurement of the K_d's of **2** to AUAU and AAUU give values of 210 and 320 nM, respectively, and stoichiometries of 2.9 and 3.7, respectively (Supplementary Fig. 4). These data suggests that **2** is a high affinity binder to stretches of AU base pairs and that the compound interacts with between 3 and 4 base pairs in each of the model hairpins. Previous studies have suggested that the aminoglycoside tobramycin recognizes model poly(rI) · poly(rC) RNA duplexes and that the compound interacts with approximately 4 bp, or a similar number of interacting sites that are proposed for **2** (ref. 28). Diphenylfuran amidine was previously reported to bind polyr(A) · polyr(U) duplex via intercalation, as determined from viscosity and circular dichroism studies[29,30]. These observations were further supported by docking studies in which the intercalation of **2** is stabilized through stacking interactions with the positively charged amidine residing in the major groove; minor groove binding could not be accommodated[29,30]. Further, the substituents in this class of compounds affect the thermal stability of polyr(A) · polyr(U), with imidazoline providing the largest enhancement[29,30].

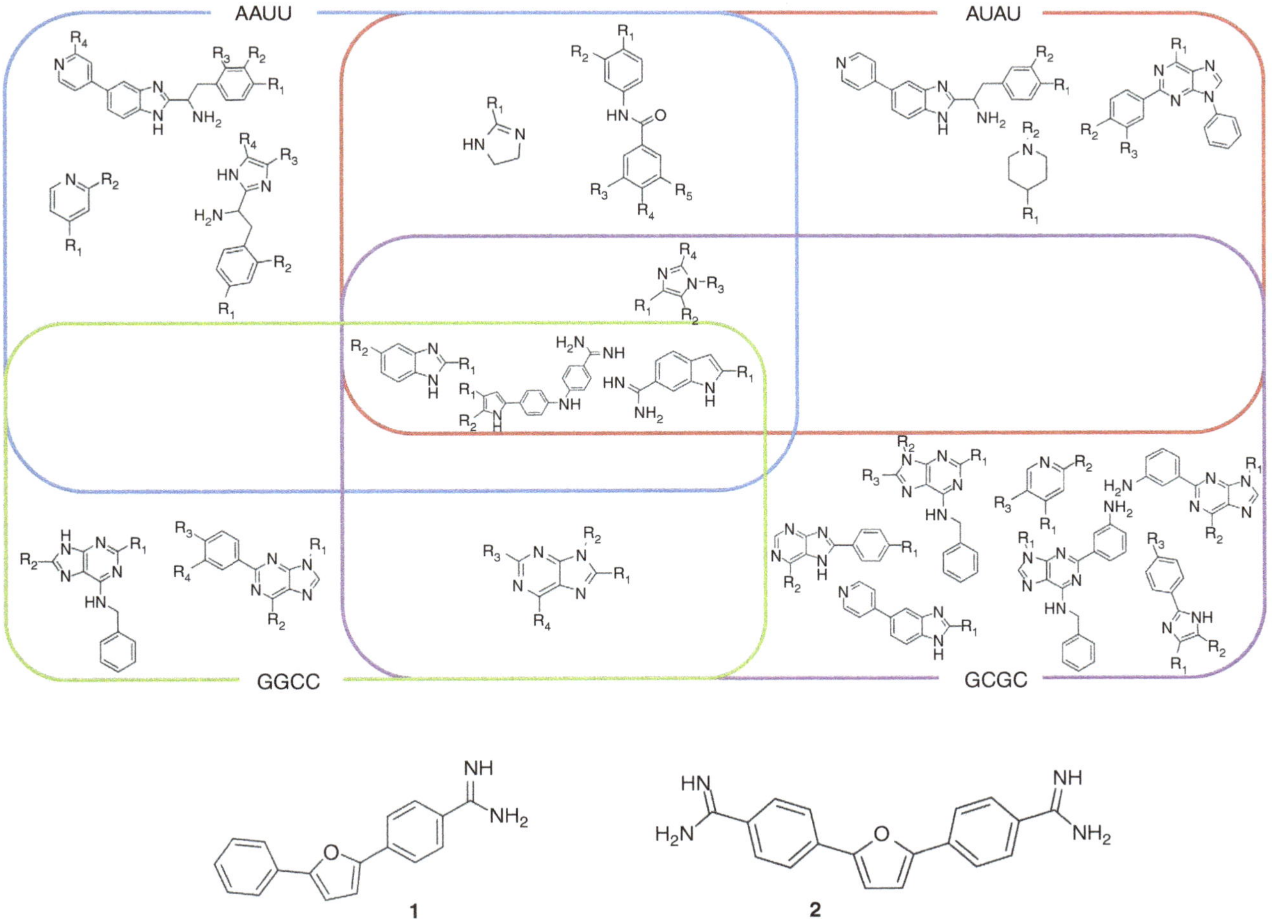

Figure 2 | Analysis of compounds identified to bind RNA base pairs. Top, Venn diagram of substructures in compounds that were found to bind to RNA from the fluorescence screening assay showed in Fig. 1c. Data were compiled by using compounds that had a *P* value of <0.001 for binding to the RNA hairpins. Bottom, structures of compounds **1** and **2** that were the most avid for binding to AUAU and AAUU RNA hairpins.

Table 1 | EC_{50}s (nM) and Hill coefficients (shown in parentheses) of compounds binding to the base paired RNAs shown in Fig. 1.

Compound	AAUU	AUAU	GGCC	GCGC
1*	170 ± 10 (3.1 ± 0.79)	45 ± 1 (1.5 ± 0.32)	390 ± 20 (1.4 ± 0.34)	240 ± 10 (0.92 ± 0.34)
2†	170 ± 40 (1.5 ± 0.24)	190 ± 20 (1.6 ± 0.28)	8,550 ± 250 (0.85 ± 0.08)	6,950 ± 250 (0.77 ± 0.16)
AU-azide†	45 ± 6 (1.0 ± 0.17)	31 ± 4 (1.0 ± 0.13)	>6,000	>2,000

*[Compound] = 3 μM.
†[Compound] = 1 μM.

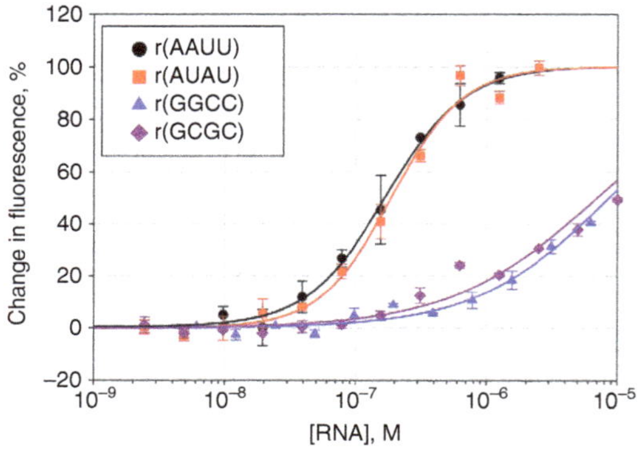

Figure 3 | Binding of compound 2 to four different RNAs Fluorescence binding assays of compound 2 to RNAs with different base pairs show that 2 binds AU base pairs selectively over GC base pairs by >40-fold.

Compounds 1 and 2 bind r(AUUCU) repeats that cause SCA10. The ultimate goal of identifying small molecules that bind RNA motifs *in vitro* is to apply these identified interactions to target an RNA that causes disease. Fortuitously, the expanded repeating r(AUUCU) RNA ($r(AUUCU)^{exp}$) that causes spinocerebellar ataxia type 10 (SCA10) contains stretches of AU base pairs[10], in particular repeating 5′AU/3′UA base pair steps (Fig. 4b)[31]. SCA10 is an incurable neuromuscular disorder that is mainly found in Latin America[32]. It is a slowly progressive disease that results in poor balance followed by loss of control over upper limbs. Previous experiments have shown that the disease is due to an RNA gain-of-function in which $r(AUUCU)^{exp}$, located within spliced intron 9 of the ataxin 10 (*ATX10*) mRNA, binds to and sequesters proteins involved in RNA biogenesis such as heterogeneous nuclear ribonucleoprotein K (hnRNP K; Fig. 4a)[33]. Sequestration of hnRNP K causes a host of cellular defects that include the formation of RNA nuclear foci, translocation of protein kinase C-δ (PKCδ) in mitochondria resulting in mitochondrial dysfunction, and activation of caspase 3 and subsequent apoptosis[33]. The binding of the repeats to RNA-binding proteins causes the transcript to be retained in nuclear foci in patient-derived cells and model cellular systems[33].

We assessed the selectivities of compounds **1** and **2** for binding r(AUUCU) repeats over other disease-associated RNA repeats including $r(CUG)_{12}$ (DM1)[9], $r(CGG)_{12}$ (FXTAS and FXS)[8,34], and $r(CCUG)_{12}$ (DM2)[11]. Compound **1** has a similar EC_{50} for all RNA repeats (36–87 nM), indicating that **1** binds to RNA internal loops as well as to AU base pairs with similar binding affinity (Supplementary Fig. 5). Compound **2** selectively recognizes $r(AUUCU)_{11}$ with 5–15-fold selectivity over the other repeats (Table 2 and Supplementary Fig. 6). Compound **2** bound $r(AUUCU)_{11}$ with a K_d of 300 nM and a stoichiometry of ca. 11:1 (**2**:$r(AUUCU)_{11}$). Because $r(AUUCU)_{11}$ contains 10 AU base pairs, it indicates that **2** is binding to each AU base pair in the target. Indeed, a nuclease protection assay revealed that **2** protects each AU base pair in $r(AUUCU)_{11}$ from cleavage (Fig. 5). Interestingly, calculated Hill coefficients indicate that **2** binds to $r(AUUCU)_{11}$ with positive cooperativity ($n = 1.7$; Table 2), suggesting that **2** could be an ideal module to design a polyvalent compound to target multiple adjacent sites in $r(AUUCU)^{exp}$ simultaneously.

An AU base pair-binding module to target $r(AUUCU)^{exp}$. Previously, our group has developed modularly assembled small molecules that target various repeating RNAs[18,19,35–38]. In this approach, an RNA-binding module or modules that recognize different motifs in an RNA target are displayed on a single molecule. These polyvalent compounds allow for simultaneous recognition of multiple motifs in an RNA target, thereby increasing affinity and selectivity relative to monomeric binders (Fig. 6).

To enable this approach for **2** and $r(AUUCU)^{exp}$, a derivative of **2**, **AU-azide** (Fig. 6), was synthesized to install an orthogonally reactive group. The azide is used for conjugation onto peptoid polyvalent scaffolds that display alkynes via a Cu-catalysed Huisgen cycloaddition reaction. Dibenzimidate (**3**) was synthesized from the furan via two reaction steps as reported previously[39,40], followed by two amidation reactions to obtain **AU-azide** (Supplementary Fig. 19; see Supplementary Information for chemical synthesis details and compound characterization). After obtaining the desired compound, it was tested for selective recognition of AU over GC base pairs (Table 1 and Supplementary Fig. 7). Interestingly, **AU-azide** has enhanced selectivity of AU base pair than **2**, >45-fold selective for AU over GC base pairs (Table 1). The selectivity of **AU-azide** for $r(AUUCU)_{11}$ over other RNA repeats compared with **2** was also improved (Table 2 and Supplementary Fig. 8).

Development of dimeric compounds to target $r(AUUCU)^{exp}$. We next synthesized a small library of **AU** dimers (Fig. 6) by using a previously published approach[19,35–37]. A peptoid backbone was used as a polyvalent scaffold that contains two propargylamine submonomers separated by different distances afforded by varying the number of propylamine spacers inserted into the backbone. The **AU-azides** (RNA-binding modules) were then conjugated by using a Cu-catalysed click reaction (Supplementary Fig. 21). The nomenclature used for these compounds is **2AU-n** where **AU** indicates the RNA-binding module; the number before **AU** indicates valency; and the number after the dash indicates the number of propylamine spacing modules between **AU** RNA-binding modules.

The library of dimeric compounds was then tested for binding to $r(AUUCU)_{11}$ by using a filtre-binding assay (Supplementary Fig. 10). After incubation of radioactively labelled $r(AUUCU)_{11}$ with dimeric compound, the compound-bound RNA was separated from free RNA by using a Dot-Blot apparatus. These studies showed that **2AU-2** bound to the RNA to the greatest extent, 2–20-fold greater than the other dimers. Additional filtre-binding assays were completed with 35-fold excess transfer RNA (tRNA) to gain insight into selectivity. Only a modest

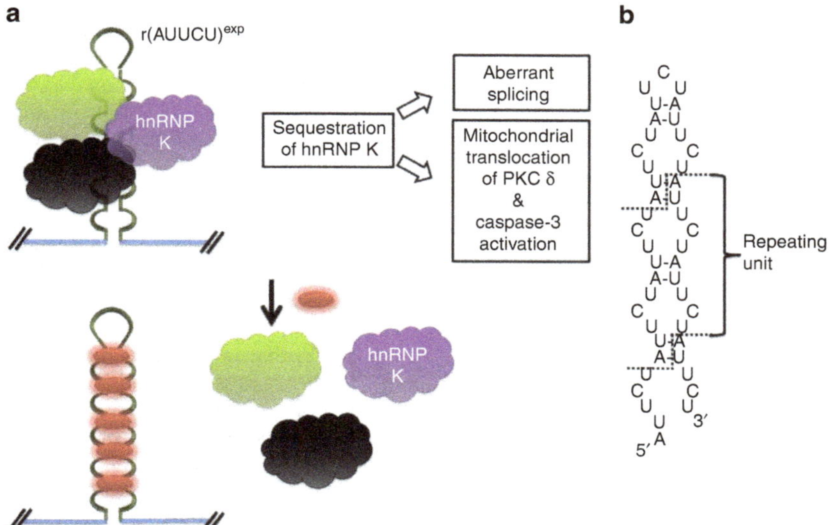

Figure 4 | Schematic of the pathogenic mechanism of SCA10 and a therapeutic approach by targeting the secondary structure of r(AUUCU) repeats. (**a**) r(AUUCU)^{exp}, located within intron 9 of ataxin 10 (*ATX10*) mRNA, sequesters proteins including hnRNP K. Sequestration of hnRNP K results in aberrant splicing of transcripts, mitochondrial translocation of PKCδ and caspase-3 activation, leading to apoptosis (top). A possible therapeutic approach is using small molecules that bind r(AUUCU) repeats and displace sequestered proteins (bottom). (**b**) secondary structure of r(AUUCU) repeats with periodically repeating 5′AU/3′UA base pair steps.

Table 2 | K_ds, Hill coefficients (shown in parentheses) and stoichiometries of 2, AU-azide and 2AU-2 binding to RNA repeats.

RNA repeats	$r(AUUCU)_{11}$		$r(CUG)_{12}$*		$r(CGG)_{12}$*		$r(CCUG)_{12}$*	
Compound	K_d, nM	Stoichiometry	K_d, nM	Stoichiometry	K_d, nM	Stoichiometry	K_d, nM	Stoichiometry
2	300 ± 47 (1.7 ± 0.2)	11 ± 0.5	~4,000	~7	~2,000	~6	~4,000	~11
AU-azide	375 ± 34 (1.3 ± 0.1)	13 ± 0.9	~5,000	~11	~3,000	~9	~5,000	~16
2AU-2	185 ± 1.0 (1.4 ± 0.4)	7 ± 0.1	~4,000	~9	~4,000	~6	~4,000	~6

*The stoichiometry from unsaturated binding curves was estimated from data fit by equation (1). The K_d was calculated by using the estimated stoichiometry.

decrease (~20%) of **2AU-2** binding was observed, suggesting the compound is selective.

To further confirm the results of the filtre binding assays, we developed an assay that evaluates the potency of small molecules for inhibiting protein loading onto $r(AUUCU)_{11}$. It is known that DiGeorge syndrome critical region 8 (DGCR8), a protein that is involved in microRNA biogenesis, binds a wide variety of RNAs[41] and thus could be of potential use as the protein component in this assay. To establish that DGCR8Δ binds $r(AUUCU)_{11}$, a gel mobility shift assay was completed, affording a dissociation constant of 1.6 μM for the RNA–protein interaction (Supplementary Fig. 11). Such affinity is similar to those found between other RNA repeats and proteins, including r(CUG)^{exp}-MBNL1 (muscleblind-like 1), r(CAG)^{exp}-MBNL1, and r(CGG)^{exp}-DGCR8 (refs 20–22).

Time-resolved fluorescence resonance energy transfer (TR-FRET) assays have been developed to screen for inhibitors of each RNA–protein complexes mentioned above[20–22]. Thus, we developed a TR-FRET assay for $r(AUUCU)_{11}$ and DGCR8Δ analogously. Screening results showed that dimers are better inhibitors than the monomer and that **2AU-2** is the most potent inhibitor amongst them (Fig. 7a). At 1.5 μM concentration, **AU-azide** only inhibits ~25% of $r(AUUCU)_{11}$-DGCR8Δ complex formation while **2AU-2** inhibits ~70%. Further, the IC_{50} of **2AU-2** was 2.7-fold less than that of **AU-azide** (Supplementary Fig. 12). Thus, both the TR-FRET and filtre-binding assays establish that **2AU-2** is the most potent binder of $r(AUUCU)_{11}$ and that there is considerable enhancement for the dimer relative to the monomer.

Consistent with results from filtre binding and TR-FRET assays, selective binding of **2AU-2** to $r(AUUCU)_{11}$ over other RNA repeats was observed (Table 2 and Supplementary Fig. 9). The stoichiometry and the K_d of dimer **2AU-2** to $r(AUUCU)_{11}$ was measured. The number of **2AU-2** per $r(AUUCU)_{11}$ was approximately half that of **AU-azide** ($n = 7$ and $n = 13$, respectively), suggesting that each RNA-binding module interacts with each AU pair. The affinity of **2AU-2** for $r(AUUCU)_{11}$ is twofold greater than the monomer and **AU-azide** and **2AU-2** maintained positively cooperative binding to $r(AUUCU)_{11}$. Similar increases in affinity when increasing valency from $n = 1$ to $n = 2$ have been observed with other repeats[19,35]. Furthermore, we studied the binding of **2AU-2** and $r(AUUCU)_{11}$ under molecular crowding conditions that mimic a cellular environment by adding 20% (w/v) PEG 8000. A ninefold enhancement in binding was observed (EC_{50} of 16 ± 4 nM) relative to non-molecular crowding conditions (EC_{50} of 146 ± 8 nM; Supplementary Fig. 13).

The binding of **2AU-2** to a DNA hairpin that contains a stretch of four consecutive AT pairs was studied. Saturable binding was not observed (K_d > 10 μM; Supplementary Fig. 14). Interestingly, **AU-azide** binds to the DNA hairpin (EC_{50} = 116 ± 15 nM) with similar affinity as the AU-rich RNAs (EC_{50} = 111 ± 3 and 113 ± 8 nM for AAUU and AUAU, respectively; Supplementary Figs 14 and 15). Thus, a monomeric binding module with modest selectivity can be reprogrammed to afford highly selective compounds for repetitive sequences by linking the binding modules together.

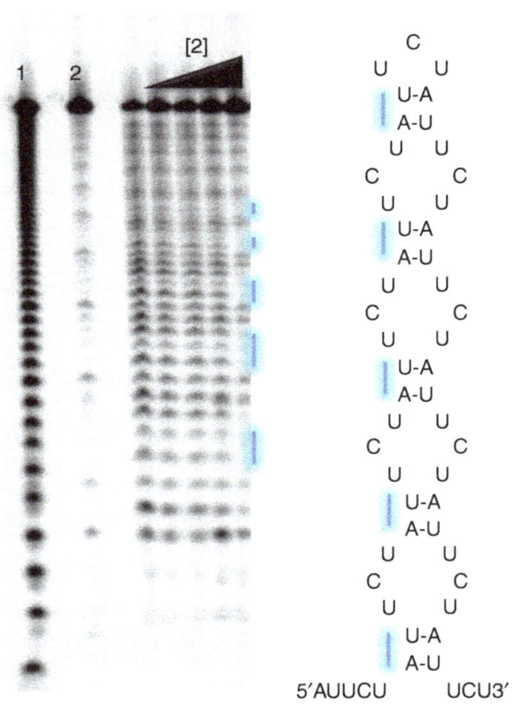

Figure 5 | Compound 2 protects r(AUUCU)$_{11}$ from cleavage by RNase V1. Left, representative gel image of the RNase protection assay. Lane 1, alkaline hydrolysis of r(AUUCU)$_{11}$; lane 2, r(AUUCU)$_{11}$ + No RNase V1; lanes 3-7, r(AUUCU)$_{11}$ + RNase V1 + **2** (0, 0.02, 0.2, 2 and 20 μM). Lines indicate sites of protection. Right, secondary structure of r(AUUCU)$_{11}$. Protected nucleotides are indicated with blue lines.

Recognition of r(AUUCU)$_{500}$ by 2AU-2 in cellular lysates. To investigate whether the designer dimer binds to r(AUUCU)$_{500}$, we developed a method named Chem-Quant-Seq. To enable Chem-Quant-Seq a biotinylated derivative, **2AU-2-Biotin**, was synthesized (Fig. 7b and Supplementary Fig. 23). After incubation of 250 nM of **2AU-2-Biotin** with total RNA isolated from cells that express r(AUUCU)$_{500}$ (ref. 33), bound RNAs were isolated with streptavidin resin. After extensive washing and elution of bound RNAs, the amount of r(AUUCU)$_{500}$ bound to **2AU-2-Biotin** was quantified by using quantitative PCR with reverse transcription (qRT–PCR). Results show that there is a significant enrichment of the r(AUUCU)$_{500}$ in the pulled-down material, as compared to 18S rRNA, showing that the compound indeed recognizes that target in the presence of cellular RNAs (Fig. 7c). To further assess the ability of the compound to recognize r(AUUCU)$_{500}$ over shorter repeats of non-pathogenic length, various concentrations of r(AUUCU)$_{11}$ in excess of r(AUUCU)$_{500}$ were added to the lysate and enrichment of r(AUUCU)$_{500}$ in the pulled-down fraction was quantified. Results from this competition experiment showed that 100-fold excess of r(AUUCU)$_{11}$ was required to decrease enrichment of r(AUUCU)$_{500}$ in the pulled-down fraction (Fig. 7d). Thus, **2AU-2-Biotin** recognizes long repeats over shorter ones. Furthermore, these data also point to cooperative binding of **2AU-2** to r(AUUCU) repeats as being a manner in which longer repeats are preferred over shorter ones. Positive cooperativity for binding to **2AU-2** was also observed *in vitro* (Hill coefficients; Table 2).

We further profiled target selectivity amongst 93 highly abundant transcripts in the pulled-down fraction via qRT–PCR. The RNAs span the diverse biology in the transcriptome, including rRNAs, mRNAs, small RNAs (sRNAs) and tRNAs. The rRNAs included all four rRNA subunits (18S, 28S 5S and 5.8S) and 45S rRNA. The 50 mRNAs were chosen from the most abundant mRNAs in HeLa cells for which there are established qRT–PCR primers[42]. The 17 sRNAs were selected from different structural and functional classes[43]: small nucleolar RNAs (HBII-85, HBII-420, U105 C/D Box snoRNAs, and ACA-16, ACA-44,

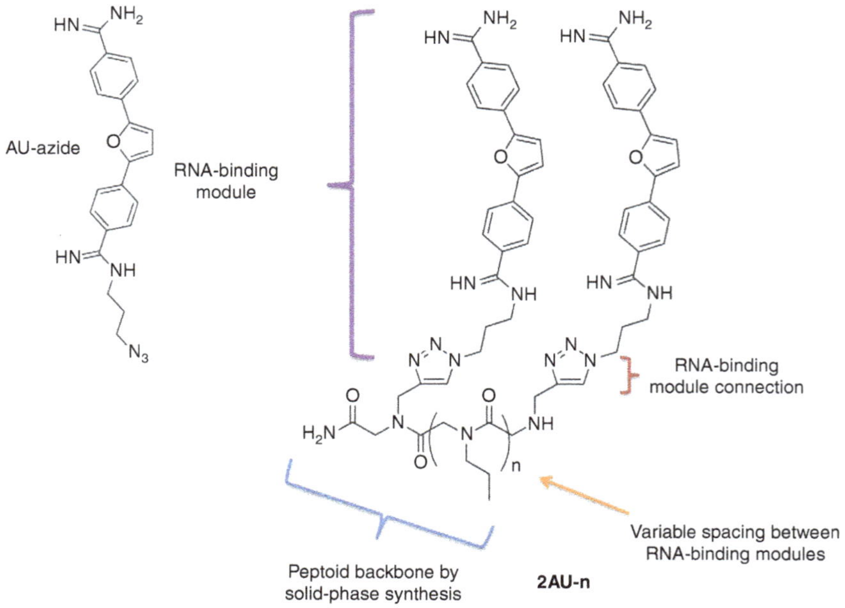

AU-azide
RNA-binding module
RNA-binding module connection
Variable spacing between RNA-binding modules
Peptoid backbone by solid-phase synthesis
2AU-n

Figure 6 | Design of dimeric compounds to target r(AUUCU)^{exp}. The RNA-binding module, **AU-Azide** (left) was assembled onto various peptoid backbones to afford dimeric compounds (right). The **AU-azides** were separated by different distances by varying the number of spacing modules (n) to generate a series of compounds named **2AU-n**, where **2AU** denotes two RNA-binding modules and n denotes the number of spacing modules.

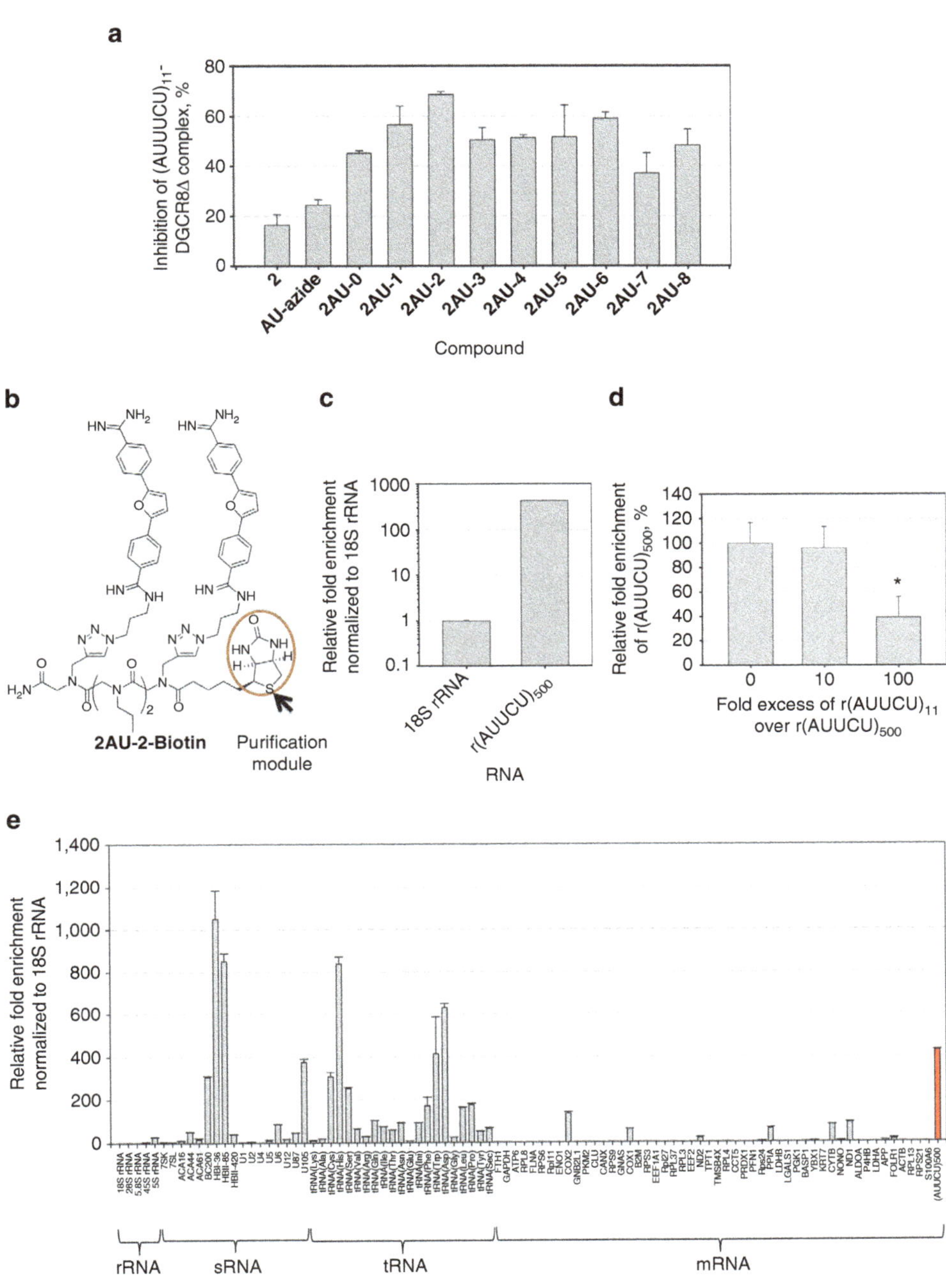

Figure 7 | 2AU-2 binds r(AUUCU) repeats *in vitro* and *in vivo* and inhibits protein binding. (**a**) quantification of inhibition of the r(AUUCU)$_{11}$-DGCR8Δ complex by monomeric and dimeric compounds (1.5 μM). (**b**) structure of **2AU-2-Biotin**. (**c**) relative fold enrichment of r(AUUCU)$_{500}$ pulled down by **2AU-2-Biotin** from total cellular RNAs. (**d**) **2AU-2-Biotin** selectively binds r(AUUCU)$_{500}$ over r(AUUCU)$_{11}$ as determined by a competition experiment. r(AUUCU)$_{500}$ levels were normalized to 18S rRNA. (**e**) Profiling of 93 highly abundant RNAs to determine whether they bind **2AU-2-Biotin** in the context of total cellular RNA.

ACA-61, HBI-36 H/ACA box snoRNAs), small cajal body-specific RNA (U87 scaRNA), small nuclear RNAs (U1, U2, U4, U5, U6 and U12 snRNAs), BC200 RNA, 7SK RNA and 7SL RNA. The 21 tRNAs profiled were randomly selected.

Only a fraction of these RNAs were enriched comparably to r(AUUCU)$_{500}$, showing **2AU-2** it possesses reasonable selectivity for the desired target (Fig. 7e). Of the nine RNAs that show significant enrichment, most are tRNAs. Since **2AU-2** was shown to pull down tRNAs, we studied its effect on translation in two different ways in HeLa cells: (i) by transfecting a plasmid that encodes green fluorescent protein (GFP); and (ii) co-transfecting plasmids that encode GFP and r(AUUCU)$_{500}$. GFP is a commonly used gene reporter in translational studies because of its visually identifiable characteristics[44]. After 24 h incubation, the fluorescence intensity of GFP was measured (Supplementary Fig. 16). Importantly, no change in the expression of GFP was observed in either system after treatment with **2AU-2**, as compared with an untreated control (Supplementary Fig. 16). Thus, **2AU-2** does not affect translation at its active concentrations where it improves SCA10-associated defects, 50 and 100 nM, *vide infra*. Interestingly, 40% of the amino acids in GFP are encoded by seven of the tRNAs pulled down by **2AU-2**. Taken together with the lack of toxicity in healthy and SCA10 patient-derived cells (*vide infra*), these data suggest that binding to tRNAs in a pull-down is not sufficient to elicit a biological effect.

Bioactivity of 2AU-2 in SCA10 patient-derived fibroblasts. Encouraged by these results, the bioactivity of **2AU-2** was assessed by measuring the ability of the compound to improve three downstream disease-associated defects in SCA10 patient-derived fibroblasts[33]. As mentioned above, caspase 3 is abnormally activated in SCA10 fibroblasts by greater than twofold[33]. Thus, the effect of **2AU-2** on the caspase-3 activity in control and SCA10 fibroblasts was measured. When SCA10-affected cells were treated with 50 and 100 nM of **2AU-2** for 48 h, caspase-3 activity was reduced to levels observed in healthy cells (Fig. 8a). For comparison, we also tested the monomer **AU-azide** and two dimers with reduced *in vitro* potencies, **2AU-3 and 2AU-4**. In contrast to **2AU-2**, treatment with 100 nM **AU-azide** reduced levels of over-activated caspase-3 activity by only ~30% while **2AU-3 and 2AU-4** were inactive up to 100 nM dosage despite showing activity *in vitro* (Supplementary Fig. 17). These results suggest that **2AU-3** and **2AU-4**, which have suboptimal distances between binding modules, may bind off-targets in cells. Thus, optimal bioactivity of **2AU-2** is a function of valency and the spacing between RNA-binding modules, which affords affinity and selectivity.

In agreement with the downregulated caspase-3 activity, **2AU-2** also reduced the mitochondrial abundance of PKCδ in SCA10 fibroblasts (Fig. 8c). PKCδ translocated to 70–80% of mitochondria in SCA10 cells, whereas only 10–15% mitochondria included PKCδ after treatment with 50 nM **2AU-2**, similar to levels observed in healthy fibroblasts. Next, the ability of **2AU-2** to disrupt formation of nuclear foci was measured. After 48 h incubation, **2AU-2** (50 nM) diminished ca. 70% of nuclear foci in SCA10 cells (Fig. 8b).

To confirm that improvement of SCA10-associated defects was due to binding of the compound to r(AAUCU)^{exp} and not toxicity, we studied the cytotoxicity of **2AU-2** in healthy and SCA10 fibroblasts by measuring released lactate dehydrogenase (LDH)[45]. No significant toxicity of the compound was observed at its active concentration, 50 nM, in either healthy or SCA10 fibroblasts (Supplementary Fig. 18). Thus, the observed downregulation of caspase-3 activity and reduction of the mitochondrial abundance of PKCδ in SCA10 fibroblasts does not result from compound toxicity. Likewise, these results are consistent with our observation that caspase-3 activity is unchanged in healthy fibroblasts upon **2AU-2** treatment.

Further, the observed bioactivity of **2AU-2** is not due to reduced abundance of the mutant *ATXN10* transcript carrying expanded AUUCU repeats as determined by qRT–PCR analysis (Fig. 8d). That is, the compound works at the RNA level, not at the transcriptional level. Interestingly, previous studies have shown that silencing of the *ATXN10* transcript improves

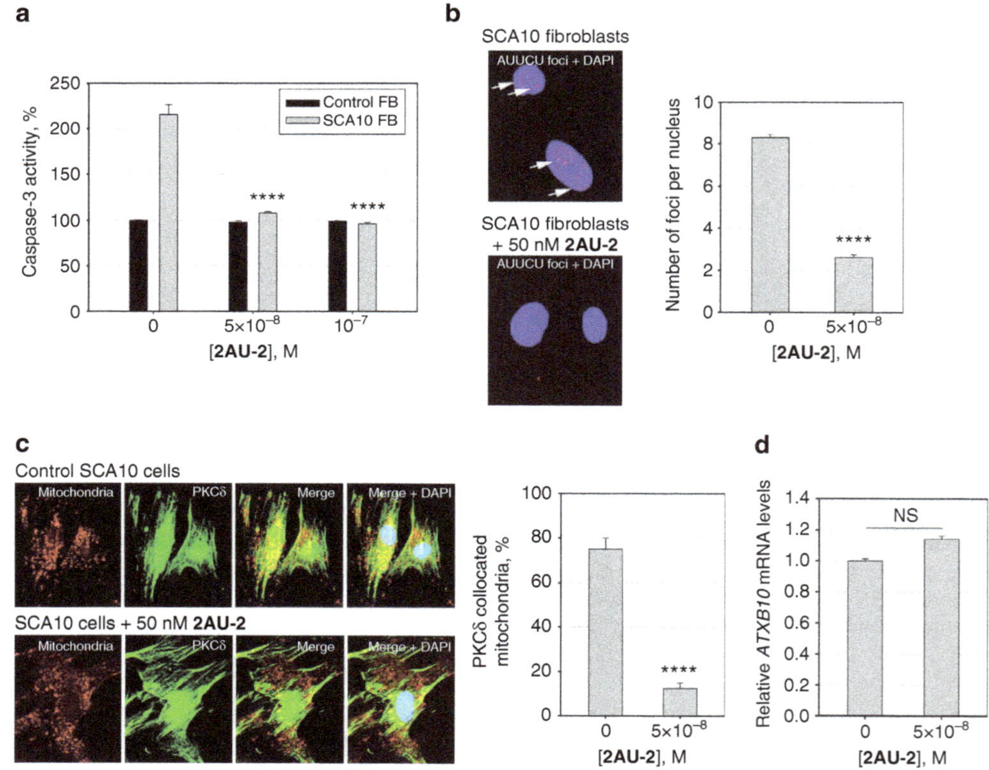

Figure 8 | Studying the bioactivity of 2AU-2 in SCA10 patient-derived fibroblasts. (**a**) Relative caspase-3 activities in normal and SCA10 fibroblasts before and after treatment with compound **2AU-2**. Caspase-3 in SCA10 was reduced to normal levels when cells were treated with 50 nM compound. (**b**) Confocal images showing r(AUUCU)^{exp}-containing nuclear foci in SCA10 cells without treatment (left, top) and after treatment with 50 nM **2AU-2** (left, bottom). Quantification of the number of r(AUUCU)^{exp}-containing nuclear foci (right) in treated and untreated cells. (**c**) confocal images showing mitochondrial translocation of PKCδ after treatment with 50 nM **2AU-2** (left, bottom) compared with control, untreated SCA10 cells (left, top). Quantification of PKCδ collocated to mitochondria in treated and untreated cells (right). (**d**) Real-time RT-PCR analysis of *ATXN10* mRNA expression levels after treatment with **2AU-2**. The amount of mRNA was normalized relative to *GAPDH* mRNA. Values are reported as the mean ± s.e. ($n = 6$). ****$P < 0.0001$ and 'ns' denotes $P > 0.05$, as compared with the untreated sample with a two-tailed Student *t*-test.

SCA10-associated defects[33] and some small molecules that improve microsatellite disease-associated defects work at the transcriptional level[46].

Taken together, **2AU-2** markedly improves defects from hnRNP K sequestration by $r(AUUCU)^{exp}$ in SCA10 patient-derived cells, suggesting that the compound binds to the cellular target, $r(AUUCU)^{exp}$, and frees sequestered proteins. **2AU-2** is the most potent inhibitor known for a traditional non-covalent binder to repeat expansions.

Conclusion

To identify selective RNA base pair binders, we screened small molecules that have RNA-binding scaffolds. The *bis*-benzamidine compound **2** is a selective AU base pair binder, as it binds AU base pairs 40-fold more strongly than GC base pairs. This compound was applied to target the pentanucleotide r(AUUCU) expansion that causes SCA10. The repeat periodically displays 5′AU/UA3′ base pair steps in its secondary structure. To improve affinity and selectivity, we modularly assembled **2** and determined that the optimal distance between RNA-binding modules was afforded by two propylamine spacing modules, or **2AU-2**. **2AU-2** significantly improves SCA10-associated defects to wild-type levels when patient-derived fibroblasts are treated with 50 nM compound. It is the first bioactive small molecule targeting $r(AUUCU)^{exp}$. The potent bioactivity of **2AU-2** suggests that base pair-targeting RNA modules could have broad utility to provide bioactive compounds targeting other RNAs in the transcriptome.

Methods

Instrumentation. All pH measurements were performed at room temperature using a Mettler Toledo SG2 pH metre that was standardized at pH 4.0, 7.0, and 10.0. Absorption and emission spectra were measured using SpectraMax M5 plate reader (Molecular Devices, Inc.). Sigma Plot (version 11.0) was used for all curve fitting.

Small molecules. All small modules were procured from the National Cancer Institute (NCI) or The Scripps Research Institute. Emission spectra (excitation: 300 nm, cutoff: 325 nm, emission: 330–600 nm) of all compounds were measured in a 384-well plate (Greiner Low-Volume 784076) to select fluorescent compounds for screening (50 µM compound in 1 × Screening Buffer (8 mM Na_2HPO_4, pH 7.0, 185 mM NaCl, 0.1 mM EDTA)).

Compound purification and analysis. Preparative HPLC was performed using a Waters 1525 Binary HPLC pump equipped with a Waters 2487 dual-absorbance detector system and a Waters Sunfire C18 OBD 5-µm 19 × 150 mm column. Absorbance was monitored at 220 and 345 nm. A gradient of 20–100% methanol in H_2O with 0.1% trifluoroacetic acid (TFA) over 60 min was used for compound purification. Analytical HPLC was performed using a Waters Symmetry C18 5 µm 4.6 × 150 mm column. Compounds were analysed using a gradient of 20–60% MeOH in H_2O with 0.1% TFA over 30 min. All compounds evaluated had ≥95% purity as determined by analytical HPLC. Mass spectrometry was performed with an Applied Biosystems MALDI ToF/ToF Analyzer 4800 Plus and Microflex (Bruker) using an α-hydroxycinnamic acid matrix. See the Supplementary Information for details of compound synthesis and compound characterization.

Oligonucleotide preparation and purification. The RNAs used in fluorescence binding assays, nuclease mapping, and filtre-binding assays were purchased from Dharmacon. The ACE protecting groups were cleaved by using Dharmacon's deprotection buffer by incubating at 60 °C for 30 min. The samples were lyophilized, resuspended in water and gel purified. Concentrations were determined by absorbance using a Beckman Coulter DU800 ultraviolet–visible spectrophotometer at 85 °C. Extinction coefficients (at 260 nm) were calculated using the HyTher server, which uses nearest-neighbour parameters[47–49].

Initial screen for small molecules that bind RNA base pairs. RNAs were folded in 1 × Screening Buffer at 95 °C for 2 min followed by slowly cooling to room temperature on the bench top. A 10-µl aliquot of a 1 µM RNA solution was dispensed into each well of a black 384-well plate (Greiner Low-Volume 784076) using an Aurora Discovery FRD-1B liquid dispenser. A 10-nl aliquot of a 2.5 mM stock of small molecule was pinned into each well using Biomek NXP Laboratory Automation Workstation that was equipped with a 384-pin head. The solution was incubated at room temperature for 30 min. Fluorescence intensity was measured using the maximum excitation/emission wavelength for each compound and the change in fluorescence was calculated by the ratio of F/F_0 where F is the fluorescence intensity in the presence of RNA and F_0 is the fluorescence intensity in the absence of RNA.

Compounds were scored as hits if a >20% change in emission (either enhancement or quenching) was observed upon incubation with RNA. The selectivity of a small molecule was computed by comparing the relative change in emission when incubated different RNAs. Statistically significant differences were calculated by using one-way analysis of variance function in Sigma Plot (version 11.0); compounds that had a P value of <0.05 (95% confidence) were chosen as selective binders.

Chemoinformatic analysis. To identify the chemical substructures that facilitate binding, hit compounds were tested by an automated R-group analysis (Tripod Development; Division of preclinical Innovation, National Center for Advancing Translational Sciences: http://tripod.nih.gov/?p=46). The functional groups that provided recognition for each type of RNA were then compared.

Fluorescence binding assays. Direct binding assays for all selective binders were performed. RNAs were folded as described above. Binding assays were performed with a constant compound concentration (1 or 3 µM) and serial dilutions of RNA or DNA in 1 × Screening Buffer. For molecular crowding experiments, PEG 8000 was added to a final concentration of 20% (w/v) to the folded RNA and to the solution used for serial dilutions. After a 20 min incubation, fluorescence intensity was measured. The resulting curves were fit to the following equation to determine EC_{50} values:

$$y = B + \frac{A - B}{1 + \left(\frac{EC50}{x}\right)^{\text{hillslope}}} \tag{1}$$

where y is fluorescence intensity, x is the concentration of RNA, B is the minimum fluorescence; A is the maximum fluorescence; and the EC_{50} is the concentration of RNA where half of the compound is bound.

Two types of plots were constructed to determine stoichiometries and K_d's: fluorescence versus [nucleic acid]/[ligand] to determine stoichiometry and fraction-bound/[nucleic acid] versus fraction bound to determine K_d's. Stoichiometries were determined from the former plots by fitting each of the two slopes (pre-saturated and saturated portions of the curves) to a line[50]. For unsaturated binding curves, the saturated portions of the curves were estimated by the fitted data from equation (1). The point at which the two equations intersect affords the stoichiometry. The K_d's were determined by fitting fraction bound/[nucleic acid] versus fraction bound to equation (2):

$$\frac{v}{[L]} = \frac{N(1 - lv/N)}{k}\left(\frac{1 - lv/N}{1 - (l - 1)v/N}\right)^{l-1} \tag{2}$$

where v is the moles of RNA lattice bound per moles of ligand, $[L]$ is the concentration of ligand, N is the number of repeating units on the RNA, l is the number of consecutive lattice units occupied by the ligand, and k is the microscopic dissociation constant.

Nuclease mapping of the small molecule-binding site. $r(AUUCU)_{11}$ was radioactively labelled at the 5′ end with [γ-^{32}P] ATP (Perkin Elmer) and T4 polynucleotide kinase (New England Biolabs) using standard methods and gel purified to homogeneity[51]. The RNA was folded by incubation at 60 °C for 5 min in 1 × RNA Structure Buffer (Ambion) followed by slow cooling to room temperature. Serially diluted concentrations of the inhibitor was added to the RNA solution and incubated at room temperature for 15 min. RNase V1 (Ambion) was added to the RNA-inhibitor complex to a final concentration of 5 µU μl^{-1} and the samples were incubated at room temperature for 60 min. RNase V1 was then inactivated by heating at 95 °C for 1 min, and cleavage products were separated on a denaturing 20% polyacrylamide gel. A hydrolysis ladder was prepared by using Alkaline Hydrolysis Buffer (Ambion) and the manufacturer's protocol.

Chemical syntheses of dimeric compounds. Details of compound syntheses and characterization are provided in Supplementary Figs 19–24 and Supplementary Table 4.

Screening of dimeric compounds for binding to $r(AUUCU)_{11}$ by filtre binding. To determine the optimal distance between RNA-binding modules, a library of dimers was synthesized and screened by using a filtre-binding assay. Radioactively labelled $r(AUUCU)_{11}$ (100 nM) was folded in 1 × PBS buffer (pH 7.4) containing 1 mM $MgCl_2$ by incubation at 60 °C for 5 min followed by slow cooling to room temperature. BSA was added to a final concentration of 50 µg ml^{-1} followed by addition of 1 µM compound. The samples were incubated at room temperature for 15 min. Nitrocellulose and nylon membranes were incubated in 1 × filtre binding assay buffer (1 × PBS buffer (pH 7.4) containing 1 mM $MgCl_2$ and 50 µg ml^{-1} BSA). Bound and unbound RNA were separated using a Dot-Blot apparatus followed by washing with 1 × filtre binding assay buffer. The membranes were exposed to a phosphorimager screen and imaged using a Molecular Dynamics Typhoon phosphorimager. The amount of $r(AUUCU)_{11}$ bound to each membrane was quantified using QuantityOne software (BioRad).

Mobility shift assay of $r(AUUCU)_{11}$ with DGCR8Δ. $r(AUUCU)_{11}$ was 5′-end labelled as described above and folded in 1 × Folding Buffer (20 mM HEPES, pH 7.5, 110 mM KCl, and 110 mM NaCl) by incubation at 60 °C for 5 min followed by slow cooling to room temperature on the bench top. The buffer was adjusted to 1 × TR-FRET Assay Buffer (20 mM HEPES pH 7.5, 110 mM KCl, 110 mM NaCl, 0.1% BSA, 2 mM $MgCl_2$, 2 mM $CaCl_2$, 0.05% Tween-20 and 5 mM DTT) and various concentrations of DGCR8Δ were added. The samples were incubated at room temperature for 15 min and loaded onto a pre-chilled native 5% polyacrylamide gel. The gel was imaged and quantified as described above.
The resulting curves were fit to equation (3):

$$y = \frac{xB_{max}}{K_d + x} \quad (3)$$

where y is percentage of bounded DGCR8Δ, x is the concentration of protein, B_{max} is maximum percentage of protein bound (restrained to equal 100%) and k_d is dissociation constant.

Determination of compound potency via a TR-FRET assay. TR-FRET assays were completed as previously described[21] with the following modifications. After folding the RNA, compound was added and incubated for 15 min at room temperature followed by addition of DGCR8Δ. The final concentrations of $r(AUUCU)_{11}$ and DGCR8Δ were 60 and 40 nM, respectively. TR-FRET was measured after an additional 30-min incubation at room temperature. IC_{50} values were calculated by curve fitting using equation (1).

Pull-down of 2AU-2's cellular targets. HeLa cells were maintained as monolayers in growth medium (1 × DMEM, 10% fetal bovine serum and 1 × GlutaMax (Invitrogen)). Cells were plated in 10-cm dishes and grown to ~90% confluency and then transfected with a plasmid encoding $(AUUCU)_{500}$ using Lipofectamine 2,000 (Invitrogen) per the manufacturer's recommended protocol. Cells were collected 18–24 h post-transfection and total RNA was extracted by using Trizol reagent (Ambion) according to the manufacturer's protocol. After RQ1 DNase (Promega) treatment, the DNase was removed by phenol:chloroform extraction and total RNA was ethanol precipitated. Next, 100 μg of total RNA was folded in 1 × Screening Buffer by heating at 75 °C for 5 min and cooling to room temperature slowly. The folded RNAs were incubated with **2AU-2-Biotin** for 30 min at room temperature. The solution was then incubated with streptavidin beads (250 μl of slurry, Sigma-Aldrich) for 30 min at room temperature with gentle shaking. The supernatant (containing unbound RNAs) was removed, and the beads were washed with 250 μl 1 × Screening Buffer after gentle shaking for 5 min at room temperature. Bound RNA was released from the beads by heating the beads in 300 μl H_2O at 80 °C for 3 min twice. The solution containing bound RNAs was concentrated to 5–50 μl by vacuum concentration. Complementary DNA (cDNA) was generated from 40 ng of RNA using a qScript cDNA Synthesis Kit (Quanta Biosciences) per the manufacturer's protocol. qPCR was performed on an ABI 7900 HT Real-Time PCR System using the following primers to detect the $r(AUUCU)_{500}$-containing RNA: 5′-AGTCTCTCT ATGTTGCCCAGG-3′ and 5′-ACTTCCCGAAACACCGTCTC-3′. The relative fold enrichment of the RNA pulled by the compound was calculated by normalization to 18S rRNA.

Profiling of cellular RNAs pulled down by 2AU-2-Biotin. Profiling was completed by qRT-PCR as described above. The 93 highly abundant RNAs, including rRNAs, sRNA, tRNAs and mRNAs, were selected based on a previous report[42]. Primer sets for mRNAs were obtained from RTPrimerDB[52] (www.rtprimerdb.org) and qPrimerDepot (http://primerdepot.nci.nih.gov). The DNA sequences of tRNAs were obtained from tRNAdb[53] (http://trna.bioinf.uni-leipzig.de/) and primer sets were designed by using Primer 3 software (http://frodo.wi.mit.edu/primer3/). All sequences of primers are listed in Supplementary Table 3.

Cell culture of SCA10 fibroblasts. SCA10 fibroblasts[33] were cultured in MEM with Eagle–Earle salt and 2 mM L-glutamine containing 15% fetal bovine serum and antibiotic in 5% CO_2 at 37 °C in 75-cm^2 flasks. Compounds were dissolved in 50% DMSO and added to the SCA10 cells at the indicated concentrations. Fresh medium with drug was added to the cells after every 12 h and cells were collected after 48 h for the caspase-3 assay, detection of AUUCU RNA foci, or for analysing the subcellular translocation of protein kinase C δ (PKCδ).

Translocation of PKCδ after drug treatment. SCA10 fibroblasts (2×10^4 cells) were seeded in chamber slides. When cells were 80–90% confluent, fresh cell culture medium containing compound was added to the cells and incubated for 48 h. The drug-treated and control cells were then incubated with mitotracker deep red 633 (Invitrogen, USA) at a concentration of 250 nM in cell culture medium and incubated at 37 °C for 30 min. The cells were then washed three times with ice-cold 1 × PBS, fixed with 4% paraformaldehyde for 30 min at room temperature, washed three times with 1 × PBS and stored in 70% ethanol for up to 24 h. Cells were blocked with DAKO antibody blocking solution (serum free) and later double stained with anti-PKCδ 1:500 in DAKO antibody diluent. Goat anti-mouse 488 was used to identify PKCδ. Fluorescent photomicrographs were taken using an Hamamatsu Camera Controller using DP controller software.

Fluorescent *in situ* hybridization to detect AUUCU RNA foci. SCA10 and control fibroblasts (2×10^4 cells) were seeded in chamber slides. When the cells were 60–70% confluent, cell culture medium containing compound was added to the cells and incubated for 48 h. After incubating with compound, the cells were fixed with 4% paraformaldehyde for 30 min at room temperature, and washed three to four times with ice-cold 1 × PBS. The AUUCU RNA foci were detected using a Cy3-labelled $(AGAAU)_{10}$ RNA oligonucleotide probe as described previously[33]. In brief, the control and SCA10 cells were pre-hybridized at 65 °C in RNA Hybridization Buffer for 1.5 h, and hybridized overnight in hybridization buffer containing 250 ng of $(AGAAU)_{10}$ Cy3-labelled RNA oligo at 45 °C. Slides were rinsed with 1 × PBS three times and extensively washed 4 × 5 min to remove all non-specific binding of Cy3-labelled RNA probes. Slides were then mounted with DAPI mounting medium and fluorescent images were taken using a confocal microscope.

Cytotoxicity of 2AU-2. SCA10 and healthy fibroblasts were treated either with **2AU-2** (50, 100 and 500 nM) or vehicle for 24 h. Later, the culture medium containing LDH was collected and the amount of LDH in the medium was quantified using TOX7 cell toxicity assay kit (Sigma-Aldrich).

References

1. Bartel, D. P. MicroRNAs: genomics, biogenesis, mechanism, and function. *Cell* **116,** 281–297 (2004).
2. Tenson, T. & Mankin, A. Antibiotics and the ribosome. *Mol. Microbiol.* **59,** 1664–1677 (2006).
3. Winkler, W., Nahvi, A. & Breaker, R. R. Thiamine derivatives bind messenger RNAs directly to regulate bacterial gene expression. *Nature* **419,** 952–956 (2002).
4. Winkler, W. C., Cohen-Chalamish, S. & Breaker, R. R. An mRNA structure that controls gene expression by binding FMN. *Proc. Natl Acad. Sci. USA* **99,** 15908–15913 (2002).
5. Harries, L. W. Long non-coding RNAs and human disease. *Biochem. Soc. Trans.* **40,** 902–906 (2012).
6. Shen, L. X., Basilion, J. P. & Stanton, Jr. V. P. Single nucleotide polymorphisms can cause different structural folds of mRNA. *Proc. Natl Acad. Sci. USA* **96,** 7871–7876 (1999).
7. Sierakowska, H., Agrawal, S. & Kole, R. Antisense oligonucleotides as modulators of pre-mRNA splicing. *Methods Mol. Biol.* **133,** 223–233 (2000).
8. Brunberg, J. A. *et al.* Fragile X premutation carriers: characteristic MR imaging findings of adult male patients with progressive cerebellar and cognitive dysfunction. *Am. J. Neuroradiol.* **23,** 1757–1766 (2002).
9. Brook, D. *et al.* Molecular basis of myotonic dystrophy: expansion of a trinucleotide (CTG) repeat at the 3′ end of a transcript encoding a protein kinase family member. *Cell* **68,** 799–808 (1992).
10. Matsuura, T. *et al.* Large expansion of the ATTCT pentanucleotide repeat in spinocerebellar ataxia type 10. *Nat. Genet.* **26,** 191–194 (2000).
11. Liquori, C. L. *et al.* Myotonic dystrophy type 2 caused by a CCTG expansion in intron 1 of *ZNF9*. *Science* **293,** 864–867 (2001).
12. The Huntington's Disease Collaborative Research Group. A novel gene containing a trinucleotide repeat that is expanded and unstable on Huntington's disease chromosomes. *Cell* **72,** 971–983 (1993).
13. Gallego, J. & Varani, G. Targeting RNA with small-molecule drugs: therapeutic promise and chemical challenges. *Acc. Chem. Res.* **34,** 836–843 (2001).
14. Poehlsgaard, J. & Douthwaite, S. The bacterial ribosome as a target for antibiotics. *Nat. Rev. Microbiol.* **3,** 870–881 (2005).
15. Johnson, L. F., Williams, J. G., Abelson, H. T., Green, H. & Penman, S. Changes in RNA in relation to growth of the fibroblast. III. Posttranscriptional regulation of mRNA formation in resting and growing cells. *Cell* **4,** 69–75 (1975).
16. Blount, K. F., Wang, J. X., Lim, J., Sudarsan, N. & Breaker, R. R. Antibacterial lysine analogs that target lysine riboswitches. *Nat. Chem. Biol.* **3,** 44–49 (2007).
17. Schramm, V. L. Enzymatic transition states, transition-state analogs, dynamics, thermodynamics, and lifetimes. *Annu. Rev. Biochem.* **80,** 703–732 (2011).

18. Childs-Disney, J. L., Hoskins, J., Rzuczek, S., Thornton, C. & Disney, M. D. Rationally designed small molecules targeting the RNA that causes myotonic dystrophy type 1 are potently bioactive. *ACS Chem. Biol.* **7,** 856–862 (2012).
19. Lee, M. M., Pushechnikov, A. & Disney, M. D. Rational and modular design of potent ligands targeting the RNA that causes myotonic dystrophy 2. *ACS Chem. Biol.* **4,** 345–355 (2009).
20. Parkesh, R. *et al.* Design of a bioactive small molecule that targets the myotonic dystrophy type 1 RNA via an RNA motif-ligand database & chemical similarity searching. *J. Am. Chem. Soc.* **134,** 4731–4742 (2012).
21. Disney, M. D. *et al.* A small molecule that targets r(CGG)^{exp} and improves defects in fragile X-associated tremor ataxia syndrome. *ACS Chem. Biol* **7,** 1711–1718 (2012).
22. Kumar, A. *et al.* Chemical correction of pre-mRNA splicing defects associated with sequestration of muscleblind-like 1 protein by expanded r(CAG)-containing transcripts. *ACS Chem. Biol.* **7,** 496–505 (2012).
23. Thomas, J. R. & Hergenrother, P. J. Targeting RNA with small molecules. *Chem. Rev.* **108,** 1171–1224 (2008).
24. Guan, L. & Disney, M. D. Recent advances in developing small molecules targeting RNA. *ACS Chem. Biol.* **7,** 73–86 (2012).
25. Mathews, D. H. *et al.* Incorporating chemical modification constraints into a dynamic programming algorithm for prediction of RNA secondary structure. *Proc. Natl Acad. Sci. USA* **101,** 7287–7292 (2004).
26. Carlson, C. B., Vuyisich, M., Gooch, B. D. & Beal, P. A. Preferred RNA binding sites for a threading intercalator revealed by in vitro evolution. *Chem. Biol.* **10,** 663–672 (2003).
27. Luedtke, N. W. *et al.* The DNA and RNA specificity of eilatin Ru(II) complexes as compared to eilatin and ethidium bromide. *Nucleic Acids Res.* **31,** 5732–5740 (2003).
28. Jin, E. *et al.* Aminoglycoside binding in the major groove of duplex RNA: the thermodynamic and electrostatic forces that govern recognition. *J. Mol. Biol.* **298,** 95–110 (2000).
29. Wilson, W. D., Ratmeyer, L., Zhao, M., Strekowski, L. & Boykin, D. The search for structure-specific nucleic acid-interactive drugs: effects of compound structure on RNA versus DNA interaction strength. *Biochemistry* **32,** 4098–4104 (1993).
30. Zhao, M. *et al.* Small changes in cationic substituents of diphenylfuran derivatives have major effects on the binding affinity and the binding mode with RNA helical duplexes. *Bioorg. Med. Chem.* **3,** 785–794 (1995).
31. Handa, V., Yeh, H. J. C., McPhie, P. & Usdin, K. The AUUCU repeats responsible for spinocerebellar ataxia type 10 form unusual RNA hairpins. *J. Biol. Chem.* **280,** 29340–29345 (2005).
32. Teive, H. A. G. *et al.* Spinocerebellar ataxia type 10 – A review. *Parkinsonism Relat. Disord.* **17,** 655–661 (2011).
33. White, M. C. *et al.* Inactivation of hnRNP K by expanded intronic AUUCU repeat induces apoptosis via translocation of PKCδ to mitochondria in spinocerebellar ataxia 10. *PLoS Genet.* **6,** e1000984 (2010).
34. Jin, P., Alisch, R. S. & Warren, S. T. RNA and microRNAs in fragile X mental retardation. *Nat. Cell Biol.* **6,** 1048–1053 (2004).
35. Pushechnikov, A. *et al.* Rational design of ligands targeting triplet repeating transcripts that cause RNA dominant disease: application to myotonic muscular dystrophy type 1 and spinocerebellar ataxia type 3. *J. Am. Chem. Soc.* **131,** 9767–9779 (2009).
36. Childs-Disney, J. L., Tsitovich, P. B. & Disney, M. D. Using modularly assembled ligands to bind RNA internal loops separated by different distances. *Chembiochem* **12,** 2143–2146 (2011).
37. Lee, M. M. *et al.* Controlling the specificity of modularly assembled small molecules for RNA via ligand module spacing: targeting the RNAs that cause myotonic muscular dystrophy. *J. Am. Chem. Soc.* **131,** 17464–17472 (2009).
38. Rzuczek, S. G. *et al.* Features of modularly assembled compounds that impart bioactivity against an RNA target. *ACS Chem. Biol.* **8,** 2312–2321 (2013).
39. Fu, H. Y. & Doucet, H. Methyl 2-furoate: an alternative reagent to furan for palladium-catalysed direct arylation. *Eur. J. Org. Chem.* **2011,** 7163–7173 (2011).
40. Das, B. P. & Boykin, D. W. Synthesis and antiprotozoal activity of 2,5-bis (4-guanylphenyl)furans. *J. Med. Chem.* **20,** 531–536 (1977).
41. Roth, B. M., Ishimaru, D. & Hennig, M. The core microprocessor component DiGeorge syndrome critical region 8 (DGCR8) is a nonspecific RNA-binding protein. *J. Biol. Chem.* **288,** 26785–26799 (2013).
42. Nagaraj, N. *et al.* Deep proteome and transcriptome mapping of a human cancer cell line. *Mol. Syst. Biol.* **7,** 548 (2011).
43. Galiveti, C. R., Rozhdestvensky, T. S., Brosius, J., Lehrach, H. & Konthur, Z. Application of housekeeping npcRNAs for quantitative expression analysis of human transcriptome by real-time PCR. *RNA* **16,** 450–461 (2010).
44. Chalfie, M., Tu, Y., Euskirchen, G., Ward, W. & Prasher, D. Green fluorescent protein as a marker for gene expression. *Science* **263,** 802–805 (1994).
45. Decker, T. & Lohmann-Matthes, M.-L. A quick and simple method for the quantitation of lactate dehydrogenase release in measurements of cellular cytotoxicity and tumor necrosis factor (TNF) activity. *J. Immunol. Methods* **115,** 61–69 (1988).
46. Coonrod, L. A. *et al.* Reducing levels of toxic RNA with small molecules. *ACS Chem. Biol.* **8,** 2528–2537 (2013).
47. Peyret, N., Seneviratne, P. A., Allawi, H. T. & SantaLucia, Jr. J. Nearest-neighbor thermodynamics and NMR of DNA sequences with internal A.A, C.C, G.G, and T.T mismatches. *Biochemistry* **38,** 3468–3477 (1999).
48. SantaLucia, Jr. J. A unified view of polymer, dumbbell, and oligonucleotide DNA nearest-neighbor thermodynamics. *Proc. Natl Acad. Sci. USA* **95,** 1460–1465 (1998).
49. Puglisi, J. D. & Tinoco, Jr. I. Absorbance melting curves of RNA. *Methods Enzymol.* **180,** 304–325 (1989).
50. Tse, W. C. & Boger, D. L. A fluorescent intercalator displacement assay for establishing DNA binding selectivity and affinity. *Acc. Chem. Res.* **37,** 61–69 (2004).
51. Sambrook, J., Fritsch, E. F. & Maniatis, T. *Molecular Cloning* 2nd edn. (Cold Spring Harbor Laboratory, 1989).
52. Lefever, S., Vandesompele, J., Speleman, F. & Pattyn, F. RTPrimerDB: the portal for real-time PCR primers and probes. *Nucleic Acids Res.* **37,** D942–D945 (2009).
53. Juhling, F. *et al.* tRNAdb 2009: compilation of tRNA sequences and tRNA genes. *Nucleic Acids Res.* **37,** D159–D162 (2009).

Acknowledgements

This work was funded by the National Institutes of Health (DP1 NS096898) to M.D.D., a John Sealy Grant to P.S.S., a FRAXA postdoctoral fellowship to W-Y.Y. and The Scripps Research Institute. M.D.D. is a Camille & Henry Dreyfus Teacher-Scholar.

Author contributions

M.D.D. provided conceptual framework. M.D.D., W-Y.Y., R.G. and P.S.S. designed the experiments. W-Y.Y. and R.G. performed the experiments and statistical analysis. M.S. performed chemical similarity searching. M.D.D., W-Y.Y., R.G. and P.S.S. wrote the manuscript. All authors reviewed the final version of the manuscript.

Additional information

Competing financial interests: The authors declare no competing financial interests.

19

CETSA screening identifies known and novel thymidylate synthase inhibitors and slow intracellular activation of 5-fluorouracil

Helena Almqvist[1,*], Hanna Axelsson[1,*], Rozbeh Jafari[2,†], Chen Dan[3], André Mateus[4], Martin Haraldsson[1], Andreas Larsson[5], Daniel Martinez Molina[2], Per Artursson[4,6,7], Thomas Lundbäck[1] & Pär Nordlund[2,3,8]

Target engagement is a critical factor for therapeutic efficacy. Assessment of compound binding to native target proteins in live cells is therefore highly desirable in all stages of drug discovery. We report here the first compound library screen based on biophysical measurements of intracellular target binding, exemplified by human thymidylate synthase (TS). The screen selected accurately for all the tested known drugs acting on TS. We also identified TS inhibitors with novel chemistry and marketed drugs that were not previously known to target TS, including the DNA methyltransferase inhibitor decitabine. By following the cellular uptake and enzymatic conversion of known drugs we correlated the appearance of active metabolites over time with intracellular target engagement. These data distinguished a much slower activation of 5-fluorouracil when compared with nucleoside-based drugs. The approach establishes efficient means to associate drug uptake and activation with target binding during drug discovery.

[1] Laboratories for Chemical Biology, Karolinska Institutet, Science for Life Laboratory Stockholm, Division of Translational Medicine & Chemical Biology, Department of Medical Biochemistry & Biophysics, Karolinska Institutet, Tomtebodavägen 23A, Solna 171 65, Sweden. [2] Department of Medical Biochemistry & Biophysics, Division of Biophysics, Karolinska Institutet, Scheeles väg 2, Stockholm 171 77, Sweden. [3] School of Biological Sciences, Nanyang Technological University, 61 Biopolis Drive (Proteos), Singapore 138673, Singapore. [4] Department of Pharmacy, Uppsala University, BMC, Box 580, Uppsala SE-751 23, Sweden. [5] School of Biological Sciences, Nanyang Technological University, SBS-04s-45, 60 Nanyang Drive, Singapore 639798, Singapore. [6] Uppsala University Drug Optimization and Pharmaceutical Profiling Platform (UDOPP), Department of Pharmacy, Uppsala University, BMC, Box 580, Uppsala SE-751 23, Sweden. [7] Science for Life Laboratory Drug Discovery and Development platform, Uppsala University, Uppsala SE-751 23, Sweden. [8] Institute of Cellular and Molecular Biology, ASTAR, 61 Biopolis Drive (Proteos), Singapore 138673, Singapore. * These authors contributed equally to this work. † Present address: Clinical Proteomics Mass Spectrometry, Department of Oncology-Pathology, Science for Life Laboratory and Karolinska Institutet, Stockholm, Sweden. Correspondence and requests for materials should be addressed to T.L. (email: thomas.lundback@ki.se) or to P.N. (email: par.nordlund@ki.se).

Therapeutic efficacy is achieved when drugs bind their relevant molecular targets in the physiologically relevant setting. Despite this known fact, insufficient control of target engagement is surprisingly common and contributes to high failure rates in clinical trials[1–3]. Methods that allow for robust measurements of drug target engagement in primary cells, tissues and patient biopsies are thus urgently needed, but have been hard to establish[4,5].

Ligand-induced changes in protein thermal stability are frequently used to monitor binding to isolated proteins in thermal shift assays[6–9]. The recently developed cellular thermal shift assay (CETSA; see Supplementary Note 1 for a list of abbreviations) builds on the discovery that ligand induced thermal shifts can also be measured in the context of cell lysates, whole cells or tissues[10]. This finding effectively allows for biophysical binding studies in native environments—preserving expression levels, posttranslational modifications and the local environment for the endogenous protein. Whereas the original CETSA study included multiple case studies, recent work extends this method to include melting transitions for a significant portion of the proteome, thus expanding the putative use of the methodology to a large number of protein families[11–13]. Of practical importance is that the melting transitions are established for individual proteins by the use of protein affinity reagents[10,14] or quantitative mass spectrometry (MS)[11–13]. As a consequence these measurements are amenable to either high-throughput measurements or proteome-wide multiplexing.

To improve current strategies for drug development, stringent control of target engagement should ideally be established from initial hit identification, through preclinical and clinical development. The same demands apply to the validation of chemical probes discovered in academic settings[2,4,15]. To probe the value of CETSA in earlier stages of the discovery process we applied it for primary screening of thymidylate synthase (TS) in live human myelogenous leukemia cells. TS is a pivotal enzyme in production of thymidine monophosphate and a well validated cancer target[16,17]. Inhibition of TS leads to thymineless death characterized by DNA-damage, chromosomal fragmentation and concomitant induction of apoptosis. Novel classes of TS inhibitors with improved efficacy and resistance profiles could provide important complements to current TS directed drugs, for which there are reports of resistance[18,19].

Here, we show for the first time that a CETSA-based screen for direct physical target engagement constitutes an attractive high throughput screening (HTS) strategy, which allows for the detection of known and novel TS inhibitors with cellular activity. Furthermore, we establish a hit validation strategy, in which time-dependent target engagement is explored in parallel with measurement of intracellular compound concentration. Taken together this provides a sound and efficient strategy to establish control of target engagement from an early stage of the drug discovery process, and which is likely to minimize problems in subsequent stages.

Results

Microplate-based CETSA measuring target engagement of TS. CETSA is based on measurements of remaining soluble target protein against a background of thermally denatured and precipitated proteins following a heat challenge[10,14]. To enable large-scale screening and automation we developed a no-wash immunoassay for TS using AlphaScreen technology in 384-well plates (see Supplementary Figs 1–6 and Supplementary Table 1). As outlined in Fig. 1a the assay workflow starts with a pre-incubation of K562 cells with library compounds or controls to allow cellular uptake, potential compound metabolism and binding to TS. The treated samples in the plates are next transiently heated in a PCR machine, resulting in denaturation and precipitation of intracellular TS unless stabilized by ligand. After cooling to room temperature the cells are lyzed and the remaining (stabilized) levels of TS are measured.

We validated the assay by investigating the response to two drugs of structurally different classes, that is, floxuridine and raltitrexed. Both drugs require intracellular enzymatic conversion prior to high-affinity TS binding[17]. Pyrimidine-based inhibitors, such as floxuridine, bind to TS as the corresponding monophosphate, whereas folate-based drugs, such as raltitrexed, are polyglutamylated and bind TS in a ternary complex with 2′-deoxyuridine 5′-monophosphate (dUMP). Two assay formats were employed for validation. First, the heating was done at a series of different temperatures at a fixed compound concentration to establish aggregation temperature (T_{agg}) curves (Fig. 1b). As expected both drugs resulted in substantial shifts of the thermal stability of TS, thus confirming cellular uptake and intracellular enzymatic conversion to the active forms that bind TS. Based on these curves, 50 °C was selected for further characterization in isothermal dose-response fingerprint ($ITDRF_{CETSA}$) experiments. In these experiments the compound concentration is titrated during the pre-incubation, after which all samples are heated to the same temperature (Fig. 1c,d). Both drugs showed dose-dependent stabilization of TS with half maximal effective concentration (EC_{50}) values in the sub-nM range. Data from parallel experiments using quantitative western blots for assessment of stabilized TS confirmed a significant shift in T_{agg} in the presence of 5 μM of either of these drugs as well as potent dose-dependent stabilization (Supplementary Fig. 7). No change in total TS levels was observable at 5 μM concentration following a 2 h pre-incubation time in the K562 cells, demonstrating that the thermal stabilization data were not influenced by drug-induced changes in total protein levels under these conditions.

Small molecule library screening and hit confirmation. We screened a library of 10,928 compounds at Chemical Biology Consortium Sweden (CBCS; www.cbcs.se) using the TS assay described above. The library includes a structurally-diverse selection of lead-like compounds[20], nucleosides and known drugs (see Methods section for details on the library). These latter subsets include folate and nucleoside-based drugs known to act on TS, suppress thymidine incorporation into DNA and reduce cell proliferation[16,21]. A schematic outline of the screen logistics is available in Supplementary Fig. 8. Screening was performed at a compound concentration of 50 μM and resulted in a reproducible response to the controls and the appearance of several stabilizing compounds (Fig. 2a). Additional graphs illustrating the screen performance and statistics are available in Supplementary Fig. 9 and Supplementary Table 2, respectively. The campaign involved one day of screening, with the AlphaScreen readings done the following morning to ensure equilibration of the antibody recognition.

The threshold for active solutions was calculated at 11.7% stabilization and resulted in 65 hits (Supplementary Table 3). Solutions for 63 of these were available for cherry-picking from our vial-based compound stores, that is, a different source intended for long-term storage. The activities of these solutions were examined in $ITDRF_{CETSA}$ experiments to confirm the screen results (Supplementary Table 3). The majority of compounds with an apparent stabilization above 30% in the primary screen confirmed activity. We also found that 12 out of the 15 vial-based solutions that failed to reproduce activity (highlighted at the bottom of Supplementary Table 3) had been contaminated with

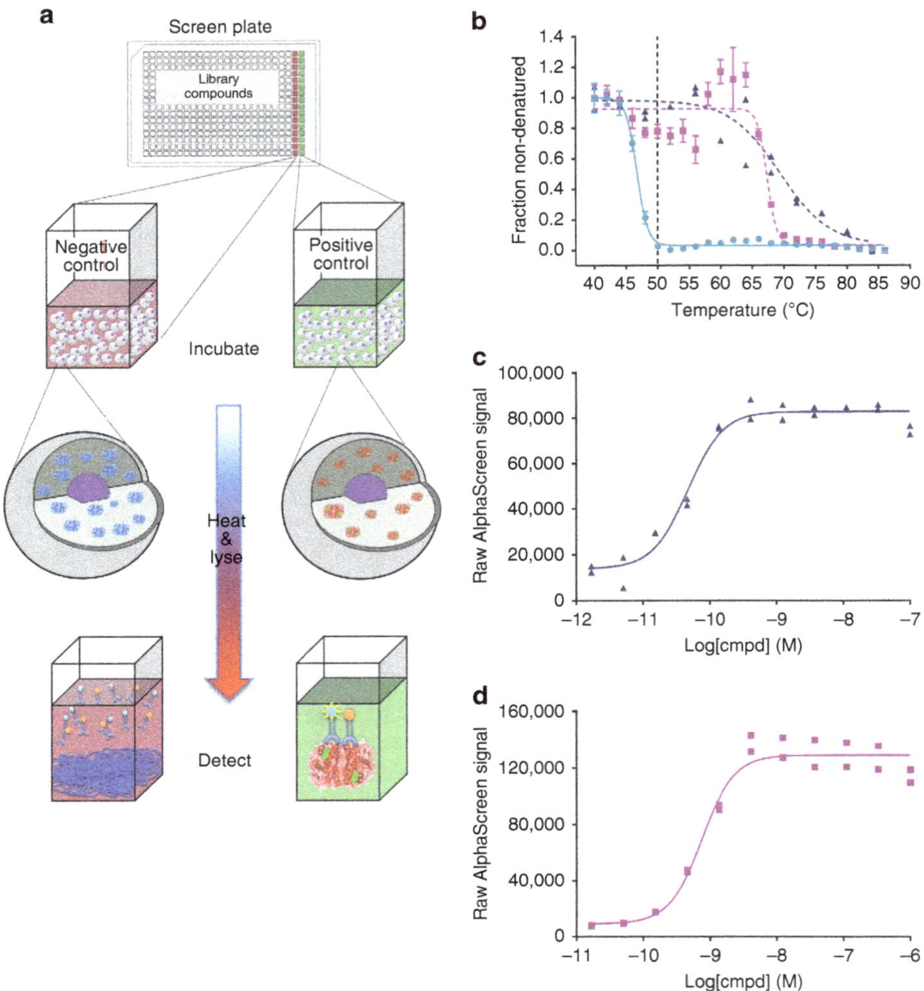

Figure 1 | Development of a no-wash CETSA for human TS. (**a**) Overview of the assay principle with live K562 cells seeded into a 384-well PCR plate. The plate contains controls or library compounds that are taken up by the cells. Following a pre-incubation period the plate is transiently heated for 3 min followed by cooling and cell lysis. Part of the cell lysate is transferred to a detection plate, to which antibodies and AlphaScreen beads are added to allow measurements of remaining soluble TS. (**b**) CETSA derived T_{agg} curves for TS in K562 cells in the presence of DMSO (0.5%) (green circle), 15 μM floxuridine (blue triangle) or 1 μM raltitrexed (magenta square). All data were normalized to the response observed for each treatment condition at the lowest test temperature. The solid line represents the best fit to the Boltzmann sigmoid equation resulting in an apparent T_{agg} of 46.7 ± 0.2 °C for the DMSO control, whereas both floxuridine and raltitrexed stabilized TS above 65 °C (we do not consider higher T_{agg} values reliable as these temperatures influence cell membrane integrity[10]). The vertical dotted line is at 50 °C, the temperature selected for the isothermal screen. Data are provided as the average and standard error of mean (s.e.m.) from two independent experiments performed in duplicate for raltitrexed and as individual data points from one experiment in duplicate for floxuridine. (**c**) $ITDRF_{CETSA}$ of floxuridine (blue triangle) at 50 °C based on raw data from the AlphaScreen readings. The solid line represents the best fit to a saturation binding curve resulting in an EC_{50} of 47 ± 16 pM. Data are provided as two individual data points from one test occasion. (**d**) The corresponding $ITDRF_{CETSA}$ for raltitrexed (magenta square) at 50 °C resulting in an EC_{50} of 0.75 ± 0.2 nM. Data are provided as two individual data points from one test occasion.

highly active compounds because of insufficient tip washing during the transfer from vials to screen library plates (Supplementary Fig. 10). Consequently these hits reproducibly confirmed activity when tested from the contaminated source plates, while the original solutions were inactive. Taken together the confirmation rate was 90% for hits yielding more than 30% apparent thermal stabilization of TS in the original screen.

Fluoropyrimidines, anti-folates and their analogs. The majority of confirmed hits were pyrimidine-based nucleosides and analogs thereof. At the top of the list were substituted 2′-deoxyuridines, including floxuridine (three independent occurrences in the library), 5-trifluoro-2′-deoxythymidine (TFT), and 5-ethynyl-2′-deoxyuridine (EdU) (Fig. 2b and Supplementary Table 3). All of these are known to be taken up and metabolized intracellularly to the active monophosphate forms that interact with TS[16,17]. Novel findings among the nucleosides included the two drugs azacitidine and its deoxyribose analog decitabine, as well as two purine nucleosides (8-bromoadenosine and 8-allyloxy-N2-isobutyryl-2′-deoxyguanosine).

With regards to folate analogs, methotrexate was present at two instances in the library, both as a racemate and as its L form. As expected both appeared as strong hits. The CETSA screen also identified two other marketed drugs, triamterene, a sodium channel inhibitor used to treat hypertension, and pyrimethamine, an inhibitor of dihydrofolate reductase from *Plasmodium falciparum* that is used to treat malaria. They have related

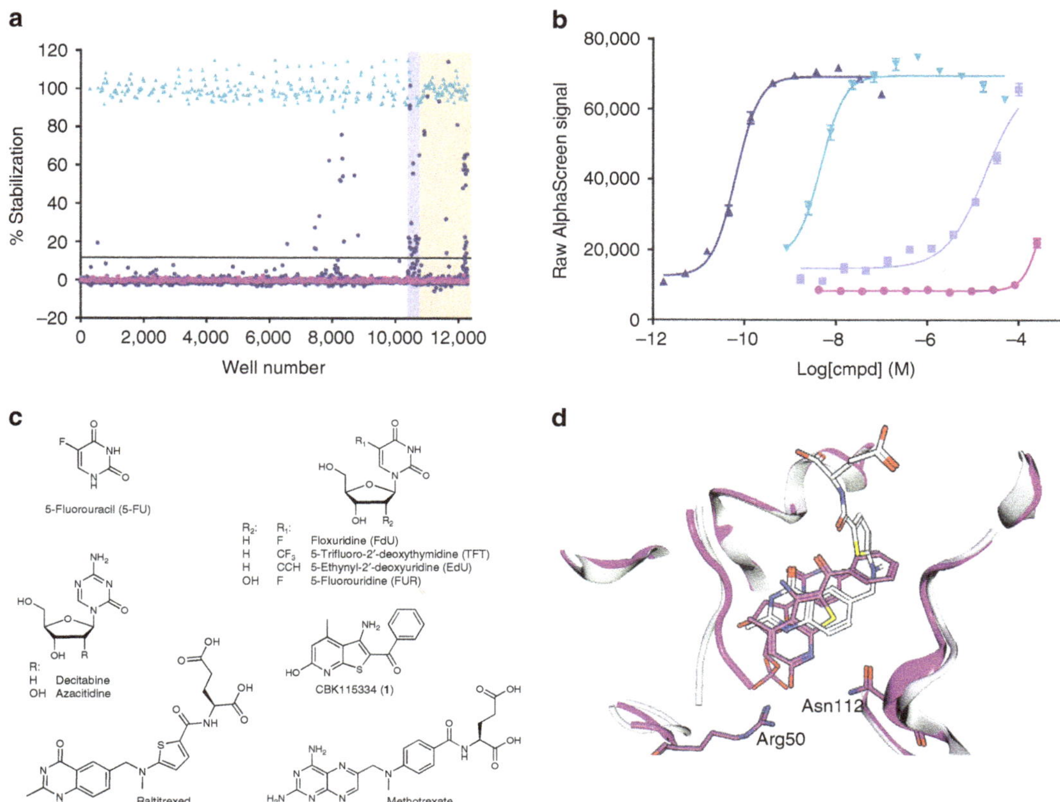

Figure 2 | Primary screen using CETSA to measure target engagement of human thymidylate synthase. (**a**) Scatter plot illustrating normalized screen data, where 0% corresponds to the TS signal observed in the presence of DMSO only (magenta square) and 100% corresponds to the TS signal observed in the presence of 100 nM raltitrexed (green triangle). Data for library compounds at a concentration of 50 μM are shown in blue (blue circle). The hit limit was calculated based on the average plus three standard deviations for the library compounds and is illustrated as a black solid line at 11.7%. The locations of the Prestwick drug set (yellow) and a nucleoside subset (purple) are highlighted. (**b**) $ITDRF_{CETSA}$ data illustrating the ranking of floxuridine (blue upwards triangle), 5-fluorouridine (FUR) (green downwards triangle), and 5-FU (lavender blue square) after 2 h of preincubation time. Data are also included for CBK115334 (magenta circle).The solid lines represent best fits to a saturation binding curve resulting in an apparent EC_{50} of TS at a concentration of 65 ± 9 pM, 47 ± 15 nM, 19 ± 4 μM and 0.46 ± 0.08 mM, respectively. Data are provided as the average and s.e.m. from one independent hit confirmation experiment done in quadruplicate. (**c**) Structures of known drugs and hit compounds discussed in the main text. (**d**) Structure of CBK115334 (magenta) and dUMP bound to TS, shown overlayed on the structure of the complex of raltitrexed (white) and dUMP (PDB 1HVY).

structures and can potentially act as folic acid antagonists[22], but they have not been previously shown to bind TS. Given the scarcity of anti-folates in the hit list we also looked whether there were any obvious false negatives in the screen and confirmed this was not the case (Supplementary Tables 4 and 5).

CBK115334 as a novel TS inhibitor. Besides the pyrimidine- and folate-based inhibitors there were 17 additional weak hits of different chemical classes (Supplementary Table 3). We investigated one of these, CBK115334 or 3-amino-2-benzoyl-4-methylthieno(2,3-b)pyridin-6-ol (**1**), which was chemically distinct from known TS inhibitors (Fig. 2c and Supplementary Fig. 11). It also appeared for the first time as a hit in our screens (Supplementary Table 6). Confirmatory data were obtained using CETSA on K562 cell lysates, which demonstrated a 3.7 °C shift at 200 μM (Supplementary Fig. 12). When applied to isolated recombinant human TS, **1** showed a 2.6 °C shift at 25 μM and a 5.2 °C shift at 100 μM and confirmed binding in the low μM range using surface plasmon resonance (Supplementary Fig. 12). We tested whether binding affected enzymatic activity of TS *in vitro* and observed 60% inhibition at 10 μM concentration and near complete inhibition at 100 μM (Supplementary Fig. 12). A crystal structure of TS with **1** revealed that the compound binds the active site of TS occupying the folate-binding pocket (Fig. 2d). The binding involves π–π stacking interactions with the substrate dUMP and polar interactions with residues lining the catalytic cavity (Asn112 and Arg50 in particular). This constitutes a novel mode of binding as compared with other anti-folates occupying this space[23,24]. Finally, we investigated the impact on cell proliferation in K562 cells. A clear impact was seen with a half-maximal inhibitory concentration (IC_{50}) value just below 100 mM (Supplementary Fig. 12), in line with the weak CETSA response.

Addressing kinetics of compound transport and metabolism. We performed time-traces of the $ITDRF_{CETSA}$ experiments, that is, by varying the time during which cells were exposed to compound prior to the heating step. $ITDRF_{CETSA}$ data obtained after various pre-incubation times are shown in Fig. 3a,b for 5-fluorouracil (5-FU) and floxuridine, demonstrating several orders of magnitude lower potency for 5-FU. The corresponding data on additional nucleosides are available in Supplementary Fig. 13. To examine whether the observed target engagement coincides with appearance of the active forms of these compounds, we monitored levels of compounds and their anticipated active metabolites using liquid chromatography

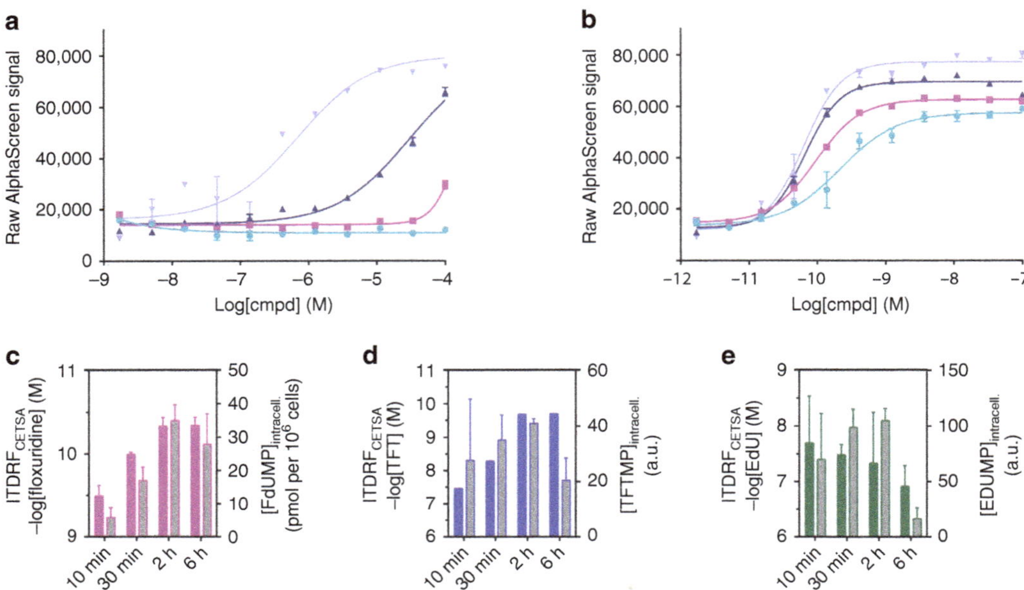

Figure 3 | Time dependence of target engagement and correlation with the appearance of intracellular active metabolites. (**a**) Representative $ITDRF_{CETSA}$ curves for 5-fluorouracil as a function of preincubation time in K562 cells; 10 min (green circle), 30 min (magenta square), 2 h (blue upwards triangle) and 6 h (lavender blue downwards triangle). The solid lines represent best fits to a saturation binding curve function to yield $ITDRF_{CETSA}$ values for half-maximal stabilization of TS. Data are provided as the average and s.e.m. from experiments done in quadruplicate at a single test occasion. (**b**) The corresponding $ITDRF_{CETSA}$ data for floxuridine. (**c**) Half-maximal stabilization of TS (magenta) and intracellular concentration of FdUMP (grey) as a function of preincubation time with floxuridine. The CETSA data are presented as the average and range from two independent experiments. The LC-MS/MS data are provided as the average and s.e.m. from experiments done at three different occasions. (**d**) The corresponding data for TFT (blue) and TFTMP (grey). (**e**) The corresponding data for EdU (green) and EdUMP (grey).

coupled to tandem mass spectrometry (LC–MS/MS)[25,26]. Intracellular and extracellular concentrations as a function of incubation time are shown in Supplementary Fig. 14 for selected nucleosides and their corresponding monophosphate species.

The cellular import and metabolic activation of floxuridine and 5-FU to generate the common active species 5-fluoro-2′-deoxyuridine 5′-monophosphate (FdUMP) require different enzymatic pathways[16,17,27]. CETSA data for floxuridine showed stabilization at low nM concentrations after only 10 min of pre-incubation (Fig. 3b). The potency improved during the first 2 h and persisted throughout the experiment. This time trace was consistent with the intracellular appearance of FdUMP, which was measureable already after 10 min and increased during the first hours of incubation (Fig. 3c). However, for 5-FU the CETSA response increased slowly in the first 6 h (Fig. 3a), with undetectable intracellular levels of FdUMP (Supplementary Fig. 14). Meanwhile the concentration of 5-FU in cells and media remained relatively constant at all time points, thus demonstrating a fast cellular uptake (Supplementary Fig. 14). We hence conclude that the enzymatic conversion of 5-FU to FdUMP is much slower than for floxuridine in K562 cells under these conditions and that the enzymatic conversion to the active species is mirrored by the CETSA responses.

EdU and TFT are structurally related to floxuridine differing only at position 5 of the uracil moiety (Fig. 2c). Although their primary activity on cell viability is believed to result from their misincorporation into DNA, they are also known to inhibit TS following intracellular phosphorylation[28,29]. The uptake and metabolism of TFT, as well as its CETSA time trace, was similar to that observed for floxuridine (Fig. 3d). This was consistent with a build-up of 5-trifluoro-2′-deoxythymidine 5′-monophosphate (TFTMP) and binding to TS in the first hours, generating full target engagement after 2 h of incubation. TFTMP is known to be a tight-binding inhibitor that forms covalent complexes with TS also in absence of the folate-based cofactor[30–32], in line with the observation of a persistent target engagement as measured by CETSA. EdU behaved differently with a more rapid uptake and faster decay of both the extracellular nucleoside and the active form 5-ethynyl-2′-deoxyuridine 5′-monophosphate (EdUMP) (Fig. 3e). The CETSA response was consistent with the fast uptake and activation with an early maximal response that then decayed slightly after the first 2 h, presumably due to the disappearance of the active species.

Phosphorylation and deamination of decitabine. An unexpected hit in the screen was decitabine, which primarily acts as an inhibitor of DNA methyltransferase[33]. The identification of a 2′-deoxycytidine analog as a hit was surprising, but reinforced by the concurrent appearance of the corresponding ribose azacitidine (Fig. 2c). To shed further light on the generation of the active compound, TS stabilization by decitabine itself was first investigated in K562 cell lysates, where activating metabolism is lower because of significant dilution of intracellular enzymes and their substrates. As shown in Supplementary Fig. 15 TS was not stabilized by decitabine in treated lysates. Likewise decitabine did not stabilize recombinant TS in a thermal shift assay, in line with observations for other nucleosides including deoxyuridine, floxuridine and TFT (Supplementary Fig. 15).

The structural analogy to the known nucleoside-based inhibitors of TS triggered the question as to whether decitabine is also phosphorylated, and potentially also deaminated, to generate a TS ligand (Fig. 4a). To investigate the importance of phosphorylation we performed $ITDRF_{CETSA}$ experiments in the presence of DI-82 (ref. 34). This compound is a potent inhibitor of deoxycytidine kinase (DCK) (Fig. 4b), which is required for formation of decitabine monophosphate[35,36]. Dose-dependent stabilization of TS was confirmed in the absence of DI-82,

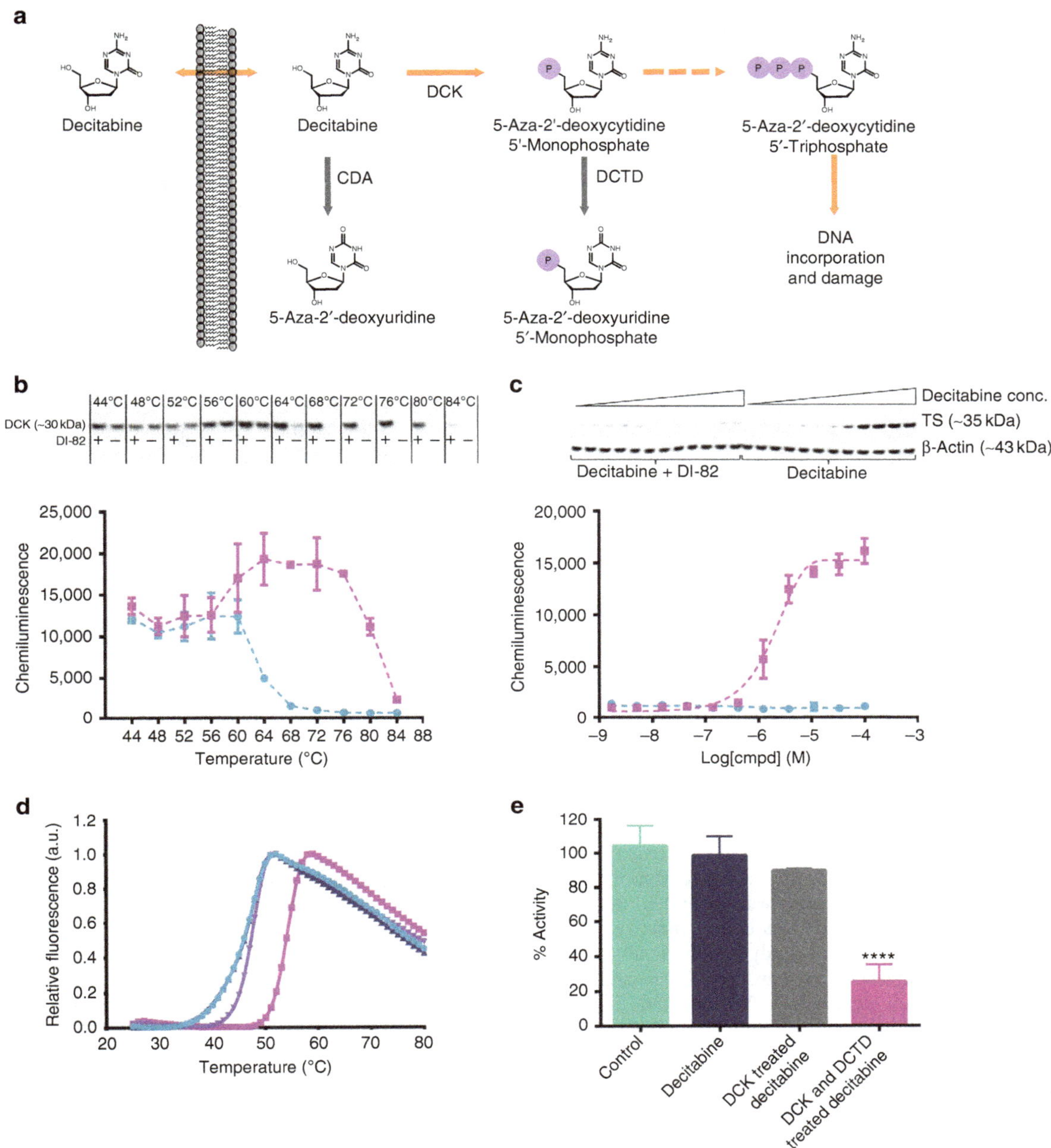

Figure 4 | Target engagement by decitabine is dependent on its metabolic activation. (**a**) Schematic overview of decitabine treatment, cellular uptake and intracellular metabolic conversion. After uptake decitabine is phosphorylated to form 5-aza-2′-deoxycytidine 5′-monophosphate by DCK. This compound is further phosphorylated in two steps to yield the triphosphate that is incorporated into DNA. Cytidine deaminase (CDA) and DCTD are known to be involved in the metabolism and clearance of decitabine[39]. (**b**) T_{agg} experiments for CDK in the absence (green circle) and presence of 200 μM of the DCK inhibitor DI-82 (magenta square). Above the graphs are the chemiluminescence data (full blots are available in Supplementary Fig. 16). The experiments were performed in K562 cells at two independent occasions. (**c**) $ITDRF_{CETSA}$ data for decitabine in the absence (magenta square) and presence of 200 μM of the DCK inhibitor DI-82 (green circle). Full blots are available in Supplementary Fig. 16. The experiments were performed in K562 cells at two independent occasions. (**d**) Normalized thermal shift assay response for recombinant human TS in the absence (magenta square) and presence of 1 mM decitabine without prior enzyme treatment (blue upwards triangle), following DCK treatment (lavender blue downwards triangle) and following treatment with both DCK and DCTD (magenta square). The data are shown as the average and s.e.m. from triplicate samples at one test occasion. (**e**) Enzyme inhibition data for TS in the presence of control and enzymatically treated decitabine samples. The data are shown as the average and s.e.m. from triplicate samples at one test occasion.

whereas its presence at 200 μM completely blunted the ability of decitabine to bind TS (Fig. 4c). However, studies using recombinant DCK to generate decitabine monophosphate resulted in only a marginal stabilization of TS (Fig. 4d). The sample was therefore additionally treated with deoxycytidylate deaminase (DCTD), which is known to deaminate decitabine monophosphate[37], resulting in a thermal shift of nearly 10 °C (Fig. 4d). The inhibitory capacity of these samples mirrored these data, that is, minor inhibition was observed after DCK treatment in the TS enzymatic assay, whereas near full inhibition appeared after treatment with both DCK and DCTD (Fig. 4e). Taken together with the structural analogy to the natural substrate of TS these data strongly infer that the TS ligand is 5-aza-2′-deoxyuridine 5′-monophosphate, that is, the expected product of phosphorylation and deamination of decitabine.

Discussion

Target engagement is essential for efficacy of targeted therapies and validation of new chemical probes[2,4,15]. These validating experiments are ideally performed for many representatives within a chemical series to allow comparisons of structure–activity relationships. To push towards the goal of having a procedure amenable to automation and screening we applied CETSA for assessment of intracellular target engagement at the stage of primary screening. Prior to this work the methodology had been applied on a growing number of drugs and chemical probes[10–14], but it remained challenging to apply to large chemical libraries.

To achieve this evaluation, we developed a homogeneous CETSA and applied it to screening in live, non-engineered cells expressing thymidylate synthase, which is targeted by several different chemical classes of drugs in clinical use[16,17]. Importantly, the screen identified all drugs within the test library that act on TS, as well as novel compounds capable of binding and inhibiting this enzyme. Collectively the known drugs and new inhibitors span over a broad range of affinities. Amongst the new hits was **1**, a μM inhibitor of the purified enzyme with sufficient cell penetration to result in intracellular target engagement and anti-proliferative effects in the high μM range. The binding mode of **1** to TS is partly new and it thus provides a potential starting point for further chemistry optimization.

Several other marketed drugs not previously known to inhibit TS emerged as hits, including triamterene, pyrimethamine and decitabine. As these are clinically-used compounds it is of interest to understand whether there are instances where the interaction with TS plays a role in either efficacy or toxicity. The identification of decitabine illustrates the relevance of monitoring target binding in live cells as this finding was dependent on active cellular metabolism. Decitabine itself was largely inactive on the protein such that, in analogy to the already known uridine-based inhibitors, enzymatic conversion to an active species is a prerequisite for observation of binding. We showed that this conversion does not take place to a significant extent in cell lysates, but can be reproduced with the *in vitro* application of enzymes for phosphorylation and deamination to yield the substrate analog 5-aza-2′-deoxyuridine 5′-monophosphate. Although our data give strong support that a metabolite of decitabine yield significant cellular inhibition of TS, further studies are required to determine whether this is relevant for polypharmacology or toxicity at typical therapeutic doses.

Time-traces of $ITDRF_{CETSA}$ were used to analyze different scenarios for cellular target engagement, thereby integrating aspects of drug transport and metabolism. Combination of these results with measurements of intracellular drug and metabolite concentrations allowed for a comprehensive dissection of cellular drug kinetics. Overall, the intracellular concentrations of the active species of the drugs correlated with the observed target engagement, consistent with the notion that CETSA directly reports on target binding. The combination of high-throughput target engagement studies with LC–MS/MS measurements of intracellular concentrations of drugs and metabolites constitutes a new paradigm for hit validation and optimization in the discovery of chemical probes and drugs. Importantly, CETSA is applicable to studies in native cells and tissue samples[10,14]. Thus the basic scenarios for compound metabolism and target engagement derived from these cell culture studies should be possible to translate towards studies of activities and resistance development to drugs in man. Of particular interest in this regard was the observation that we nearly missed the identification of 5-FU in the screen because of the relatively slow appearance of target engagement. It will be interesting to extend these experiments to patient cells.

The present work demonstrates that CETSA constitutes a robust high-throughput screening strategy that allows for target proteins to be approached in their natural cellular environment. This is in contrast to the majority of targeted cellular HTS assays as these rely on overexpressed and tagged proteins. Since CETSA does not require engineered cells or compounds, it could be particularly attractive for screening in primary cells, tissues or patient-derived material. Our approach can be applied to a large number of different proteins, with the generic assay development path being established in this work. The work also introduces the combination of time-dependent $ITDRF_{CETSA}$ and measurement of intracellular concentrations of metabolites as a stringent approach for hit validation, where the same assay format can be utilized and provide value throughout the drug discovery process.

Methods

Cell culture conditions in AlphaScreen-based experiments. Human myelogenous leukemia cell line K562 (ATCC no. CCL-243) were cultured in RPMI-1640 (SH30027.01, HyClone) supplemented with 10% fetal bovine serum (SV30160.03, HyClone), 0.3 g l^{-1} L-glutamine (G7513, Sigma-Aldrich) and 100 units ml^{-1} Penicillin-Streptomycin (P4333, Sigma-Aldrich). The same cell medium composition was used for all experiments unless otherwise stated.

Development of an AlphaScreen-based assay for TS. Measurements of remaining levels of soluble TS in cell lysates were achieved based on an AlphaScreen-based assay. Establishment of this assay required the identification of a pair of antibodies that simultaneously recognize TS (Supplementary Fig. 1). Combinations of four mouse-derived and three rabbit-derived antibodies directed towards different epitopes of TS (see Supplementary Table 1) were tested for this ability. Four different conditions were tested for each pair, with two of those being the absence and presence of target protein. Given our previous experience of ligand induced quenching of protein target recognition by the antibody pair[14] we also included a control containing an excess of dUMP with and without the additional presence of raltitrexed, which are known binders to the active sites of TS. Recombinant TS, diluted in 1 × AlphaLISA buffer (AL000F, PerkinElmer), was preincubated at room temperature in the presence of buffer only, 100 μM dUMP or 100 μM dUMP and 10 μM raltitrexed in a total volume of 4 μl in a ProxiPlate (#6008280, PerkinElmer). After this preincubation all 12 possible combinations of antibody pairs were added to the sample in a volume of 4 μl followed by incubation for 30 min at room temperature. A mix of AlphaScreen acceptor and donor beads was finally added in a volume of 4 μl under subdued light and allowed to incubate at room temperature for 2 h before reading in an Envision plate reader (PerkinElmer). Final concentrations of the reagents in the detection step were 2 nM recombinant TS, 2 nM of each antibody, 40 μg ml^{-1} AlphaScreen anti-mouse donor beads (#AS104D, PerkinElmer) and 10 μg ml^{-1} AlphaScreen anti-rabbit acceptor beads (#AL104C, PerkinElmer). The plates were sealed with TopSeal-A PLUS (6050185, PerkinElmer). The data were analyzed using microsoft excel and GraphPad Prism 6.

Four different antibody pair combinations based on sc-376161, WH0007298M1, 15047-1-AP and D5B3 (Supplementary Table 1) were selected from the antibody screen to study the kinetics of their recognition of TS in cell lysate. Two batches of 7.5 million K562 cells per ml in supplemented cell culture medium were prepared to serve as max and min controls. One culture was left at room temperature and the other was heated to 52 °C for 3 min in a PCR machine (TECHNE TC-PLUS thermal cycler). Both batches of cells were then lysed by the addition of an equal volume of 2X AlphaScreen SureFire Lysis Buffer (TGRLB100ML, PerkinElmer). After thorough mixing, 4 μl aliquots of the lysates were transferred to a ProxiPlate and detected and analyzed as described above except that the bead incubation was performed at 2 h, 6 h and overnight.

The sc-376161 and 15047-1-AP antibodies were titrated to match their concentrations with the AlphaScreen bead concentrations, that is, to ensure they do not exceed concentrations where hook effects are observed. Fifteen million K562 cells per ml were prepared in supplemented cell culture medium and lysed as described above. Aliquots of 4 μl were transferred to a ProxiPlate followed by the addition of 4 μl of a mix of different concentrations of the two antibodies (final concentrations of each antibody in the detection varied between 0 and 10 nM). Detection and analysis was done as described above, except the bead incubation was performed overnight.

Optimization of cell numbers was achieved by serial dilution of a cell suspension of K562 cells in supplemented cell culture medium. Each sample was then split into two aliquots, which were either kept at room temperature or heated to 52 °C as described above. Both aliquots were then lysed as described above. After thorough mixing, 3 µl of the lysates were transferred to a ProxiPlate followed by the addition of 6 µl of a mix of antibodies and AlphaScreen acceptor and donor beads in AlphaLISA buffer under subdued light. Detection and analysis was achieved as described above except the antibody concentrations were modified to 1 nM 15047-1-AP and 0.4 nM sc-376161.

The control experiment, in which recombinant TS was seeded to cell lysates was prepared based on a serial dilution of recombinant human TS. Dilutions were done in equal volumes of supplemented cell medium and 2 × AlphaScreen SureFire Lysis Buffer. K562 cells at a cell density of 2 million cells per ml were lysed as described above and split in two samples, which were either kept at room temperature or heated to 52 °C as described above. A 10 µl aliquot of each TS dilution was then added to the same volume of each of the two lysates as well as to the mixture of cell medium and lysis buffer. A 3 µl aliquot of each sample was then transferred to a ProxiPlate and detected and analyzed as described above.

Thermal aggregation experiments using AlphaScreen. Floxuridine and raltitrexed were diluted from dimethyl sulfoxide (DMSO) stock solutions to concentrations of 30 µM and 20 µM respectively in supplemented cell culture medium (final DMSO content 1%). These solutions were transferred in a volume of 10 µl to a skirted Twin.tec PCR 96-wellplate (0030 128 672, Eppendorf). A suspension of K562 cells in a volume of 10 µl and a density of 10 million cells per ml were then added to all wells. The PCR plates containing the compounds and cells were sealed with a breathable plate seal (3345, Corning) and incubated for 2 h in a humidified incubator at 37 °C and 5% CO_2. The cells were then transiently heated to different temperatures ranging from 40 °C to 86 °C for 3 min, followed by a controlled cooling to 20 °C for 1 min using a real-time PCR machine (ProFlex, Applied Biosystems). After the heating step the plate was centrifuged briefly (1,000 × *g* for 1 min) followed by lysis of the heated cells by the addition of 20 µl of 2 × AlphaScreen SureFire Lysis Buffer using a Flexdrop IV (PerkinElmer). To ensure sufficient lysis the cell lysates were mixed by 10 repetitive aspiration and dispensing cycles using a Bravo liquid handling platform (Agilent). The lysates (3 µl) were then transferred to 384-well ProxiPlates followed by the addition of 6 µl of a mix of antibodies and AlphaScreen acceptor and donor beads in AlphaLISA buffer under subdued light. Final concentrations of the assay reagents in the detection step were 1 nM rabbit polyclonal anti-TS IgG (15047-1-AP, Proteintech), 0.4 nM mouse monoclonal anti-TS IgG (sc-376161, Santa Cruz), 40 µg ml^{-1} AlphaScreen anti-mouse donor beads and 10 µg ml^{-1} AlphaScreen anti-rabbit acceptor beads. The plates were sealed with TopSeal-A PLUS and incubated over night at room temperature prior to detection in an Envision plate reader. The data were analyzed using microsoft excel and GraphPad Prism 6.

Composition and storage of the primary screening set. The library of compounds applied in this screening campaign consists of 10,928 compounds and is part of the primary screening set at CBCS. The majority of these compounds was donated by Biovitrum AB and originates from both in-house and commercial sources. Compounds included in the primary screening set were selected to represent a diverse selection of a larger set of 65,000 compounds, while keeping a certain depth to allow crude structure–activity relationship studies. The selection was also biased towards lead-like and drug-like profiles with regards to molecular weight, hydrogen bond donors/acceptors and LogP[20]. The library also includes a nucleoside set from Berry & Associates and a set of approved drugs from Prestwick. Compound stock solutions at 10 mM in DMSO are stored frozen at approximately − 20 °C in individual capped tubes in REMP 96 Storage Tube Racks. The racks are stored in a REMP Small-Size Store, which allows cherrypicking while the solutions are still frozen to minimize repetitive freeze-thaw cycles. For screening purposes the compound solutions have been replicated from the REMP racks to Labcyte 384 LDV plates (LP-0200) and then further into Labcyte 1536 HighBase plates (LP-03730) to enable dispensing using acoustic liquid handling equipment.

Compound handling. Assay ready plates were prepared by transferring 200 nl of the 10 mM DMSO solutions of compounds and controls by means of acoustic dispensing (Echo 550, Labcyte) to 384-well polypropylene plates (784201, Greiner). Compounds were placed in columns 1–22. DMSO controls were placed in column 23 and raltitrexed controls were placed in column 24. The assay ready plates were heat sealed with a Peelable Aluminium seal (24210-001 Agilent) using a thermal microplate sealer (PlateLoc, Agilent) and stored at − 20 °C until use. At the day of the experiment the plates were allowed to thaw for 30 min followed by a brief centrifugation step (1,000 × *g* for 1 min) prior to removal of the seal. The compounds were then diluted with 20 µl supplemented cell culture medium using a Multidrop Combi reagent dispenser (Thermo Scientific). Finally 5 µl of the diluted compounds were transferred to a 384 well hardshell PCR plate (HSR480, BIORAD) using a Bravo liquid handling platform equipped with a 384-well head (Agilent). The final concentrations in the incubation with cells (see below) were 50 µM of test compounds and 100 nM of the positive control raltitrexed. The final concentration of DMSO in the assay was 0.5% in all samples.

For the $ITDRF_{CETSA}$ experiments 11-point dose-response curves with three-fold difference in concentration between wells were generated using the Bravo liquid handling system (all serial dilutions were done in 100% DMSO). The final highest concentrations of the test compounds in the incubation with cells were ranging from 100 nM–50 µM depending on estimated potency. The concentration of DMSO was 0.5% in all samples. The final concentration of the positive control raltitrexed was 100 nM. The assay ready plates were prepared as outlined above for the screen.

Screening and dose-response characterization by AlphaScreen. The screen procedure started with the addition of 5 µl of a suspension of K562 cells at a density of 10 million cells per ml to all wells of a 384 well hardshell PCR plate (HSR480, BIORAD) using an electronic multichannel pipette (Biohit). The plates were then heat sealed with Peelable Aluminium seal in a thermal microplate sealer (PlateLoc, Agilent) and allowed to incubate for 2 h in an incubator at 37 °C and 5% CO_2. For the time-course experiments the incubation times were altered to include also 10 min, 30 min and 6 h. To allow gas exchange during the longer incubation times these plates were instead sealed with at breathable plate seal (3345, Corning). After the incubation step the plates were transiently heated at 50 °C for 3 min followed by a controlled cooling to 20 °C for 1 min using a real-time PCR machine (LightCycler480 system, Roche). Plate handling was then as described above for the thermal aggregation experiments. The data were analyzed using microsoft excel and GraphPad Prism 6.

Screen and $ITDRF_{CETSA}$ data analysis. Screen data were imported into microsoft excel and normalized for each compound based on the negative and positive controls on each plate, that is, with the response in the presence of DMSO defining 0% stabilization and the response in the presence of 100 nM raltitrexed defining 100% stabilization. A calculation of the average and standard error of means for each set of controls also allowed an illustration of how these responses varied over the 32 screening plates. The Z′ factor[38] is commonly used as a measure of how well the assay separates between the controls and this was calculated as described based on the calculated averages and standard deviations of the controls on a per plate basis. For the T_{agg} shift and the $ITDRF_{CETSA}$ experiments the data were analyzed in GraphPad Prism using the Boltzmann sigmoid equation and the saturation binding curve (rectangular hyperbola; binding isotherm) function, respectively. As already discussed[14] these methods make use of equilibrium models for data analysis although the methodology depends on the irreversible aggregation of denatured material. For this reason we refer to the observed responses as apparent and isothermal dose-response fingerprints and are careful with any quantitative interpretations, being well aware of their dependency on experimental conditions. Experiments are on-going to address the quantitative interpretation of CETSA data.

Measurements of identity and purity of test compound solutions. Assessments of identity and purity of the test solutions that were used for hit confirmation purposes, that is, those being stored in REMP vials, was done by means of high-pressure liquid chromatography coupled to mass spectrometry (HPLC–MS). A small aliquot of each test solution (2 µl of a 10 mM solution) was placed in a 96-well plate (267245, Nunc) and diluted with 20 µl of methanol. The plate was then placed in an Agilent 1,100 HPLC UV/MS with electrospray ionization (ESI +). The HPLC method was based on an ACE C8 3 µm column (3.0 × 50 mm) and a mobile phase (CH_3CN)/(0.1% TFA/H_2O). All solvents were HPLC grade and absorbance was monitored at 220 nm. Compounds that did not give satisfactory data were re-analyzed using a method based on a Waters XBridge C18 3.5 µm column (3.0 × 50 mm), 3.5 min gradient mobile phase (CH_3CN)/(10 mM NH_4HCO_3/H_2O). The instrument software was used to integrate the UV response for each peak and provided a list of the peaks and their associated masses. The estimated purity was calculated based on the integrated area for the expected mass compared with the areas of all other peaks. The result was manually controlled and if there were deviations from the expected outcome a meticulous investigation of the UV-response and MS was performed.

Cell viability assay. A concentration–response curve of CBK115334 was generated using the Bravo liquid handling system (serial dilution of a 50 mM stock solution was done in 100% DMSO). A total of 150 nl of the serially diluted solutions and controls (positive control 0.67 mM staurosporine and negative control DMSO) were transferred to a white 384-well assay plate (3570, Corning) by means of acoustic dispensing (Echo 550, Labcyte). A Multidrop reagent dispenser (Thermo Scientific) was used to dispense 30 µl of a K562 cell suspension at a density of 33 × 10^3 cells per ml in supplemented cell culture medium. The cells were incubated at 37 °C in the presence of 5% CO_2 for 72 h before addition of 30 µl CellTiter-Glo Luminescent Cell Viability Assay reagent (Promega) using a Multidrop Combi reagent dispenser (Thermo Scientific). The plate was placed on a plate shaker for 15 min prior to detection of the luminescence signal in an Envision plate reader (PerkinElmer). The final highest concentration of CBK115334 in the incubation with cells was 250 µM and the final concentration of the positive control staurosporine was 3 µM. All samples contained 0.5% DMSO. The data were analyzed using microsoft excel and GraphPad Prism 6.

Chemicals and buffers in western blot-based experiments. The cell lysis buffer contained 100 mM 4-(2-hydroxyethyl)-1-piperazineethanesulfonic acid (HEPES, pH 7.5), 1 mM Tris-(2-carboxyethyl)phosphine hydrochloride (TCEP) and 10 mM magnesium chloride (Sigma-Aldrich) supplemented with complete (EDTA-free) protease inhibitor cocktail from Roche (Switzerland). Tris-buffered saline with tween (TBST) buffer (150 mM NaCl, 0.05% (v/v) Tween-20, 50 mM Tris-HCl buffer at pH 7.6) was prepared by dissolving TBS-TWEEN tablets obtained from Merck KGaA (Darmstadt, Germany) in ddH_2O. The blocking buffer consisted of 5% (w/v) non-fat milk (Semper AB, Sundbyberg, Sweden) diluted in tris-buffered saline with tween. Hank's Balanced Salt Solution (HBSS) was from Gibco/Life Technologies. Raltitrexed monohydrate, dUMP and decitabine was purchased from Sigma-Aldrich and Selleckchem, respectively. DI-82 was kindly provided by Prof. Caius G. Radu and Raymond M. Gipson at the Department of Molecular and Medical Pharmacology, University of California, Los Angeles.

Cell lines and cultures in western blot-based experiments. Human cell line K562 (ATCC no. CCL-243) was cultured in RPMI-1640 medium (Sigma-Aldrich) supplemented with $0.3\,g\,l^{-1}$ L-glutamine and 10% fetal bovine serum (FBS, Gibco/Life Technologies, Carlsbad, CA, USA), 100 units per ml penicillin and 100 units per ml streptomycin (Gibco/Life Technologies). Short-term passages (<20) were used for experiments.

Cell lysate thermal shift experiments. For the cell lysate thermal shift experiments, cultured K562 cells were harvested and washed with Hank's Balanced Salt Solution. The cells were diluted in lysis buffer supplemented with complete protease inhibitor cocktail. The cell suspensions were freeze-thawed three times using liquid nitrogen and passed through a 27″ gauge needle five times. The soluble fraction (lysate) was separated from the cell debris by centrifugation at $20,000 \times g$ for 20 min at 4 °C. For the thermal aggregation curve experiments cell lysates were diluted with lysis buffer supplemented with 200 µM dUMP and divided into two aliquots, with one aliquot being treated with ligand and the other aliquot with vehicle (control). After 10 min incubation at room temperature the respective lysates were divided into smaller (50 µl) aliquots and heated individually at different temperatures for 3 min in a Veriti thermal cycler (Applied Biosystems/Life Technologies) followed by cooling for 3 min at room temperature. The heated lysates were centrifuged at $20,000 \times g$ for 20 min at 4 °C in order to separate the soluble fractions from precipitates. The supernatants containing the remaining soluble proteins were transferred to new 0.2 ml microtubes and analyzed by sodium dodecyl sulfate polyacrylamide gel electrophoresis (SDS-PAGE) followed by western blot analysis.

For the in-cell experiments K562 cells were harvested and resuspended with culture medium to a cell density of 5 million cells per ml and seeded into T25 flasks. Cells were treated with either raltitrexed, floxuridine, DI-82 or vehicle (DMSO) for 2 h in an incubator at 37 °C and 5% CO_2. The cell suspensions were then divided into 100 µl aliquots in 0.2 ml tubes and heated at designated temperatures ranging from 40 to 84 °C for 3 min in a Veriti thermal cycler (Life Technologies) followed by 3 min of cooling at room temperature. The heat-treated cell suspensions were freeze-thawed three times using liquid nitrogen and a heating block set at 25 °C. Tubes were gently vortexed between the freeze-thaw cycles. The resulting cell lysates were centrifuged at $20,000 \times g$ for 20 min at 4 °C. The supernatant was removed from the cell debris and aggregates and the remaining soluble TS was analyzed using western blot.

For the $ITDRF_{CETSA}$ in cell experiments, raltitrexed and floxuridine were serially diluted to generate an 11 point dose–response curve with three-fold difference in concentration between each point. K562 cells were treated with each respective compound concentrations and one vehicle as control in 100 µl aliquots in 0.2 ml tubes for 2 h in an incubator at 37 °C and 5% CO_2. The cell aliquots were heated at 50 °C and analyzed with western blot following the procedure described above.

For the decitabine metabolism, decitabine was serially diluted to generate an 11 point dose–response curve and an $ITDRF_{CETSA}$ experiment was performed as described above in absence and presence of 200 µM of the DCK inhibitor DI-82 (referred to as 12R in the main text of the original publication and DI-82 in the Supplementary Material)[34].

SDS-PAGE and western blot. NuPage Novex Bis-Tris 4–12% polyacrylamide gels with NuPAGE MES SDS running buffer (Life Technologies) were used for separation of proteins in the samples. Proteins were transferred to nitrocellulose membranes using the iBlot2 blotting system (Life Technologies). Primary antibodies anti-TS (D5B3) XP (Cell Signaling), anti-dCK (sc-393099), anti-β-actin (sc-69879); secondary goat anti-mouse HRP-IgG (sc-2055) and bovine anti-rabbit HRP-IgG (sc-2374) antibodies (Santa Cruz Biotechnology, Santa Cruz, CA, USA) were used for immunoblotting. All membranes were blocked with blocking buffer; standard transfer and western blot protocols recommended by the manufacturers (listed above) were used. All antibodies were diluted in blocking buffer. The membranes were developed using Clarity Western ECL substrate HRP-Substrate (Bio-Rad) according to the manufacturer's recommendations. Chemiluminescence intensities were detected and quantified using a ChemiDoc XRS+ imaging system (Bio-Rad) with Image Lab software (Bio-Rad).

Expression and purification of human thymidylate synthase. The gene encoding human TS (NM_001071.2) was subcloned into the pNIC28-Bsa4 vector and expressed in Rosetta BL21-DE3 Escherichia coli (Novagen) in Terrific Broth media supplemented with $50\,\mu g\,ml^{-1}$ of kanamycin and $34\,\mu g\,ml^{-1}$ chloramphenicol. Cells were grown at 37 °C until $OD_{600\,nm}$ reached about 2.0 and induced with 0.5 mM isopropyl-beta-D-1-thiogalactopyranoside (IPTG) at 18 °C overnight. The cells were harvested by centrifugation at $4,500 \times g$ for 15 min at 15 °C. The cell pellet was re-suspended in lysis buffer (100 mM HEPES, 500 mM NaCl, 10 mM imidazole, 10% (v/v) glycerol and 1 mM TCEP at pH 8.0) supplemented with 1:1,000 (v/v) EDTA-free protease inhibitor cocktail (Calbiochem) and $125\,U\,ml^{-1}$ of Benzonase (Merck). Cells were lysed by sonication on ice at 70% amplitude, 3 s on/off for 3 min. The lysate was clarified by centrifugation at $47,000 \times g$ for 25 min at 4 °C, and the supernatant was filtered through a 1.3 µm syringe filter to remove cell debris. The cell-free extract was loaded on a pre-equilibrated HisTrapTM HP column (GE Healthcare) in IMAC wash buffer 1 (20 mM HEPES, 500 mM NaCl, 10 mM imidazole, 10% (v/v) glycerol and 1 mM TCEP at pH 7.5) and subsequently washed with 20 column volumes (CVs) of IMAC wash buffer 1 and 15 CVs of IMAC wash buffer 2 (20 mM HEPES, 500 mM NaCl, 25 mM imidazole, 10% (v/v) glycerol and 1 mM TCEP at pH 7.5). Bound protein was eluted with 5 CVs of elution buffer (20 mM HEPES, 500 mM NaCl, 500 mM imidazole, 10% (v/v) glycerol and 1 mM TCEP at pH 7.5) and loaded onto a HiLoad 16/60 Superdex-200 column (GE Healthcare) pre-equilibrated with buffer (20 mM HEPES, 300 mM NaCl, 10% (v/v) glycerol, and 1 mM TCEP at pH 7.5). Based on Nu-PAGE gel results pure protein fractions were pooled and concentrated using a 50 kDa cutoff centrifugal driven filter concentrator (Sartorius Stedium Biotech). The protein concentration was determined by the absorbance at 280 nm using a Nanodrop spectrophotometer (Thermo Scientific).

Thermal shift *in vitro* assay on recombinant protein. The assay was performed on the iCycler iQ Real Time PCR Detection System (Bio-Rad), using the 96-well thin-wall PCR plate (Bio-Rad). The experiment was conducted in a buffer containing 20 mM HEPES at pH 7.5 and 150 mM NaCl. A total volume of 25 µl solution containing $0.2\,mg\,ml^{-1}$ protein, compounds and $\times 5$ Sypro Orange dye (Invitrogen) diluted from $5,000\times$ stock was dispensed into the 96-well plate. The same amount of DMSO was added in the control wells. The plates were sealed with Microseal B adhesive sealer (Bio-Rad) and heated in iCycler from 25 to 80 °C (56 heating cycles in 28 min). Fluorescent filter used for Sypro Orange measurements was $\lambda_{excitation} = 492$ nm and $\lambda_{emission} = 610$ nm. The calculation of

Table 1 | X-ray diffraction data and refinement statistics.

	TS-dUMP-CBK115334
Data collection	
Space group	$P4_32_12$
Cell dimensions	
a, b, c (Å)	108.2, 108.2, 313.9
α, β, γ (°)	90, 90, 90
Resolution (Å)	30-3.1 (3.2-3.1)*
R_{merge}	0.147 (0.619)
$I/\sigma I$	15.56 (4.98)
Completeness (%)	99.9 (99.9)
Redundancy	11.9 (10.9)
Refinement	
Resolution (Å)	30-3.1 (3.2-3.1)
No. reflections	34,453
R_{work}/R_{free}	18.0/26.8
No. atoms	
Protein	13,596
Ligand dUMP	186
Ligand CBK115334	96
Water	11
B-factors	
Protein	45.3
Ligand dUMP	45.1
Ligand CBK115334	51.9
Water	30.9
R.m.s. deviations	
Bond lengths (Å)	0.014
Bond angles (°)	1.096

*Highest resolution shell is shown in parenthesis.

the midpoint of the curves (T_m) was performed using the software package XLfit from IDBS within microsoft excel.

TS enzyme inhibition assay. Enzymatic activity of recombinant human TS was measured spectrophotometrically at 340 nm by monitoring the absorbance change during the conversion of 5,10-methylenetetrahydrofolate to dihydrofolate using an Infinite M200 spectrometer (Tecan). Measurements were carried out at room temperature and in a buffer of 50 mM Tris at pH 7.5 and 150 mM NaCl. Initial velocities were measured with 250 nM of purified protein, 100 μM 5,10-methylenetetrahydrofolate and 100 μM dUMP in the presence of compounds using the same amount of DMSO as control. Initial rates and activity were analyzed with the software package Prism (GraphPad Software).

Surface plasmon resonance. Recombinant human TS protein (25 μg ml^{-1} in a buffer of 10 mM sodium acetate at pH 5.0, 1 mM dUMP and 200 μM methotrexate) were captured on Sensor Chip S-CM5 via amine coupling to a level of ~5,000 resonance units using Biacore T-200. Raltitrexed was used as a positive control to ensure that the protein remained active after immobilization and during the run. A concentration series (20 nM to 10 μM) of CBK115334 was injected over the prepared surface for 60 s and allowed to dissociate for 60 s with a flow rate of 70 μl min^{-1} at 25 °C. The assay buffer was 20 mM HEPES, 150 mM NaCl, pH 7.5 and 0.005% Tween-20 supplemented with 1% DMSO and 200 μM dUMP. Response data was processed using the BIAevaluation software. Responses were double referenced and solvent-corrected. The data sets were fitted to 1:1 steady-state model for determination of binding constants.

Decitabine treatment with DCK and DCTD. Decitabine at a concentration of 1 mM was incubated with 1 mg ml^{-1} of recombinant DCK and 2.5 mM ATP in a buffer of 50 mM Tris at pH 7.5, 150 mM NaCl and 0.5 mM $MgCl_2$ at room temperature for 60 min to generate the corresponding monophosphates. To probe for nucleotide deamination the samples were further treated with 1 mg ml^{-1} of recombinant DCTD in the presence of 1 mM ATP and 10 μM $ZnCl_2$ for 20 min at room temperature. After incubation, the samples were heated at 95 °C for 10 min and centrifuged for 10 min at the highest speed at 4 °C using a benchtop centrifuge. The supernatant was tested without dilution in thermal shift *in vitro* assays and the TS enzyme inhibition assay. The supernatants from samples without nucleoside were used as the treatment controls.

Crystallization and structure determination. TS protein crystallized in sitting drops comprising equal volume of protein (about 24 mg ml^{-1}) and reservoir solution at 20 °C. The crystallization condition was composed of 0.1 M sodium cacodylate at pH 6.5 and 15% PEG 4,000. Crystals were soaked with 1 mM compound and 2 mM dUMP in cryo-protectant buffer containing 0.1 M sodium cacodylate at pH 6.5 and 25% PEG 4,000 and 10% DMSO for 15 min, followed by flash frozen in liquid nitrogen. Data collection was performed on beamline MX1 at Australian Synchrotron. X-ray diffraction data was collected at 100 K with a wavelength of 0.9537 Å. It should be noted that CBK115334 is subject to keto–enol isomerization. While the resolution is not sufficient to distinguish between these, the included illustrations are based on the enol form (both forms make interactions with Asn112 and Arg50, but with different donor–acceptor pairs). The structure was solved by molecular replacement using Phaser with the hTS-dUMP-raltitrexed structure (PDB code 1HVY) as the search model. Structure was refined with phenix refine. Ligand structures and restraints files were generated using eLBOW. In the TS-dUMP-CBK115334 complex structure, 90.43% of residues were in favoured regions and 7.92% of residues were in allowed regions. The data collection parameters and refinement statistics are summarized in Table 1. An image of the electron density map of the active site in the co-crystal structure is available in Supplementary Fig. 17.

Table 2 | Monitored LC-MS/MS transitions.

Compound/Metabolite	Parent and daughter ions
5-FU	128.8>41.9
FdU	244.9>155.0
FdUMP	324.9>195.0
FUR	260.9>171.0
EdU	250.9>135.8
EdUMP	330.9>195.0
TFT	249.9>179.7
TFTMP	374.9>179.4
Decitabine	227.0>93.8
Decitabine-MP	307.0>195.0
Pyrimethamine*	248.8>176.9
CBK115334*	284.9>188.9

*Analyzed with electrospray ionization in positive mode.

Intracellular compound and metabolite concentrations. Intracellular concentrations of compounds were measured as previously described[25,26]. Briefly, K562 cells were incubated with the compounds for a predefined time at 37 °C in a 5% CO_2 atmosphere. After incubation, the cells were centrifuged (300 × *g* for 5 min) and a medium sample (supernatant) was collected and diluted 1:10 in a 50 nM warfarin solution (internal standard). The cells were washed with phosphate buffered salt solution and lysed with methanol. Methanol was evaporated and the cell samples were reconstituted in 50 nM warfarin. Samples were analyzed with LC-MS/MS with electrospray ionization in negative mode with transitions monitored as listed in Table 2.

References

1. Morgan, P. *et al.* Can the flow of medicines be improved? Fundamental pharmacokinetic and pharmacological principles toward improving Phase II survival. *Drug Discov. Today* **17,** 419–424 (2012).
2. Bunnage, M. E., Chekler, E. L. P. & Jones, L. H. Target validation using chemical probes. *Nat. Chem. Biol.* **9,** 195–199 (2013).
3. Cook, D. *et al.* Lessons learned from the fate of AstraZeneca's drug pipeline: a five-dimensional framework. *Nat. Rev. Drug Discov.* **13,** 419–431 (2014).
4. Simon, G. M., Niphakis, M. J. & Cravatt, B. F. Determining target engagement in living systems. *Nat. Chem. Biol.* **9,** 200–205 (2013).
5. Durham, T. B. & Blanco, M.-J. Target engagement in lead generation. *Bioorg. Med. Chem. Lett.* **25,** 998–1008 (2015).
6. Pantoliano, M. W. *et al.* High-density miniaturized thermal shift assays as a general strategy for drug discovery. *J. Biomol. Screen.* **6,** 429–440 (2001).
7. Ericsson, U. B., Hallberg, B. M., DeTitta, G. T., Dekker, N. & Nordlund, P. Thermofluor-based high-throughput stability optimization of proteins for structural studies. *Anal. Biochem.* **357,** 289–298 (2006).
8. Senisterra, G. A. *et al.* Screening for ligands using a generic and high-throughput light-scattering-based assay. *J. Biomol. Screen* **11,** 940–948 (2006).
9. Niesen, F. H., Berglund, H. & Vedadi, M. The use of differential scanning fluorimetry to detect ligand interactions that promote protein stability. *Nat. Protoc.* **2,** 2212–2221 (2007).
10. Martinez Molina, D. *et al.* Monitoring drug target engagement in cells and tissues using the cellular thermal shift assay. *Science* **341,** 84–87 (2013).
11. Savitski, M. M. *et al.* Tracking cancer drugs in living cells by thermal profiling of the proteome. *Science* **346,** 1255784 (2014).
12. Franken, H. *et al.* Thermal proteome profiling for unbiased identification of direct and indirect drug targets using multiplexed quantitative mass spectrometry. *Nat. Protoc.* **10,** 1567–1593 (2015).
13. Huber, K. V. M. *et al.* Proteome-wide drug and metabolite interaction mapping by thermal-stability profiling. *Nat. Methods* **12,** 1055–1057 (2015).
14. Jafari, R. *et al.* The cellular thermal shift assay for evaluating drug target interactions in cells. *Nat. Protoc.* **9,** 2100–2122 (2014).
15. Arrowsmith, C. H. *et al.* The promise and peril of chemical probes. *Nat. Chem. Biol.* **11,** 536–541 (2015).
16. Longley, D. B., Harkin, D. P. & Johnston, P. G. 5-fluorouracil: mechanisms of action and clinical strategies. *Nat. Rev. Cancer* **3,** 330–338 (2003).
17. Wilson, P. M., Danenberg, P. V, Johnston, P. G., Lenz, H.-J. & Ladner, R. D. Standing the test of time: targeting thymidylate biosynthesis in cancer therapy. *Nat. Rev. Clin. Oncol.* **11,** 282–298 (2014).
18. Assaraf, Y. G. Molecular basis of antifolate resistance. *Cancer Metastasis Rev.* **26,** 153–181 (2007).
19. Gonen, N. & Assaraf, Y. G. Antifolates in cancer therapy: Structure, activity and mechanisms of drug resistance. *Drug Resist Updat.* **15,** 183–210 (2012).
20. Lipinski, C. A. Lead- and drug-like compounds: the rule-of-five revolution. *Drug Discov. Today Technol.* **1,** 337–341 (2004).
21. Houghton, J. A., Tillman, D. M. & Harwood, F. G. Ratio of 2′-deoxyadenosine-5′-triphosphate/thymidine-5′-triphosphate influences the commitment of human colon carcinoma cells to thymineless death. *Clin. Cancer Res.* **1,** 723–730 (1995).
22. Lambie, D. G. & Johnson, R. H. Drugs and folate metabolism. *Drugs* **30,** 145–155 (1985).
23. Almog, R., Waddling, C. A., Maley, F., Maley, G. F. & Van Roey, P. Crystal structure of a deletion mutant of human thymidylate synthase Δ (7-29) and its ternary complex with Tomudex and dUMP. *Protein Sci.* **10,** 988–996 (2001).
24. Sayre, P. H. *et al.* Multi-targeted antifolates aimed at avoiding drug resistance form covalent closed inhibitory complexes with human and Escherichia coli thymidylate synthases. *J. Mol. Biol.* **313,** 813–829 (2001).
25. Mateus, A., Matsson, P. & Artursson, P. Rapid measurement of intracellular unbound drug concentrations. *Mol. Pharm.* **10,** 2467–2478 (2013).
26. Mateus, A., Matsson, P. & Artursson, P. A high-throughput cell-based method to predict the unbound drug fraction in the brain. *J. Med. Chem.* **57,** 3005–3010 (2014).

27. O'Connor, O. A. in *Cancer Drug Discovery and Development: Combination Cancer Therapy: Modulators and Potentiators* (ed. Schwartz, G. K.) 133–174 (Humana Press Inc., 2005).
28. De Clercq, E. *et al.* Thymidylate synthetase as target enzyme for the inhibitory activity of 5-substituted 2′-deoxyuridines on mouse leukemia L1210 cell growth. *Mol. Pharmacol.* **19,** 321–330 (1981).
29. Temmink, O. H., Comijn, E. M., Fukushima, M. & Peters, G. J. Intracellular thymidylate synthase inhibition by trifluorothymidine in FM3A cells. *Nucleosides Nucleotides Nucleic Acids* **23,** 1491–1494 (2004).
30. Danenberg, P. V, Langenbach, R. J. & Heidelberger, C. Structures of reversible and irreversible complexes of thymidylate synthetase and fluorinated pyrimidine nucleotides. *Biochemistry* **13,** 926–933 (1974).
31. Danenberg, P. V & Lockshin, A. Fluorinated pyrimidines as tight-binding inhibitors of thymidylate synthetase. *Pharmac. Ther.* **13,** 69–90 (1981).
32. Eckstein, J. W., Foster, P. G., Finer-Moore, J., Wataya, Y. & Santi, D. V. Mechanism-based inhibition of thymidylate synthase by 5-(trifluoromethyl)-2′-deoxyuridine 5′-monophosphate. *Biochemistry* **33,** 15086–15094 (1994).
33. Stresemann, C. & Lyko, F. Modes of action of the DNA methyltransferase inhibitors azacytidine and decitabine. *Int. J. Cancer* **123,** 8–13 (2008).
34. Nomme, J. *et al.* Structure-Guided Development of Deoxycytidine Kinase Inhibitors with Nanomolar Affinity and Improved Metabolic Stability. *J. Med. Chem.* **57,** 9480–9494 (2014).
35. Momparler, R. L. Molecular, cellular and animal pharmacology of 5-aza-2′-deoxycytidine. *Pharmacol. Ther.* **30,** 287–299 (1985).
36. Momparler, R. L. Pharmacology of 5-aza-2′-deoxycytidine (decitabine). *Semin. Hematol.* **42,** S9–S16 (2005).
37. Momparler, R. *et al.* Kinetic interaction of 5-AZA-2′-deoxycytidine-5′-monophosphate and its 5′-triphosphate with deoxycytidylate deaminase. *Mol. Pharmacol.* **25,** 436–440 (1984).
38. Zhang, J.-H., Chung, T. D. Y. & Oldenburg, K. R. A simple statistical parameter for use in evaluation and validation of high throughput screening assays. *J. Biomol. Screen.* **4,** 67–73 (1999).
39. Chabot, G. G., Bouchard, J. & Momparler, R. L. Kinetics of deamination of 5-aza-2′-deoxycytidine and cytosine arabinoside by human liver cytidine deaminase and its inhibition by 3-deazauridine, thymidine or uracil arabinoside. *Biochem. Pharmacol.* **32,** 1327–1328 (1983).

Acknowledgements

T.L., H.Al., M.H. and H.Ax. acknowledge Karolinska Institutet, SciLifeLab and the Swedish Research Council (Vetenskapsrådet), which funds Chemical Biology Consortium Sweden. P.N. acknowledges funding from Karolinska Institutet (DPA), the Swedish Research Council, the Swedish Cancer Society, the Knut and Alice Wallenberg foundation, as well as a startup grant from Nanyang Technological University. P.A. acknowledges the Swedish Research Council and SciLifeLab. A.M. acknowledges the Portuguese Research Council (Fundação para a Ciência e Tecnologia). R.J. acknowledges Magnus Bergvalls Stiftelse, The Lars Hierta Memorial Foundation and Helge Ax:son Johnsons stiftelse. We are very grateful to Caius G. Radu and Raymond M. Gipson for providing the DCK inhibitor DI-82. We would also like to thank Protein Science Facility (PSF) at Karolinska Institutet for providing DCTD and Staffan Eriksson from the Swedish University of Agricultural Sciences for providing the plasmid for DCK. We are also grateful to Carlo Zaniol at PerkinElmer for valuable support in development of the AlphaScreen assays. Brinton Seashore-Ludlow is acknowledged for careful reviewing and commenting on the manuscript.

Author contributions

H.Al., H.Ax., R.J., D.M.M., T.L. and P.N. conceived the study. H.Al., H.Ax. and T.L. developed the homogenous TS CETSA assay supported by R.J. and D.M.M. and ran the screen. R.J. generated the western blot CETSA data. A.M. and P.A. planned and generated the intracellular concentration data. C.D. generated the *in vitro* thermal shift and surface plasmon resonance data, and solved the crystal structure of CBK115334 together with A.L. M.H. performed the cheminformatics and metabolic pathway analysis. P.N., P.A. and T.L. lead the project. T.L. and P.N. wrote the first draft of the manuscript. All co-authors contributed to the final draft of the manuscript.

Additional information

Accession codes: The crystal structure of CBK115334 and dUMP in complex with TS has been deposited with the RCSB Protein Data Bank under the accession code 5HS3.

Competing financial interests: D.M.M. and P.N. are founders of the company Pelago Bioscience AB. D.C., A.L., A.M., P.A, R.J., T.L., H.Al., M.H. and H.Ax. declare no competing financial interests.

Applying medicinal chemistry strategies to understand odorant discrimination

Erwan Poivet[1,*], Zita Peterlin[2,*], Narmin Tahirova[1], Lu Xu[1], Clara Altomare[1], Anne Paria[1], Dong-Jing Zou[1] & Stuart Firestein[1]

Associating an odorant's chemical structure with its percept is a long-standing challenge. One hindrance may come from the adoption of the organic chemistry scheme of molecular description and classification. Chemists classify molecules according to characteristics that are useful in synthesis or isolation, but which may be of little importance to a biological sensory system. Accordingly, we look to medicinal chemistry, which emphasizes biological function over chemical form, in an attempt to discern which among the many molecular features are most important for odour discrimination. Here we use medicinal chemistry concepts to assemble a panel of molecules to test how heteroaromatic ring substitution of the benzene ring will change the odour percept of acetophenone. This work allows us to describe an extensive rule in odorant detection by mammalian olfactory receptors. Whereas organic chemistry would have predicted the ring size and composition to be key features, our work reveals that the topological polar surface area is the key feature for the discrimination of these odorants.

[1] Department of Biological Sciences, Columbia University, New York, New York 10027, USA. [2] Corporate Research and Development, Firmenich Incorporated, Plainsboro, New Jersey 08536, USA. * These authors contributed equally to this work. Correspondence and requests for materials should be addressed to S.F. (email: sjf24@columbia.edu).

A comprehensive system for classifying odours has been an elusive goal of olfactory inquiry for centuries. The root of the problem, which can be stated most simply as biology versus chemistry, can be seen even in the earliest attempts to bring order to odours. Linnaeus, the master classifier, developed an odour classification scheme using seven primary percepts along a scale of pleasant to unpleasant[1]. Following him, Zwaardemaker[2] proposed the most comprehensive organization of odours, using 9 or 10 perceptual groupings. With the 19th century development of atomic and organic chemistry, numerous researchers attempted to correlate chemical characteristics with odours[3,4]. Perfumers and other fragrance purveyors implemented their own, sometimes less scientific schemes[5]. In the past century more modern attempts generated schemes that encompassed psychophysical descriptors and behavioural responses to complex mixtures[6–8]. However, with the landmark discovery of the unexpectedly large odorant receptor (OR) family of GPCRs by Buck and Axel[9], these efforts largely came to a halt, replaced by the promise of a molecular basis for odour perception. Because typical mammalian odour gene families number over a thousand different receptors, it seemed that the coding problem would soon be solved with high-throughput screening technologies[10].

Mature olfactory sensory neurons (OSNs) are believed to express only one OR gene[11–13]. This property, combined with the unexpectedly large number of receptors, has given rise to the widely accepted proposal that peripheral discrimination works through a reciprocal combinatorial code in which one chemical can be detected by different ORs and one OR can detect a group of different chemicals[14,15]. Additionally, the axons of all OSNs expressing a particular OR project to the same glomerulus in the olfactory bulb, suggesting a labelled line-style 'odour-map' in the brain[16–18]. Taken together, these properties seemed to reduce the odour-coding problem to simply matching particular receptors to their cognate odours. Thus, recent efforts have mainly been directed at identifying ligands for various ORs by screening large sets of supposedly diverse odours[19–21]. However, this programme has run into several obstacles.

First, only a handful of ORs have been successfully de-orphaned, severely limiting the possibility of uncovering hypothesized combinatorial rules. Additional confusion arose when an unexpectedly large repertoire of chemically different molecules were identified as ligands of the single mouse OR, SR1 (ref. 22), complicating the idea of an 'odour-map' and re-opening the question of broadly versus narrowly tuned receptors. Finally, several psychophysical odour paradoxes remain, such as the diversity of compounds that give rise to identical musk percepts. The enormity of the issue was further emphasized by a recent publication claiming that the human olfactory system could discriminate over 1 trillion odours[23]. Absent a systematic understanding of odour detection and discrimination at the periphery, it is difficult to imagine how higher brain centres process the sensory input to develop perceptions and regulate behaviour.

To address these issues from a new perspective, we here take an alternate approach to receptor ligand interactions that is based on medicinal chemistry principles. Medicinal chemistry emphasizes biological function—in this case receptor activation—over chemical form. Similarity between odorants is defined not by strict chemical characteristics but rather by their ability to activate the same receptor or receptors. We use a panel of compounds based on the common odorant acetophenone to investigate the effect of heteraromatic ring substitution for benzene rings on its odour percept. Using both single cell responses and behavioural tests in mice we find that the classification of the odorants is significantly different from the one expected when classified using classical organic chemical rules. From these results it appears that this approach, based on medicinal chemistry and the related concept of bioisosterism, may reveal a novel strategy for comprehending odour discrimination.

Results

Responses of OSNs to aromatic odorants. Odorants are multi-dimensional stimuli but not all features are necessarily equally weighted by ORs. Here, in a calcium imaging assay, we challenged dissociated mouse OSNs with a panel of related heteroaromatic odorants to investigate whether the ring's sterics (size) or its toplogical polar surface area (TPSA) are better correlated with odorant co-detection.

Panel 1 consisted of acetophenone [1] and five derivatives that replaced the apolar, 6-membered benzene ring with heteroaromatic rings of different sizes and atomic composition (Fig. 1a). Ten per cent of viable OSNs (276/2,750) responded to at least one panel member. Thirty-six distinct patterns were observed when responses were conservatively scored in a binary fashion (Fig. 1c). The analogues varied in their ability to mimic [1] in terms of activation. Of the OSNs detecting [1], 72% also detected 2-acetylthiophene [2], 38% detected 2-acetylpyridine [4], 30% 2-acetylthiazole [5], 25% 2-acetylfuran [3] and 13% 2-acetylpyrazine [6]. [1] and [2] have similar TPSAs but different ring sizes. In contrast, [1], [4] and [6] have the same ring size but different TPSAs. That [1] and [2] are far more frequently co-detected than are [1] and [4] or [6] suggests that TPSA is a more heavily weighted 'epitope' than ring size.

The prioritization of TPSA over ring size appears to be a general trend shaping OSN response patterns. [1], [4] and [6] preserve the same ring size, but as the TPSA increased, the extent of co-detection with [1] decreased. Among OSNs responding to [2], 65% co-detect the similar TPSA but larger-sized ring [1], while only 32% co-detect the higher TPSA but similar-sized ring [5]. Likewise, among OSNs responding to [4], 50% co-detect the similar TPSA but smaller-size ring [5], while only 37% co-detect the higher TPSA but similar-sized ring [6]. This further reinforces that although the geometry of the molecule may be most salient, the TPSA seems to be the driver of these co-recognition patterns.

Strikingly, we found that the diversity of response patterns was constrained by two extensible rules. The first rule is that, at the assay concentration of 30 μM, every OSN that detects both [1] and [3] will also detect [2]. Even when assayed at a higher (150 μM) concentration (Supplementary Fig. 1), this same 'if [1] and [3] then [2]' rule applies, suggesting that there is a conserved biological constraint among OR-binding pockets. At 30 μM, we also note that [5], a five-membered ringed odorant with similar TPSA to [3], can substitute for [3] 95% of the time in this rule, making the relationship 'if [1] and [5] then [2]' a highly predictive one. The second extensible rule is that if an OSN detects [1], [3] and [6] then it will detect all the odorants of Panel 1. Although at first surprising, this rule may be considered to be a fusion of the rule 'If [1] and [3] then [2]' with how OSNs respond to a graded increase in TPSA within a fixed ring size among [1], [4] and [6].

Although the TPSA-based rule was strict for [1], [2] and [3], discrimination based on TPSA partly breaks down when considering [1], [4] and [6]. One might expect that an OSN responding to both [1] and [6] would never reject the intermediate TPSA [4], and yet this occurs 12% of the time. One possibility may be how the appended ketone group interacts with the dual nitrogens of [6]. The benzene ring in [1] has neither a dipole nor a polar constituent. The pyrazine ring in [6] has no dipole (that of the two oppositely situated nitrogens cancelling out), but it is still highly polar (hence its high TPSA). The ketone group, while preferring to lie in plane with the aromatic ring, has

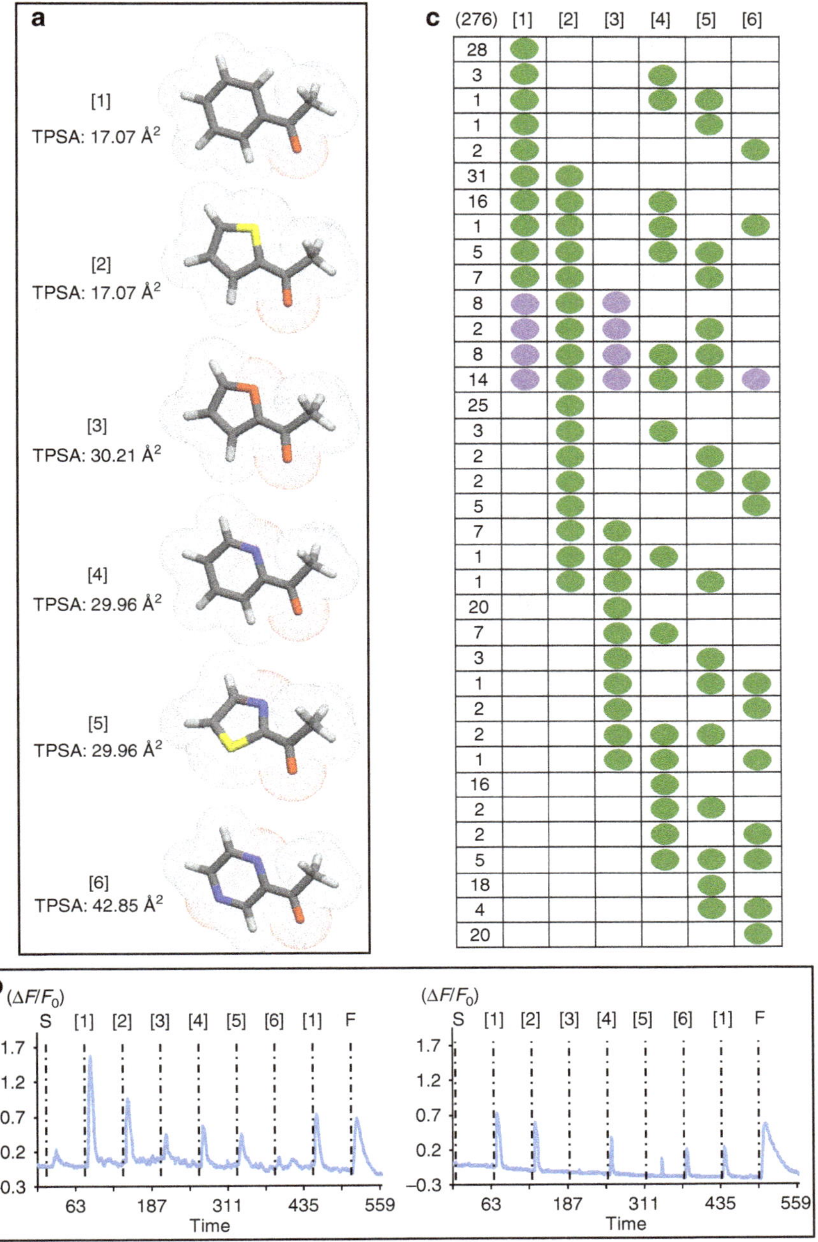

Figure 1 | Reponses of dissociated OSNs to Panel 1 odorants in calcium imaging. (**a**) Three-dimensional (3D) representations of Panel 1 odorants. The vertices of the tubes symbolize atoms—grey, carbon; blue, nitrogen; yellow, sulfur; red, oxygen. The dotted red surface around the atoms represents polar regions of the surface area. 3D-representations of these and all odorants used in the study were made using Galaxy 3D Structure Generator free software (www.molinspiration.com.) and TPSA were calculated according to ref. 36. (**b**) Calcium imaging traces of two different OSNs responding to Panel 1 odorants. (**c**) A total of 276 OSNs out of 2,750 viable OSNs responded to at least one Panel 1 odorant, leading to 36 distinct binary response patterns. The numbers indicate how often a particular response pattern was observed. Green dot: activation of the OSN by the corresponding odorant. The OSNs that respond to [1] and [3] always respond to [2] (Purple dot). OSN that respond to [1], [3] and [6] always respond to all the odorants of the panel (Purple dot). S, dimethyl sulfoxide; F, forskolin.

freedom to rotate in [1], but less so in [6], where the two polar nitrogens tend to mutually repulse it. With just one nitrogen to interact with the appended ketone, [4] should then co-activate 50% of ORs detecting [1] and 50% of ORs detecting [6]. This is indeed the response pattern observed in the OSNs: 50% of ORs detecting [1] co-detect [4], and 41% of ORs detecting [4] co-detect [6].

To investigate if the rule of 'If [1] and [3] then [2]' transferred to other contexts, we tested two manipulations. A second panel of odorants (Panel 2) included molecules that were also ketones, but had an extra benzene ring fused to their far end. This manipulation increases the total surface area and affords an extended aromatic system while preserving the TPSA and relationship of the heteroatom to the carbonyl group. Thus, the Panel 2 odorants included 2-acetonaphtone [7] as an analogue to [1], 2-acetylbenzothiophene [8] to [2] and 2-benzofuranyl-methyl-ketone [9] to [3] (Supplementary Fig. 2). Another panel of odorants (Panel 3) replaced the ketone group with a carboxylic acid group. This change allows us to sample a markedly different chemical space as judged by the low frequency of co-recognition of the ketone [1] versus its acid version 2-naphthoic acid [10] (Fig. 1d). Panel 3 includes three acids and their ketone analogues: [10] as the acid analogue to [7], benzo[b]thiophene-2-carboxilic acid [11] to [8] and benzo[b]furan-2-carboxilic acid [12] to [9] (Supplementary Fig. 3).

Twenty-six per cent of OSNs (245/926) responded to at least one Panel 2 member, generating 26 distinct binary OSN response patterns. Consistent with the prior study, OSNs detecting [1] co-detected [2] more frequently than [3] (59% versus 17%, respectively). The benzene-fused analogues showed the same trend; OSNs detecting [7] co-detected [8] more frequently than [9] (83% versus 64%, respectively). The strict co-detection rule that was seen for the single ring [1], [2] and [3] also extended to the benzene-fused [7], [8] and [9]. That is, if an OSN responded to both [7] and [9] it always responded to [8] (Fig. 2; Supplementary Fig. 2). Thus, the 'TPSA rule' is robust among both ketone scaffolds.

Intriguingly, the benzene-fused analogues of Panel 2 activated markedly more OSNs than did their single ring counterparts. Eighteen per cent of OSNs were activated by [7] versus 9% by [1], 18% [8] versus 8% [2] and 13% [9] versus 3% [3] (Supplementary Fig. 2). This suggests that increased surface area and/or extended aromaticity could be a stabilizing factor, perhaps by improving pi–pi stacking with aromatic amino-acid side chains in the binding pocket. This may form the basis of a strategy to rationally design an aromatic odorant to increase the breadth of ORs it targets.

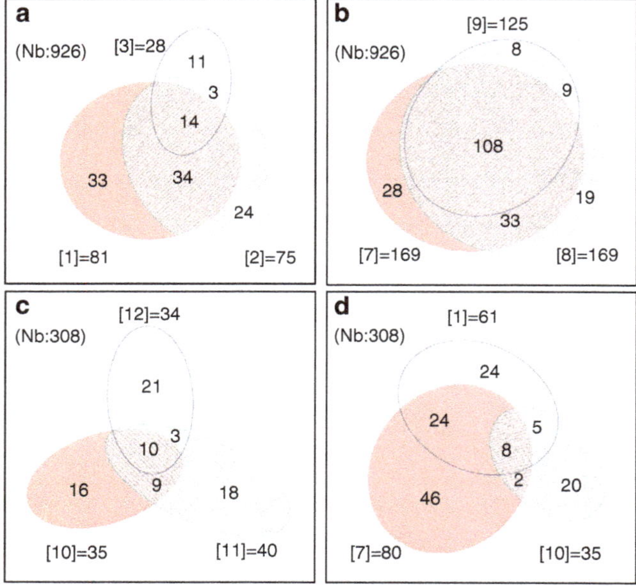

Figure 2 | Transferability of the intra-ring TPSA rule. (**a**) Venn diagram of OSNs responding to the single-ring ketones [1], [2] and [3]. If an OSN responds to [1] and [3] it always responds to [2]. (**b**) Venn diagram of OSNs responding to the double-ring ketones [7], [8] and [9]. If an OSN responds to [7] and [9], it always responds to [8]. (**c**) Venn diagram of OSNs responding to the double-ring acids [10], [11] and [12]. If an OSN responds to [10] and [12] it always responds to [11]. (**d**) Venn diagram of OSNs responding to the single-ringed ketone [1], the double-ringed ketone [7] and the double-ringed acid [10]. Note that OSNs co-detecting the acid make up just a small portion of the overall responses. OSNs were counted and converted into surface area for each response combination using the eulerAPE free software. The number of OSNs responding with that pattern is indicated in that sector. All odorants were tested at 30 μM. Nb, total number of viable OSNs screened.

Among the acids of Panel 3, we again observed conservation of the 'TPSA rule' with all OSNs that responded both to [10] and [12] also responding to [11] (Fig. 2c). Twenty-two distinct patterns were observed when responses were conservatively scored in a binary fashion (Supplementary Fig. 3). Of the 308 OSNs recorded, 45% responded to at least one Panel 3 member; for the ketones 26% responded to [7] and 20% to [1]. For the acids only 11% responded to [10], 13% to [11] and 11% to [12]. These results indicate that acids are generally weaker odorants than ketones. Interestingly the OSNs recognizing the acid [10] were mostly distinct from the population responding to either the single-ringed ketone [1] or the double-ringed ketone [7] (Fig. 2d), lending further support to the transferability of the 'TPSA rule'.

Comparing odorant classifications. Medicinal chemistry substitutions can be discrepant in form but they nevertheless preserve similar biological functionality across multiple targets. In our panels, several of the heteroaromatic substitutions from the 'lead' odorant [1] were inspired by medicinal chemistry substitutions. We thus compared the classification of the Panel 1 odorants using both traditional chemistry-centric and biology-centric approaches.

For the chemistry-centric approach, we used the e-Dragon software to obtain 1,666 molecular descriptors for each odorant. We generated a dendrogram (Fig. 3a) which revealed two clearly distinguishable branches. The segregation was driven by ring size with the 6-membered ring [1], [4] and [6] forming one cluster, and the 5-membered ring [2], [3] and [5] forming a second cluster. The two families were further fractionated by atomic composition via the presence of nitrogen in the 6-membered ring family and sulfur in the 5-membered ring family. In the 5-membered ring family, [3] and [5] are split apart despite their similar TPSA, leaving [5] to cluster with [2]. This clustering pattern underscores that in the traditional chemistry-centric classification atomic composition is given pre-eminence over TPSA.

For the biology-centric classification the response patterns of the OSNs formed the basis for the hierarchical cluster analysis. The resulting dendrogram has striking differences (Fig. 3b). Notably, in the dendrogram for Panel 1, [1] and [2] are tightly linked, as determined from their biological activity profiles. This branch, which contains the two low TPSA rings, segregates from the odorants with larger TPSA values. TPSA, however, is not the sole determinant of the remaining organization as [5] clusters with the higher TPSA [6] instead of the matched TPSA [4]. When Panel 2 odorants were clustered via their OSN response patterns, the major split was along the lines of total surface area with all the double-ringed odorants segregating from the single-ringed odorants (Fig. 3c). Within each family, however, clustering reflected the division of low TPSA from high TPSA that was seen in the Panel 1 odorants. That is, [1] was tightly linked to [2] and separate from [3], whereas [7] was tightly linked with [8] and separate from [9].

Similarly, biology-centric classification separates Panel 3 odorants according to their TPSA. The three acids segregate from the ketone [7], and [10] was tightly linked to [11] and separated from [12] (Supplementary Fig. 4). A chemistry-centered approach on the other hand separates once again Panel 3 odorants according to their ring size and composition: [7] and [10] group together despite their functional group difference, and separate from [11] and [12].

Behavioural response of mice to the odorants. Having examined how OSNs parse heteroaromatic odorants, we turned to a habituation–dishabituation test to investigate how readily a

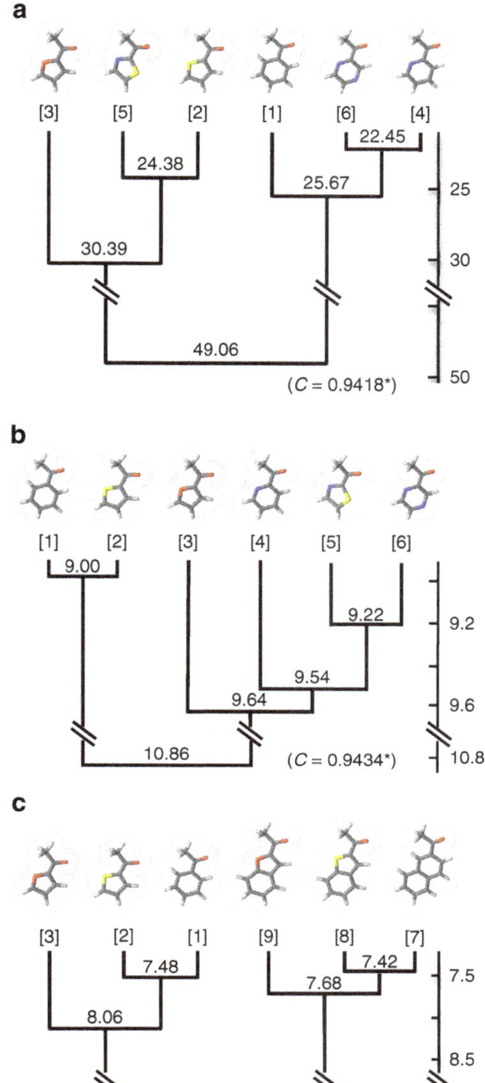

Figure 3 | Hierarchical clustering analysis of Panel 1 and Panel 2 odorants. (**a**) Panel 1 odorants clustered according to chemical similarity as evaluated by 1,666 molecular descriptors downloaded through the e-dragon applet. (**b**) Panel 1 odorants clustered according to biological response similarity based on calcium imaging of dissociated OSNs. Note that in the chemical-based clustering the major division is on ring size while in the biological-based clustering the major division is on the TPSA. (**c**) Panel 2 odorants clustered according to their biological responses, as in **b**. Although there is a major division based on the presence of a double-ring scaffold, within each branch further subdivisions follow the TPSA rule as in **b**. *Cophenetic correlation coefficient. All distances in the dendrograms are Euclidian. See online methods for details of dendrogram generation.

mouse could discriminate between select pairings of Panel 1 and Panel 2 odorants. Habituation is defined by a progressive decrease in olfactory investigation towards repeated presentation of the same odour stimulus. Dishabituation is defined by reinstatement of olfactory investigation when a novel odour is presented.

Many of the trends seen in the behavioural assay paralleled those seen in the response patterns of OSNs. Notably, there was robust acceptance for a carbon-to-sulfur swap; mice that habituated to [1] remained habituated to [2] (Fig. 4). This habituation also occurred when odorants were presented in the reverse order (i.e., habituation to [2] then probed with [1]). Reciprocal habituation also occurred when mice were challenged with [7] and [8], the double-ringed analogues of [1] and [2].

Mice also demonstrated reciprocal habituation to [4] and [5] (Table 1). Like [1] and [2], [4] and [5] are related by a carbon-to-sulfur swap but in an overall more polar background. Although [1] and [2] cluster tightly in the OSN response-based dendrogram, [4] and [5] are admittedly more distant (Fig. 3b). Still, they are far closer in the OSN-based response dendrogram than in the molecular descriptor-based dendrogram. This supports that OSN response patterns are indeed a better predictor of olfactory-guided behaviour.

Clear reciprocal dishabituation was noted for certain carbon-to-oxygen and carbon-to-nitrogen swaps. Mice stimulated by [1] failed to generalize to the oxygen-containing [3]. This behaviour may find its basis in that OSNs show a far lower degree of co-detection between [3] and [1] as opposed to [2] and [1]. Dishabituation was also seen when the mouse was stimulated by [7] but probed with [9], the double-ring analogues of [1] and [3], or stimulated by [10] but probed with [12] (their acids analogues) (Fig. 4). For carbon-to-nitrogen swaps, reciprocal dishabituation was observed between [2] followed by [5] and by [1] followed by [4] (Table 1). Within both of these pairings, the ring size is preserved but TPSA changes. This further reinforces the relative pre-eminence of TPSA from a biological standpoint.

Interestingly, not all the habituations were reciprocal. Habituation was observed when the mouse was stimulated with [4] then probed with [3] but not if stimulated with [3] then probed with [4]. The same situation occurred between [5] and [6]. Cases of asymmetrical habituation have been previously reported in the psychophysical literature and are suggestive of non-overlapping sets of receptors that bind the same ligands.

Discussion

The classification of the vast number and diversity of odorant molecules has been a controversial topic in psychophysics and more recently in molecular physiology and systems biology of the olfactory system[23,24]. Here, our work reveals an extensible rule of odorant detection by OSNs.

In colour perception there is a generally agreed-upon set of rules determining how wavelengths mix to produce millions of hues. In the auditory system the combination of frequencies and amplitudes produces a predictable perception of tonality. No such agreement or scheme is available in olfaction and it remains virtually impossible to predict, from looking at a chemical structure, whether a molecule will have an odour or not, let alone what that quality may be.

One obstacle to gaining this understanding may be that we have adopted a physical and organic chemistry scheme of molecular description and classification. Chemists classify molecules according to characteristics that are useful in synthesis or isolation, features that may be of no importance to a biological sensory system, either at the olfactory receptor level or at higher perceptual levels.

It has been shown that among all molecular features that describe a compound, some are more important than others for odorant perception by receptors[25,26]. Learning how features of odorants are weighted by ORs could clarify the fundamental structure of the stimulus space and help predict similarity of odour quality. Computational models such as the 3D-QSAR can already efficiently identify a few key descriptors common to all the ligands of an OR and then predict and design new ligands for

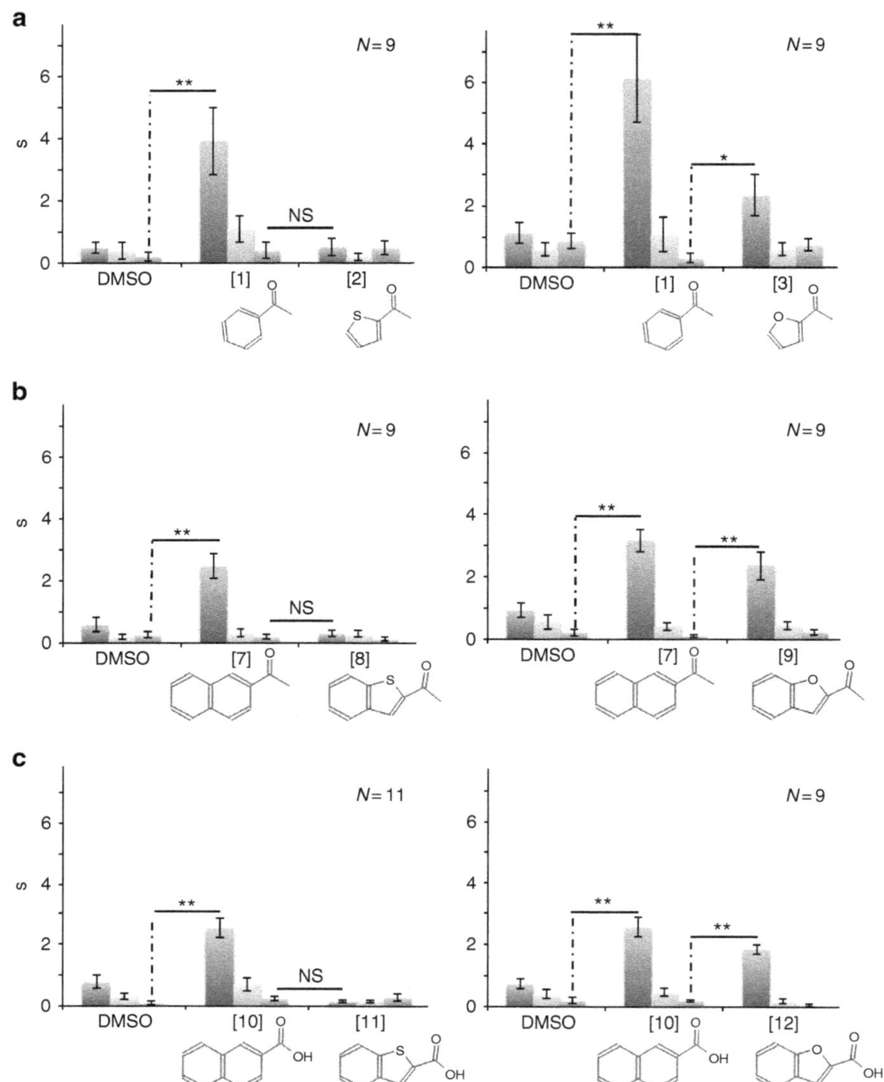

Figure 4 | Habituation-dishabituation olfactory test. The average olfactory investigation time (s) by mice during repetitive 2 min exposures to odorant pairs or DMSO (solvent). (**a**) Mice that habituated to [1] remained habituated to [2] but dishabituated to [3]. (**b**) Mice that habituated to [7] remained habituated to [8] but dishabituated to [9]. (**c**) Mice that habituated to [10] remained habituated to [11] but dishabituated to [12]. In all cases, the analogue with the low TPSA thiophene ring was not discriminated from the lead, low TPSA benzene-ringed version, but the analogue with the higher TPSA furan ring was. Behaviour tests were analysed using ANOVA test followed by a *post hoc* paired *t*-test (*$P<0.05$, **$P<0.005$ paired *post hoc t*-test). NS, not significant, *P-value <0.05, **P-value <0.005 paired *t*-test. Error bars: s.e.m. *N*, number of animals.

that OR[26,27]. But this model depends on already partially deorphanized ORs, and these key descriptors appear to be different for every OR. Recently Sobel's lab[28], correctly identified the problem of odour perception as one of quantifying odour characteristics, has taken a mathematical approach to reduce complex odour structures to a small number of vectors. Unfortunately, a reliance on chemical descriptors means elements of the vectors cannot often be identified with any empirical odour structure. (Examples from their Table 1 include, 'the molecular multiple path count number', the 'spectral moment from edge adj. matrix weighted by dipole moments' and 19 other similarly esoteric descriptors).

We have instead taken an approach that is more bio-centric using principles developed in the practice of medicinal chemistry to identify biologically relevant features of an odour stimulus[29]. This is sometimes known as bioisosterism—the practice of exchanging molecular fragments that subtly tweak but largely preserve chemical structure and performance at a variety of enzyme and receptor targets.

As a proof of principle we assessed one type of bioisosteric exchange, that of heteroaromatic rings for benzene, against the suite of mouse ORs. Starting from acetophenone as the 'lead' odorant, we found that several of the predicted exchanges were, indeed, well tolerated. Acetophenone possesses a benzene ring that can be replaced by alternative ring structures. The most common prediction would be that odour quality varies according to ring steric size and shape or atomic composition. On the contrary, our analysis revealed that the overall TPSA was of greater importance, such that having a ring component with a high TPSA was a generally disfavoured epitope for OSNs responding to acetophenone. These findings at the sensory neuron/receptor level transferred to behavioural testing

A second panel, which included benzene-fused double-ringed versions of the analogues, surprisingly revealed that the

Table 1 | OSNs discrimination and behaviour response to Panel 1 odorants.

Odorant pairs	Changes	Co-activation	Exclusion (%)	Behaviour
[1] versus [2]	C->S, polarity and ring size change	72%/66%	30	Habituated
[1] versus [3]	C->O, polarity, ring size and TPSA changes	25%/41%	69	Dishabituated**
[1] versus [4]	C->N, polarity and ring TPSA change	38%/55%	71	Dishabituated*
[1] versus [5]	C->S, C->N, dipolarity, ring size and TPSA changes	30%/49%	55	—
[1] versus [6]	C->N (2 ×), ring TPSA changes	13%/29%	74	Dishabituated*
[2] versus [3]	S->O, polarity and ring TPSA changes	30%/53%	62	—
[2] versus [4]	Polarity, ring size and TPSA changes	35%/55%	57	—
[2] versus [5]	C->N, dipolarity and ring TPSA change	37%/65%	53	Dishabituated**
[2] versus [6]	Polarity, ring size and TPSA changes	16%/37%	81	—
[3] versus [4]	Polarity, ring size change	43%/38%	60	Dishabituated*
[3] versus [5]	O->N, C->S, dipolarity	40%/40%	60	—
[3] versus [6]	Ring size and TPSA changes	23%/30%	73	—
[4] versus [5]	C->S, dipolarity, ring size change	42%/47%	55	Habituated
[4] versus [6]	C->N, polarity, ring size and TPSA changes	26%/39%	68	—
[5] versus [6]	Dipolarity, ring size and TPSA changes	33%/44%	62	Habituated

TPSA, topological polar surface area.
This table recapitulates co-activation among the OSNs and behavioural responses observed with Panel 1 odorant pairs. 'Changes' gives the substitutions and transformations from one odorant to the other. The first co-activation number gives the percentage of OSNs responding to the first odorant of the pair that were co-activated by the second odorant. The second co-activation number gives the percentage of OSNs responding to the second odorant of the pair that were co-activated by the first odorant. 'Exclusion' numbers give the percentage of OSNs that respond exclusively to one odorant of the pair among the total number of OSNs that respond to those two odorants. 'Behaviour' recapitulates the results observed during the habituation/dishabituation olfactory tests with the odorants of the pair. Behaviour results were analysed using ANOVA test followed by a *post hoc* paired *t*-test (*$P<0.05$, **$P<0.005$ paired *post hoc* *t*-test).

double-ringed odorants activated far more OSNs than did the single-ringed ones. The added benzene ring not only increased the breadth of activation across the suite of ORs but it also often led to an increased breadth of tuning for a given single OR. This strategy could be exploited to probe binding pocket accommodation.

A third panel used acid analogues of the double-ringed ketones of Panel 2. We observed only minor levels of co-recognition between the single-ring acid [10] and the analogous single-ringed ketone [1] or the double-ring ketone [7], demonstrating that the acids of Panel 3 likely cover distinct sectors of chemical space than do the ketones of Panel 1 and Panel 2. Yet despite this, the 'TPSA rule' translated well, demonstrating its robustness as a predictive tool.

An important caveat to this work is that we used a simple binary accounting for whether an OSN was activated or not, and each panel was conducted at a single concentration (with the exception of a control experiment run at 150 μM, Supplementary Fig. 1). Thus, we did not measure affinity or efficacy as variables. Increasing concentration would likely activate additional receptors and alter the patterns of overlap, although it has been shown that increasing concentration only rarely alters odorant perceptual quality[30]. Although these effects are not uninteresting they would have clouded the main purpose of the present study—to determine the biologically most relevant attribute of related molecules among a group of receptors. In this regard the olfactory system offers a novel forum for evaluating medicinal chemistry strategies because we are not testing various molecules on a single receptor, as is the case in pharmaceutical experiments. In the olfactory system we have a large number (>1,000 in mouse) of G-protein-coupled receptors that are being tested simultaneously with a panel of carefully altered odour compounds. In a sense we are using the receptors simply to 'take a vote,' which is necessarily binary, on the biologically relevant characteristics of a molecule.

Although we can draw no conclusion as to why TPSA should be of special importance there are several interesting speculations. The TPSA is effectively a measure of the solvent accessible surface area presented by a molecule. Given that odorants must pass through both aqueous and lipid environments to access the presumptive binding regions of the receptors, the surface area could raise or lower the entropic cost of accessing that activating region[31]. Access to the receptor, or specific parts of it, may be more crucial in determining the efficacy of a molecule than the particular fit it may make in a presumptive binding pocket. The popular lock and key model of receptor ligand interactions is too naive to capture the biophysical requirements that play a role in how a molecule may interact with and stabilize an activated conformation of the receptor. Bioisosterism is an empiric method for probing and understanding those functional details.

As a bonus, this approach also revealed an extensible rule—that if an OSN accepted both the low TPSA, 6-membered benzene ring and the high TPSA, 5-membered furan ring, then it will always accept the 'intermediate challenge' of a low TPSA, 5-membered thiophene ring. We witnessed this for ketone odorant sets [1], [3], [2] and [7], [9], [8] and acids [10], [11], [12]. This rule joins the electronegativity rule of 'if an OSN accepts a n-alcohol and the homologous n-acid, it will always accept the electronegative intermediate homologous n-aldehyde'[32], and the backbone continuity rule of 'if an OSN accepts a chain length of N and N + 2 in an n-odorant, then it will always accept a chain length of N + 1' (refs 15,33,34). These three rules show that constraints in detection exist, despite the wide diversity of odorants and receptors.

We anticipate that there are other rules to be discovered through application of this medicinal chemistry strategy, and that these rules may be extended to other, non-olfactory, GPCRs. Notions such as broad versus narrow tuning of receptors could be revisited in terms of sensitivity to molecular features rather than molecular compounds. Indeed it might well be worth revisiting the idea of odour primaries (as in colours or fundamentals in sound) that are recombined in innumerable, but comprehensible, ways to provide a rich odour world.

Methods

Chemicals. Two panels of six ketone odorants (Panel 1 and Panel 2) and a panel of three acid odorants (Panel 3) were designed to test the hypothesis that, among odorants, heteroaromatic rings can substitute for benzene rings with ORs exhibiting a predictable preference between them. All panels are derived around a lead odorant, acetophenone [1]. Panel 1 consisted of acetophenone [1], 2-acetylthiophene [2], 2-acetylfuran [3], 2-acetylpyridine [4], 2-acetylthiazole [5] and acetylpyrazine [6]. Panel 2 consisted of acetophenone [1], 2-acetylthiophene [2], 2-acetylfuran [3], 2-acetonaphthone [7], 2-acetyl-benzothiofene [8] and 2-benzofuranyl-methyl-ketone [9]. Panel 3 consisted of acetophenone [1], 2-acetonaphthone [7], 2-naphthoic acid [11], benzo[b]thiophene-2-carboxylic acid [11] and benzo[b]furan-2-carboxylic acid [12]. Odorants [1]–[9] were purchased from Sigma-Aldrich (St Louis, MO, USA). Odorants [10]–[12] were purchased from Acrōs Organics (Thermo Fisher Scientific, New Jersey, USA). Odorant stocks were made in >99% dimethyl sulfoxide (DMSO) (Sigma-Aldrich) and were diluted in freshly prepared Ringer's solution to a final concentration of 30 or 150 μM just before experiments.

Animals and tissue collection. All animal procedures conformed to Columbia University guidelines for care and use of animals. *OMP-Cre*-driven *GCaMP3* mice used in this work were generated by crossing the *OMP-Cre* line (*JAX 006668*) with the *Ai38* line (*RCL-GCaMP3, JAX014538*). In these compound mutant mice, the expression of the genetically encoded calcium sensor GCaMP3 is restricted to the mature olfactory sensory neurons. All mice were reared and maintained in the department animal facility.

Olfactory sensory neurons were isolated from 5 to 8-week old *OMP-Cre*-driven *GCaMP3* male mice with a genotype of $OMP\text{-}Cre^{+/-}$ $GCaMP3^{-/-}$. The mice were overdosed with anaesthetics (ketamine 90 mg kg^{-1}; xylazine 10 mg kg^{-1}, i.p.) and decapitated. The head was cut open sagitally and the septum was removed to expose the medial surface of the olfactory epithelium and turbinates. The olfactory epithelium and turbinates were dissected and collected in divalent-free Ringer's solution (mM: 145 NaCl, 5.6 KCl, 10 Hepes, 10 Glucose, 4 EGTA, pH 7.4). The tissue was incubated at 37 °C for 45 min in 5 ml of divalent-free Ringer's solution containing 0.5 mg ml^{-1} collagenase, 5 mg ml^{-1} bovine serum albumin (Sigma-Aldrich), 8 U ml^{-1} dispase (Roche, Bassel, Switzerland) and 50 μg ml^{-1} deoxyribonuclease II (Sigma). The tissue was then transferred to a clean tube of culture medium and washed. The OSNs were dissociated by tapping the tube containing the tissue. The OSNs (50 μl volume) were split onto four concanavalin-coated glass coverslips (Sigma-Aldrich, 10 mg ml^{-1}), placed in 35 mm Petri dishes. After allowing the cells to settle for 20 min, 2 ml of culture medium was added to each dish and the dishes were placed at 37 °C for at least 1 h. Culture medium consisted of DMEM/F12 (Gibco BRL, Grand Island, NY, USA) supplemented with 10% fetal bovine serum, 1 × insulin-transferrin-selenium (Gibco BRL), 100 U ml^{-1} penicillin and 100 μg ml^{-1} streptomycin (Gibco BRL) and 100 μM ascorbic acid (Sigma-Aldrich).

Calcium imaging recording. After being washed with fresh Ringer's solution, the coverslips were mounted on a recording chamber. Imaging was carried out at room temperature on an inverted fluorescence microscope (IMT-Olympus, Tokyo, Japan) equipped with a SIT camera (C10600, Hamamatsu Photonics, Hamamatsu, Japan), a Lambda XL light source (Sutter Instrument, Novato, CA, USA), and Lamba-10B optical filter changer (Sutter Instrument). Using a 1260 Infinity HPLC system (Agilent Technologies, Santa Clara, CA, USA) the dissociated OSNs were stimulated with the odorants in random order between two flanking stimulations with the lead odorant, [1]. A final stimulation with a 10 μM Forskolin (Sigma-Aldrich) solution was made to assess the viability of the OSNs. Recordings were made at 490 nm excitation and 520 nm emission. Images were taken every 4 s and there was a 4 min delay between stimulations. The images were then computed using Metamorph Premier software (Molecular Device LLC, Downingtown, PA, USA) and the cells were manually counted.

Data analysis of calcium imaging recording. 1,666 molecular descriptors for the P1 and P2 odorants were downloaded through e-dragon free applet (http://www.vcclab.org/)[35]. Normalized descriptors were used for calculating Euclidean distances and for generating dendrograms using Matlab (MathWorks, Boston, MA, USA). Neuron responses to Panel 1 or Panel 2 odorants in calcium imaging were transformed to an *m*n* bool matrix where '*m*' is the number of neurons responding to at least one chemical, and '*n*' is the number of chemicals used; '1' means 'response' and '0' means 'no response'. This matrix was used to calculate Euclidean distances and generate dendrograms of the odorants using Matlab. A Coshran's *Q* test comparison followed by *post hoc* McNemar tests was performed to compare the odorant 'response', 'No response' heatmaps using Statview (SAS institute, Cary, NC, USA).

Habituation–dishabituation behavioural test. Similarities in perceptual odour quality among the Panel 1 odorants were evaluated by a habituation–dishabituation olfactory test in the mouse. Thirty minutes before experimentation, 5–8 weeks old $OMP\text{-}Cre^{+/-}$ $GCaMP3^{-/-}$ male mice were placed individually into a hood in an empty mouse cage containing a cotton swab soaked in 1/1,000 DMSO/Ringer's solution. Each animal was then stimulated three consecutive times over 2 min with the DMSO/Ringer's solution soaked cotton swab as a negative control. Then they received three consecutive presentations of a cotton swab soaked in the first odorant solutions at 30 μM. Each presentation lasted 2 min with a 1 min interval between presentations. Following a 1 min rest, animals were then given three presentations of the second odour in a similar manner. Following a final 1-min break, a 30 μM solution of propyl-valerate was given in a 2-min single stimulation as a positive control. The cumulative sniffing time of the cotton swab was recorded using a silent clock. An analysis of variance (ANOVA) statistic comparison, followed by *post hoc* Paired *t*-test, was performed on the results using Statview. Each mouse was used only once with the same odorant. Mice that were unable to detect the first odorant stimulation or that responded to the negative control were removed from further analysis.

References

1. Linnaeus, C. Odores medicamentorum. *Amoen. Acad.* **3,** 183–201 (1756).
2. Zwaardemaker, H. *Die Physiologie des Geruchs* (Рипол Классик, 1895).
3. Dumas, M. J. Ueber die vegetabilischen Substanzen welche sich dem Kampfer nähern, und über einige ätherische Oele. *Annalen der Pharmacie* **6,** 245–258 (1833).
4. Perkin, W. H. VI. On the artificial production of coumarin and formation of its homologues. *J. Chem. Soc.* **21,** 53–63 (1868).
5. Ohloff, G., Pickenhagen, W. & Kraft, P. Scent and chemistry, the molecular world of odors. *Chem. Listy* **106,** 685–692 (2012).
6. Guillot, M. Physiologie des sensations-anosmies partielles et odeurs fondamentales. *C. R. Acad. Sci.* **226,** 1307–1309 (1948).
7. Amoore, J. E. Specific anosmia: a clue to the olfactory code. *Nature* **214,** 1095–1098 (1967).
8. Wise, P. M., Olsson, M. J. & Cain, W. S. Quantification of odor quality. *Chem. Senses* **25,** 429–443 (2000).
9. Buck, L. & Axel, R. A novel multigene family may encode odorant receptors: a molecular basis for odor recognition. *Cell* **65,** 175–187 (1991).
10. Zhang, X., Zhang, X. & Firestein, S. Comparative genomics of odorant and pheromone receptor genes in rodents. *Genomics* **89,** 441–450 (2007).
11. Chess, A., Simon, I., Cedar, H. & Axel, R. Allelic inactivation regulates olfactory receptor gene expression. *Cell* **78,** 823–834 (1994).
12. Serizawa, S. *et al.* Mutually exclusive expression of odorant receptor transgenes. *Nat. Neurosci.* **3,** 687–693 (2000).
13. Serizawa, S., Miyamichi, K. & Sakano, H. One neuron–one receptor rule in the mouse olfactory system. *Trends Genet.* **20,** 648–653 (2004).
14. Zhao, H. *et al.* Functional expression of a mammalian odorant receptor. *Science* **279,** 237–242 (1998).
15. Malnic, B., Hirono, J., Sato, T. & Buck, L. B. Combinatorial receptor codes for odors. *Cell* **96,** 713–723 (1999).
16. Stewart, W. B., Kauer, J. S. & Shepherd, G. M. Functional organization of rat olfactory bulb analysed by the 2-deoxyglucose method. *J. Comp. Neurol.* **185,** 715–734 (1979).
17. Ressler, K. J., Sullivan, S. L. & Buck, L. B. A zonal organization of odorant receptor gene expression in the olfactory epithelium. *Cell* **73,** 597–609 (1993).
18. Mori, K., Nagao, H. & Yoshihara, Y. The olfactory bulb: coding and processing of odor molecule information. *Science* **286,** 711–715 (1999).
19. Touhara, K. *et al.* Functional identification and reconstitution of an odorant receptor in single olfactory neurons. *Proc. Natl Acad. Sci. USA* **96,** 4040–4045 (1999).
20. Fukuda, N., Yomogida, K., Okabe, M. & Touhara, K. Functional characterization of a mouse testicular olfactory receptor and its role in chemosensing and in regulation of sperm motility. *J. Cell Sci.* **117,** 5835–5845 (2004).
21. Saito, H., Chi, Q., Zhuang, H., Matsunami, H. & Mainland, J. D. Odor coding by a mammalian receptor repertoire. *Sci. Signal.* **2,** ra9–ra9 (2009).
22. Grosmaitre, X. *et al.* SR1, a mouse odorant receptor with an unusually broad response profile. *J. Neurosci.* **29,** 14545 (2009).
23. Bushdid, C., Magnasco, M. O., Vosshall, L. B. & Keller, A. Humans can discriminate more than 1 trillion olfactory stimuli. *Science* **343,** 1370–1372 (2014).
24. Meister, M. On the dimensionality of odor space. *eLife* **4,** 1–12 (2015).
25. Bieri, S., Monastyrskaia, K. & Schilling, B. Olfactory receptor neuron profiling using sandalwood odorants. *Chem. Senses* **29,** 483–487 (2004).
26. Schmuker, M., de Bruyne, M., Hahnel, M. & Schneider, G. Predicting olfactory receptor neuron responses from odorant structure. *Chem. Cent. J.* **1,** 11 (2007).
27. Sanz, G. *et al.* Relationships between molecular structure and perceived odor quality of ligands for a human olfactory receptor. *Chem. Senses* **33,** 639–653 (2008).
28. Snitz, K. *et al.* Predicting odor perceptual similarity from odor structure. *PLoS Comput. Biol.* **9,** e1003184 (2013).
29. Sheridan, R. P. The most common chemical replacements in drug-like compounds. *J. Chem. Inf. Comput. Sci.* **42,** 103–108 (2002).
30. Furudono, Y., Sone, Y., Takizawa, K., Hirono, J. & Sato, T. Relationship between peripheral receptor code and perceived odor quality. *Chem. Senses* **34,** 151–158 (2009).
31. Lee, B. & Richards, F. M. The interpretation of protein structures: estimation of static accessibility. *J. Mol. Biol.* **55,** 379–IN374 (1971).
32. Araneda, R. C., Peterlin, Z., Zhang, X., Chesler, A. & Firestein, S. A pharmacological profile of the aldehyde receptor repertoire in rat olfactory epithelium. *J. Physiol.* **555,** 743–756 (2004).
33. Sato, T., Hirono, J., Tonoike, M. & Takebayashi, M. Tuning specificities to aliphatic odorants in mouse olfactory receptor neurons and their local distribution. *J. Neurophysiol.* **72,** 2980–2989 (1994).
34. Kaluza, J. F. & Breer, H. Responsiveness of olfactory neurons to distinct aliphatic aldehydes. *J. Exp. Biol.* **203,** 927–933 (2000).

35. Tetko, I. *et al.* Virtual computational chemistry laboratory—design and description. *J. Comput. Aided Mol. Des.* **19,** 453–463 (2005).
36. Ertl, P., Rohde, B. & Selzer, P. Fast calculation of molecular polar surface area as a sum of fragment-based contributions and its application to the prediction of drug transport properties. *J. Med. Chem.* **43,** 3714–3717 (2000).

Acknowledgements

This research was supported by the NIDCD, R01DC013553. The authors want to thank Christian Margot for his comments on the chemistry and Cen Zhang for her help with the animal facility and lab managing.

Authors contributions

S.F. conceived and supervised the project. E.P. and Z.P. designed the experiments. E.P. conducted the experiments and analysed the results. Z.P. and L.X. helped with chemical classification and analyzes. N.T., A.P. and C.A. helped with behaviour experiment and cell counting. D.-J.Z. developed and maintained mouse line. E.P., Z.P. and S.F. wrote the manuscript. All authors refined the manuscript.

Additional information

Competing financial interests: The authors declare no competing financial interests.

Orthogonal ring-closing alkyne and olefin metathesis for the synthesis of small GTPase-targeting bicyclic peptides

Philipp M. Cromm[1,2], Sebastian Schaubach[2,3], Jochen Spiegel[1,2], Alois Fürstner[2,3], Tom N. Grossmann[2,4,5] & Herbert Waldmann[1,2]

Bicyclic peptides are promising scaffolds for the development of inhibitors of biological targets that proved intractable by typical small molecules. So far, access to bioactive bicyclic peptide architectures is limited due to a lack of appropriate orthogonal ring-closing reactions. Here, we report chemically orthogonal ring-closing olefin (RCM) and alkyne metathesis (RCAM), which enable an efficient chemo- and regioselective synthesis of complex bicyclic peptide scaffolds with variable macrocycle geometries. We also demonstrate that the formed alkyne macrocycle can be functionalized subsequently. The orthogonal RCM/RCAM system was successfully used to evolve a monocyclic peptide inhibitor of the small GTPase Rab8 into a bicyclic ligand. This modified peptide shows the highest affinity for an activated Rab GTPase that has been reported so far. The RCM/RCAM-based formation of bicyclic peptides provides novel opportunities for the design of bioactive scaffolds suitable for the modulation of challenging protein targets.

[1] Department of Chemical Biology, Max-Planck-Institute of Molecular Physiology, Otto-Hahn-Strasse 11, D-44227 Dortmund, Germany. [2] Technische Universität Dortmund, Fakultät für Chemie and Chemische Biologie, Otto-Hahn-Strasse 6, D-44227 Dortmund, Germany. [3] Max-Planck-Institut für Kohlenforschung, Kaiser-Wilhelm-Platz 1, D-45470 Mülheim/Ruhr, Germany. [4] Chemical Genomics Centre of the Max Planck Society, Otto-Hahn-Strasse 15, D-44227 Dortmund, Germany. [5] Department of Chemistry and Pharmaceutical Sciences, VU University Amsterdam, De Boelelaan 1083, 1081 HV Amsterdam, The Netherlands. Correspondence and requests for materials should be addressed to A.F. (email: fuerstner@kofo.mpg.de) or to T.N.G. (email: tom.grossmann@cgc.mpg.de) or to H.W. (email: herbert.waldmann@mpi-dortmund.mpg.de).

Macrocyclic peptides exhibit unique surface recognition properties and allow the stabilization of bioactive peptide conformations resulting in ligands with increased bioactivity and bioavailability[1–5]. Such scaffolds already proved useful for the modulation of biological targets which are intractable by typical small molecules, such as transcription factors and small GTPases[6–12]. Recently, structurally rigid bicyclic peptides obtained mainly by epitope grafting on disulfide-rich frameworks[13,14] or by phage-display screening[15,16] have emerged as particularly interesting inhibitor types. Given the potential of this new chemical modality as scaffold for next-generation therapeutics, the development of efficient synthetic methods that enable the introduction of non-natural fragments into peptidic bicycles is in high demand. This is particularly true for approaches that allow the design of scaffolds that go beyond the size of small epitopes.

For the synthesis of monocyclic peptides, a variety of methods is available[17–25]. Notably, in such peptides, the crosslink itself can directly contribute to bioactivity[26–28]. In this respect, hydrocarbon crosslinks formed by ruthenium-catalysed ring-closing olefin metathesis (RCM) proved particularly successful owing to the hydrophobic and inert character of those crosslinks[2,29]. Prominent examples involve hydrogen bond surrogates[8,30,31] and hydrocarbon stapling[32–35], which have provided a number of potent inhibitors of protein—protein interactions[2]. In these cases, the synthesis of bicyclic architectures requires the presence of multiple olefins, which causes selectivity problems during cyclization[36,37]. Undesired side reactions can be reduced by the selection of appropriate ring sizes and distances[38], by functional group transformations[39] and by tedious fine tuning of olefin reactivity[39]. Thus, only a small set of scaffolds is accessible by multiple RCM reactions[36–40]. This creates the need for synthesis methods that integrate two consecutive, chemically orthogonal metathesis reactions thereby enabling efficient chemo- and regioselective construction of complex bicyclic peptides. Ideally, such methods would be compatible with solid-phase peptide synthesis (SPPS).

Molybdenum-catalysed ring-closing alkyne metathesis[41] (RCAM) shares many of the advantageous properties of RCM, and is in principle chemically orthogonal to ruthenium-catalysed RCM. RCAM has been applied for peptide macrocyclizations in solution[42–44]. However, the synthesis of bicyclic peptides by orthogonal ring-closing olefin and alkyne metathesis has not been explored so far. Here, we report the solid-phase synthesis of bicyclic peptides by means of orthogonal ring-closing olefin- and alkyne-metathesis reactions. We demonstrate that the alkyne macrocycle can be further functionalized selectively. The orthogonal RCM/RCAM system was successfully used to evolve a monocyclic peptide inhibitor of the small GTPase Rab8 into a bicyclic ligand with increased target affinity.

Results

RCAM and functionalization on solid support. To explore RCAM-based macrocyclization of peptides on solid support (Fig. 1a), two α-methyl-α-alkynyl building blocks (**1–4**) of varying linker length and configuration (Fig. 1b) were introduced into model peptides using Fmoc-based SPPS. Peptide sequences, architectures and relative spacing of non-natural amino acids ($i,i+3$, $i,i+4$ and $i,i+7$) were selected by analogy to previously explored RCM-based peptide macrocyclizations[33]. As proof-of-concept and to test the robustness of the reaction, we designed model peptides that contain all functionalities present among the 20 proteinogenic amino acids and yield macrocyclic peptides **7–9** after RCAM (Fig. 2a). Investigation of various RCAM conditions including the latest generation of stable Mo-complexes[45,46] (Supplementary Table 1) revealed efficient conversions after 3 h at 40 °C in toluene if Tentagel rink amide resin and complex **5** (Fig. 1a) were used (Supplementary Figs 2–5, Supplementary Table 2). Under these conditions, macrocycles were formed for all three architectures (**7–9**) with the best results obtained for an $i,i+4$ geometry and a final crosslink of nine carbon atoms (**8**). Shortening the hydrocarbon bridge from nine to eight carbon atoms reduces the efficiency of the reaction presumably due to increased ring strain (Supplementary Fig. 4).

Selective functionalization of the alkyne linker embedded in the macrocycle was achieved, after treatment of macrocyclic peptide **11** with $CuBr_2$ in dry acetonitrile on solid support to yield dibrominated olefin **12** (Fig. 2b). Notably, the reaction can be performed conveniently with different resin-bound peptides (for all tested architectures: $i,i+3$, $i,i+4$ and $i,i+7$) using standard syringe reactors (Supplementary Figs 6–8, Supplementary Table 2). Full conversion in the dibromination reaction is only achieved after multiple treatments with $CuBr_2$ and for peptides that lack the two N-terminal sulfur containing amino acids (Cys and Met).

Bicyclic peptide synthesis via orthogonal RCM and RCAM. To determine whether RCM and RCAM can be performed orthogonally within one peptide sequence (Fig. 3a), peptide **16** was synthesized which embodies two alkyne-functionalized building blocks (**1** and **2**) in $i,i+4$-position at the carboxy (C) terminus, and two olefin-containing amino acids (**6**, Fig. 1b) in $i,i+4$-position at the amino (N) terminus (Fig. 3b). In peptide **16**, an olefin macrocycle can be formed next to an alkyne-bearing macrocycle (Fig. 3b). The treatment of immobilized precursor peptide **13** (blue peak) with either complex **5** or Grubbs first-generation catalyst leads to selective formation of the alkyne (**14**, red peak) and olefin macrocycle (**15**, orange peak), respectively (Fig. 3b, Supplementary Figs 9 and 10). HPLC-MS analyses of the alkyne and olefin crosslinked intermediates (**14** and **15**) reveal highly selective formation of the desired macrocycle without formation of an alternative cyclization product (Supplementary Fig. 10). Both monocycles can be converted into the bicyclic product **16** by means of the second metathesis reaction. This result is remarkable since previous attempts of orthogonal macrocycle formation within peptides failed[44], but were successful only for the assembly of simple building blocks[47]. In an even more demanding set-up, the simultaneous closure of both macrocycles in a one-pot reaction was tested (instead of the previous sequential synthesis). Strikingly, treatment of the open peptide precursor **13** with a mixture of complex **5** and Grubbs first-generation catalyst also yields the desired bicyclic peptide **16** (green peak, Fig. 3b and Supplementary Fig. 10).

In peptide **16**, the two individual macrocycles are sequentially arranged along the amino acid chain, that is, the two individual macrocycles are linked by a linear amino acid sequence. A synthetically more challenging setup involves the synthesis of two entangled macrocyles resulting in more constrained peptide scaffolds (for example, peptide **17**, Fig. 4). In this architecture, an edge-on bimacrocycle structure is generated as opposed to a linear macrocycle arrangement as in peptide **16**. Most notably, entangled bicyclic peptide **17** (Fig. 4) was also efficiently formed in both the sequential as well as the one-pot synthesis (Supplementary Figs 11 and 12).

Bicyclic ligands of the small GTPase Rab8. To demonstrate the potential of this robust orthogonal RCM/RCAM macrocyclization, we aimed at the improvement of a monocyclic bioactive peptide targeting a challenging protein. Small GTPases comprise a protein superfamily with clinically highly relevant, yet

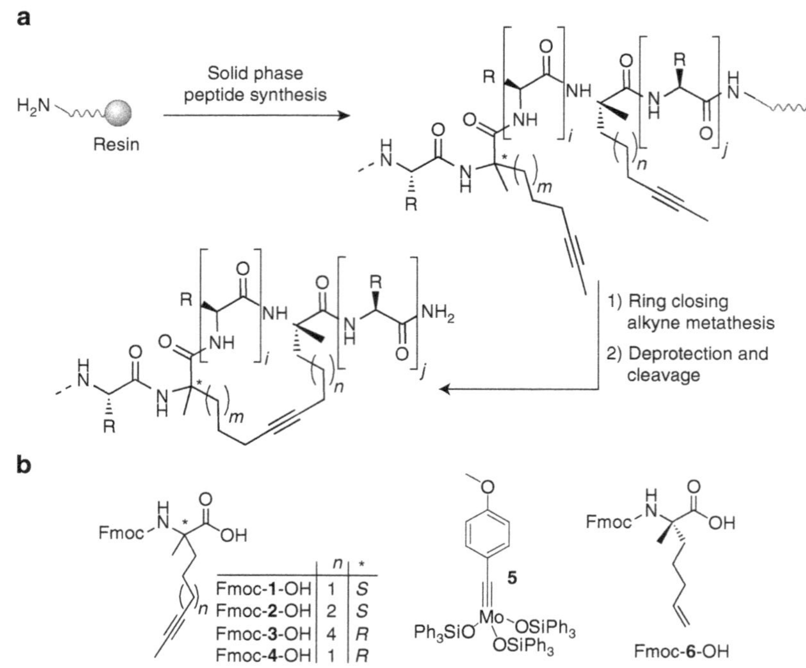

Figure 1 | Alkyne macrocyclization. (**a**) The linear peptide is assembled via SPPS including the incorporation of two α-methylated-α-alkynylated building blocks (**1-4**). The C-terminal building block is always (*S*)-configured, the configuration of the N-terminal building block varies between the different architectures. Complex **5** is used to perform the RCAM reaction. ($i = 2, 3, 6$, number of amino acids between non-natural building blocks; $j = 3, 6$; $m = 1, 2, 4$; $n = 1, 2$; R = side chain of a proteinogenic amino acid) (**b**) Fluorenylmethoxycarbonyl (Fmoc) protected non-natural amino acids incorporated into the peptide sequence (alkyne: **1-4**, olefin: **6**). The alkyne building blocks **1-4** are either used in the (*S*)- or (*R*)-configuration depending on the macrocycle architecture. Mo-complex (**5**) used for RCAM.

particularly challenging, drug targets[48–54]. Despite enormous efforts, no efficient inhibitors of small GTPases have reached clinical trials. Importantly, the target affinity of small molecule modulators typically does not exceed the low-to-medium micromolar range[50,51]. Among the small GTPase superfamily, Rab proteins (Ras-related in brain) constitute key regulators of intracellular vesicular transport and trafficking[55,56]. As starting point for the generation of a bicyclic peptide, we selected the hydrocarbon-stapled monocyclic peptide **StRIP3,** which binds the small GTPase Rab8a with moderate affinity (dissociation constant (K_d) = 20.7 μM, Table 1, entry 2)[12]. **StRIP3** resembles the only known inhibitor of a Rab protein–protein interaction[12] and is based on the interaction motif of Rab6-interacting protein 1 (**wt-R6IP**, Table 1, entry 1)[57]. Initially, alkyne-bearing macrocycles based on **StRIP3** were explored in which the $i,i+4$ olefin crosslink was replaced by alkynes with varying crosslink length (9–10 carbon atoms, Table 1, entry 3–5). The 10-carbon crosslink requires double incorporation of building block **2** (entry 3). A nine-carbon crosslink is generated by incorporation of two different building blocks (**1** and **2**), which results in two different architectures (entry 4: **1/2**, entry 5: **2/1**). The synthesis of an eight-carbon crosslinked **StRIP3** derivative containing building block **1** twice was not possible, most likely due to high ring strain caused by the linear geometry of the triple bond.

In addition, dibrominated (entry 6–8) and bicyclic peptides (entry 9–14) were synthesized resulting in a total of 12 **StRIP3** derivatives grouped into four subfamilies (Table 1, Supplementary Table 3): (i) alkyne mono-macrocyclic peptides **18–20** (entry 3–5); (ii) dibrominated olefin macrocyclic peptides **21–23** (entry 6–8); (iii) orthogonally macrocyclized peptides **24–26** carrying the original olefin crosslink and an additional alkyne crosslink at the C terminus (entry 9–11); and (iv) bicyclic peptides **27–29** with exchanged positions for the alkyne and the olefin crosslink (entry 12–14). Since the N-terminal part of parent peptide **StRIP3** is already constrained by the olefin macrocycle, we aimed for the introduction of a new macrocycle in the C-terminal part. We reasoned that additional constraint could further stabilize the bioactive peptide conformation. Owing to a lack of structural information, it is not obvious which amino acids are directly involved in Rab-binding. For this reason, we selected two amino acids with hydrophobic side chains (L911 and A915) for macrocycle introduction as their non-polar side chains are potentially mimicked by the hydrocarbon macrocycle. All the peptides were synthesized via SPPS and modified with an N-terminal fluorescein–polyethyleneglycol label (Supplementary Table 3) to enable determination of their binding affinity towards activated Rab8a$_{6\text{-}176}$(GppNHp) in a fluorescence polarization (FP) assay (Supplementary Fig. 13). After initial ranking of the peptides by means of relative K_d values (rel. K_d, Table 1, Supplementary Table 4), the affinity of the best binders (peptide **21**, **25** and **28**) was determined in an independent FP assay run in triplicates (Table 1, Supplementary Fig. 14). Replacement of the olefin by an alkyne crosslink yields peptides **18–20** with affinities comparable to **StRIP3**. In contrast, the dibrominated olefin derivatives **21–23** show improved affinity towards Rab8a$_{6\text{–}176}$ with peptide **21** being the most potent binder within this subfamily (K_d = 10.7 μM, Table 1). Peptide **21** shows a 2-fold increased binding affinity when compared with **StRIP3.** Notably, an even higher improvement in binding affinity to Rab8a$_{6\text{–}176}$(GppNHp) is observed for two of the bicyclic peptides **24–29,** namely peptide **25** and **28** (Table 1 and Supplementary Table 4). In both the cases, the nine-carbon alkyne crosslink

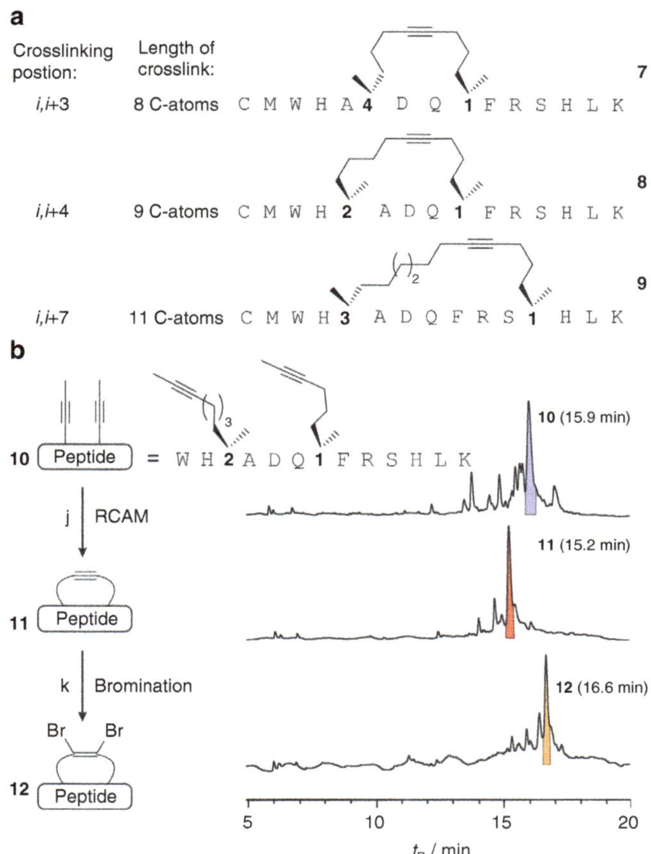

Figure 2 | Ring-closing alkyne metathesis on solid support. (**a**) Sequences of peptides **7-9** containing different macrocylic architectures. (**b**) Sequence of peptide **10** with non-natural amino acids **1** and **2** at position *i* and *i* + 4 (nine-carbon crosslink) with corresponding chromatograms of crude reaction mixtures before (**10**, top) and after RCAM (**11**, middle) and after dibromination (**12**, bottom). Corresponding product peaks are highlighted: open (**10**, blue), closed (**11**, red) and dibrominated (**12**, orange) macrocycle. Chromatograms were obtained after deprotection and release of intermediates from the resin. 'j' represents Complex **5**, dry toluene, 40 °C, 2 × 1.5 h; 'k' represents $CuBr_2$, dry MeCN, 3 × 1 h.

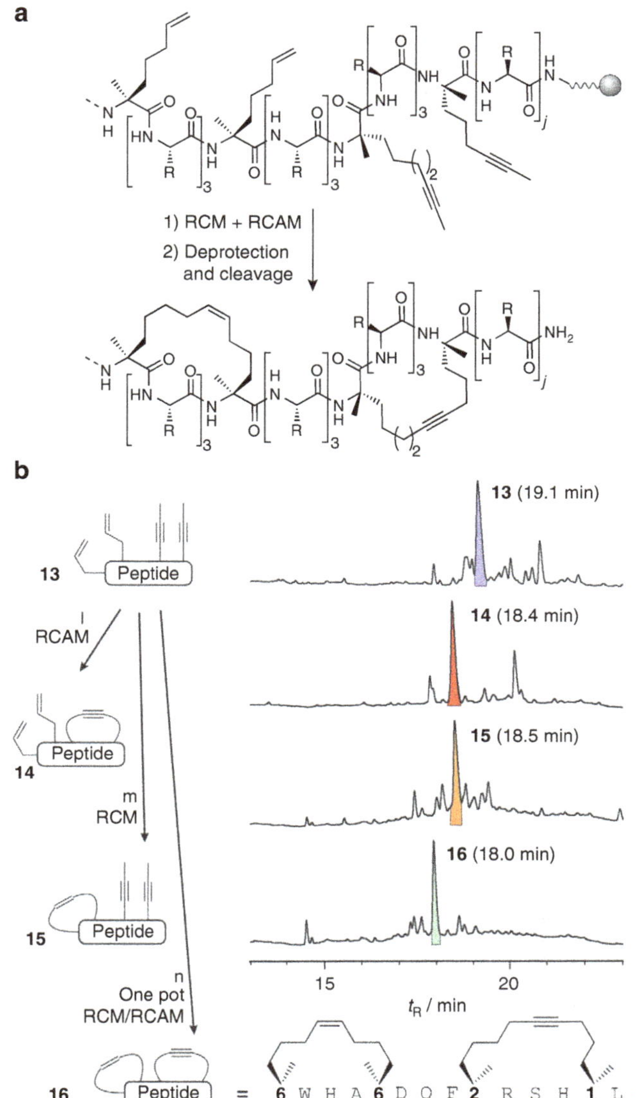

Figure 3 | Solid phase synthesis of bicyclic peptides by means of the RCM/RCAM method. (**a**) General scheme for the synthesis of bicyclic peptides obtained by means of RCM and RCAM of the acyclic precursor peptides. (j = 2, number of C-terminal amino acids; R = side chain of a proteinogenic amino acid except Cys or Met). (**b**) Sequence of bicyclic test peptide **16** bearing an $i,i+4$ olefin crosslink (eight C-atoms) and an $i,i+4$ alkyne crosslink (nine C-atoms). Chromatograms of crude reaction mixtures of peptide **16** before macrocyclization (**13**, top), after RCAM (**14**, second) and RCM (**15**, third), respectively, and after simultaneous (one-pot) RCM and RCAM (**16**, bottom). Corresponding product peaks are highlighted: fully open (**13**, blue), alkyne monocycle (**14**, red), olefin monocycle (**15**, orange) and bicyclic peptide (**16**, green). Chromatograms were obtained after deprotection and cleavage of resin-bound intermediates. 'l' represents Complex **5**, dry toluene, 40 °C, 2 × 1.5 h; 'm' represents Grubbs first-generation catalyst, DCE, 3 × 2 h; 'n' represents Complex **5**, Grubbs first-generation catalyst, dry toluene, 40 °C, 2 × 1.5 h.

(with **1** at N-terminal and **2** at C-terminal position within the sequence) provides the most potent architecture resulting in two significantly improved ligands for activated Rab8a$_{6-176}$ (K_d[**25**] = 6.6 μM; K_d[**28**] = 9.6 μM). Bicyclic peptide **25** (Fig. 5a) is more than three times more potent than the parent hydrocarbon stapled peptide **StRIP3** and displays a more than 15-fold increased binding affinity compared with the unmodified wild-type peptide **wt-R6IP**. Binding affinity of peptide **25** was confirmed in microscale thermophoresis measurements. On the basis of fluorescence intensity, an affinity for Rab8a$_{6-176}$(GppNHp) was observed (K_d[**25**] = 11 μM, Supplementary Table 5, Supplementary Figs 15 and 16), which is in the range of our FP measurements (K_d[**25**] = 6.6 μM, see above). In addition, FP competition experiments were performed using a complex between labelled peptide **25** and Rab8a$_{6-176}$(GppNHp), which was treated with an excess of acetylated **StRIP3**. In this setup, we observed full displacement of peptide **25** (IC_{50} = 33 μM, red Fig. 5b). As one would expect, the acetylated low-affinity peptide **wt-R6IP** does not compete with peptide **25** (black, Fig. 5b). These results verify reversible binding of peptide **25** to the same site on Rab8 as parent peptide **StRIP3**.

Discussion

We identified conditions that enable the performance of RCAM reactions in conjunction with SPPS allowing alkyne-based macrocyclization of peptide sequences involving all natural side-chain functionalities. Subsequent functionalization of the alkyne allows further modification of the macrocycle, which opens new perspectives in the design of macrocyclic scaffolds. In addition, we report the chemo- and regioselective synthesis of bicyclic peptides bearing an alkyne as well as an olefin crosslink accessible via orthogonal ring-closing olefin and alkyne metathesis on solid support. This approach allows direct control of the individual macrocyclization reaction and enables the formation of bicyclic peptides with novel architectures combining two different macrocycles within the same peptide sequence. The applicability of such scaffolds for highly challenging targets, such as small GTPases, was demonstrated via identification of the currently most potent binder of an activated Rab GTPase (peptide **25**, $K_d = 6.6\,\mu M$). Since the bioactivity of a peptide is mainly determined by its secondary structure[1,2], alkyne macrocyclization and the orthogonal introduction of bicyclic alkyne/olefin macrocycles within the same peptide sequence give rise to novel constrained peptide architectures with high potential for the targeting of currently intractable proteins.

17 Peptide = W H **2** A **6** D **1** Q **6** F R S H L K

Figure 4 | Sequence and chemical structure of the engulfed bicyclic peptide 17. R, side chain of a proteinogenic amino acid except Cys or Met.

a

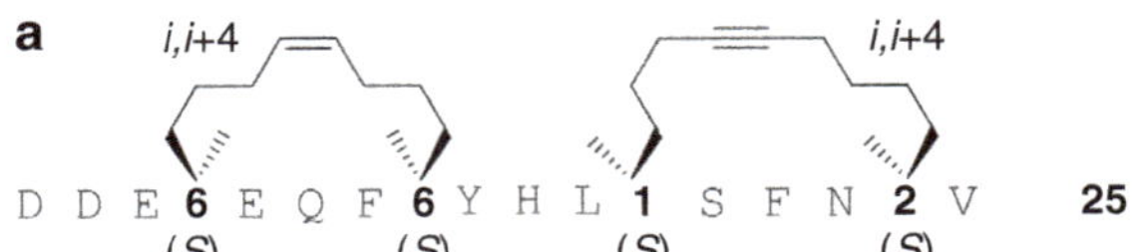

b

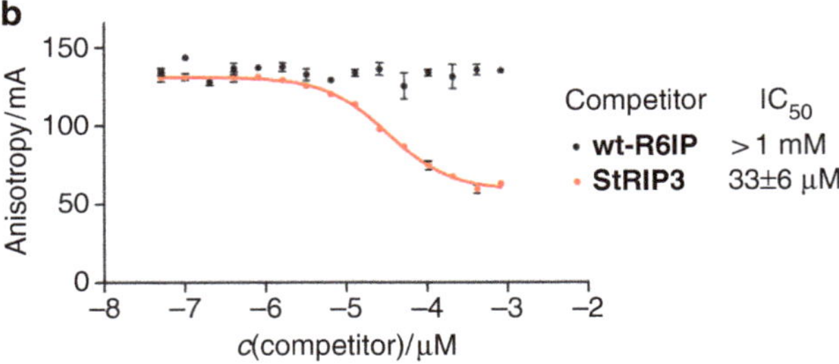

Figure 5 | Sequence and binding studies of peptide 25. (**a**) Sequence of bicyclic peptide **25** showing highest affinity for Rab8a$_{6-176}$(GppNHp). (**b**) Competition of fluorescein-labelled peptide **25** (60 nM) bound to Rab8a(GppNHp; 15 μM) with increasing concentrations of acetylated peptides **StRIP3** and **wt-R6IP** (competitors). Errors represent 1σ of triplicates.

Methods

General. For abbreviations and detailed information about the experimental procedures, analytical data and FP binding curves, see Supplementary Figs 1–16, Supplementary Tables 1–5, Supplementary Note 1 and Supplementary Methods.

Synthesis of building blocks 1-4. Synthesis of the Fmoc protected building blocks **1–4** was performed according to adapted protocols using Ni(II)-BPB ((*R/S*)-2-[N-(N′-benzylpropyl)amino]benzophenone) complexes[58,59]. For a detailed description of building block synthesis and analytical data, see Supplementary Methods.

Peptide synthesis. Peptides were synthesized according to standard Fmoc-chemistry for SPPS using HCTU (*O*-(6-chlorobenzotriazol-1-yl)-*N,N,N′*,

Table 1 | Small GTPase targeting peptides.

900 905 910 915
D D E [K] E Q F [L] Y H L [L] S F N [A] V **wtR6IP**

Entry	Peptide	aa 903	aa 907	aa 911	aa 915	Rel. K_d	K_d (μM)
1	**wt-R6IP**	K	L	L	A	ND	>100
2	**StRIP3**	6	6	L	A	1.00	20.7 ± 0.7
3	**18**	2	2	L	A	0.92	ND
4	**19**	1	2	L	A	0.99	ND
5	**20**	2	1	L	A	0.89	ND
6	**21***	2	2	L	A	0.40	10.7 ± 0.5***
7	**22***	1	2	L	A	0.46	ND
8	**23***	2	1	L	A	0.52	ND
9	**24**	6	6	2	2	0.43	ND
10	**25**	6	6	1	2	0.27	6.6 ± 0.4***
11	**26**	6	6	2	1	0.44	ND
12	**27**	2	2	6	6	0.44	ND
13	**28**	1	2	6	6	0.42	9.6 ± 0.4***
14	**29**	2	1	6	6	0.56	ND

ND, not determined. Wild-type sequence of linear starting sequence **wtRIP** (aa 900-916 of Rab6 interacting protein) with table of mono- and bicyclic peptide derivatives. Peptides were synthesized using SPPS, macrocyclized and N-terminally labelled with a fluorescein-polyethylene glycol conjugate. Affinities towards Rab8a$_{6-176}$(GppNHp) were determined via fluorescence polarization (FP) assays (rel. $K_d = K_d$ [Peptide]/K_d [StRIP3] (these K_d-values are single point measurements)). Given K_d-values are average of triplicate measurements (errors account for 1σ). ***$P < 0.001$.
*Dibrominated olefin.

N′-tetramethyluronium hexafluorophosphate) and COMU (1-[(1-(cyano-2-ethoxy-2-oxoethylidenaminooxy)-dimethylaminomorpholino)]-uronium hexafluorophosphate) as coupling reagents (Supplementary Fig. 1). For more detailed information about peptide synthesis, see Supplementary Methods and Supplementary Tables 2 and 3.

Ring-closing alkyne metathesis. The dried resin was swollen and shrunken under argon alternating in dry diethyl ether and dry toluene (3 × each). Afterwards 0.5 ml of a solution of the alkyne-metathesis complex **5** (2 mg ml^{-1}) in dry toluene was added and the reaction mixture was stirred at 40 °C for 1.5 h. During the reaction time, argon was bubbled through the reaction mixture to evaporate the 2-butyne. After addition of 0.5 ml of fresh complex **5** solution, the mixture was stirred at 40 °C for 1.5 h.

Ring-closing olefin metathesis. The dried resin was swollen in 1,2-dichloroethane (DCE) for 15 min. Subsequently, 0.5 ml of a solution of Grubbs first-generation catalyst (2 mg ml^{-1}) in DCE was added to the resin and reacted for 2 h at room temperature. During the reaction time, argon was bubbled through the reaction mixture to remove ethene. The procedure was repeated twice.

One-pot ring-closing alkyne and olefin metathesis. The dried resin was swollen and shrunken under argon alternating in dry diethyl ether and dry toluene (3 × each). Afterwards 0.5 ml of a solution of the alkyne-metathesis complex **5** (2 mg ml^{-1}) and Grubbs first-generation catalyst (2 mg ml^{-1}) in dry toluene was added and the reaction mixture stirred at 40 °C for 1.5 h. During the reaction time, argon was bubbled through the reaction mixture to evaporate 2-butyne and ethene. After the addition of 0.5 ml of fresh complex solution (alkyne complex **5** and Grubbs first-generation catalyst), the mixture was stirred at 40 °C for 1.5 h.

Dibromination of alkyne macrocycles. The dried resin was swollen in dry MeCN for 15 min and treated with a mixture of $CuBr_2$ in dry MeCN (2 mg ml^{-1}) for 2 h. The reaction was performed in a Syringe reactor and the procedure was repeated twice.

Protein expression and purification. The expression and purification of Rab8a$_{6-176}$ was performed by analogy to full-length Rab8a according to established protocols[60,61].

Nucleotide exchange. Nucleotide exchange was performed according to previously established protocols[60,62]. Briefly, for nucleotide removal, Mg^{2+} was removed by the addition of a 5-fold excess of EDTA and reacted for 1 h at room temperature. The protein solution was desalted using a PD-10 desalting column Sephadex G-25 DNA Grade (GE Healthcare) with elution buffer consisting of 20 mM HEPES (pH 7.5), 50 mM NaCl, 1 mM TCEP. After removal of Mg^{2+}, the protein was diluted to 80–100 μM before the addition of $ZnCl_2$ (500 μM) and $(NH_4)_2SO_4$ (200 mM). After the addition of alkaline phosphatase (5 U mg^{-1}Rab protein), the mixture was incubated for 16 h at 4 °C. For nucleotide exchange, the mixture contained a 5-fold excess of GppNHp during alkaline phosphatase incubation. Afterwards, the mixture was desalted using a PD-10 desalting column Sephadex G-25 DNA Grade (GE Healthcare) with elution buffer consisting of 25 mM HEPES (pH 7.5) 150 mM NaCl, 1 mM TCEP, 1 mM $MgCl_2$ and 1 μM GppNHp.

Fluorescence polarization assay. Rab8a$_{6-176}$(GppNHp) was serially diluted in a buffer containing 25 mM HEPES (pH 7.5), 150 mM NaCl, 1 mM $MgCl_2$, 1 mM TCEP, 0.01% Tween 20 and 1 μM GppNHp, treated with 66 nM fluorescein-labelled peptides and incubated for 4 h at room temperature. Fluorescence polarization values ($\lambda_{ex} = 470$ nm, $\lambda_{em} = 525$ nm) were determined at room temperature. Initial studies for alkyne macrocyclized peptides were performed as single measurements. Final affinity measurements of a subset of peptides were performed in triplicates. After correction for changes in fluorescence intensity upon binding, the fluorescence anisotoropy data were converted into fraction bound of the FITC-labelled peptide and fitted to a one-site binding model derived from the law of mass action using K_d as the only fitting parameter (for details, see Supplementary Methods)[63]. Nonlinear regression was performed in Prism 5.0 (Graphpad)[64].

Competition fluorescence polarization assay. Acetylated peptides were serially diluted and incubated with a mixture of the fluorescein-labelled peptide and Rab8a$_{6-176}$ (GppNHp) at room temperature for 1 h. Fluorescence polarization was determined and IC_{50} values were calculated by nonlinear regression analysis using Prism 5.0 software (GraphPad)[64].

References

1. Bock, J. E., Gavenonis, J. & Kritzer, J. A. Getting in shape: controlling peptide bioactivity and bioavailability using conformational constraints. *ACS Chem. Biol.* **8,** 488–499 (2013).
2. Pelay-Gimeno, M., Glas, A., Koch, O. & Grossmann, T. N. Structure-based design of inhibitors of protein-protein interactions: mimicking peptide binding epitopes. *Angew. Chem. Int. Ed.* **54,** 8896–8927 (2015).
3. Hill, T. A., Shepherd, N. E., Diness, F. & Fairlie, D. P. Constraining cyclic peptides to mimic protein structure motifs. *Angew. Chem. Int. Ed.* **53,** 13020–13041 (2014).
4. Mas-Moruno, C., Rechenmacher, F. & Kessler, H. Cilengitide: the first anti-angiogenic small molecule drug candidate. design, synthesis and clinical evaluation. *Anticancer Agents Med. Chem.* **10,** 753–768 (2010).
5. Srinivas, N. *et al.* Peptidomimetic antibiotics target outer-membrane biogenesis in *Pseudomonas aeruginosa. Science* **327,** 1010–1013 (2010).
6. Leshchiner, E. S. *et al.* Direct inhibition of oncogenic KRAS by hydrocarbon-stapled SOS1 helices. *Proc. Natl Acad. Sci. USA* **112,** 1761–1766 (2015).
7. Moellering, R. E. *et al.* Direct inhibition of the NOTCH transcription factor complex. *Nature* **462,** 182–188 (2009).
8. Patgiri, A., Yadav, K. K., Arora, P. S. & Bar-Sagi, D. An orthosteric inhibitor of the Ras-Sos interaction. *Nat. Chem. Biol.* **7,** 585–587 (2011).
9. Grossmann, T. N. *et al.* Inhibition of oncogenic Wnt signaling through direct targeting of β-catenin. *Proc. Natl Acad. Sci. USA* **109,** 17942–17947 (2012).
10. Upadhyaya, P. *et al.* Inhibition of Ras signaling by blocking Ras-effector interactions with cyclic peptides. *Angew. Chem. Int. Ed.* **54,** 7602–7606 (2015).
11. Giordanetto, F. & Kihlberg, J. Macrocyclic drugs and clinical candidates: what can medicinal chemists learn from their properties? *J. Med. Chem.* **57,** 278–295 (2014).
12. Spiegel, J. *et al.* Direct targeting of Rab-GTPase-effector interactions. *Angew. Chem. Int. Ed.* **53,** 2498–2503 (2014).
13. Northfield, S. E. *et al.* Disulfide-rich macrocyclic peptides as templates in drug design. *Eur. J. Med. Chem.* **77,** 248–257 (2014).
14. Poth, A. G., Chan, L. Y. & Craik, D. J. Cyclotides as grafting frameworks for protein engineering and drug design applications. *Biopolymers* **100,** 480–491 (2013).
15. Heinis, C., Rutherford, T., Freund, S. & Winter, G. Phage-encoded combinatorial chemical libraries based on bicyclic peptides. *Nat. Chem. Biol.* **5,** 502–507 (2009).
16. Baeriswyl, V. & Heinis, C. Polycyclic peptide therapeutics. *Chem. Med. Chem.* **8,** 377–384 (2013).
17. White, C. J. & Yudin, A. K. Contemporary strategies for peptide macrocyclization. *Nat. Chem.* **3,** 509–524 (2011).
18. Montalbetti, C. A. & Falque, V. Amide bond formation and peptide coupling. *Tetrahedron* **61,** 10827–10852 (2005).
19. Góngora-Benítez, M., Tulla-Puche, J. & Albericio, F. Multifaceted roles of disulfide bonds. peptides as therapeutics. *Chem. Rev.* **114,** 901–926 (2014).
20. Assem, N., Ferreira, D. J., Wolan, D. W. & Dawson, P. E. Acetone-linked peptides: a convergent approach for peptide macrocyclization and labeling. *Angew. Chem. Int. Ed.* **54,** 8665–8668 (2015).
21. Wang, Y. & Chou, D. H.-C. A thiol-ene coupling approach to native peptide stapling and macrocyclization. *Angew. Chem. Int. Ed.* **54,** 10931–10934 (2015).
22. Lau, Y. H., Andrade, P., de McKenzie, G. J., Venkitaraman, A. R. & Spring, D. R. Linear aliphatic dialkynes as alternative linkers for double-click stapling of p53-derived peptides. *ChemBioChem.* **15,** 2680–2683 (2014).
23. Lau, Y. H. *et al.* Double strain-promoted macrocyclization for the rapid selection of cell-active stapled peptides. *Angew. Chem. Int. Ed.* **54,** 15410–15413 (2015).
24. Mendive-Tapia, L. *et al.* New peptide architectures through C-H activation stapling between tryptophan-phenylalanine/tyrosine residues. *Nat. Commun.* **6,** 7160 (2015).
25. Lau, Y. H., Andrade, P., de Wu, Y. & Spring, D. R. Peptide stapling techniques based on different macrocyclisation chemistries. *Chem. Soc. Rev.* **44,** 91–102 (2015).
26. Baek, S. *et al.* Structure of the stapled p53 peptide bound to Mdm2. *J. Am. Chem. Soc.* **134,** 103–106 (2012).
27. Phillips, C. *et al.* Design and structure of stapled peptides binding to estrogen receptors. *J. Am. Chem. Soc.* **133,** 9696–9699 (2011).
28. Glas, A. *et al.* Constrained peptides with target-adapted cross-links as inhibitors of a pathogenic protein-protein interaction. *Angew. Chem. Int. Ed.* **53,** 2489–2493 (2014).
29. Pérez de Vega, M. J., García-Aranda, M. I. & González-Muñiz, R. A role for ring-closing metathesis in medicinal chemistry: mimicking secondary architectures in bioactive peptides. *Med. Res. Rev.* **31,** 677–715 (2011).
30. Wang, D., Chen, K., Kulp, J. L. & Arora, P. S. Evaluation of biologically relevant short alpha-helices stabilized by a main-chain hydrogen-bond surrogate. *J. Am. Chem. Soc.* **128,** 9248–9256 (2006).
31. Mahon, A. B. & Arora, P. S. End-capped α-helices as modulators of protein function. *Drug Discov. Today Technol.* **9,** e57–e62 (2012).

32. Cromm, P. M., Spiegel, J. & Grossmann, T. N. Hydrocarbon stapled peptides as modulators of biological function. *ACS Chem. Biol.* **10,** 1362–1375 (2015).
33. Kim, Y.-W., Grossmann, T. N. & Verdine, G. L. Synthesis of all-hydrocarbon stapled α-helical peptides by ring-closing olefin metathesis. *Nat. Protoc.* **6,** 761–771 (2011).
34. Blackwell, H. E. & Grubbs, R. H. Highly efficient synthesis of covalently cross-linked peptide helices by ring-closing metathesis. *Angew. Chem. Int. Ed.* **37,** 3281–3284 (1998).
35. Schafmeister, C. E., Po, J. & Verdine, G. L. An all-hydrocarbon cross-linking system for enhancing the helicity and metabolic stability of peptides. *J. Am. Chem. Soc.* **122,** 5891–5892 (2000).
36. Ghalit, N., Rijkers, D. T. S., Kemmink, J., Versluis, C. & Liskamp, R. M. J. Pre-organization induced synthesis of a crossed alkene-bridged nisin Z DE-ring mimic by ring-closing metathesis. *Chem. Commun.* 192–194 (2005).
37. Slootweg, J. C., Kemmink, J., Liskamp, R. M. J. & Rijkers, D. T. Synthesis and structural characterization of the individual diastereoisomers of a cross-stapled alkene-bridged nisin DE-ring mimic. *Org. Biomol. Chem.* **11,** 7486–7496 (2013).
38. Bird, G. H. *et al.* Hydrocarbon double-stapling remedies the proteolytic instability of a lengthy peptide therapeutic. *Proc. Natl Acad. Sci. USA* **107,** 14093–14098 (2010).
39. Robinson, A. J. *et al.* Regioselective formation of interlocked dicarba bridges in naturally occurring cyclic peptide toxins using olefin metathesis. *Chem. Commun.* **28,** 4293–4295 (2009).
40. Hilinski, G. J. *et al.* Stitched α-helical peptides via bis ring-closing metathesis. *J. Am. Chem. Soc.* **136,** 12314–12322 (2014).
41. Fürstner, A. Alkyne metathesis on the rise. *Angew. Chem. Int. Ed.* **52,** 2794–2819 (2013).
42. Aguilera, B. *et al.* Synthesis of diaminosuberic acid derivatives via ring-closing alkyne metathesis. *J. Org. Chem.* **66,** 3584–3589 (2001).
43. IJsselstijn, M. *et al.* Ring-closing alkyne metathesis mediated synthesis of cyclic β-turn mimetics. *Tetrahedron Lett.* **45,** 4379–4382 (2004).
44. Ghalit, N., Poot, A. J., Fürstner, A., Rijkers, D. T. S. & Liskamp, R. M. J. Ring-closing alkyne metathesis approach toward the synthesis of alkyne mimics of thioether A-, B-, C-, and DE-ring systems of the lantibiotic nisin Z. *Org. Lett.* **7,** 2961–2964 (2005).
45. Heppekausen, J. *et al.* Optimized synthesis, structural investigations, ligand tuning and synthetic evaluation of silyloxy-based alkyne metathesis catalysts. *Chem. Eur. J.* **18,** 10281–10299 (2012).
46. Heppekausen, J., Stade, R., Goddard, R. & Fürstner, A. Practical new silyloxy-based alkyne metathesis catalysts with optimized activity and selectivity profiles. *J. Am. Chem. Soc.* **132,** 11045–11057 (2010).
47. Burnley, J., Jackson, W. R. & Robinson, A. J. One-pot selective homodimerization/hydrogenation strategy for sequential dicarba bridge formation. *J. Org. Chem.* **80,** 9057–9063 (2015).
48. Wennerberg, K., Rossman, K. L. & Der, C. J. The Ras superfamily at a glance. *J. Cell Sci.* **118,** 843–846 (2005).
49. McCormick, F. KRAS as a therapeutic target. *Clin. Cancer Res.* **21,** 1797–1801 (2015).
50. Spiegel, J., Cromm, P. M., Zimmermann, G., Grossmann, T. N. & Waldmann, H. Small-molecule modulation of Ras signaling. *Nat. Chem. Biol.* **10,** 613–622 (2014).
51. Cromm, P. M., Spiegel, J., Grossmann, T. N. & Waldmann, H. Direct modulation of small GTPase activity and function. *Angew. Chem. Int. Ed.* **54,** 13516–13537 (2015).
52. Stephen, A. G., Esposito, D., Bagni, R. K. & McCormick, F. Dragging ras back in the ring. *Cancer Cell* **25,** 272–281 (2014).
53. Ostrem, J. M., Peters, U., Sos, M. L., Wells, J. A. & Shokat, K. M. K-Ras(G12C) inhibitors allosterically control GTP affinity and effector interactions. *Nature* **503,** 548–551 (2013).
54. Agola, J. O. *et al.* A competitive nucleotide binding inhibitor: *in vitro* characterization of Rab7 GTPase inhibition. *ACS Chem. Biol.* **7,** 1095–1108 (2012).
55. Bhuin, T. & Roy, J. K. Rab proteins: the key regulators of intracellular vesicle transport. *Exp. Cell Res.* **328,** 1–19 (2014).
56. Hutagalung, A. H. & Novick, P. J. Role of Rab GTPases in membrane traffic and cell physiology. *Physiol. Rev.* **91,** 119–149 (2011).
57. Recacha, R. *et al.* Structural basis for recruitment of Rab6-interacting protein 1 to Golgi via a RUN domain. *Structure* **17,** 21–30 (2009).
58. Belokon', Y. N., Tararov, V. I., Maleev, V. I., Savel'eva, T. F. & Ryzhov, M. G. Improved procedures for the synthesis of (S)-2-[N-(N'-benzylprolyl)amino] benzophenone (BPB) and Ni(II) complexes of Schiff's bases derived from BPB and amino acids. *Tetrahedron* **9,** 4249–4252 (1998).
59. Bird, G. H., Crannell, W. C. & Walensky, L. D. Chemical synthesis of hydrocarbon-stapled peptides for protein interaction research and therapeutic targeting. *Curr. Protoc. Chem. Biol.* **3,** 99–117 (2011).
60. Hou, X. *et al.* A structural basis for Lowe syndrome caused by mutations in the Rab-binding domain of OCRL1. *EMBO J.* **30,** 1659–1670 (2011).
61. Bleimling, N., Alexandrov, K., Goody, R. & Itzen, A. Chaperone-assisted production of active human Rab8A GTPase in Escherichia coli. *Protein Expr. Purif.* **65,** 190–195 (2009).
62. Simon, I., Zerial, M. & Goody, R. S. Kinetics of interaction of Rab5 and Rab7 with nucleotides and magnesium ions. *J. Biol. Chem.* **271,** 20470–20478 (1996).
63. Huang, X. & Aulabaugh, A. Application of fluorescence polarization in HTS assays. *Methods Mol. Biol.* **565,** 127–143 (2009).
64. Motulsky, H. & Christopoulos, A. *Fitting Models to Biological Data Using Linear and Nonlinear Regression. A Practical Guide to Curve Fitting* (Oxford Univ. Press, 2004).

Acknowledgements

We thank N. Bleiming for protein expression/purification and technical assistance. P.M.C. is grateful to the Studienstiftung des Deutschen Volkes for a Fellowship. S.S. and J.S. acknowledge financial support by the Fonds der Chemischen Industrie. T.N.G. thanks the Deutsche Forschungsgemeinschaft (Emmy Noether program GR3592/2-1), AstraZeneca, Bayer CropScience, Bayer HealthCare, Boehringer Ingelheim, Merck KGaA and the Max-Planck Society for their support.

Author contributions

P.M.C. designed and carried out the building block synthesis, peptide synthesis, as well as FP assays and analysed the data. S.S. supported alkyne-metathesis reactions and analysed the data. J.S. supported the design and performance of experiments. A.F., T.N.G. and H.W. designed the experiments and supervised the project. All the authors discussed the results and commented on the manuscript. P.M.C., T.N.G. and H.W. wrote the manuscript.

Additional information

Competing financial interests: The authors declare no competing financial interests.

Perfluorocarbon nanoparticles enhance reactive oxygen levels and tumour growth inhibition in photodynamic therapy

Yuhao Cheng[1,*], Hao Cheng[1,*], Chenxiao Jiang[1], Xuefeng Qiu[1], Kaikai Wang[1], Wei Huan[1], Ahu Yuan[1], Jinhui Wu[1] & Yiqiao Hu[1,2]

Photodynamic therapy (PDT) kills cancer cells by converting tumour oxygen into reactive singlet oxygen ($^1O_2$) using a photosensitizer. However, pre-existing hypoxia in tumours and oxygen consumption during PDT can result in an inadequate oxygen supply, which in turn hampers photodynamic efficacy. Here to overcome this problem, we create oxygen self-enriching photodynamic therapy (Oxy-PDT) by loading a photosensitizer into perfluorocarbon nanodroplets. Because of the higher oxygen capacity and longer $^1O_2$ lifetime of perfluorocarbon, the photodynamic effect of the loaded photosensitizer is significantly enhanced, as demonstrated by the accelerated generation of $^1O_2$ and elevated cytotoxicity. Following direct injection into tumours, *in vivo* studies reveal tumour growth inhibition in the Oxy-PDT-treated mice. In addition, a single-dose intravenous injection of Oxy-PDT into tumour-bearing mice significantly inhibits tumour growth, whereas traditional PDT has no effect. Oxy-PDT may enable the enhancement of existing clinical PDT and future PDT design.

[1] State Key Laboratory of Pharmaceutical Biotechnology, Medical School, Nanjing University, Nanjing 210093, China. [2] Jiangsu Key Laboratory for Nano Technology, Nanjing University, Nanjing 210093, China. * These authors contributed equally to this work. Correspondence and requests for materials should be addressed to J.W. (email: wuj@nju.edu.cn) or to Y.H. (email: huyiqiao@nju.edu.cn).

Photodynamic therapy (PDT) depends on the ability of photosensitizers (PS) to transfer energy from lasers to tumour-dissolved oxygen (O_2) to generate cytotoxic singlet oxygen ($^1O_2$) for cancer treatment[1,2]. However, the effectiveness of PDT is impaired by an inadequate oxygen supply in tumours[3,4]. In most solid tumours, hypoxia is common because the oxygen supply is reduced by disturbed microcirculation and deteriorated diffusion[5]. Moreover, PDT worsens hypoxia through oxygen consumption and vascular shutdown effects[6]. Low oxygen content can reduce the photodynamic efficacy of PS, preventing PDT from achieving its full therapeutic potential[7].

Traditional methods have attempted to optimize tumour oxygenation to ensure PDT efficacy. For example, dividing irradiation into light–dark circles[8] and extending irradiation with a low fluence rate[9] have both been investigated as techniques for better tumour reoxygenation by the blood. However, these approaches only affect PDT-induced oxygen depletion, whereas the pre-existing hypoxia cannot be reversed; moreover, vascular shutdown due to PDT would also result in severe hypoxia[10]. Hyperbaric oxygen inhalation has also been used to actively increase the level of tumour oxygen[11–14]. However, vascular damage during PDT still prevents further oxygenation from hyperbaric blood[15]; moreover, the potential toxic effects of excessive oxygen are an impediment to its clinical use[16,17]. To our knowledge, no existing techniques can effectively reverse the tumour oxygen content during PDT. Therefore, optimizing the efficacy with limited oxygen is of great importance for photodynamic therapy.

To address this challenge, herein we load photosensitizer into perfluorocarbon nanodroplets to develop a novel oxygen self-enriched photodynamic therapy (Oxy-PDT). Because of its high oxygen capacity[18], perfluorocarbon can maintain a higher oxygen content than the tumour matrix at a given oxygen partial pressure (Supplementary Fig. 1). Thus, although the tumour oxygen content remains limited during PDT, sufficient O_2 can always be enriched in the PFC droplet for photodynamic consumption by the loaded PS, thus obtaining improved efficacy (Fig. 1a). This type of enhancement is possible regardless of pre-existing hypoxia, photodynamic consumption, or vascular damage; moreover, it has been reported that the $^1O_2$ lifetime in perfluorocarbon is much longer than in the cellular environment or in water[19], which results in long-lasting photodynamic effects. Therefore, Oxy-PDT might help PS to achieve its full therapeutic potential. In this study, we assessed the therapeutic efficacy of Oxy-PDT as a novel form of PDT in cancer models. First, we studied the photodynamic effect of Oxy-PDT on the generation of $^1O_2$ and its cytotoxicity by incubating tumour cells with Oxy-PDT, which were then irradiated with laser beams. Next, we assessed the effect of Oxy-PDT on tumour growth by intratumoural injections *in vivo*. Last, we examined the passive targeting of Oxy-PDT by intravenous injections *in vivo*. We envision that this new approach may guide improvements in the clinical use of PDT.

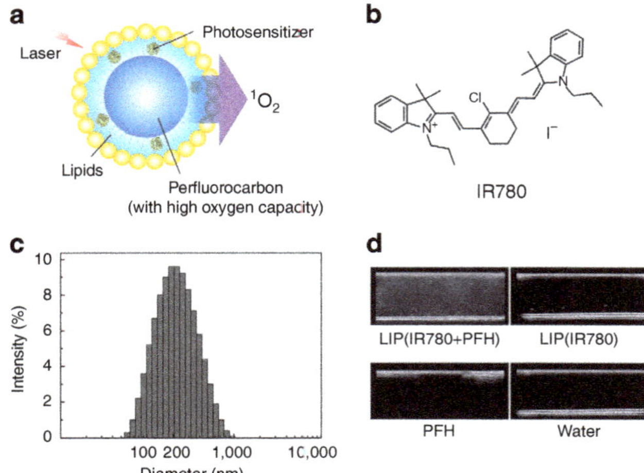

Figure 1 | Characterization of the Oxy-PDT agent. (**a**) Structure and design of the Oxy-PDT agent. Photosensitizer and perfluorocarbon are coencapsulated by lipids. Photosensitizer is uniformly dispersed inside the lipid monolayer and PFC in the core of the nanoparticle. When irradiated by laser, PS transfers energy to the oxygen enriched in PFH, producing $^1O_2$, resulting in enhanced tumour inhibition. (**b**) Structure of IR780. (**c**) Dynamic light scattering of the Oxy-PDT agent. (**d**) Ultrasound images of the Oxy-PDT agent and other groups tested in 5-ml plastic test tubes.

Results

Synthesis of the Oxy-PDT agent. The near-infrared photosensitizer IR780 (Fig. 1b) and perfluorohexane (PFH) were used in this manuscript to prepare the Oxy-PDT agent LIP(IR780 + PFH). IR780 is uniformly dispersed in a lipid monolayer (composed of lecithin, cholesterol, and DSPE-PEG2000), and the average diameter of the resulting nanodroplets is 200 nm (Fig. 1c). As the Oxy-PDT agent is irradiated by a near-infrared (NIR) 808-nm laser, IR780 transfers energy to the oxygen enriched in the PFH, producing cytotoxic singlet oxygen (Fig. 1a). The existence of IR780 in the Oxy-PDT agent was confirmed by the absorption peak in the NIR region (Supplementary Fig. 2). The existence of PFH in the Oxy-PDT agent was confirmed by the contrast enhancement in the ultrasound image, whereas LIP(IR780), pure PFH, and water produced blank echo signals (Fig. 1d). PFH in Oxy-PDT agent was also confirmed by GC-Mass (Supplementary Fig. 2b,c). The stability and self-quenching capability of the Oxy-PDT agent were then evaluated (Supplementary Fig. 3). The results indicate that Oxy-PDT can increase the dark stability of IR780 and reduce its self-quenching.

Characterization of photodynamic efficacy. We compared the $^1O_2$ generation by Oxy-PDT with traditional PDT, as determined by the fluorescence intensity of oxidized SOSG (an indicator of $^1O_2$). In the presence of $^1O_2$, the oxidation of SOSG results in increased fluorescence and therefore provides a means of monitoring $^1O_2$ production. We measured the varying extent of fluorescence gain in water in the presence of LIP(IR780 + PFH) or LIP(IR780) irradiated by an 808-nm laser for 5-s intervals (Fig. 2a). The presence of LIP(IR780 + PFH) resulted in the highest rate of fluorescence gain, and the total accumulation was also significantly higher than in the presence of LIP(IR780), which resulted in only a marginal fluorescence gain ($P < 0.05$, two-sided Student's *t*-test). The singlet oxygen quantum yields (Φ_{so}) of both LIP(IR780) and LIP(IR780 + PFH) were also calculated (Supplementary Table 1). The Φ_{so} value of LIP(IR780 + PFH) is higher than for LIP(IR780) or IR780, indicating that the Oxy-PDT platform can increase the quantum yield of photosensitizer. Moreover, this phenomenon can also be achieved using other photosensitizers, suggesting that the enhancement is not specific to IR780 (Supplementary Fig. 4).

To determine whether such fluorescence gain is a result of the presence of PFH, we diluted LIP(IR780 + PFH) and LIP(IR780) to a series of solutions with concentrations of PFH ranging from 30 v/v% to 1.88 v/v% (Fig. 2b). The dilution caused a marked relative reduction in the fluorescence between 20 s continually irradiated LIP(IR780 + PFH) and LIP(IR780), from 12.2- to 0.84-fold. Moreover, the enhancement was proven to be independent

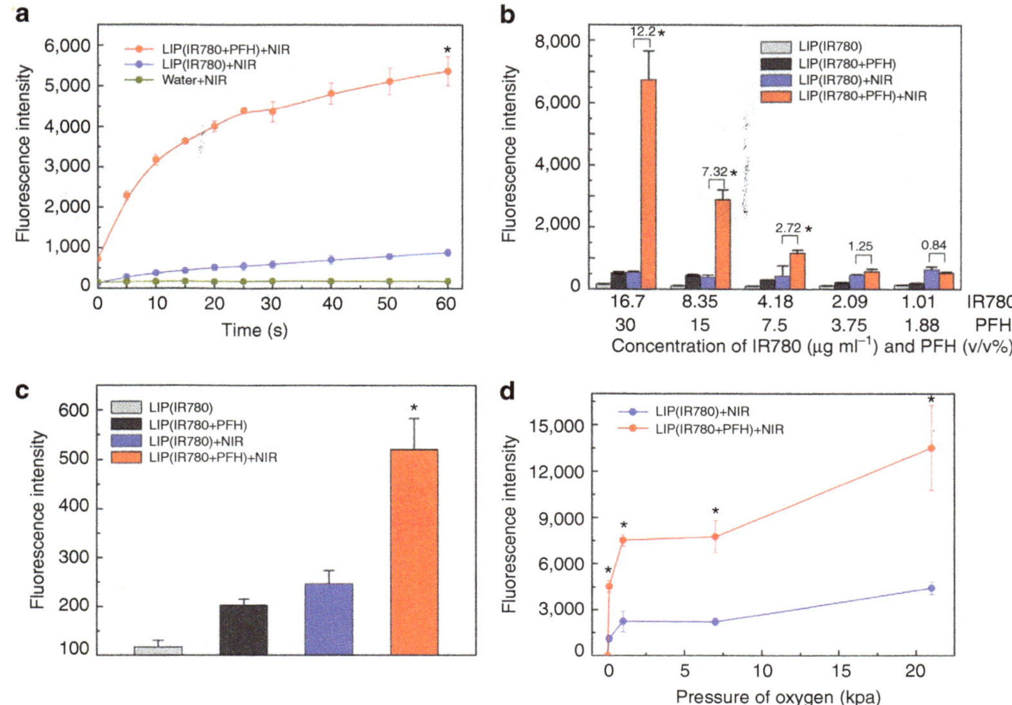

Figure 2 | $^1O_2$ production of different samples under NIR laser irradiation as determined by the accumulated fluorescence intensity of oxidized SOSG. (**a**) $^1O_2$ production of LIP(IR780 + PFH) (16.7 μg ml^{-1} IR780, 30 v/v% PFH), LIP(IR780) (16.7 μg ml^{-1} IR780), and water under different laser irradiation exposures. Values are the means ± s.d. ($n = 3$, *$P < 0.05$, versus LIP(IR780) + NIR, two-sided Student's *t*-test); (**b**) $^1O_2$ production in different diluted samples. The concentrations of IR780 and PFH varied from 16.7 to 1.01 μg ml^{-1} and 30% to 1.88% (v/v%), respectively. Values are the means ± s.d. ($n = 3$, *$P < 0.05$, versus LIP(IR780) + NIR, two-sided Student's t-test). Irradiation was performed by an 808 nm laser (2 W cm^{-2}) for 20 s. (**c**) $^1O_2$ production of LIP(IR780 + PFH) with a low concentration of IR780 and a high concentration of PFH (1.01 μg ml^{-1} IR780, 30 v/v% PFH). Values are the means ± s.d. ($n = 3$). Irradiation was performed by an 808-nm laser (2 W cm^{-2}) for 20 s, (*$P < 0.05$, versus LIP(IR780) + NIR, two-sided Student's *t*-test); (**d**) $^1O_2$ production after 20-s irradiation in different hypoxic conditions (0.1, 1, 7, or 21 kPa O_2), for LIP(IR780 + PFH) (16.7 μg ml^{-1} IR780, 15 v/v% PFH) and LIP(IR780) (16.7 μg ml^{-1} IR780). Values are the means ± s.d. ($n = 3$, *$P < 0.05$, versus LIP(IR780) + NIR, two-sided Student's *t*-test).

of IR780 concentration (Supplementary Fig. 5), indicating that the presence of PFH is a key factor in the enhanced PDT effect. Then, when we added enough PFH (resulting in 30 v/v% PFH) to the diluted LIP(IR780 + PFH), the relatively reduced fluorescence recovered (Fig. 2c), confirming the participation of PFH in the generation of $^1O_2$.

We then tested the photodynamic efficacy of both LIP(IR780) and LIP(IR780 + PFH) in different hypoxic conditions (Fig. 2c). The samples were exposed to different atmospheres (containing 0.1, 1, 7 and 21 kPa O_2) and then received 20 s irradiation. The results suggested that LIP(IR780 + PFH) significantly enhanced $^1O_2$ production under different oxygen pressures. Meanwhile, LIP(IR780 + PFH) in extremely hypoxic conditions (0.1 kPa O_2) showed higher $^1O_2$ generation than LIP(IR780) in non-hypoxic conditions (21 kPa O_2), indicating that during Oxy-PDT treatment, the PFC can successfully enrich oxygen to accelerate $^1O_2$ generation.

Cell assays. Assays were performed on both MCF-7 human breast cancer cells and CT26 murine colon adenocarcinoma cells. First, we examined the production of reactive oxygen species (ROS) such as $^1O_2$ from Oxy-PDT and traditional PDT in live cells using carboxy-H_2DCFDA as a fluorogenic marker for ROS. Carboxy-H_2DCFDA permeates cell membranes to be oxidized, emitting bright green fluorescence in the presence of $^1O_2$. The resulting oxidatively stressed cells showed green fluorescence, indicating increased $^1O_2$ gain. We treated cells with PBS, LIP(IR780) or LIP(IR780 + PFH), with and without 20 s continual 808-nm laser irradiation. Without laser irradiation, MCF-7 cells treated with PBS, LIP(IR780) or LIP(IR780 + PFH) showed negligible fluorescence (Fig. 3a,b). After irradiation, cells treated with LIP(IR780 + PFH) showed significant green fluorescence, whereas cells treated with PBS and LIP(IR780) still showed negligible fluorescence. Similar results can also be observed in treated CT26 cells (Supplementary Fig. 6). To verify the results, flow cytometry was used to analyse the percentage of cells stained with green fluorescence (Fig. 3c). Cells treated with PBS, LIP(IR780) and LIP(IR780 + PFH) showed a relatively low percentage (2.84%, 9.69% and 13.2%, respectively) of green fluorescent cells, whereas cells treated with LIP(IR780) showed an increased percentage (24.7%) after irradiation. More notably, the percentage (41.0%) in cells treated with LIP(IR780 + PFH) and an 808-nm laser was much higher than in cells treated with LIP(IR780), indicating the better performance of LIP(IR780 + PFH) as the $^1O_2$ producer.

After comparing their performances as $^1O_2$ producers, we tested Oxy-PDT and traditional PDT for their photodynamic effects on inducing cell death. Without laser irradiation, we found no significant cytotoxicity in MCF-7 cells treated with LIP(IR780) or LIP(IR780 + PFH) (Fig. 4a). After 20 s continual irradiation by an 808-nm laser, we detected a reduction in the viability of cells treated with both LIP(IR780) and LIP(IR780 + PFH). It is notable that the reductions in viability were higher in cells treated with LIP(IR780 + PFH) than in cells treated with LIP(IR780) when the concentrations of IR780 were higher than 2.09 μg ml^{-1} ($P < 0.05$,

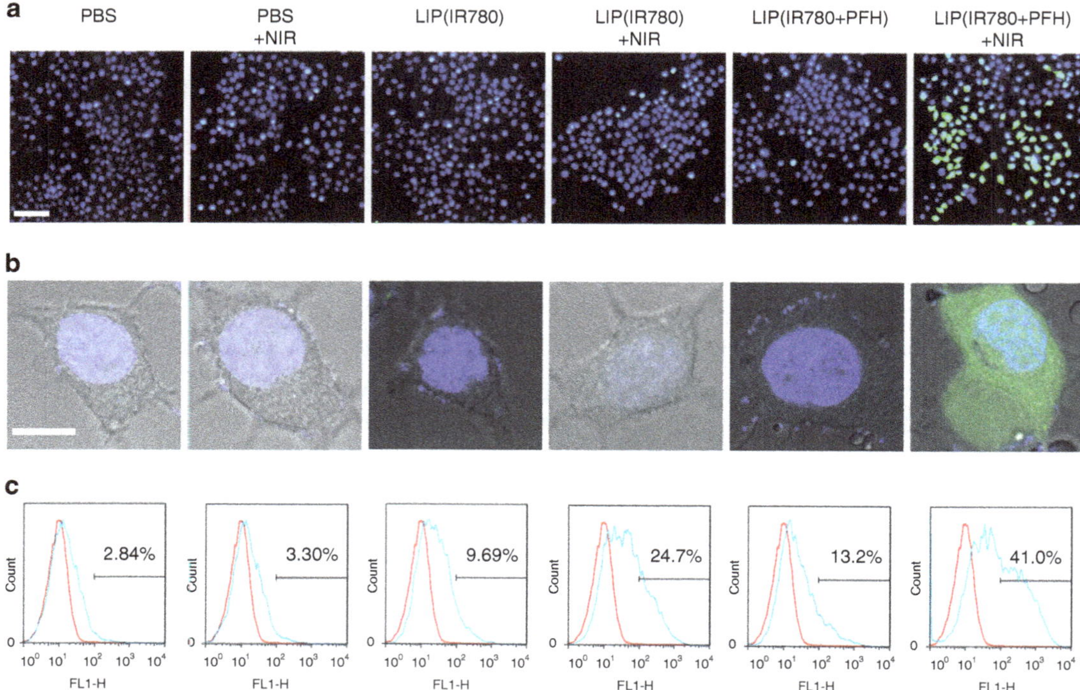

Figure 3 | Enhanced $^1O_2$ production by Oxy-PDT in cells. (**a**) Cells were treated with different agents and then exposed to an 808-nm laser (2 W cm^{-2} for 20 s). ROS generation was detected using carboxy-H_2DCFDA. Confocal images showing green fluorescence indicate positive staining for ROS; the positions of the cells are shown by blue fluorescence indicative of nuclear counterstaining with Hoechst 33342 (scale bar, 50 μm). (**b**) Magnified images (scale bar, 10 μm). (**c**) Flow-cytometry analysis of ROS generation in cells treated with different agents and then exposed to an 808-nm laser (2 W cm^{-2} for 20 s) detected using carboxy-H_2DCFDA.

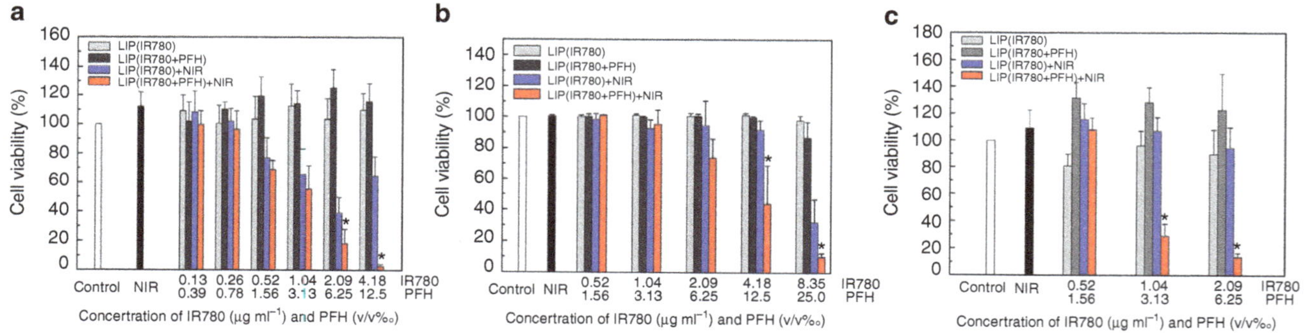

Figure 4 | Enhanced cytotoxicity by Oxy-PDT agents in normal and hypoxic conditions. Cells were exposed to 2 W cm^{-2} of an 808-nm NIR laser for 20 s, and viability was measured by the CCK-8 assay. (**a**) MCF-7 cells; (**b**) CT-26 cells; (**c**) CT-26 cells in hypoxic conditions. Values are the means ± s.d. ($n = 3$, $^*P < 0.05$ versus LIP(IR780) + NIR, two-sided Student's t-test).

two-sided Student's t-test). Similar results were also observed in CT26 murine colon adenocarcinoma cells (Fig. 4b). In addition, cell death induced by photothermal effects was not evident in the minimal IR780 and irradiation dosages (Supplementary Fig. 7a).

The effects of Oxy-PDT in hypoxia were also studied (Fig. 4c). CT26 cells were placed in a hypoxic transparent box for 4 h before irradiation. Then, laser irradiation and a further 1-h incubation were performed. Interestingly, in hypoxic conditions, Oxy-PDT still maintained superior cytotoxicity to traditional PDT ($P < 0.05$, two-sided Student's t-test), indicating that Oxy-PDT can improve the efficacy of PDT in both normal and hypoxic conditions.

***In vivo* PDT using intratumoural injection.** The *in vivo* $^1O_2$ generation of both LIP(IR780) and LIP(IR780 + PFH) was measured. SOSG was also used as an indicator because of its green fluorescence after oxidization by the generated $^1O_2$. Without laser irradiation, tumours treated with LIP(IR780) or LIP(IR780 + PFH) showed negligible fluorescence. After laser irradiation, tumours treated with LIP(IR780 + PFH) showed significant green fluorescence, whereas tumours treated with LIP(IR780) showed weak fluorescence (Fig. 5a). This result indicated that higher $^1O_2$ generation by Oxy-PDT can also be achieved *in vivo*.

We further compared the efficacy of Oxy-PDT and traditional PDT *in vivo* on CT26 tumour-bearing mice via intratumoural injections. The mice were divided into five groups, including a

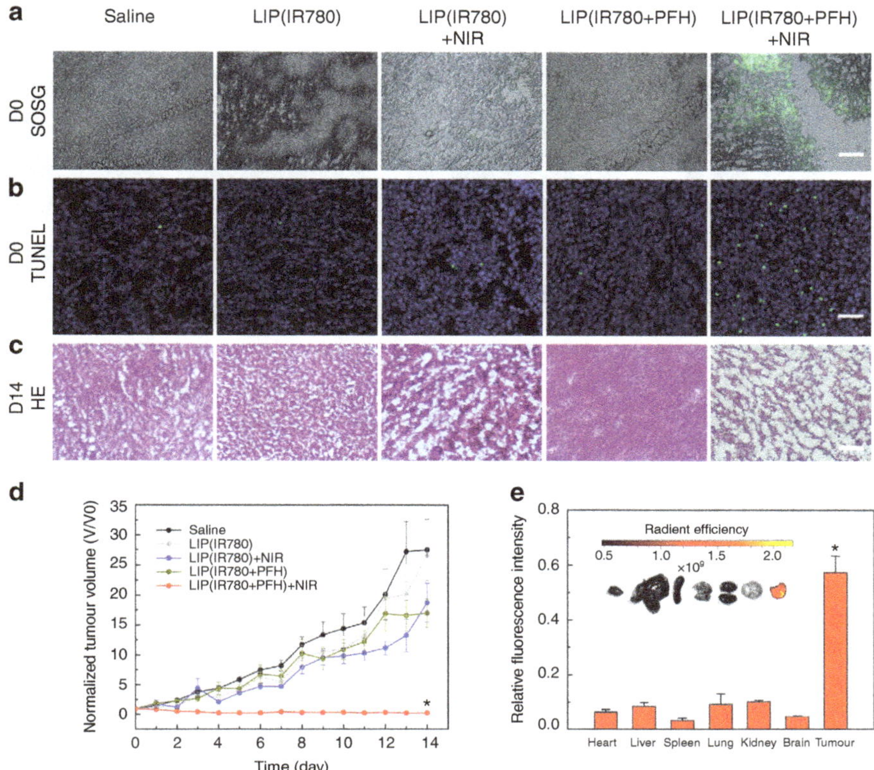

Figure 5 | *In vivo* photodynamic therapy of Oxy-PDT by intratumoural injection in a subcutaneous tumour model. (**a**) SOSG staining in tumour sections for $^1O_2$ determination (scale bar, 100 μm). Before sectioning, a mixture of SOSG with saline, LIP(IR780), or LIP(IR780 + PFH) was injected into the tumours, followed by laser irradiation. (**b**) TUNEL staining for apoptosis in tumour sections from each group to determine the effectiveness of Oxy-PDT. DAPI counterstaining indicates the tumour nuclear region (scale bar, 50 μm). (**c**) H&E staining for pathological changes in tumour sections from each group to determine the effectiveness of Oxy-PDT (scale bar, 50 μm). (**d**) Changes in tumour volumes used to assess the effectiveness of Oxy-PDT in tumour-bearing mice by intratumoural injection. Values are the means ± s.e.m. ($n = 6$, $^*P < 0.05$ versus LIP(IR780) + NIR, two-sided Student's *t*-test). (**e**) Biodistribution of intratumourally injected LIP(IR780 + PFH) in organs of mice at 14 days after initial treatment. Organs were isolated and quantified by near-infrared imaging (based on IR780 content). Values are the means ± s.e.m. ($n = 6$).

saline control group and LIP(IR780) and LIP(IR780 + PFH) groups with and without 808-nm laser irradiation. To avoid the additional efficacy induced by photothermal effects, the temperature of the tumour during irradiation was controlled by dividing the irradiation time into two consecutive 10 s applications with a 1-min interval in between (Supplementary Fig. 7b). We first evaluated the efficacy of the treatment in terms of tumour cell apoptosis by performing TUNEL staining on histological sections from the different treatment groups immediately after drug administration. We found a greater number of apoptotic cells in histological sections from the group receiving LIP(IR780 + PFH) and irradiation (Fig. 5b), which suggested the successful destruction of tumour cells by Oxy-PDT.

We then assessed the photodynamic effects of each group by monitoring the tumour volumes over a period of 2 weeks (Fig. 5d, Supplementary Data 1). The tumour volumes in mice receiving LIP(IR780 + PFH) with 808-nm laser irradiation were significantly inhibited, whereas no significant differences in tumour volumes were found between the saline control group and other treatment groups, including LIP(IR780 + PFH) and LIP(IR780) with and without laser irradiation. We then performed H&E staining on tissue sections from each group at 14 days after treatment. We found that most tumour cells were severely damaged or destroyed in mice treated with LIP(IR780 + PFH) and irradiation by an 808-nm laser (Fig. 5c). In the other groups, there was incomplete tumour cell death, suggesting the successful destruction of tumour cells by Oxy-PDT. At 14 days after treatment, a biodistribution study of the mice receiving only the intratumoural injection of LIP(IR780 + PFH) and irradiation showed the presence of IR780 only in the tumour tissues (Fig. 5e), suggesting that IR780 remained primarily in the tumour mass after administration and that the diffusion from tumour tissue to other tissues was negligible.

***In vivo* PDT using intravenous injection.** After the study of intratumoural injection, we examined the efficacy of Oxy-PDT by intravenous injection. Because of the enhanced permeability and retention effect, nanoparticles in the range of 10–400 nm can accumulate in tumour tissue at levels 70 times higher than in normal tissue[20,21]. Accordingly, LIP(IR780 + PFH) with a mean particle size of 200 nm showed passive tumour targeting, as demonstrated by the NIR (Supplementary Fig. 8) and the ultrasound imaging of tumour accumulation after intravenous injection. The tumour accumulation of IR780 reached its maximum at 24 h after intravenous injection (Fig. 6a); meanwhile, ultrasound imaging confirmed the existence of PFH in the tumours at 24 h (Fig. 6b). Therefore, 24 h after intravenous injection was chosen for 808-nm laser irradiation.

Mice were divided into five groups, including the saline control group and the LIP (IR780) and LIP (IR780 + PFH) groups with and without laser irradiation. To avoid the confounding effects

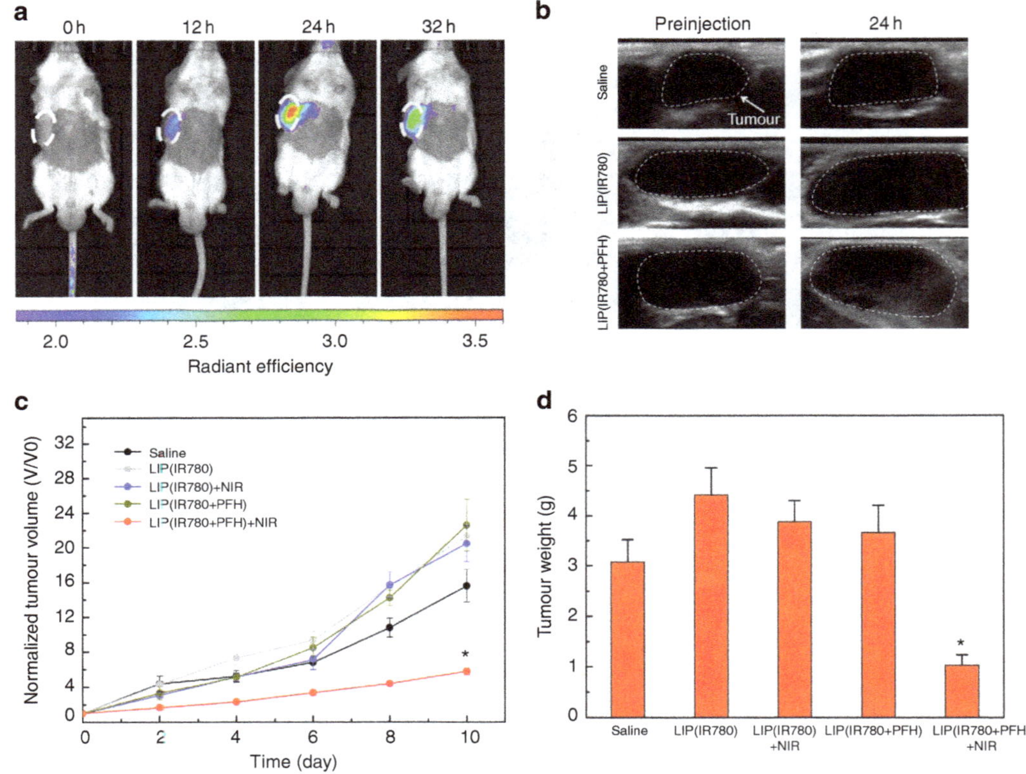

Figure 6 | *In vivo* photodynamic therapy of Oxy-PDT by intravenous injection in a subcutaneous tumour model. (**a**) Near-infrared imaging of tumour accumulation of IR780 in tumour-bearing mice after intravenous injection of LIP(IR780 + PFH). Images were taken at 0, 12, 24 and 32 h postinjection. Tumours are circled with white dashed lines. (**b**) Ultrasound imaging of tumours on mice before (0 h) and after intravenous injection (24 h) of LIP(IR780 + PFH) (0.2 ml, 60 μg ml^{-1} IR780, 10 v/v% PFH), LIP(IR780) (0.2 ml, 60 μg ml^{-1} IR780), and saline. Tumours are circled with white dashed lines. (**c**) Changes in tumour volumes used to assess the effectiveness of Oxy-PDT in tumour-bearing mice by intravenous injection. Treatments were performed only once. Values are the means ± s.e.m. ($n = 6$, *$P < 0.05$ versus LIP(IR780) + NIR, two-sided Student's *t*-test). (**d**) Average weights of tumours at day 10. Mice were killed, and tumours were isolated for weighing. Values are the means ± s.e.m. ($n = 6$, *$P < 0.05$ versus LIP(IR780) + NIR, two-sided Student's *t*-test).

induced by photothermal radiation, the temperature of the tumour during irradiation was controlled within a safe range by dividing the irradiation time into two consecutive 10-s applications with a 1-min interval (Supplementary Fig. 7b). Monitoring the change in tumour volume as a function of time after treatment revealed a significant reduction in the tumour growth rate of mice receiving LIP(IR780 + PFH) and laser irradiation ($P < 0.05$, versus LIP(IR780) + NIR, two-sided Student's *t*-test, Fig. 6c, Supplementary Data 2). No significant reduction was found in the tumour growth rate of mice receiving LIP(IR780) and laser irradiation. At the end point of day 10, the tumours from each mouse were excised and weighed (Fig. 6d). The mean tumour weight in the mice receiving LIP(IR780 + PFH) and laser irradiation was approximately fourfold lower than in mice receiving LIP(IR780) and laser irradiation ($P < 0.05$, two-sided Student's *t*-test), suggesting the improved efficacy of Oxy-PDT.

Although the tumours were significantly inhibited, they were not completely regressed as a result of intravenous injection plus laser irradiation. Indeed, significant tumour inhibition was obtained by a mere single-dose injection and 20-s irradiation, compared with traditional PDT, in which the dosage was too low to show any therapeutic effect. In light of the current results, further optimization of administration frequency is warranted to exploit the full potential of Oxy-PDT-enhanced photosensitizer as a new PDT clinical approach

Discussion

In this study, we demonstrate a novel Oxy-PDT platform for achieving enhanced efficacy. PDT depends strongly on $^1O_2$ to kill cancer cells, and thus the $^1O_2$ generation rate determines PDT efficacy. In the Oxy-PDT agent, both PS and oxygen are enriched in the nanodroplet, and thus the oxygen available for the photodynamic reaction are increased compared with traditional PDT in the tumour matrix. Moreover, the lifetime of $^1O_2$ varies with the polarity of the solvent: the half-life of $^1O_2$ is $\sim 6 \times 10^{-7}$ s in the cellular environment, 5×10^{-6} s in water, and 5×10^{-2} s in PFH[19]. Therefore, by using a PFC nanodroplet as the PS carrier, the lifetime of $^1O_2$ is extended. These phenomena may be two major reasons that Oxy-PDT can enhance the reactive oxygen level.

NIR dyes (such as IR780) typically have a lower $^1O_2$ quantum yield (Φ_{so}) than visible dyes because the wavelength of NIR light (> 800 nm) is longer than the wavelength of visible light and may have insufficient energy to excite oxygen to its singlet state[1,2,22]. However, in this study, Φ_{so}LIP(IR780 + PFH) was found to be higher than Φ_{so}LIP(IR780), demonstrating that the Oxy-PDT platform can increase the $^1O_2$ quantum yield of NIR dyes. Furthermore, our results showed that Oxy-PDT could increase the dark stability of IR780 and reduce its self-quenching.

The results also showed a higher therapeutic efficacy of Oxy-PDT than traditional PDT both *in vitro* and *in vivo*. With direct injection into tumours, the *in vivo* studies showed complete tumour growth inhibition in Oxy-PDT mice treated with a low photosensitizer dosage and 20-s laser irradiation, whereas traditional PDT showed negligible tumour inhibition. These results suggested that in Oxy-PDT, PFH can help the photosensitizer achieve improved effects. The ultraviolet–visible absorption of the NIR dye is reduced after laser irradiation, possibly due to the degradation of the NIR dye by exposure to $^1O_2$. Although the degradation products might also be toxic to cells, the enhanced tumour growth effect of LIP(IR780 + PFH) is still attributed to PFH because the possible degradation product is also present in LIP(IR780). Interestingly, with only a single-dose intravenous injection into tumour-bearing mice, Oxy-PDT still exhibited significant tumour inhibition, indicating that passive targeting plays an important role in the therapeutic efficacy. It should be noted that in all our experiments, the influence of photothermal therapy has been excluded to examine only photodynamic effects. Moreover, previous studies have already confirmed the high oxygen content in perfluorocarbons, which are used as artificial blood in clinical applications and can be used as ultrasonography[23] and MRI[24,25] contrast agents to monitor the behaviour of Oxy-PDT agents *in vivo*.

As previously discussed, Oxy-PDT is considered to be the first PDT design that can realize high efficacy in hypoxic conditions. This Oxy-PDT approach with self-enriching oxygen offers a simple yet effective treatment option for cancer patients. We have provided a proof of concept for the PFC/photosensitizer-loaded emulsion as an agent of improved PDT *in vivo* and anticipate its wide clinical application after dose optimization.

Methods

Chemicals and reagents. Lecithin and cholesterol were purchased from Aladdin Industrial Corporation, and DSPE-PEG2000 was obtained from A.V.T. Pharm. Ltd. (Shanghai, China). The 99% perfluorohexane was purchased from Bailingwei Tech Co., Ltd. (Beijing, China). IR780 was purchased from Sigma-Aldrich Chemical Corporation (St Louis, MO, USA). Singlet Oxygen Sensor Green was obtained from Molecular Probes, Inc. Carboxy-H2DCFDA was purchased from Invitrogen (USA). Cell counting kit-8 (CCK-8) was supplied by Dojindo Laboratories (Japan). MCF-7 and CT-26 cells were purchased from the Cell Bank of Shanghai Institutes for Biological Sciences, Chinese Academy of Sciences (Shanghai, China). All of the BALB/c mice were purchased from Yangzhou University Medical Centre (Yangzhou, China). All of the chemicals were used as supplied without further purification.

Synthesis of the Oxy-PDT agent. First, 24.65 mg lecithin, 4.28 mg cholesterol, 3.79 mg DSPE-PEG2000, and the specified IR780 were dissolved in 5 ml dichloromethane. The dichloromethane was removed from a 25-ml round flask by rotary evaporation to form lipid films. Using 10-min sonication, 1.4 ml pure water was added, and the film was peeled off. Next, 0.6 ml PFH was added gradually under high-speed dispersion (IKA, T25, German) at 24,000 r.p.m. in an ice bath for 10 min to form 2 ml LIP(IR780 + PFH) (30 v/v% PFH). LIP(IR780) can be formed by the addition of pure water instead of PFH.

Detection of singlet oxygen *in vitro*. First, 0.1 ml samples and 0.02 ml of 50 µM SOSG were mixed in black 96-well plates (Costar). After irradiation (808-nm, 2 W cm^{-2}), the oxidized SOSG was quantified by measuring the fluorescence intensity (excited at 504 nm and measured at 525 nm) using a multifunctional microplate reader (Safire, TECAN). As for the production of singlet oxygen in hypoxia, samples were kept in transparent box with different hypoxic air (0.1, 1, 7 or 21 kpa O_2). After laser irradiation (808-nm, 2 W cm^{-2}), the oxidized SOSG was quantified by measuring the fluorescence intensity. All operations were performed without light exposure. The experiments for each group were run in triplicate.

The MCF-7 cells were seeded with a density of 2×10^5 per well in 12-well plates. After the cells were incubated for 24 h, the medium was replaced with 700 µl fresh culture medium. Then, 350 µl PBS, LIP(IR780) or LIP(IR780 + PFH) was added to the well. The cells were further incubated for 30 min at 37 °C and 5% CO_2. The final concentration of IR780 was 4 µg ml^{-1}. After washing once with PBS, the cells were incubated with 600 µl carboxy-H_2DCFDA (25 µM) for 10 min. Subsequently, the cells were washed once with PBS and irradiated by an 808-nm laser (2 W cm^{-2}) for 20 s per well. Then, the cells were fixed by 4% formaldehyde polymer for 10 min and labelled with 600 µl Hoechst 33342 (1 µM) for 5 min. Finally, the cells were replaced with 1 ml PBS. The fluorescence emission spectrum of carboxy-DCF (Ex/Em = 495/529 nm) and Hoechst 33342 (Ex/Em = 350/461 nm) were immediately captured on a confocal fluorescence microscope (OLYMPUS FV1000).

Flow cytometry. The MCF-7 cells were seeded with a density of 5×10^5 per well in 12-well plates. After incubation for 24 h, the medium was replaced with 1.4 ml fresh culture medium. Then, 700 µl PBS, LIP(IR780), or LIP(IR780 + PFH) was added to each well, as appropriate. The cells were further incubated for 50 min at 37 °C in an atmosphere containing 5% CO_2. The final concentration of IR780 was 4 µg ml^{-1}. After washing once with PBS, the cells were incubated with 550 µl carboxy-H_2DCFDA (25 µM) for 10 min. Subsequently, the cells were washed once with PBS and irradiated by an 808-nm laser (2 W cm^{-2}) for 20 s per well. The cells were then centrifuged, resuspended in 500 µl PBS, and analysed by flow cytometry (FACS-Calibur, BD Corp.). Green fluorescence was collected on the FL1 channel due to intracellular carboxy-DCF. Data were obtained and analysed using the CELL QUEST and FLOWJO programs.

Cytotoxicity. The MCF-7 or CT26 cells were seeded into 96-well plates at a density of 4×10^4 cells per well. After incubation for 24 h, the cells were treated with LIP(IR780) or LIP(IR780 + PFH) at different concentrations (final concentrations of 20 µl samples mixed with 100 µl culture medium). For cytotoxicity in hypoxia, the cells were put into a GENbox Jar, where GENbox anaer and anaerobic atmosphere indicator were included. As the oxygen was consumed by GENbox anaer, the indicator changed its colour from blue to colourless. The Jar was approximately oxygen-free 4 h later. Then, the cells were immediately irradiated by an 808-nm laser (2 W cm^{-2}) for 20 s per well. After co-incubation for 2 h, the drugs were removed, and fresh culture medium was added. After further incubation for 24 h, a mixed solution consisting of CCK-8 (10 µl) and fresh culture medium (100 µl) was added to each well and incubated for an additional 2 h at 37 °C and 5% CO_2. Finally, the absorbance was measured at 450 nm using the microplate reader. Cells without any drugs or NIR irradiation were used as a negative control.

Animals. BALB/C male mice aged 4–6 weeks were purchased from Yangzhou University Medical Centre (Yangzhou, China) and were used in accordance with the regulations of the Institutional Animal Care and Use Committee (IACUC) of Nanjing University. During the study, animals were observed for any clinically relevant abnormalities daily or once every other day. If any animal was moribund due to treatment-associated toxicity, tumour over-growth ($\geq$3,000 mm^3), then the loss of 20% of body weight relative to the start of the study, or the appearance of large or open ulceration in the xenograft before scheduled killing, it was killed by CO_2 inhalation. In several instances, however, tumour volumes were allowed to exceed the stated limit of 3,000 mm^3 because the affected mice appeared otherwise healthy and had lost <5% of their original body weight. This implementation of the protocol has been confirmed by NJU-IACUC. Hairs on the flanks of the mice were removed before further treatments. Tumours were first developed in BALB/C mice by subcutaneously implanting 1×10^7 CT26 cells suspended in 100 µl of serum-free DMEM in the lower flanks of the mice. When the tumour volume reached ~200 mm^3, the tumour mass was removed and cut into small pieces of approximately 2–6 mm^3, which were subcutaneously implanted into other mice.

Detection of singlet oxygen *in vivo*. Tumours were developed in 4- to 6-week-old BALB/C male mice. When the tumour volume reached ~1,000 mm^3, the following study was performed. A mixture of 25 µl SOSG (50 µM), 25 µl saline, and LIP(IR780) (156 µg ml^{-1} IR780) or LIP(IR780 + PFH) (156 µg ml^{-1} IR780, 30 v/v% PFH) was directly injected into tumours. Subsequently, laser treatment (with an 808-nm laser (2 W cm^{-2}) for two consecutive exposures of 10 s each, with a 1-min interval between the two irradiations) was performed on the LIP(IR780) + NIR and LIP(IR780 + PFH) + NIR groups to generate $^1O_2$. Then, tumours from the five groups were collected and cryosectioned onto slides at a 7-µm thickness. The fluorescence emission of the oxidized SOSG (Ex/Em = 504/525 nm) was captured by fluorescence microscope.

***PDT* in tumour-bearing mice by intratumoural injection.** PDT treatments were then performed on 4- to 6-week-old BALB/C male mice 7 days after inoculation of the 2–6 mm^3 tumour pieces. The groups were as follows: group 1: saline; group 2: LIP(IR780); group 3: LIP(IR780) + NIR; group 4: LIP(IR780 + PFH); group 5: LIP(IR780 + PFH) + NIR. First, 50 µl of LIP(IR780) (156 µg ml^{-1} IR780), LIP(IR780 + PFH) (156 µg ml^{-1} IR780, 30 v/v% PFH) or saline alone was directly injected into the tumour mass. Then, laser treatment was immediately performed on groups 3 and 5 by irradiating the tumour regions with an 808-nm laser (2 W cm^{-2}) for two consecutive exposures of 10 s each, with a 1-min interval between exposures for tumour cooling. At day 0, tumours from the five groups were cryosectioned at 5-µm thickness onto slides and stained with TUNEL (Roche, Basel, Switzerland) according to the manufacturer's instructions. Tumour size was measured daily using a vernier calliper for 14 days after the first PDT treatment. The maximum width (X) and length (Y) of the tumours were measured, and the tumour volumes (V) were calculated using the formula $V = (X^2Y)/2$. Changes in tumour volume as a function of time were determined for each mouse by normalizing the tumour volume at day X to their respective tumour volume at day 0 after treatment. Mice were randomly selected in each group, and the tumours were photographed at days 7 and 14. At 14 days after treatment, the tumour, heart, liver, spleen, lung, kidney and brain tissues of mice from group 5 were collected and detected under *in vivo* small animal imaging for the biodistribution study.

Tumours from the five groups were cryosectioned at 7-μm thickness onto slides and stained with H&E according to the manufacturer's instructions.

***PDT* in tumour-bearing mice by intravenous injection.** The CT26 subcutaneous tumours were first developed in the mice as described above. PDT treatment was then performed at 8 days after inoculation of the tumour pieces. The average initial tumour volume was 144.4 mm^3. The testing groups were as follows: group 1: saline; group 2: LIP(IR780); group 3: LIP(IR780) + NIR; group 4: LIP(IR780 + PFH); group 5: LIP(IR780 + PFH) + NIR. First, 200 μl of LIP(IR780) (60 μg ml^{-1} IR780), LIP(PFH + IR780) (60 μg ml^{-1} IR780, 10 v/v% PFH) or saline alone was intravenously injected. NIR images of IR780 accumulation in the tumours of the mice in the LIP(IR780 + PFH) group were taken at 0, 12, 24 and 32 h, and ultrasound images of the tumour accumulation of PFH were taken pre- and 24-h postinjection. Twenty-four hours later, laser treatment was performed on groups 3 and 5 by irradiating the tumour region with an 808-nm laser (2 W cm^{-2}) for two consecutive exposures of 10 s each, with a 1-min interval between the two irradiations for tumour cooling. Tumour size was measured every two days using a vernier calliper for 10 days after the first PDT treatment. The tumours were measured for the maximum width (X) and length (Y) and the tumour volumes (V) were calculated using the formula: $V = (X^2Y)/2$. Changes in tumour volume as a function of time were determined for each mouse by normalizing the tumour volume at day X to the respective tumour volume at day 0 after treatment. Mice were randomly selected in each group, and the tumours were photographed at day 0, 5 and 10. At 10 days after treatment, the mice in each group were killed, and the tumours were removed, photographed and weighed.

Statistical analysis. Statistical analysis was performed by two-sided Student's t-test for two groups, and one-way analysis of variance for multiple groups. A value of $P < 0.05$ was considered statistically significant.

References

1. Agostinis, P. *et al.* Photodynamic therapy of cancer: an update. *CA. Cancer J. Clin.* **61,** 250–281 (2011).
2. Celli, J. P. *et al.* Imaging and photodynamic therapy: mechanisms, monitoring, and optimization. *Chem. Rev.* **110,** 2795–2838 (2010).
3. Maas, A. L. *et al.* Tumour vascular microenvironment determines responsiveness to photodynamic therapy. *Cancer Res.* **72,** 2079–2088 (2012).
4. Henderson, B. W. & Fingar, V. H. Relationship of tumour hypoxia and response to photodynamic treatment in an experimental mouse tumour. *Cancer Res.* **47,** 3110–3114 (1987).
5. Hockel, M. & Vaupel, P. Tumour hypoxia: definitions and current clinical, biologic, and molecular aspects. *J. Natl Cancer Inst.* **93,** 266–276 (2001).
6. Wang, W., Moriyama, L. T. & Bagnato, V. S. Photodynamic therapy induced vascular damage: an overview of experimental PDT. *Laser Phys. Lett.* **10,** 023001–023008 (2013).
7. Henderson, B. W. & Dougherty, T. J. How does photodynamic therapy work. *Photochem. Photobiol.* **55,** 145–157 (1992).
8. Curnow, A., McIlroy, B. W., Postle-Hacon, M. J., MacRobert, A. J. & Bown, S. G. Light dose fractionation to enhance photodynamic therapy using 5-aminolevulinic acid in the normal rat colon. *Photochem. Photobiol.* **69,** 71–76 (1999).
9. Sitnik, T. M., Hampton, J. A. & Henderson, B. W. Reduction of tumour oxygenation during and after photodynamic therapy *in vivo*: effects of fluence rate. *Br. J. Cancer* **77,** 1386–1394 (1998).
10. Busch, T. M., Wang, H. W., Wileyto, E. P., Yu, G. Q. & Bunte, R. M. Increasing damage to tumour blood vessels during motexafin lutetium-pdt through use of low fluence rate. *Radiat. Res.* **174,** 331–340 (2010).
11. Tomaselli, F., Maier, A., Pinter, H., Stranzl, H. & Smolle-Juttner, F. M. Photodynamic therapy enhanced by hyperbaric oxygen in acute endoluminal palliation of malignant bronchial stenosis (clinical pilot study in 40 patients). *Eur. J. Cardiothorac. Surg.* **19,** 549–554 (2001).
12. Jirsa, Jr M., Pouckova, P., Dolezal, J., Pospisil, J. & Jirsa, M. Hyperbaric oxygen and photodynamic therapy in tumour-bearing nude mice. *Eur. J. Cancer* **27,** 109 (1991).
13. Maier, A. *et al.* Hyperbaric oxygen and photodynamic therapy in the treatment of advanced carcinoma of the cardia and the esophagus. *Lasers Surg. Med.* **26,** 308–315 (2000).
14. Maier, A. *et al.* Does hyperbaric oxygen enhance the effect of photodynamic therapy in patients with advanced esophageal carcinoma? A clinical pilot study. *Endoscopy* **32,** 42–48 (2000).
15. Fingar, V. H., Mang, T. S. & Henderson, B. W. Modification of photodynamic therapy-induced hypoxia by fluosol-DA (20%) and carbogen breathing in mice. *Cancer Res.* **48,** 3350–3354 (1988).
16. Dong, G. C., Hu, S. X., Zhao, G. Y., Gao, S. Z. & Wu, L. R. Experimental study on cytotoxic effects of hyperbaric oxygen and photodynamic therapy on mouse transplanted tumour. *Chin Med. J. (Engl)* **100,** 697–702 (1987).
17. Thom, S. R. Hyperbaric oxygen: its mechanisms and efficacy. *Plast. Reconstr. Surg.* **127,** 131s–141s (2011).
18. Castro, C. I. & Briceno, J. C. Perfluorocarbon-based oxygen carriers: review of products and trials. *Artif. Organs* **34,** 622–634 (2010).
19. Fuchs, J. & Thiele, J. The role of oxygen in cutaneous photodynamic therapy. *Free Radic. Biol. Med.* **24,** 835–847 (1998).
20. Davis, M. E., Chen, Z. G. & Shin, D. M. Nanoparticle therapeutics: an emerging treatment modality for cancer. *Nat. Rev. Drug Discov.* **7,** 771–782 (2008).
21. Alexis, F., Pridgen, E., Molnar, L. K. & Farokhzad, O. C. Factors affecting the clearance and biodistribution of polymeric nanoparticles. *Mol. Pharm.* **5,** 505–515 (2008).
22. Juzeniene, A., Nielsen, K. P. & Moan, J. Biophysical aspects of photodynamic therapy. *J. Environ. Pathol. Toxicol. Oncol.* **25,** 7–28 (2006).
23. Zhou, Y. *et al.* Microbubbles from gas-generating perfluorohexane nanoemulsions for targeted temperature-sensitive ultrasonography and synergistic HIFU ablation of tumours. *Adv. Mater.* **25,** 4123–4130 (2013).
24. Srinivas, M., Boehm-Sturm, P., Figdor, C. G., de Vries, I. J. & Hoehn, M. Labeling cells for *in vivo* tracking using F-19 MRI. *Biomaterials* **33,** 8830–8840 (2012).
25. Ahrens, E. T. & Bulte, J. W. M. Tracking immune cells *in vivo* using magnetic resonance imaging. *Nat. Rev. Immunol.* **13,** 755–763 (2013).

Acknowledgements

This project was supported by National Natural Science Foundation (No. 81202474, 81273464 and 81473146), Changzhou Special Project of Biotechnology and Biopharmacy (No.CE20105006) and Social Development of Natural Science Foundation of Jiangsu Province (No. BE2015674). J.W. is sponsored by Qing Lan Project.

Author contributions

Y.C.,J.W. and Y.H. designed the study; H.C.and K.W. performed the animal experiment; C.J. and W.H. performed the cell experiment; J.W. and Y.C. wroted the paper. H.C.,X.Q.,A.Y.and Y.H. edited the manuscript; J.W. and Y.H. supervised the whole project.

Additional information

Competing financial interests: The authors declare no competing financial interests.

23

Target engagement and drug residence time can be observed in living cells with BRET

Matthew B. Robers[1], Melanie L. Dart[1], Carolyn C. Woodroofe[2,†], Chad A. Zimprich[1], Thomas A. Kirkland[2], Thomas Machleidt[1], Kevin R. Kupcho[1], Sergiy Levin[2], James R. Hartnett[1], Kristopher Zimmerman[1], Andrew L. Niles[1], Rachel Friedman Ohana[1], Danette L. Daniels[1], Michael Slater[1], Monika G. Wood[1], Mei Cong[1], Yi-Qiang Cheng[3] & Keith V. Wood[1]

The therapeutic action of drugs is predicated on their physical engagement with cellular targets. Here we describe a broadly applicable method using bioluminescence resonance energy transfer (BRET) to reveal the binding characteristics of a drug with selected targets within intact cells. Cell-permeable fluorescent tracers are used in a competitive binding format to quantify drug engagement with the target proteins fused to Nanoluc luciferase. The approach enabled us to profile isozyme-specific engagement and binding kinetics for a panel of histone deacetylase (HDAC) inhibitors. Our analysis was directed particularly to the clinically approved prodrug FK228 (Istodax/Romidepsin) because of its unique and largely unexplained mechanism of sustained intracellular action. Analysis of the binding kinetics by BRET revealed remarkably long intracellular residence times for FK228 at HDAC1, explaining the protracted intracellular behaviour of this prodrug. Our results demonstrate a novel application of BRET for assessing target engagement within the complex milieu of the intracellular environment.

[1] Promega Corporation, 2800 Woods Hollow Road, Fitchburg, Wisconsin 53711, USA. [2] Promega Biosciences Incorporated, 277 Granada Drive, San Luis Obispo, California 93401, USA. [3] UNT System College of Pharmacy, Department of Pharmaceutical Sciences, University of North Texas Health Science Center, Fort Worth, Texas, USA. † Present address: National Institutes of Health, 9800 Medical Center Drive, Rockville MD 20850, USA. Correspondence and requests for materials should be addressed to M.B.R. (email: Matt.robers@promega.com).

Deciphering how small molecule modulators bind their intracellular targets is fundamental to understanding pharmacological mechanism. In addition to the specificity and affinity of target engagement, binding dynamics under non-equilibrium conditions may also underlie the therapeutic potential of new drug candidates[1–3]. These parameters are routinely assessed through biochemical means, which may fail to adequately mimic the complexity of the intracellular environment. Proteins reside in structurally intricate settings within the cells and typically function as components of extended molecular complexes, and thus they may exhibit significantly different behaviours than they would as isolated polypeptides[4–7]. It is not surprising that biochemical analysis of target engagement often fails to correlate with compound potency measured by cellular phenotype. Preferably, correlations between binding interactions and physiological outcomes should be made within a common physiological context. For this reason, the pharmaceutical industry has directed increased efforts towards assessing target engagement within intact cells[8–10].

While quantitation of compound binding to purified proteins or surface receptors (in particular G-protein coupled receptors) is well established[11–13], similar analysis for intracellular targets has been more difficult. Indirect approaches are often used instead, relying on deconvolution of cellular responses to infer target engagement[14]. For example, expression profiling may be used as an indicator of altered target activity in response to agonists or antagonists. However, compounds typically bind to multiple targets within cells, where only a few are mechanistically associated with the relevant phenotype. Unambiguously resolving the molecular targets of compounds within complex pathways and establishing that a cellular response serves as an adequate proxy for physical binding by the compound can be challenging.

More recently, various qualitative approaches based on ligand-induced protein stabilization have been used to characterize target engagement[9,10,15,16]. Such methods can be limited by the incremental stability imparted by compound binding relative to the inherent stability of the intracellular target. Consequently, these methods are prone to false negative results as many targets fail to exhibit measurable stabilization upon ligand binding[17]. For some of these techniques, elevated temperatures are required for the analysis, and thus may not represent physiological conditions for compound binding. Importantly, these methods are limited to end point analysis, complicating the application of such methods for measurements of binding kinetics or compound residence time.

Assessments of target engagement are especially challenging for prodrug inhibitors that require intracellular activation for maximal potency[18–20]. Mechanistic studies for such prodrug inhibitors may not be adequately represented in a biochemical framework, and may require analysis in cells to be physiologically meaningful. For example, the clinically approved histone deacetylase (HDAC) prodrug FK228 (depsipeptide, romidepsin, Istodax) as well as the related natural product thailandepsin A (TDP-A) utilize a unique mechanism that require intracellular reduction to achieve maximal potency[18,19,21]. It has been recently demonstrated that pulse-treatment of cells with FK228 results in highly potent and persistent inhibition of pan-HDAC activity[22–24]. Although various alternate intracellular mechanisms have been proposed for this observation[24], it has not been determined whether the sustained potency of FK228 is mechanistically associated with the intracellular residence time at HDAC isozymes. Biophysical methods compatible with living cells are therefore needed to interrogate target engagement and residence time for this compound class.

Bioluminescence resonance energy transfer (BRET) can reveal real-time molecular interactions within intact cells without cell lysis or non-physiological temperatures[25]. Energy transfer techniques such as BRET or fluorescence resonance energy transfer (FRET) are well established for quantifying intracellular protein–protein interactions within cells; however, BRET is often preferred owing to increased detection sensitivity[26–28]. While both energy transfer techniques have been utilized to measure compound binding to extracellular or lysate-derived analytes[12,13,29,30], neither has been successfully applied to the interrogation of target engagement and compound residence time within intact cells.

In contrast to previous applications of energy transfer, the approach presented here utilizes live cells expressing an intracellular target protein genetically fused to NanoLuc luciferase and a cell-permeable fluorescent tracer derived from a suitable drug or tool compound. BRET is achieved inside intact cells by reversible binding of the fluorescent tracer to the intracellular target. The binding characteristics of an interacting compound are revealed by its ability to compete with the tracer and thus influence the production of BRET. The general applicability of this approach for intracellular proteins is supported by our ability to quantify intracellular engagement by inhibitors of HDACs, bromodomains (BRDs) and kinases. Our analysis focused on target engagement at HDACs because this new capability should enable the biophysical characterization of target engagement and residence time for a diverse set of HDAC inhibitors, including the prodrugs FK228 and TDP-A. The BRET approach enabled a mechanistic interrogation on the enhanced potency and sustained efficacy of FK228, allowing us to directly measure both target engagement and residence time against target HDACs within intact cells. Using BRET, we were able to determine that the prolonged phenotypic effects of FK228 and TDP-A prodrugs in non-equilibrium conditions are due to the remarkably stable complexes formed between these molecules and HDAC protein within cells.

Results

BRET enables target engagement analysis for HDACs. We used a small luciferase (NanoLuc/Nluc, 19 kDa) as a BRET donor, which has been recently demonstrated to produce extraordinarily intense and stable luminescence with a relatively narrow spectral distribution[31]. For BRET tracers, we applied Non-Chloro-TOM dye (NCT) as a BRET acceptor, which demonstrated adequate cell-permeability and provided significant spectral resolution from Nluc[25]. Detection of tracer binding by energy transfer should be broadly applicable to intracellular proteins so long as the tracer is permeable to the cells and the proteins can be suitably tagged with Nluc. Intracellular target engagement is measured by competitive displacement of the tracer resulting in a loss of BRET (Fig. 1a).

HDACs served as the primary model system, where a single broad-coverage tracer could enable analysis of target engagement over multiple classes of HDACs. To elucidate inhibitor interactions across classes I and IIb HDACs, a broad-coverage target engagement assay was developed using a fluorescent tracer derived from SAHA coupled to NCT dye (Fig. 1b). Intracellular binding of the SAHA-NCT tracer to selected HDAC isozymes was detected by measuring the bioluminescence emission from a population of cells expressing a genetic fusion between the isozyme and Nluc. The putative targets of SAHA[32]; classes I and IIb HDACs, were included in the study to reveal isozyme-specific differences in inhibitor affinity. As HDACs coordinate binding of hydroxamic acid-based inhibitors such as SAHA via two highly conserved active-site His residues[33,34], a binding-deficient construct encoding Nluc-HDAC6 CD2 (H610A/H611A) was included in the analysis as a negative control. Furthermore, class IIa HDACs (HDACs 4, 5, 7 and 9) and class IV HDAC

(HDAC11) were also included as controls because of their expectedly low affinity to the SAHA-NCT tracer[32]. Microplate measurements of HeLa cells transiently expressing the genetic fusions confirmed both specific and concentration-dependent BRET only for classes I and IIb HDACs (Fig. 1c, Supplementary Fig. 1). To determine specific BRET signal, BRET data were background-corrected using a molar excess of unlabelled SAHA (Supplementary Fig. 1a). Both N- and C- terminal fusions were evaluated, with the orientation producing the largest BRET ratio for each isozyme shown in Fig. 1c. HDACs are known to tolerate reporter tags or purification tags larger than Nluc[35], and we found that tethering of Nluc did not significantly alter HDAC activity, using HDAC2 as a an example (Supplementary Fig. 1c).

The highest tracer affinity was evident for HDACs 1, 2, 6 and 10, with lower affinity observed for HDACs 3 and 8 (Fig. 1c). While the presence of the fluorescent moiety on SAHA impacted affinity of the tracer, the observed rank-order engagement by the SAHA-NCT tracer was in general agreement with the relative affinities reported for unmodified SAHA[32] (Supplementary Table 1). Because of the high luminescence intensity of Nluc interaction of the SAHA-NCT tracer could be detected at expression levels comparable to the endogenous protein, as demonstrated for HDAC1 in multiple cell types (Supplementary Fig. 1d). These results support that HDAC-Nluc fusions do not require overexpression to detect target engagement analysis via BRET.

In contrast to other members of the class I/IIb HDAC family, the HDAC6 isotype possesses two putative catalytic domains (CDs) as determined by homology analysis[36–38]. To determine whether the SAHA-NCT tracer binds one of the domains preferentially, we generated Nluc fusions with segregated CDs of HDAC6 and queried tracer binding in cells. BRET measurements demonstrated engagement of the tracer with the C-terminal CD (CD2) (Fig. 1c), whereas negligible BRET signal was observed at CD1 (Supplementary Fig. 1b). It has been reported that CD1 may lack deacetylase activity, and our results suggest that altered binding specificity may contribute to this[38]. As expected, the HDAC6 CD2 (H610A/H611A) mutant engaged SAHA-NCT poorly as determined via BRET (Fig. 1c).

To verify that BRET was arising from within living cells rather than from cellular debris that may be present in the culture medium, we imaged the luminescence emission from individual cells expressing Nluc fusions of HDAC6 or HDAC10. The addition of the SAHA-NCT tracer (1 μM) resulted in observable BRET clearly located within HeLa cells transiently expressing Nluc fusions of HDAC6 or HDAC10 (Fig. 1d, Supplementary Fig. 1e). Challenge with a molar excess of unmodified SAHA (10 μM) resulted in attenuation of the BRET signal, indicating that the BRET signal was generated by a specific and reversible interaction of the tracer with the Nluc fusion protein. BRET signal was observed exclusively in the cytoplasm of HeLa cells expressing Nluc-HDAC6, whereas HDAC10-Nluc expressing cells generated BRET in both the nucleus and cytosol. This is consistent with the expected localization patterns of both HDAC6 and HDAC10, and further demonstrates that the BRET signal is imposed by the placement of the luciferase even though the SAHA-NCT tracer is expected to bind multiple intracellular HDACs[36].

The ability to displace the tracer by an unlabelled compound allowed the relative binding efficiency by HDAC inhibitors to be determined for multiple intracellular isozymes. Unlabelled SAHA effectively attenuated the BRET signal in a concentration-dependent manner when added to cells in combination with the SAHA-NCT tracer (Fig. 1e). The relative binding efficiency of SAHA for different HDAC isozymes is apparent by the concentration required to displace a defined amount of the tracer. Using a fixed concentration (1 μM) of SAHA-NCT for competitive displacement, relative binding efficiencies were estimated by the Cheng-Prusoff equation[39] (see Supplementary Table 1 for observed and adjusted values). By this method, the greatest binding was observed with Nluc fusions of HDAC1, 2, 6 and 10, whereas HDACs 3 and 8 showed lower relative binding, as expected.[32] Although SAHA and the SAHA-NCT tracer share the same binding motif, this approach should be applicable to any molecule able to competitively displace the tracer from the target.

Profiling engagement and potency of HDAC inhibitors in HeLa. To demonstrate the utility of the BRET method to profile intracellular target engagement across HDACs, we used a structurally diverse set of inhibitors that included both hydroxamate- and non-hydroxamate-based compounds. Hydroxamate-based inhibitors were represented by SAHA, trichostatin A (TSA), ACY1215, M344 and panobinostat. Mocetinostat is an amino-benzamide-based inhibitor, and FK228 is a bicyclic depsipeptide prodrug. All six of the tested inhibitors engaged HDACs 1, 2 and 3, with FK228 demonstrating the highest engagement for these isozymes (Fig. 1f). Negligible binding of FK228 and mocetinostat were observed for HDAC6, HDAC8 and HDAC10 (Fig. 1f). Rank-order binding of the compounds for HDACs 1 and 2 were in agreement, likely explained by the close sequence homology between these proteins[40]. Other HDAC isozymes had more varied selectivity profiles, providing selectivity signatures that were largely in agreement with previous reports, albeit with some exceptions[32,40]. The bicyclic depsipeptide inhibitors of HDACs (including FK228 and the recently described TDP-A) are notable in that they rely on a unique mechanism of prodrug activation

Figure 1 | Measuring target engagement at intracellular HDACs. (**a**) Illustration of intracellular target engagement assay. A permeable fluorescent tracer binds in dynamic equilibrium to an intracellular target protein fused to Nluc, resulting in BRET. Introduction of compounds that bind the same target cause the tracer to be displaced, resulting in a decrease in BRET. (**b**) The HDAC tracer was derived from the adduct of a broad-coverage HDAC inhibitor (SAHA, shown in black) and the NCT dye (shown in red). (**c**) Introduction of SAHA-NCT to cell medium resulted in specific and concentration-dependent intracellular BRET with Nluc fusion of various HDACs (classes I and IIb) expressed in HeLa cells, as measured using a microplate luminometer. A control HDAC6 CD2 construct encoding a binding-deficient mutant (H610A/H611A) showed weakened engagement with the tracer. BRET values at each tracer concentration were background-corrected by parallel measurements made in the presence of an excess of unmodified SAHA (20 μM) (as described in Methods and Supplementary Fig. 1a). Apparent tracer affinities were estimated using equation (1) and reported in Supplementary Table 1. Data are mean ± s.e.m. of three independent experiments. (**d**) Luminescence images of HeLa cells expressing HDAC6 or HDAC10 fused to Nluc, shown with false colouring to represent light emission from 420–500 nm (donor) or above 590 nm (acceptor). Images were acquired in the presence of SAHA-NCT tracer alone (1 μM), or in combination with excess unlabelled SAHA (10 μM). Signal suppression caused by excess SAHA indicates specificity of the BRET signal. (**e**) Concentration-dependent attenuation of BRET from intracellular HDAC fusions with titration of SAHA in the presence of 1 μM SAHA-NCT tracer. Data were collected on a microplate luminometer and are mean ± s.e.m. of three independent experiments. See Supplementary Table 1 and equations (2) and (3) for estimation of apparent affinities of SAHA to HDACs. (**f**) BRET measurements showing the relative affinity of HDAC inhibitors in HeLa cells (1 μM SAHA-NCT). See Supplementary Table 2 for relative compound affinities to individual HDACs. Data are mean ± s.d. of four data points.

which requires intracellular reduction of a disulfide bond[18,19,41]. The ability to observe target engagement within living cells thus allows characterization of inhibitor mechanism for these compounds within the physiological environment necessary for prodrug conversion.

It is well established that upregulated HDAC 1 and 2 activities inhibit apoptosis and mediate proliferation in cervical cancer cell lineages such as HeLa[40,42,43]. To verify that our intracellular target engagement profiles measured by BRET accurately correlate with antiproliferation, we determined potencies for the

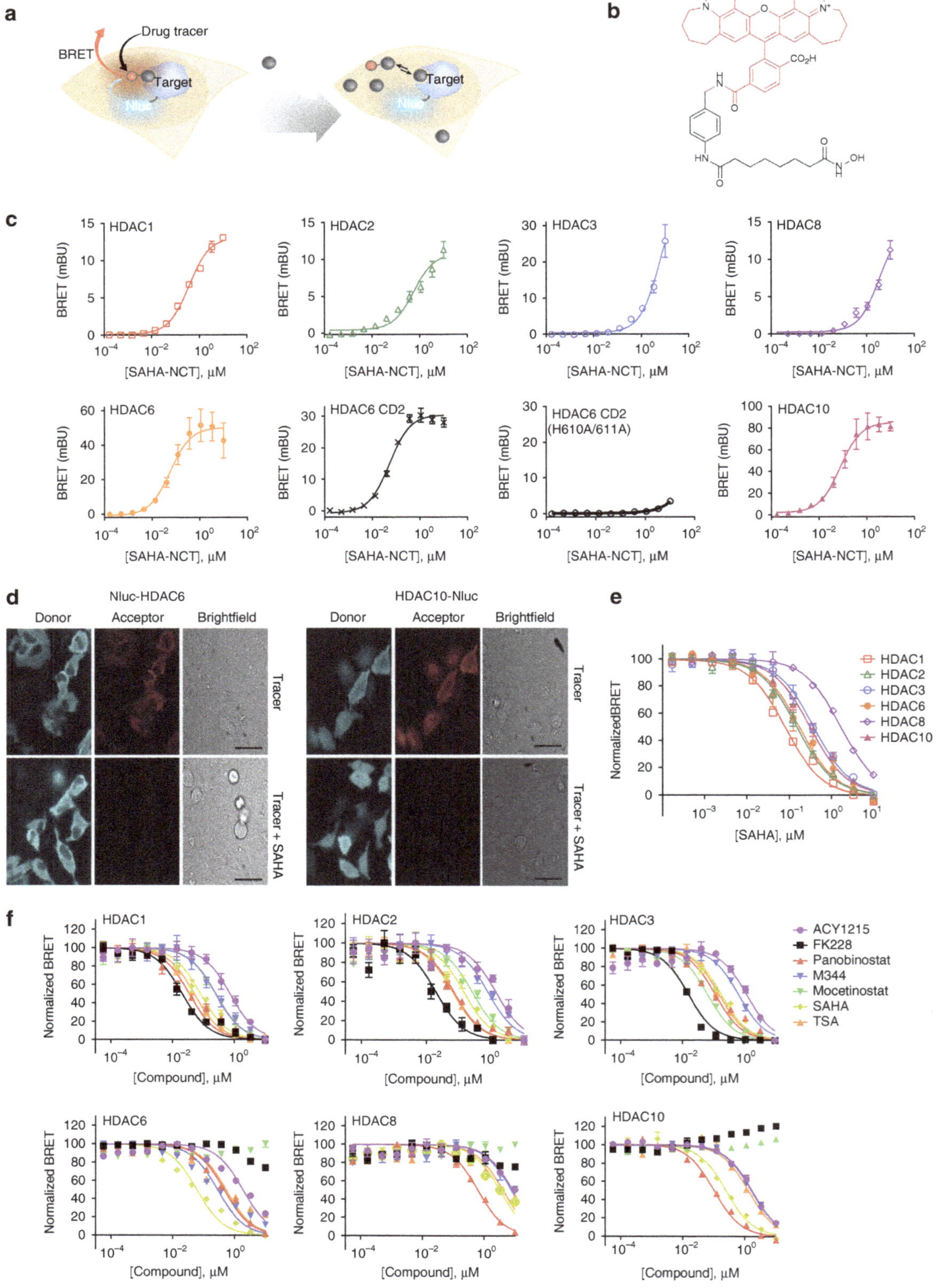

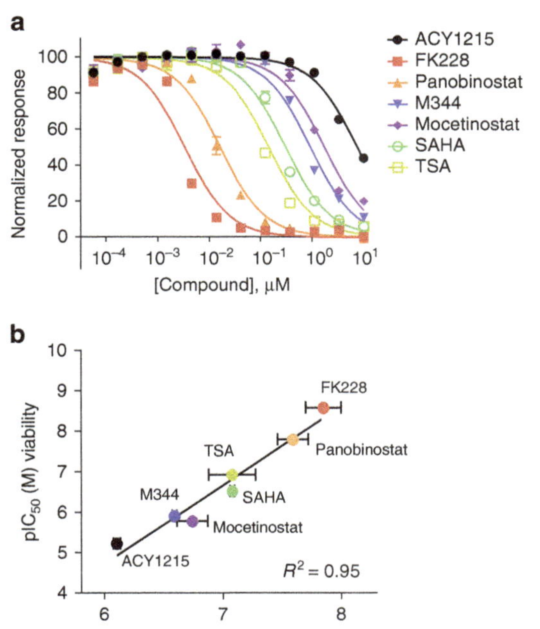

Figure 2 | Correlation of phenotypic potency with target engagement to intracellular HDAC isozymes. (**a**) 48 h treatment with HDAC inhibitors results in antiproliferative effects in HeLa cells, as measured by intracellular ATP levels. Data are the mean of three independent experiments ± s.e.m.. (**b**) Antiproliferative potency of HDAC inhibitors, as determined by cellular ATP levels in HeLa cells, is strongly correlated with target engagement to HDAC1. See Supplementary Fig. 2b and Supplementary Table 2 for the comparative correlation with other HDAC isozymes. Data are the mean of 3 independent experiments ± s.d.

panel of inhibitors using assays of apoptosis (caspase 3/7 activation) and cell proliferation (cellular ATP). A range of potencies was observed with similar rank-order produced by either method (Fig. 2a, Supplementary Fig. 2a). As expected[40], target engagement was found to strongly correlate with antiproliferation for HDAC1 and HDAC2, yielding $R^2 = 0.95$ and 0.88 respectively (Fig. 2b, Supplementary Fig. 2b and Supplementary Table 2). Unsurprisingly, the correlations with less relevant HDACs were relatively poor (Supplementary Fig. 2b, Supplementary Table 2). As HDAC1 and HDAC2 are the dominant HDACs mediating cell proliferation in many cancer cell lines, these correlations reinforce the validity of the target engagement measurements provided by BRET[40,42,43].

BRET reveals long residence times for FK228 and TDP-A. FK228 and related TDP-A require the reducing environment within cells to activate their sulfhydryl groups and achieve maximal potency[18] (Fig. 3a). Although there has been speculation regarding the possible causes for protracted efficacy of FK228 in pulse-treatment experiments[22,24], the precise mechanism has not been determined. We investigated this for FK228 and TDP-A by analysing temporal changes in the BRET measurements to characterize kinetic aspects of target engagement. As a prerequisite, it was necessary to establish that SAHA-NCT demonstrates rapid binding kinetics to ensure that dynamic interaction of the tracer with the intracellular target remains close to equilibrium over the time interval needed for engagement by the inhibitors[44]. As SAHA has fast binding kinetics, the SAHA-NCT tracer should be suitable for kinetic analysis of relatively slow-binding HDAC inhibitors in a competitive format[45].

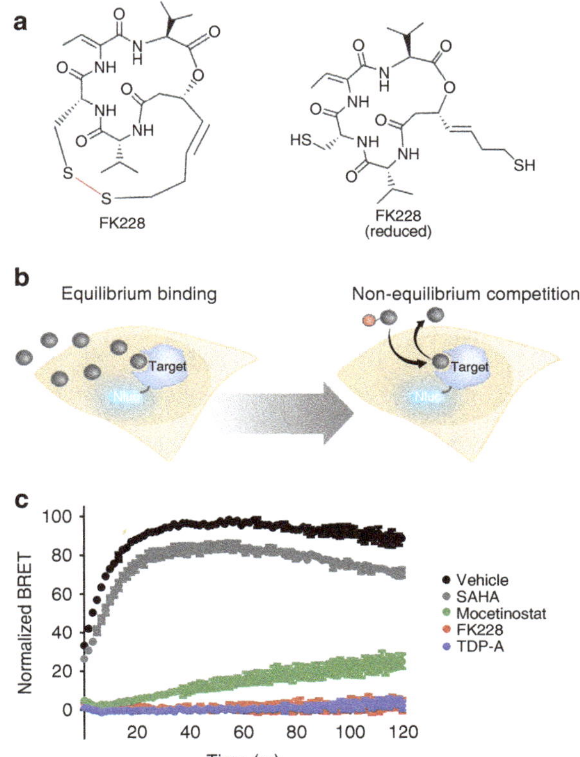

Figure 3 | Measuring the intracellular residence time of HDAC inhibitors at HDAC1. (**a**) Structure of the inhibitor FK228 in the prodrug form (left) and the form activated by intracellular reduction (right). (**b**) Illustration of assay method for measuring intracellular residence time using BRET. Live cells expressing the target protein fused to Nluc are equilibrated with a near-saturating concentration of compound. The cells are then washed to remove unbound compound and treated with a near-saturating concentration of a tracer. The profile of compound with slow dissociation kinetics from the target impedes tracer binding, which slows production of the BRET signal. (**c**) Residence time analysis by BRET reveals remarkably slow dissociation rates for FK228 (red) and TDP-A (blue), compared with mocetinostat (green), SAHA (grey) or vehicle/DMSO control (black). Data are normalized to maximum signal (vehicle/DMSO-treated) versus full-occupancy control (10 μM SAHA, no washout). The kinetic traces for FK228 and TDP-A are nearly indistinguishable from the full occupancy control (10 μM SAHA, no washout). Data are mean ± s.e.m.. of four independent experiments.

Addition of a 1 μM solution of tracer to cells expressing HDAC1-Nluc resulted in a rapid increase in BRET, reaching a plateau within ~20 min of tracer addition (Supplementary Fig. 3a). This rate is at least partially impacted by permeability across the plasma membrane, as addition of digitonin as a permeabilizing agent resulted in near-instantaneous BRET between the tracer and HDAC1-Nluc (Supplementary Fig. 3e).

Unlike hydroxamate-based inhibitors such as SAHA, it as been previously reported that prodrug inhibitors in the FK228 family possess a slow but protracted activity in cancer cell lineages[23]. Using the BRET approach, we confirmed that fast binding kinetics are observed for unmodified SAHA in HeLa cells (Supplementary Fig. 3b). In contrast to SAHA, FK228 and TDP-A equilibrated slowly, displaying an IC_{50} value that dropped continuously over the 180 min timecourse. The slow-binding kinetics of the prodrug inhibitors in cells were corroborated in an enzymatic assay using purified HDAC1 and chemically reduced FK228 or TDP-A (Supplementary Fig. 3c). Our results therefore support previous observations regarding the delayed effect of FK228 inside cancer cells.

Because of the reported functional persistence of FK228 activity, it has been suggested that these inhibitors may accumulate within cells, impact HDAC expression levels, or release slowly from their targets[22,24]. To directly assess the possibility of slow release from intracellular HDAC protein, the BRET method was reconfigured to measure the relative rates of compound dissociation from HDAC1. HeLa cells expressing HDAC1-Nluc were first equilibrated with a saturating concentration of compound. The aminobenzamide inhibitor mocetinostat was included as a control, as it has been demonstrated that inhibitors in this class possess slow dissociation kinetics with HDAC1 (refs 45–47). Cells were treated with FK228 at 100 nM, TDP-A at 10 nM, mocetinostat at 10 μM, or SAHA at 10 μM, followed by ligand removal (including an additional wash for FK228 and TDP-A) and immediate challenge with a saturating concentration of SAHA-NCT tracer. Increased BRET is indicative of tracer binding to the HDAC, which cannot occur until after the compound has dissociated (Fig. 3b, see Supplementary Fig. 3d for a detailed schematic representation of the assay). This analysis was also performed in lysed cells to address the proposed possibility that the reduced FK228 and TDP-A could accumulate and become trapped within cells, leading to residual target engagement after compound removal[22,24]. In live cells, dissociation of SAHA from HDAC1 was rapid and beyond the detection limits of the assay, whereas the reference compound mocetinostat displayed a slower dissociation rate as expected (Fig. 3c). The intracellular dissociation rate for FK228 and TDP-A were slower than the control compound mocetinostat at HDAC1, with a residence time profile similar to fully bound HDAC1 (samples without 10 μM SAHA removal, Fig. 3c). Results were corroborated in lysed cells, suggesting that intracellular trapping of FK228 is insufficient to explain the observed kinetics of dissociation (Supplementary Fig. 3e). These results indicate a remarkably slow dissociation rate (long residence time) for FK228 and TDP-A from HDAC1, and suggest that the strong binary complex between the inhibitors and HDAC protein are the cause of the prolonged phenotypic effect.

BRET for target engagement at alternate target classes. In addition to HDACs, we evaluated the BRET method for the BET family of BRDs and the lymphocyte specific protein tyrosine kinase (LCK) using BRET tracers derived from known inhibitors of these target proteins (Supplementary Fig. 4a, Supplementary Methods). An NCT tracer derived from iBET-762 engaged full-length Nluc-BRD4 proteins (Fig. 4a, Supplementary Figure 4b), as well as other members of the BET family of BRDs (Supplementary Fig. 4c). Target engagement profiles at BRD4 were then determined in competitive displacement formats with a panel of known BRD4 inhibitors (Fig. 4b) as well as segregated domains of BRD4 (Supplementary Fig. 4d). Applicability to intracellular kinases was then demonstrated at LCK using an NCT tracer derived from BIBF-1120 (Supplementary Fig. 4e,f). For both BRDs and LCK, rank-order affinities of various reference compounds observed using BRET were consistent with previous reports[48–50] Taken together, these results indicate that energy transfer to cell-permeable tracer may provide a broadly applicable means for evaluating target engagement over key intracellular target classes.

Discussion

This report describes the first method to directly assess target engagement and binding kinetics within intact mammalian cells under physiological conditions. Compound binding is detected by BRET, a biophysical process which provides significant advantages over alternative methods that rely on more complex biological proxies, operate under non-physiological or disruptive conditions, or are unsuitable for real-time analysis of compound binding and dissociation[10,15]. The simplified workflow we describe also eliminates the laborious liquid transfer steps and excessive hands-on time required of many alternative methodologies, particularly those utilizing thermal denaturation. Compared with biochemical methods, detection of intracellular target engagement provides an assessment of binding efficiency in an environment more representative of the cellular milieu where it would occur in tissues. The intracellular measurements also circumvent the need for isolated enzymes, which may be difficult to obtain by heterologous expression with sufficient purity and in a structurally appropriate form. This is the case with HDACs, for example, which generally function in protein complexes[51].

The ratiometric nature of energy transfer measurements mitigates potential assay interferences, such as variations in cell number or expression level between samples[26,27,52]. BRET was chosen as the preferred energy transfer system over FRET due to the increased detection sensitivity it provides in microplate formats[26–28,30,52,53]. NanoLuc, in particular, provides excellent sensitivity as a BRET donor because of its small and stable structure, exceptionally bright luminescence, and relatively narrow emission spectrum[31]. Corroborating the signal strength and sensitivity of this method within live cells, energy transfer between Nluc and the NCT tracers produced sufficient BRET signal to directly image target engagement at the single-cell level using bioluminescent imaging microscopy. Using this BRET technique, it may be therefore possible to study target engagement distribution over a cell population.

The binding profiles for the tracers described in this report provide evidence that the red-emitting fluorophore, NCT, can be

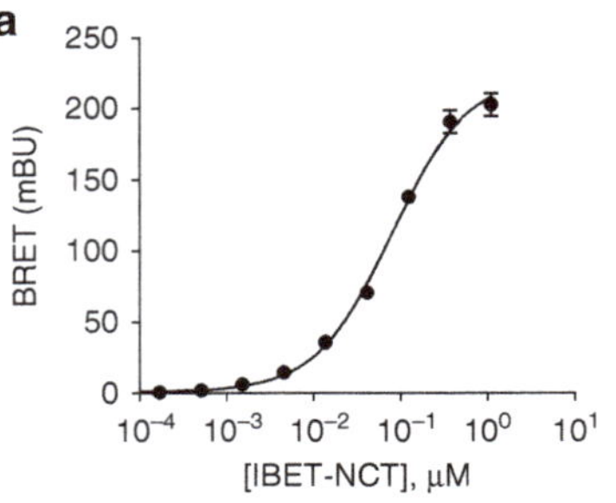

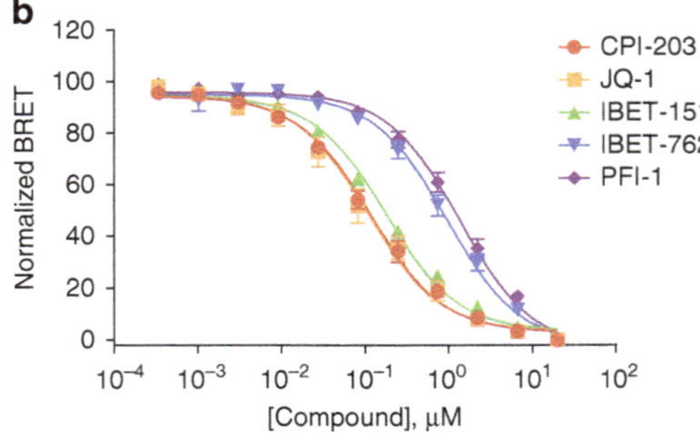

Figure 4 | Measuring intracellular target engagement at bromodomain BRD4 using BRET. (**a**) Specific and dose-dependent BRET was observed with Nluc-fusions to full-length BRD4 expressed in HeLa. BRET values at each tracer concentration were background-corrected by parallel measurements made in the presence of an excess of unmodified compound (20 μM) (described in Methods). Data are mean ± s.d. of four data points. (**b**) Use of BRET to measure rank-order affinity of BRD inhibitor panel against BRD4 within live HeLa cells (1 μM IBET-NCT held constant). Data are mean ± s.e.m. of four independent experiments.

coupled onto structurally diverse chemical probes to provide cell-permeable BRET tracers for a variety of target classes. For tracer derivatization, we utilized probes with known mechanism of action and putative target engagement profiles. Probe molecules with less established structure–activity relationships may represent additional challenge for NCT modification. In the context of phenotypic screening (when knowledge of target selectivity for a lead compound is unknown), it may be useful to explore the suitability of the BRET technique for target identification. As an extension of the principle demonstrated here, it may be possible to apply an NCT derivative of a lead compound against a diverse panel of Nluc fusion constructs as a screen for potential intracellular targets. Such an approach could serve as a complement to more traditional mass spectrometry-based methods for target identification.

Although the fluorescent moiety of the tracer may impart altered target affinity compared with the unlabelled parent compound, our results support general applicability of the method so long as the tracer is permeable to cells, specific BRET can be measured over a titratable concentration range, and that competitive displacement can reveal accurate target engagement profiles for unlabelled compounds. However, use of BRET tracers for target engagement studies may represent a limitation for mechanistic studies on allosteric ligands that occupy binding sites distinct from that of the tracer. Ligands that engage the target but fail to compete with the tracer would therefore represent false negatives. While this may represent a potential liability, it has been well-documented that allosteric ligands may bind in a mutually exclusive manner with orthosteric (active-site) tracers[54]. Future studies are warranted to determine if this BRET technique could enable target engagement studies in this context. Non-tracer-based techniques (such as those utilizing thermal stability or thermal shift) are prone to a distinct set of false negatives, as high affinity ligands may not impart a measurable increase in stability for certain target proteins[17]. As this BRET technique is independent of target stability or denaturation steps, it may be a useful complement to stability-based assessments of target engagement.

By using a broad-spectrum tracer for analysis of class I/IIb HDACs, we successfully demonstrated that a single tracer could enable a target engagement study across multiple classes of HDACs. Although our engagement results were largely in agreement with literature[32,40], small discrepancies could be attributed to the behaviour of isolated proteins versus the intracellular targets interrogated in our analysis. Indeed, there is a lack of consensus in the literature regarding the profiles of our compound set against purified HDACs[4,32,40], possibly explained by the diversity and variability of available biochemical HDAC assay components.

To evaluate the validity of our HDAC target engagement results, we performed the first systematic correlation analysis between intracellular isozyme affinity and antiproliferative potency in a common cellular context. Target engagement measured by BRET for HDAC1 and HDAC2 for the compound panel showed a strong correlation with both apoptosis and proliferation of HeLa cells. The involvement of HDACs 1 and 2 in these phenotypic outcomes is consistent with proposed models for their roles in tumorigenesis in cervical cancer cells such as HeLa. This relationship is not surprising, as HDAC1 and HDAC2 share 87% sequence similarity and form intracellular protein complexes which coordinate the transition from G1 to S-phase in the cell cycle[42,43]. They are also commonly upregulated in tumour cells, including HeLa. Consequently, it is not surprising that pharmacological inhibition of these enzymes should inhibit proliferation in this cell model[40]. While a strong correlation was observed for HDACs 1 and 2 (and to a lesser extent HDAC3), the relatively poor correlation observed at HDACs 6, 8 and 10 support that these targets are not directly implicated in the antiproliferative effects of HDAC inhibitors in this cell model. Our observed profiles for target engagement therefore corroborate the proposed link between HDAC1 and HDAC2 activities in tumour cell proliferation and inhibition of apoptosis.

Although assessments of target occupancy are often assessed under equilibrium (using affinity values such as K_d, IC_{50}), this may not be adequate for predicting target occupancy *in vivo*, where equilibrium conditions may not apply[1]. Under the dosing dynamics that are representative of *in vivo* conditions, dissociation rate, or residence time, may better characterize the ligand-receptor complex[1–3]. Furthermore, intracellular residence time may be impacted by intracellular target densitites, suggesting that binding analysis using purified analytes may not be adequate to predict drug residence time *in vivo*[7]. However, no methods currently exist to directly measure intracellular target engagement under non-equilibrium conditions. To enable a biophysical assessment of this process as it occurs inside intact cells, we explored the feasibility for using intracellular BRET to observe the kinetics of drug dissociation for a select group of HDAC inhibitors.

To mechanistically characterize the persistent effects of FK228 following inhibitor washout experiments, we configured the BRET assay to directly monitor dissociation of the prodrug inhibitors at HDAC1 inside cells. In this configuration, extremely slow apparent dissociation kinetics (long residence time) were observed for these HDAC inhibitors compared with SAHA. Moreover, the prodrug inhibitors showed even longer residence time than mocetinostat, a compound with reportedly slow dissociation rates at HDACs[45–47].

Consistent with our residence time analysis, it has been well-documented that pulse-treatment of cells with FK228 results in enhanced and persistent inhibition of intracellular HDAC activity compared with SAHA[22,24]. This enhanced duration of HDAC inhibition was concomitant with increased HIV RNA expression and virion release from infected T-cells, indicating that FK228 should be further assessed for treatment of latent viral reservoir in HIV-infected patients[22]. In the previous studies, it was not determined whether the sustained efficacy of FK228 resulted from long residence time at HDACs versus alternate mechanisms (potentially involving HDAC expression levels, cellular accumulation of the reduced drug, inhibition of HDAC complexes and so forth). For prodrug molecules such as FK228, acellular assay formats are unsuitable to explore these mechanisms. The intracellular BRET technique was able to interrogate the dynamics of FK228 target engagement because of its compatibility with equilibrium and non-equilibrium binding analysis. Results presented here enabled a mechanistic interrogation into the enhanced phenotypic effect of FK228 under such pulse-treatment conditions, and indicate that HDAC occupancy is enhanced for this class of prodrug molecules under open system conditions. In a broader context, optimizing a lead compound for increased intracellular residence time at primary targets, while decreasing residence time at collateral targets, could mitigate potential drug side effects and increase safety profiles. The ability to configure the BRET assay to interrogate binding kinetics could be used to guide medicinal chemistry efforts during the workflow of lead optimization.

In summary, we have found that BRET can provide quantitative analysis of intracellular target engagement over a diverse set of target classes. This approach can be used to assess target engagement and binding kinetics in a simplified, homogeneous assay format. We have demonstrated that intracellular binding can be correlated with phenotypic potency, potentially allowing for primary drug targets to be differentiated from targets engaged collaterally. The use of BRET for interrogating compound binding to intracellular targets should therefore advance capabilities in drug design and mechanistic analysis.

Methods

Expression plasmid construction. To produce Nluc fusions with the targets interrogated in this study, pF31K Nluc [CMV/Neo] and pF32K [CMV/Neo] were used to place Nluc at the N-terminus or the C-terminus of the target protein (respectively) using the manufacturer's protocol (Promega). For N-terminal tagging of Nluc to the target protein in pF31K, the resulting fusion encoded a flexible Gly-Ser-Ser-Gly-Ala-Ile-Ala linker connecting Nluc with the target. For C-terminal tagging of Nluc to the target protein in pF32K, the resulting fusion encoded a flexible Val-Ser-Leu-Gly-Ser-Ser-Gly linker connecting the target protein with Nluc. Complementary DNAs encoded the following target proteins, and were a 100% match to their respective NCBI reference sequence identifiers; BRD2 (NP005095), BRD3 (AB383723.1), BRD4 (NP490597), BRDT (NP001229739), Kat2b (NP003875), HDAC1 (NP004955), HDAC2 (NP001518), HDAC3 (NP003874), HDAC4 (NP006028), HDAC5 (NP005465), HDAC6 (NP006035), HDAC7 (NP056216), HDAC8 (NP060956), HDAC9 (NP848510), HDAC10 (NP114408), HDAC11 (NP079103) and LCK (NP005347). To generate Nluc fusions with segregated domains of HDAC6, ORFs encoding amino acid residues 74-455 and residues 479-845 were used for HDAC6/CD1 and HDAC6/CD2, respectively. Nluc-HDAC6 CD2 was mutated at H610A/H611A (residues represented from full-lenth HDAC6) to generate a binding-deficient mutant protein. To generate Nluc fusions with segregated domains of BRD4, ORFs encoding amino acids 44-168 and residues 333-460 were used for BRD4/BD1 and BRD4/BD2, respectively.

Cell transfection and BRET measurements under equilibrium conditions. To lower intracellular expression levels of the reporter fusion, Nluc/target fusion constructs into carrier DNA (pGEM3ZF-, Promega) at a mass ratio of 1:10 (mass/mass), before forming FuGENE HD complexes according to the manufacturer's protocol (Promega). DNA:FuGENE complexes were formed at a ratio of 1:3 (μg DNA per μl FuGENE). One part of the transfection complexes was then mixed with 20 parts (v/v) of HeLa cells (ATCC) suspended at a density of 2×10^5 in DMEM (Gibco) + 10% fetal bovine serum (FBS) (GE Healthcare), followed by incubation in a humidified, 37 °C/5% CO_2 incubator for 20 h. Cells were trypsinized and resuspended in Opti-MEM without phenol red (Life Technologies). Cells were then seeded into white, nonbinding surface plates (Corning) at a density of 2×10^4 cells/well. All chemical inhibitors were prepared as concentrated stock solutions in dimethylsulphoxide (DMSO) (Sigma-Aldrich). TDP-A was prepared by bacterial fermentation from the Cheng group, as described[19,41]. Remaining chemical inhibitors were purchased from Selleck Chemicals, with the exception of iBET, iBET-151, PFI-1 and CPI-203 (Xcessbio) and JQ-1 (EMD Biosciences). For generating tracer isotherms against targets expressed in cells, serially diluted tracer was added to cells in the presence or absence of 20 μM competing unlabelled compound (with the exception of BIBF-1120, for which Dasatinib was used). Cells were then equilibrated for 2 h before BRET measurements. For determining unlabelled compound isotherms, BRET tracers were added to the cells at fixed concentrations before test compound addition. A final concentration of 1 μM was used for SAHA-NCT and iBET-NCT. Experiments with BIBF1120-NCT utilized 3 μM. Serially diluted test compounds were then added to the cells and allowed to equilibrate for 2 h before BRET measurements. To measure BRET, NanoBRET NanoGlo Substrate-(Promega) was added, and filtered luminescence was measure on a BMG LABTECH Clariostar luminometer equipped with 450 nm BP filter (donor) and 610 nm LP filter (acceptor), using 0.5 s integration time with gain settings of 2,800 and 3,500, respectively. Background-corrected BRET ratios were determined by subtracting the BRET ratios of samples with excess competing ligand (20 μM) from the BRET ratios in the absence of competing ligand. Milli-BRET units (mBU) are the BRET values × 1,000. Apparent tracer affinity values were determined as described previously[13] using curve fits in GraphPad Prism with the equation (equation (1)):

$$Y = Bmax \times X/(Kd + X). \quad (1)$$

Competitive displacement data were then graphed with GraphPad Prism software using a three-parameter curve fit with the following equation (equation (2));

$$Y = Bottom + (Top - Bottom)/(1 + 10^{((X - LogIC50))}) \quad (2)$$

Normalized data were generated by assigning 100% to the theoretical maximum of the three-parameter curve fit and 0% for the theoretical minimum value of the three-parameter curve fit. Apparent affinity values for each compound were calculated from observed IC_{50} values according to the Cheng-Prusoff equationref. 39 (equation (3)):

$$K_i = \frac{IC_{50}}{1 + \frac{[L]}{K_D}} \quad (3)$$

where $[L]$ is the concentration of fluorescent ligand in μM and K_D is the apparent intracellular K_D of fluorescent ligand in μM. The apparent intracellular K_D values were calculated from the tracer saturation binding experiments described above.

Kinetic analysis of target engagement via BRET. For kinetic analysis of the equilibration rates of SAHA, FK228 and TDP-A, cells transfected with Nluc-HDAC fusions as described above were pre-equilibrated for 2 h with 1 μM SAHA-NCT tracer prior addition of test compound. NanoBRET NanoGlo Substrate was added to the samples and equilibrated at room temperature for 30 min before BRET measurements. Immediately after addition of the unlabelled test compound, kinetic BRET analysis was performed at room temperature over the time indicated on a Thermo Varioskan Luminometer equipped with 450 nm BP filter (donor) and 610 nm LP filter (acceptor), using 0.5 s integration times.

Kinetic analysis of ligand dissociation via BRET. For direct analysis of relative compound dissociation rates via BRET, 2×10^6 cells transfected with HDAC1-Nluc (in 10 ml of Opti-MEM) were aliquoted into 15 ml conical tubes and first pre-equilibrated with DMSO (vehicle), SAHA (10 μM), mocetinostat (10 μM), FK228 (100 nM) or TDP-A (10 nM) for 3 h at 37 °C/5% CO_2. Final concentration of DMSO was 0.1%. Cells treated with SAHA or mocetinostat were pelleted and resuspended in 10 mL of Opti-MEM in the presence of NanoBRET NanoGlo Substrate and 1 μM SAHA-NCT tracer immediately before BRET measurements. FK228 and TDP-A were subjected to an additional centrifugation and 10 ml wash step (with 5 min incubation) before BRET measurements, to ensure adequate removal of inhibitor from the cell medium. In addition to a zero-occupancy (DMSO/vehicle-treated) sample for determination of $BRET_{100}$, a full-occupancy control sample ($BRET_0$) was included, wherein 10 μM unmodified SAHA was left incubating on the cells (no washout) during the kinetic BRET analysis. To ensure that FK228 and TDP-A were not trapped within intact cells during the residence time analysis, a separate experiment was performed with digitonin added as lytic reagent (50 μg ml^{-1}) added at the time of 1 μM SAHA-NCT tracer addition. BRET data were normalized to 100% signal from the positive control (defined as the maximum BRET value observed from cells treated with 1uM SAHA-NCT in the absence of unlabelled competing compound) and 0% signal (defined as the BRET value observed from cells treated with 1 uM SAHA-NCT + 10 μM unmodified SAHA).

BRET imaging. HeLa cells were transfected with Nluc/target fusion constructs as described previously (see above). Cells suspended at a density of 2×10^5 cells per ml in DMEM (Gibco) + 10% FBS (Hyclone) were plated into 35 mm tissue culture treated imaging dishes (ibidi) at 2 ml per dish and incubated 18–24 h at 37 °C/5% CO_2. Media was removed from imaging dishes via gentle aspiration and replaced with 2 ml warm Opti-MEM without phenol red (Gibco) in the presence or absence of tracer +/− competing cold compound. Tracers and cold compound pairs used include 1 μM SAHA-NCT +/− 10 μM SAHA, 3 μM IBET-NCT +/− 10 μM IBET and 3 μM BIBF-1120-NCT +/− 10 μM Nilotinib. Cells were equilibrated for 2 h at 37 °C + 5% CO_2 before addition of NanoBRET NanoGlo Substrate. Images were captured on an Olympus LV200 microscope equipped with an environmental stage and a Hamamatsu ImagEM EMCCD camera. All images were acquired using a × 100/1.4 UPLanSApo objective and Olympus cellSens software. To image BRET events, images of donor and acceptor emission were acquired sequentially using a 460/80 bandpass filter and a 590 nm long-pass filter, respectively.

Apoptosis and cell proliferation assays. To measure induction of apoptosis, HeLa cells were seeded into 96-well plates at a density of 10^4 cells per well in DMEM + 10% FBS. Serially diluted test compounds were added to the cells and incubated for 20 h. After incubation, an equal volume of Caspase-Glo (3/7) reagent (Promega) was added to the cells, and quantified on a GloMax-Multi Microplate Luminometer (Promega) according to the manufacturer's protocol. To measure inhibition of proliferation, HeLa cells were seeded into 96-well plates at a density of 2.5×10^3 cells per well in DMEM + 10% FBS. Serially diluted test compounds were added as described above and incubated 48 h. After incubation, an equal volume of CellTiter-Glo Luminescent Cell Viability Assay (Promega) was added to the cells, and luminescence was quantified according to the manufacturer's protocol. Data were then graphed with GraphPad Prism software as described above for the BRET target engagement experiments.

Kinetic analysis of compound inhibition on purified HDAC1. Full-length human recombinant HDAC 1 was purchased from SignalChem. HDAC 1 enzymatic activity was measured using HDAC-Glo I/II Assay (Promega)[55]. To determine real-time IC_{50} values, 90 μl of 1/2,400 diluted HDAC 1 in HDAC-Glo I/II assay buffer was added to a opaque white, sterile, TC-treated 96-well assay plate (Corning). To enzyme, 100 μl of HDAC-Glo I/II detection reagent was added (190 μl total volume per well). The assay plate was mixed by a brief plate shake and the HDAC reaction was allowed to initiate and come to a steady-state luminescent signal by incubating for 20 min at room temperature. During this incubation, a serial dilution of SAHA, FK228, TDP-A was performed at a 200 × concentration in 100% DMSO in a separate master 96-well plate. A 10 µl aliquot of this master titration series was added to HDAC-Glo I/II assay buffer to generate a 20 × concentrated intermediate dilution containing 2.5 mM DTT for the prodrug inhibitors. Once the previous 20 min incubation was complete, 10 µl replicates ($n = 2$ for SAHA and $n = 3$ for FK228 and TDP-A) from this master intermediate titration series of compounds were transferred to the opaque white assay plate for a final total volume of 200 µl. The plate was then placed in a POLARstar OPTIMA (BMG LABTECH, Ortenberg, Germany) and luminescence was measured every 5 min for 120 min. For each time point, the raw luminescent signal for each test well of the appropriate compound was normalized to the no inhibition control well average (to calculate % inhibition). For each compound, the % inhibition was graphed versus inhibitor concentration for each time point to determine IC_{50}. Data were then graphed with GraphPad Prism software as described above for the BRET target engagement experiments.

Analysis of expression level of HDAC-NLuc fusions. HEK293 or HeLa cells were transfected with DNA constructs encoding HDAC1-NLuc at 0.8 µg ml^{-1} using PEI as transfection reagent as described previously[56]. To reduce expression levels the DNA was undiluted, diluted 1:10 and diluted 1:100 into a promoterless carrier DNA plasmid to generate a final total DNA concentration of 0.8 µg ml^{-1}. Control cells were transfected with the promoterless carrier DNA plasmid only. Twenty-four hours after transfection the cells were collected using Cellstriper (Corning), washed with PBS and then lysed using detergent lysis buffer (mammalian lysis buffer from Promega) supplemented with 1:50 dilution of RQ1 DNase (Promega) and 1 × RQ1 DNAase buffer and 1 × protease inhibitor cocktail (Promega). 5% of each cell lysate was analysed by SDS-PAGE and electro-transferred onto a PVDF membrane (Life Technologies). The membrane was blocked for 1 h with 5% BSA (Promega) in TBS buffer and probed overnight at 4 °C with the primary antibody in TBS supplemented with 0.1% Tween-20 (TBST). After three washes in TBST, the membrane was incubated with a secondary HRP - conjugated antibody (Jackson laboratories) in TBST for 1 h, washed five times with TBST and one time with TBS. The immune-stained proteins were detected using enhanced chemiluminescent (ECL) reagent (Promega) and detected on the LAS400 imager (GE Healthcare). Antibody source: anti-HDAC1 (Abcam; ab46985), anti-HDAC2 (Abcam; ab51832).

Activity of HDAC2 expressed in cell free expression system. HDAC2-NLuc, HDAC2 and NLuc were expressed in the S30 T7 High-Yield Protein expression system (Promega) as recommended by the manufacturer. A total of 40 µl of each expression reaction (in triplicates) were tested for HDAC2 activity using HDAC-Glo 2 assay (Promega). Luminescence was measured on a GloMAX luminometer (Promega).

References

1. Copeland, R. A., Pompliano, D. L. & Meek, T. D. Drug-target residence time and its implications for lead optimization. *Nat. Rev. Drug. Discov.* **5,** 730–739 (2006).
2. Lu, H. & Tonge, P. J. Drug-target residence time: critical information for lead optimization. *Curr. Opin. Chem. Biol.* **14,** 467–474 (2010).
3. Tummino, P. J. & Copeland, R. A. Residence time of receptor-ligand complexes and its effect on biological function. *Biochemistry* **47,** 5481–5492 (2008).
4. Bantscheff, M. *et al.* Chemoproteomics profiling of HDAC inhibitors reveals selective targeting of HDAC complexes. *Nat. Biotechnol.* **29,** 255–265 (2011).
5. Becher, I. *et al.* Chemoproteomics reveals time-dependent binding of histone deacetylase inhibitors to endogenous repressor complexes. *ACS Chem. Biol.* **9,** 1736–1746 (2014).
6. Vauquelin, G. & Charlton, S. J. Exploring avidity: understanding the potential gains in functional affinity and target residence time of bivalent and heterobivalent ligands. *Br. J. Pharmacol.* **168,** 1771–1785 (2013).
7. Vauquelin, G. Rebinding: or why drugs may act longer *in vivo* than expected from their *in vitro* target residence time. *Expert Opin. Drug Discov.* **5,** 927–941 (2010).
8. Savitski, M. M. *et al.* Proteomics. Tracking cancer drugs in living cells by thermal profiling of the proteome. *Science* **346,** 1255784 (2014).
9. Jafari, R. *et al.* The cellular thermal shift assay for evaluating drug target interactions in cells. *Nat. Protoc.* **9,** 2100–2122 (2014).
10. Martinez Molina, D. *et al.* Monitoring drug target engagement in cells and tissues using the cellular thermal shift assay. *Science* **341,** 84–87 (2013).
11. Zwier, J. M. *et al.* A fluorescent ligand-binding alternative using Tag-lite(R) technology. *J. Biomol. Screen.* **15,** 1248–1259 (2010).
12. Lebakken, C. S. *et al.* Development and applications of a broad-coverage, TR-FRET-based kinase binding assay platform. *J. Biomol. Screen.* **14,** 924–935 (2009).
13. Stoddart, L. A. *et al.* Application of BRET to monitor ligand binding to GPCRs. *Nat. Methods.* **12,** 661–663 (2015).
14. Simon, G. M., Niphakis, M. J. & Cravatt, B. F. Determining target engagement in living systems. *Nat. Chem. Biol.* **9,** 200–205 (2013).
15. Moreau, M. J., Morin, I. & Schaeffer, P. M. Quantitative determination of protein stability and ligand binding using a green fluorescent protein reporter system. *Mol. Biosyst.* **6,** 1285–1292 (2010).
16. Taipale, M. *et al.* Chaperones as thermodynamic sensors of drug-target interactions reveal kinase inhibitor specificities in living cells. *Nat. Biotechnol.* **31,** 630–637 (2013).
17. Savitski, M. M. *et al.* Tracking cancer drugs in living cells by thermal profiling of the proteome. *Science* **346,** 1255784 (2014).
18. Furumai, R. *et al.* FK228 (depsipeptide) as a natural prodrug that inhibits class I histone deacetylases. *Cancer Res.* **62,** 4916–4921 (2002).
19. Wang, C. *et al.* Thailandepsins: bacterial products with potent histone deacetylase inhibitory activities and broad-spectrum antiproliferative activities. *J. Nat. Prod.* **74,** 2031–2038 (2011).
20. Giang, I., Boland, E. L. & Poon, G. M. Prodrug applications for targeted cancer therapy. *AAPS J.* **16,** 899–913 (2014).
21. Wilson, A. J., Cheng, Y. Q. & Khabele, D. Thailandepsins are new small molecule class I HDAC inhibitors with potent cytotoxic activity in ovarian cancer cells: a preclinical study of epigenetic ovarian cancer therapy. *J. Ovarian Res.* **5,** 12 (2012).
22. Wei, D. G. *et al.* Histone deacetylase inhibitor romidepsin induces HIV expression in CD4 T cells from patients on suppressive antiretroviral therapy at concentrations achieved by clinical dosing. *PLoS Pathog.* **10,** e1004071 (2014).
23. Crabb, S. J. *et al.* Characterisation of the *in vitro* activity of the depsipeptide histone deacetylase inhibitor spiruchostatin A. *Biochem. Pharmacol.* **76,** 463–475 (2008).
24. Ito, T. *et al.* Real-time imaging of histone H4K12-specific acetylation determines the modes of action of histone deacetylase and bromodomain inhibitors. *Chem. Biol.* **18,** 495–507 (2011).
25. Machleidt, T. *et al.* NanoBRET-A novel BRET platform for the analysis of protein-protein interactions. *ACS Chem. Biol.* **10,** 1797–1804 (2015).
26. Pfleger, K. D. & Eidne, K. A. Illuminating insights into protein-protein interactions using bioluminescence resonance energy transfer (BRET). *Nat. Methods* **3,** 165–174 (2006).
27. Pfleger, K. D., Seeber, R. M. & Eidne, K. A. Bioluminescence resonance energy transfer (BRET) for the real-time detection of protein-protein interactions. *Nat. Protoc.* **1,** 337–345 (2006).
28. Dacres, H., Dumancic, M. M., Horne, I. & Trowell, S. C. Direct comparison of bioluminescence-based resonance energy transfer methods for monitoring of proteolytic cleavage. *Anal. Biochem.* **385,** 194–202 (2009).
29. Friedman Ohana, R. *et al.* Deciphering the cellular targets of bioactive compounds using a chloroalkane capture tag. *ACS Chem. Biol.* **10,** 2316–2324 (2015).
30. Griss, R. *et al.* Bioluminescent sensor proteins for point-of-care therapeutic drug monitoring. *Nat. Chem. Biol.* **10,** 598–603 (2014).
31. Hall, M. P. *et al.* Engineered luciferase reporter from a deep sea shrimp utilizing a novel imidazopyrazinone substrate. *ACS Chem. Biol.* **7,** 1848–1857 (2012).
32. Bradner, J. E. *et al.* Chemical phylogenetics of histone deacetylases. *Nat. Chem. Biol.* **6,** 238–243 (2010).
33. Finnin, M. S. *et al.* Structures of a histone deacetylase homologue bound to the TSA and SAHA inhibitors. *Nature* **401,** 188–193 (1999).
34. Wang, D. F., Helquist, P., Wiech, N. L. & Wiest, O. Toward selective histone deacetylase inhibitor design: homology modeling, docking studies, and molecular dynamics simulations of human class I histone deacetylases. *J. Med. Chem.* **48,** 6936–6947 (2005).
35. Miller, K. M. *et al.* Human HDAC1 and HDAC2 function in the DNA-damage response to promote DNA nonhomologous end-joining. *Nat. Struct. Mol. Biol.* **17,** 1144–1151 (2010).
36. Yao, Y. L. & Yang, W. M. Beyond histone and deacetylase: an overview of cytoplasmic histone deacetylases and their nonhistone substrates. *J. Biomed. Biotechnol.* **2011,** 146493 (2011).
37. Zhang, Y., Gilquin, B., Khochbin, S. & Matthias, P. Two catalytic domains are required for protein deacetylation. *J. Biol. Chem.* **281,** 2401–2404 (2006).
38. Zou, H., Wu, Y., Navre, M. & Sang, B. C. Characterization of the two catalytic domains in histone deacetylase 6. *Biochem. Biophys. Res. Commun.* **341,** 45–50 (2006).
39. Cheng, Y. & Prusoff, W. H. Relationship between the inhibition constant (K1) and the concentration of inhibitor which causes 50 per cent inhibition (I50) of an enzymatic reaction. *Biochem. Pharmacol.* **22,** 3099–3108 (1973).
40. Witt, O., Deubzer, H. E., Milde, T. & Oehme, I. HDAC family: what are the cancer relevant targets? *Cancer. Lett.* **277,** 8–21 (2009).
41. Wang, C., Flemming, C. J. & Cheng, Y. Q. Discovery and activity profiling of thailandepsins A through F, potent histone deacetylase inhibitors, from E264. *MedChemComm* **3,** 976–981 (2012).
42. Wilting, R. H. *et al.* Overlapping functions of Hdac1 and Hdac2 in cell cycle regulation and haematopoiesis. *EMBO J.* **29,** 2586–2597 (2010).

43. Yamaguchi, T. *et al.* Histone deacetylases 1 and 2 act in concert to promote the G1-to-S progression. *Genes Dev.* **24,** 455–469 (2010).
44. Neumann, L., von Konig, K. & Ullmann, D. HTS reporter displacement assay for fragment screening and fragment evolution toward leads with optimized binding kinetics, binding selectivity, and thermodynamic signature. *Methods Enzymol.* **493,** 299–320 (2011).
45. Di Micco, S. *et al.* Structural basis for the design and synthesis of selective HDAC inhibitors. *Bioorg. Med. Chem.* **21,** 3795–3807 (2013).
46. Fournel, M. *et al.* MGCD0103, a novel isotype-selective histone deacetylase inhibitor, has broad spectrum antitumor activity *in vitro* and *in vivo*. *Mol. Cancer. Ther.* **7,** 759–768 (2008).
47. Bonfils, C. *et al.* Evaluation of the pharmacodynamic effects of MGCD0103 from preclinical models to human using a novel HDAC enzyme assay. *Clin. Cancer Res.* **14,** 3441–3449 (2008).
48. Schulze, J. *et al.* Cell-based protein stabilization assays for the detection of interactions between small-molecule inhibitors and BRD4. *J Biomol. Screen.* **20,** 180–189 (2014).
49. Davis, M. I. *et al.* Comprehensive analysis of kinase inhibitor selectivity. *Nat. Biotechnol.* **29,** 1046–1051 (2011).
50. Karaman, M. W. *et al.* A quantitative analysis of kinase inhibitor selectivity. *Nat. Biotechnol.* **26,** 127–132 (2008).
51. Guenther, M. G., Barak, O. & Lazar, M. A. The SMRT and N-CoR corepressors are activating cofactors for histone deacetylase 3. *Mol. Cell. Biol.* **21,** 6091–6101 (2001).
52. Couturier, C. & Deprez, B. Setting Up a bioluminescence resonance energy transfer high throughput screening assay to search for protein/protein interaction inhibitors in mammalian cells. *Front. Endocrinol.* **3,** 100 (2012).
53. Dacres, H., Dumancic, M. M., Horne, I. & Trowell, S. C. Direct comparison of fluorescence- and bioluminescence-based resonance energy transfer methods for real-time monitoring of thrombin-catalysed proteolytic cleavage. *Biosens. Bioelectron.* **24,** 1164–1170 (2009).
54. Lebakken, C. S., Reichling, L. J., Ellefson, J. M. & Riddle, S. M. Detection of allosteric kinase inhibitors by displacement of active site probes. *J Biomol. Screen.* **17,** 813–821 (2012).
55. Halley, F. *et al.* A bioluminogenic HDAC activity assay: validation and screening. *J Biomol. Screen.* **16,** 1227–1235 (2011).
56. Ohana, R. F. *et al.* HaloTag-based purification of functional human kinases from mammalian cells. *Protein Expr. Purif.* **76,** 154–164 (2011).

Acknowledgements

We thank Frank Fan, Jennifer Wilkinson, Cesear Corona and Poncho Meisenheimer (Promega) for their thoughtful input on this manuscript.

Author contributions

M.B.R. and K.V.W. wrote the paper and designed the experiments. All authors contributed to the design and execution of the experiments.

Additional information

Competing financial interests: Besides Yi-Qiang Cheng, all authors are employees of Promega Corporation.

Permissions

All chapters in this book were first published in NC, by Nature Publishing Group; hereby published with permission under the Creative Commons Attribution License or equivalent. Every chapter published in this book has been scrutinized by our experts. Their significance has been extensively debated. The topics covered herein carry significant findings which will fuel the growth of the discipline. They may even be implemented as practical applications or may be referred to as a beginning point for another development.

The contributors of this book come from diverse backgrounds, making this book a truly international effort. This book will bring forth new frontiers with its revolutionizing research information and detailed analysis of the nascent developments around the world.

We would like to thank all the contributing authors for lending their expertise to make the book truly unique. They have played a crucial role in the development of this book. Without their invaluable contributions this book wouldn't have been possible. They have made vital efforts to compile up to date information on the varied aspects of this subject to make this book a valuable addition to the collection of many professionals and students.

This book was conceptualized with the vision of imparting up-to-date information and advanced data in this field. To ensure the same, a matchless editorial board was set up. Every individual on the board went through rigorous rounds of assessment to prove their worth. After which they invested a large part of their time researching and compiling the most relevant data for our readers.

The editorial board has been involved in producing this book since its inception. They have spent rigorous hours researching and exploring the diverse topics which have resulted in the successful publishing of this book. They have passed on their knowledge of decades through this book. To expedite this challenging task, the publisher supported the team at every step. A small team of assistant editors was also appointed to further simplify the editing procedure and attain best results for the readers.

Apart from the editorial board, the designing team has also invested a significant amount of their time in understanding the subject and creating the most relevant covers. They scrutinized every image to scout for the most suitable representation of the subject and create an appropriate cover for the book.

The publishing team has been an ardent support to the editorial, designing and production team. Their endless efforts to recruit the best for this project, has resulted in the accomplishment of this book. They are a veteran in the field of academics and their pool of knowledge is as vast as their experience in printing. Their expertise and guidance has proved useful at every step. Their uncompromising quality standards have made this book an exceptional effort. Their encouragement from time to time has been an inspiration for everyone.

The publisher and the editorial board hope that this book will prove to be a valuable piece of knowledge for researchers, students, practitioners and scholars across the globe.

List of Contributors

Santosh Rudrawar, Jeffrey C. Dyason, Faith J. Rose, Mark von Itzstein and Robin J. Thomson
Institute for Glycomics, Gold Coast Campus, Griffith University, Queensland 4222, Australia

Marie-Anne Rameix-Welti, Sylvie van der Werf and Nadia Naffakh
Institut Pasteur, Unité de Génétique Moléculaire des Virus à ARN, Département de Virologie, Paris F-75015, France
CNRS URA3015, Paris F-75015, France
Université Paris Diderot, Paris F-75013, France

Philip S. Kerry, Rupert J.M. Russell
Interdisciplinary Centre for Human and Avian Influenza Research, University of St Andrews, North Haugh, St Andrews, Fife KY16 9ST, UK

Lijun Sun
Department of Surgery, Center for Drug Discovery and Translational Research, Beth Israel Deaconess Medical Center, Harvard Medical School, 110 Francis Street, Suite 9F, Boston, Massachusetts 02215, USA.

Venkata R. Krishnamurthy, Mohammed Y. R. Sardar, Carolyn Haller, Erbin Dai, Donny Hanjaya-Putra and Elliot L. Chaikof
Department of Surgery, Center for Drug Discovery and Translational Research, Beth Israel Deaconess Medical Center, Harvard Medical School, 110 Francis Street, Suite 9F, Boston, Massachusetts 02215, USA
Wyss Institute of Biologically Inspired Engineering, Harvard University, 110 Francis Street, Suite 9F, Boston, Massachusetts 02115, USA

Yu Ying, Xuezheng Song and Richard D. Cummings
Department of Biochemistry, Emory University, Atlanta, Georgia 30322, USA

Xiaocong Wang
Complex Carbohydrate Research Center, University of Georgia, Athens, Georgia 30602, USA.

Vasilios Morikis and Scott I. Simon
Department of Biomedical Engineering, University of California Davis, Davis, California 95616, USA

Robert J. Woods
Complex Carbohydrate Research Center, University of Georgia, Athens, Georgia 30602, USA
School of Chemistry, National University of Ireland, Galway, University Road, Galway, Ireland

Zhenghuan Zhao, Zijian Zhou, Juan Hu and Kaiyuan Ni
State Key Laboratory of Physical Chemistry of Solid Surfaces, The Key Laboratory for Chemical Biology of Fujian Province, and Department of Chemical Biology, College of Chemistry and Chemical Engineering, Xiamen University, Xiamen 361005, China

Jianfeng Bao, Zhenyu Wang, Ruifang Wang and Zhong Chen
Department of Physics and Electronic Science, Fujian Key Laboratory of Plasma and Magnetic Resonance, Xiamen University, Xiamen 361005, China

Xiaoqin Chi
Fujian Provincial Key Laboratory of Chronic Liver Disease and Hepatocellular Carcinoma, Zhongshan Hospital, Xiamen University, Xiamen 361004, China

Xiaoyuan Chen
Laboratory of Molecular Imaging and Nanomedicine, National Institute of Biomedical Imaging and Bioengineering, National Institutes of Health, Bethesda, Maryland 20892, USA

Jinhao Gao
State Key Laboratory of Physical Chemistry of Solid Surfaces, The Key Laboratory for Chemical Biology of Fujian Province, and Department of Chemical Biology, College of Chemistry and Chemical Engineering, Xiamen University, Xiamen 361005, China
Center for Molecular Imaging and Translational Medicine, School of Public Health, Xiamen University, Xiamen 361005, China

Patrice Guillon, Larissa Dirr, Ibrahim M. El-Deeb, Moritz Winger, Benjamin Bailly, Thomas Haselhorst, Jeffrey C. Dyason and Mark von Itzstein
Institute for Glycomics, Gold Coast Campus, Griffith University, Gold Coast, Queensland 4222, Australia

Amit A. Vernekar, Govindasamy Mugesh and Prasath U. Paramasivam
Department of Inorganic and Physical Chemistry, Indian Institute of Science, Bangalore 560012, India

Renato Ribeiro-Viana
Department of Chemistry, University of Oxford, Chemistry Research Laboratory, 12 Mansfield Road, Oxford OX1 3TA, UK
Glycosystems Laboratory, Instituto de Investigaciones Quı´micas (IIQ), CSIC—Universidad de Sevilla, Ame´rico Vespucio 49, Seville 41092, Spain

Macarena Sa´nchez-Navarro, Julia R. Koeppe, G. Davis
Department of Chemistry, University of Oxford, Chemistry Research Laboratory, 12 Mansfield Road, Oxford OX1 3TA, UK

Joanna Luczkowiak, Rafael Delgado and Benjamin
Laboratorio de Microbiologı ´aMolecular, Instituto de Investigacio´n Hospital 12 de Octubre (imas12), Madrid 28041, Spain

Javier Rojo
Glycosystems Laboratory, Instituto de Investigaciones Quı´micas (IIQ), CSIC—Universidad de Sevilla, Ame´rico Vespucio 49, Seville 41092, Spain

Pratap S. Patil, Ting-Jen Rachel Cheng, Medel Manuel L. Zulueta, Shih-Ting Yang,
Larry S. Lico and Shang-Cheng Hung
Genomics Research Center, Academia Sinica, No. 128, Section 2, Academia Road, Taipei 115, Taiwan

Catherine Baud, Jére´my Guérin, Emmanuelle Petit, Elodie Lesne, Elian Dupré, Camille Locht and Françoise Jacob-Dubuisson
Center for Infection and Immunity of Lille, Institut Pasteur de Lille, 1 rue Calmette, Lille 59021, France
CNRS UMR8204, Lille 59021, France
INSERM U1019, Lille 59045, France
University of Lille Nord de France, Lille 59044, France

Kazuki Fukushima
IBM Almaden Research Center, 650 Harry Road, San Jose, California 95120, USA.
Department of Polymer Science and Engineering, Yamagata University, Yonezawa, Yamagata 992-8510, Japan

Amanda C. Engler, Hareem Maune, Daniel J. Coady, Alshakim Nelson, Jed Pitera and James L. Hedrick
IBM Almaden Research Center, 650 Harry Road, San Jose, California 95120, USA

Shaoqiong Liu, Hong Wu, Nikken Wiradharma, Shrinivas Venkataraman, Jackie Y. Ying and Yi Yan Yang
Institute of Bioengineering and Nanotechnology, 31 Biopolis Way, The Nanos, Singapore 138669, Singapore

Yuan Huang and Weimin Fan
State Key Laboratory for Diagnosis and Treatment of Infectious Diseases, First Affiliated Hospital, College of Medicine, Zhejiang University, Hangzhou 310003, China

Kun Xu, Thomas Gilles and Bernhard Breit
Institut für Organische Chemie, Albert-Ludwigs-Universität Freiburg, Albertstrasse 21, Freiburg im Breisgau 79104

Benjamin H. Rotstein, Nickeisha A. Stephenson, Neil Vasdev and Steven H. Liang
Division of Nuclear Medicine and Molecular Imaging, Center for Advanced Medical Imaging Sciences, Massachusetts General Hospital & Department of Radiology, Harvard Medical School, 55 Fruit Street, Boston, MA 02114, USA. * These authors contributed equally to this work

Christopher J. Vavricka
Research Network of Immunity and Health (RNIH), Beijing Institutes of Life Science (BIOLS), Beijing 100101, China
CAS Key Laboratory of Pathogenic Microbiology and Immunology, Institute of Microbiology, Chinese Academy of Sciences, Beijing 100101, China

Yue Liu, Jianxun Qi, Yan Wu, Yan Li and Jinghua Yan
CAS Key Laboratory of Pathogenic Microbiology and Immunology, Institute of Microbiology, Chinese Academy of Sciences, Beijing 100101, China

Hiromasa Kiyota and Kosuke Tanaka
Graduate School of Agricultural Science, Tohoku University, Aoba-ku Sendai 981-8555, Japan

Nongluk Sriwilaijaroen
Faculty of Medicine, Thammasat University, Pathumthani 12120, Thailand
College of Life and Health Sciences, Chubu University, Aichi 487-8501, Japan

Qing Li
CAS Key Laboratory of Pathogenic Microbiology and Immunology, Institute of Microbiology, Chinese Academy of Sciences, Beijing 100101, China
School of Life Sciences, University of Science and Technology of China, Hefei, Anhui Province 230027, China

Yasuo Suzuki5
College of Life and Health Sciences, Chubu University, Aichi 487-8501, Japan

George F. Gao
Research Network of Immunity and Health (RNIH), Beijing Institutes of Life Science (BIOLS), Beijing 100101, China
CAS Key Laboratory of Pathogenic Microbiology and Immunology, Institute of Microbiology, Chinese Academy of Sciences, Beijing 100101, China
School of Life Sciences, University of Science and Technology of China, Hefei, Anhui Province 230027, China
Chinese Center for Disease Control and Prevention (China CDC), Beijing 102206, China

Jing He, Lawrence G. Hamann and Rohan E.J. Beckwith
Department of Global Discovery Chemistry, Novartis Institutes for BioMedical Research, 250 Massachusetts Avenue, Cambridge, Massachusetts 02139, USA

Huw M.L. Davies
Department of Chemistry, Emory University, 1515 Dickey Drive, Atlanta, Georgia 30322, USA

Nghia P. Truong, Zhongfan Jia and Michael J. Monteiro
Australian Institute for Bioengineering and Nanotechnology, The University of Queensland, Brisbane Queensland 4072, Australia

Wenyi Gu
Australian Institute for Bioengineering and Nanotechnology, The University of Queensland, Brisbane Queensland 4072, Australia
Institute of Health and Biomedical Innovation, Queensland University of Technology, Kelvin Grove Campus, Brisbane Queensland 4059, Australia

Indira Prasadam, Ross Crawford and Yin Xiao
Institute of Health and Biomedical Innovation, Queensland University of Technology, Kelvin Grove Campus, Brisbane Queensland 4059, Australia

Wang-Yong Yang and Matthew D. Disney
Departments of Chemistry and Neuroscience, The Scripps Research Institute, Scripps Florida, Jupiter, Florida 33458, USA

Rui Gao and Partha S. Sarkar
Mitchell Center for Neurodegenerative Disorders, Department of Neurology, Neuroscience and Cell Biology, University of Texas Medical Branch, Galveston, Texas 77555, USA

Mark Southern
Informatics Core, The Scripps Research Institute, Scripps Florida, Jupiter, Florida 33458, USA

Helena Almqvist, Hanna Axelsson, Martin Haraldsson, Thomas Lundbäck
Laboratories for Chemical Biology, Karolinska Institutet, Science for Life Laboratory Stockholm, Division of Translational Medicine & Chemical Biology, Department of Medical Biochemistry & Biophysics, Karolinska Institutet, Tomtebodavägen 23A, Solna 171 65, Sweden

Rozbeh Jafari, Daniel Martinez Molina
Department of Medical Biochemistry & Biophysics, Division of Biophysics, Karolinska Institutet, Scheeles väg 2, Stockholm 171 77, Sweden

Chen Dan
School of Biological Sciences, Nanyang Technological University, 61 Biopolis Drive (Proteos), Singapore 138673, Singapore

André Mateus
Department of Pharmacy, Uppsala University, BMC, Box 580, Uppsala SE-751 23, Sweden

Andreas Larsson and Per Artursson
Department of Pharmacy, Uppsala University, BMC, Box 580, Uppsala SE-751 23, Sweden
School of Biological Sciences, Nanyang Technological University, SBS-04s-45, 60 Nanyang Drive, Singapore 639798, Singapore
Uppsala University Drug Optimization and Pharmaceutical Profiling Platform (UDOPP), Department of Pharmacy, Uppsala University, BMC, Box 580, Uppsala SE-751 23, Sweden

Pär Nordlund
Science for Life Laboratory Drug Discovery and Development platform, Uppsala University, Uppsala SE-751 23, Sweden
Institute of Cellular and Molecular Biology, ASTAR, 61 Biopolis Drive (Proteos), Singapore 138673, Singapore

Erwan Poivet, Narmin Tahirova, Lu Xu, Clara Altomare, Anne Paria, Dong-Jing Zou and Stuart Firestein
Department of Biological Sciences, Columbia University, New York, New York 10027, USA
Corporate Research and Development, Firmenich Incorporated, Plainsboro, New Jersey 08536, USA

Zita Peterlin
Department of Chemical Biology, Max-Planck-Institute of Molecular Physiology, Otto-Hahn-Strasse 11, D-44227 Dortmund, Germany

Philipp M. Cromm, Jochen Spiegel and Herbert Waldmann
Department of Chemical Biology, Max-Planck-Institute of Molecular Physiology, Otto-Hahn-Strasse 11, D-44227 Dortmund, Germany.
Technische Universität Dortmund, Fakultät für Chemie and Chemische Biologie, Otto-Hahn-Strasse 6, D-44227 Dortmund, Germany

Sebastian Schaubach and Alois Fürstner
Technische Universität Dortmund, Fakultät für Chemie and Chemische Biologie, Otto-Hahn-Strasse 6, D-44227 Dortmund, Germany
Max-Planck-Institut für Kohlenforschung, Kaiser-Wilhelm-Platz 1, D-45470 Mülheim/Ruhr, Germany

Tom N. Grossmann
Technische Universität Dortmund, Fakultät für Chemie and Chemische Biologie, Otto-Hahn-Strasse 6, D-44227 Dortmund, Germany
Chemical Genomics Centre of the Max Planck Society, Otto-Hahn-Strasse 15, D-44227 Dortmund, Germany
Department of Chemistry and Pharmaceutical Sciences, VU University Amsterdam, De Boelelaan 1083, 1081 HV Amsterdam, The Netherlands

Yuhao Cheng, Hao Cheng, Chenxiao Jiang, Xuefeng Qiu, Kaikai Wang, Wei Huan, Ahu Yuan, Jinhui Wu and Yiqiao Hu
State Key Laboratory of Pharmaceutical Biotechnology, Medical School, Nanjing University, Nanjing 210093, China. 2 Jiangsu Key Laboratory for Nano Technology, Nanjing University, Nanjing 210093, China

Matthew B. Robers, Melanie L. Dart, Chad A. Zimprich, Thomas Machleidt, Kevin R. Kupcho, James R. Hartnett, Kristopher Zimmerman, Andrew L. Niles, Rachel Friedman Ohana, Danette L. Daniels, Michael Slater, Monika G. Wood, Mei Cong and Keith V. Wood
Promega Corporation, 2800 Woods Hollow Road, Fitchburg, Wisconsin 53711, USA

Carolyn C. Woodroofe, Thomas A. Kirkland andSergiy Levin
Promega Biosciences Incorporated, 277 Granada Drive, San Luis Obispo, California 93401, USA.

Yi-Qiang Cheng
UNT System College of Pharmacy, Department of Pharmaceutical Sciences, University of North Texas Health Science Center, FortWorth, Texas, USA

Index

R

S

T

V

X

www.ingramcontent.com/pod-product-compliance
Lightning Source LLC
Chambersburg PA
CBHW080631200326
41458CB00013B/4584
9781682854075